# PATHOLOGY ILLUSTRATED

*Senior Content Strategist:* Jeremy Bowes
*Content Development Specialist:* Carole McMurray
*Project Manager:* Anne Collett
*Design:* Amy Buxton
*Illustration Manager:* Amy Faith Heyden
*Marketing Manager:* Deborah Watkins

Eighth Edition

# PATHOLOGY ILLUSTRATED

Edited by

**Fiona Roberts** BSc MD FRCPath

Consultant Pathologist
Queen Elizabeth University Hospital Glasgow
Honorary Senior Lecturer
Glasgow University, Glasgow, UK

**Elaine MacDuff** BSc MB ChB FRCPath

Consultant Pathologist
Queen Elizabeth University Hospital Glasgow
Honorary Senior Lecturer
Glasgow University, Glasgow, UK

*Original illustrations by*

**Robin Callander** FFPH FMAA AIMI

Formerly Director, Medical Illustrations Unit, Glasgow University, Glasgow, UK

Additional illustrations by

**Ian Ramsden**

Formerly Head of Medical Illustration, Glasgow University, Glasgow, UK

**For additional online content visit** StudentConsult.com

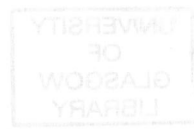

## ELSEVIER

Edinburgh London New York Oxford Philadelphia St Louis Sydney Toronto

# ELSEVIER

© 2019, Elsevier Limited All rights reserved.

First edition 1981
Second edition 1986
Third edition 1991
Fourth edition 1995
Fifth edition 2000
Sixth edition 2005
Seventh edition 2011
Eighth edition 2018

The rights of Fiona Roberts and Elaine MacDuff to be identified as authors of this work have been asserted by them in accordance with the Copyright, Designs and Patents Act 1988.

**ISBN:** 978-0-7020-7206-2 (Main edition)

**ISBN:** 978-0-7020-7205-5

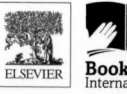
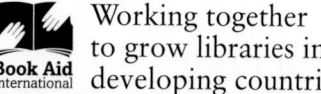

Last digit is the print number:  9  8  7  6  5  4  3  2  1

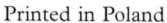

Working together
to grow libraries in
developing countries

www.elsevier.com • www.bookaid.org

# CONTENTS

'We believe that communication by verbal and written methods is the fundamental basis for study and learning. Nevertheless, in the modern setting where knowledge is increasing so rapidly and in a subject where morphological changes are a major component, we consider that the visual image has an important facilitating role'.

Since these comments were written in the preface to the first edition of 1981, undergraduate medical education has evolved greatly, notably in the widespread adoption of topic- or problem-based curricula and the generally diminished allocation of time, at least in a formal sense, to pathology.

We do not believe, however, that there has been any reduction in the importance of pathology as one of the foundations of clinical medicine.

In this eighth edition, whilst we have retained the division into general and systems-based chapters, we have increased the general chapters to include the basics of haemodynamics and shock along with a chapter outlining basic techniques in molecular biology. It is hoped that the latter will provide theory to explain significant developments that are included in the systems-based chapters. Again the aim is to be simple yet comprehensive and provide relevant information that can be assimilated in a reasonable time scale. We have concentrated on 'core' topics and on what we regard as clinically important pathology, not solely in 'Western' countries. We recognize that our attempts at simplification do not tell the whole story.

We are indebted to our predecessors, Alasdair Govan, Peter Macfarlane, Robin Reid, Robin Callander and Ian Ramsden, whose vision inspired the original concept of *Pathology Illustrated*. Much of their work from earlier editions remains with, we hope, appropriate modification. The credit for the book remains due to them; the shortcomings of this revision are our responsibility.

The most recent illustrations are the work of Graeme Chambers, to whom we are grateful. Many thanks are also owed to Carole McMurray, Content Development Specialist at Elsevier, for her considerable efforts in bringing this project to completion.

F. Roberts  
E. MacDuff  
Glasgow, May 2017

Pathology is the study of disease. It describes the effects, progress and consequences of the disease and attempts to determine the cause (aetiology) and underlying mechanisms (pathogenesis). It forms a bridge between basic science and clinical practice and has traditionally had the same role in linking pre-clinical and clinical study for medical students.

Disease occurs when there are variations of function or structure outside the normal range.

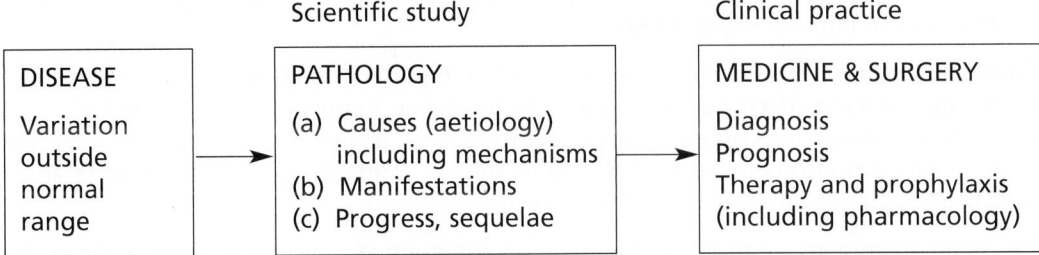

The manifestations of the disease are the sum of the damage done by the precipitating cause and the body's response (which may be helpful or unhelpful, or both). The variations in these components account for the great diversity of disease, which can then be classified into four main groups:

DEVELOPMENTAL   INFLAMMATORY   NEOPLASTIC   DEGENERATIVE

The relative importance of these groups varies with the age of the individual:

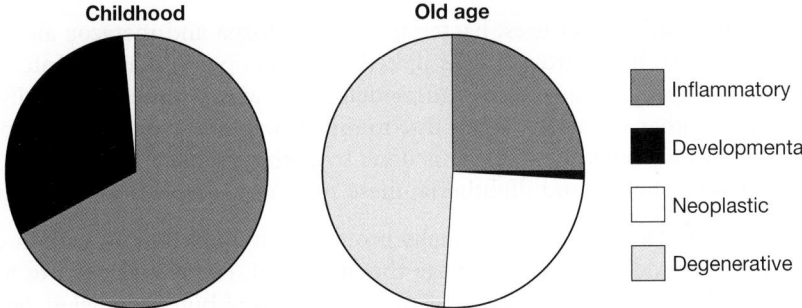

Different diseases affect different age groups. Developmental disorders and degenerative diseases affect the opposite extremes of life while tumours, in general, affect an ageing population.

Physiological ageing itself implies a gradual loss of cellular and body vitality, usually associated with atrophy of tissues and organs. This process is aggravated and mimicked by the degenerative diseases of old age so that the physiological and pathological states tend to merge. Nonetheless, the student should attempt to identify the distinctions between ageing and disease. Additionally, in old age multiple diseases often co-exist and interact with one another, and drug-induced disorders are also common in this age group.

# CAUSES OF DISEASE

The various factors involved are considered in two broad groups: (1) environmental and (2) genetic.

1. **ENVIRONMENTAL FACTORS** are numerous and can be classified under the following general headings:

**Physical agents**. Among these are trauma, radiation, both ionising and non-ionising, extremes of temperature and electrical power, i.e. the application to the body of excess (or insufficiency) of physical energy in any form.

**Chemical poisons**. Historically, these increased in importance with advances in industrial processing, but their effects have diminished by legislation to provoke safe working environments. Some, for example cyanide, are toxic to all tissues, while others target certain organs – paraquat affects the lungs and organic solvents damage especially the kidneys and liver. Others, for example strong acids and alkalis, act locally.

Iatrogenic diseases are an increasingly important subgroup as powerful drugs often have undesirable side effects, either predictably in a dose-dependent fashion or in an unpredictable idiosyncratic manner.

**Nutritional deficiencies and excesses**. These may arise from an inadequate supply, due to interference with absorption, inefficient transport within the body or defective utilisation. The effects may be general in distribution as in starvation or in severe hypoxia or they may damage specific tissues, e.g. vitamin deficiencies. Dietary excess plays an increasingly important role in Western countries, the rapidly increasing prevalence of diabetes mellitus being noteworthy.

**Infections and infestations**. Viruses, bacteria, fungi, protozoa and metazoa all cause disease. They may do so by destroying cells directly, for example in malaria. Infection with HIV destroys T cells resulting in severe immunodeficiency which renders the individual susceptible to many other infections, often due to organisms of low virulence (opportunistic infections). In other infections the damage is done by toxins produced by the infecting agent such as tetanus, cholera and diphtheria; these may have a general or local effect.

**Abnormal immune reactions**. The normally protective immune system can, in certain circumstances, become deranged and damage the individual. Hypersensitivity to foreign substances can lead to anaphylactic shock or to more localised but nonetheless potentially lethal disorders such as asthma. If the process of 'tolerance' by which the immune system recognises the body's own tissues as self breaks down, then auto-immune diseases such as thyroiditis and pernicious anaemia result.

**Psychological factors**. These cause and influence disease processes in several ways. Psychological stress may lead to mental illness, and may alter the individual's symptoms and response to somatic diseases. They are important components of diseases caused by addiction such as alcohol, tobacco and drugs. Finally, it is thought that psychological factors may be causally related to diseases such as hypertension, coronary thrombosis and, perhaps because of its effects on the immune system, to ulcerative colitis. It is worth noting, however, that the importance ascribed to stress in the pathogenesis of duodenal ulcers became much less when the pathogenic effects of *Helicobacter pylori* were discovered in the 1980s.

2.   **GENETIC FACTORS** are the results of actions of single genes or groups of genes. Research, including the human genome project, has led to a rapid expansion in our knowledge. Both variations in 'normal' genes and mutations which radically affect the function of 'abnormal genes' influence the development of disease.

**Normal genes**. There is considerable genetic variation among individuals, both within and between races and even within families. These genetic polymorphisms strongly influence SUSCEPTIBILTY and RESISTANCE to disease. For example:

a)   The susceptibility of fair skin to damage by ultraviolet light and the development of skin cancer is well known and the mechanism – lack of the protective pigment melanin – is obvious and presumably determined on evolutionary grounds.

b)   The human leucocyte antigen (HLA) system is a complex of genes on chromosome 6 in which there is great allelic variation. An individual's HLA type strongly influences the development of many disorders, especially auto-immune diseases, and of course determines whether a transplanted organ from a potential donor will be rejected or not.

**Abnormal genes**. The mutations which give rise to disease vary from point mutations which affect a single base pair (e.g. sickle cell anaemia) through chromosomal translocations found in many tumour types such as Burkitt lymphoma to the presence of an entire extra chromosome (e.g. trisomy 21 – Down syndrome). Many mutations appear to arise spontaneously while others follow exposure to irradiation (in the survivors of Chernobyl and those who have received radiotherapy) or chemicals. Some mutations arise in the somatic tissues, whilst others are transmitted in the germline. These give rise to INHERITED diseases such as cystic fibrosis where the mutation directly determines the disease. In many other diseases there is a genetic component, often contributed to by multiple genes, and an environmental contribution.

There is also variation in the rate at which mutations occur within individuals, often determined by variations in the genes responsible for DNA repair.

# METHODS IN PATHOLOGY

The traditional methods of careful naked eye and light microscopic examination of organs at autopsy have been supplemented by the much wider use in clinical practice of biopsy and cytology where tissue or cells are removed during life for diagnosis.

Endoscopic and fine needle techniques allow biopsies to be obtained from most parts of the body. In addition, technological advances have allowed examination at more detailed levels:

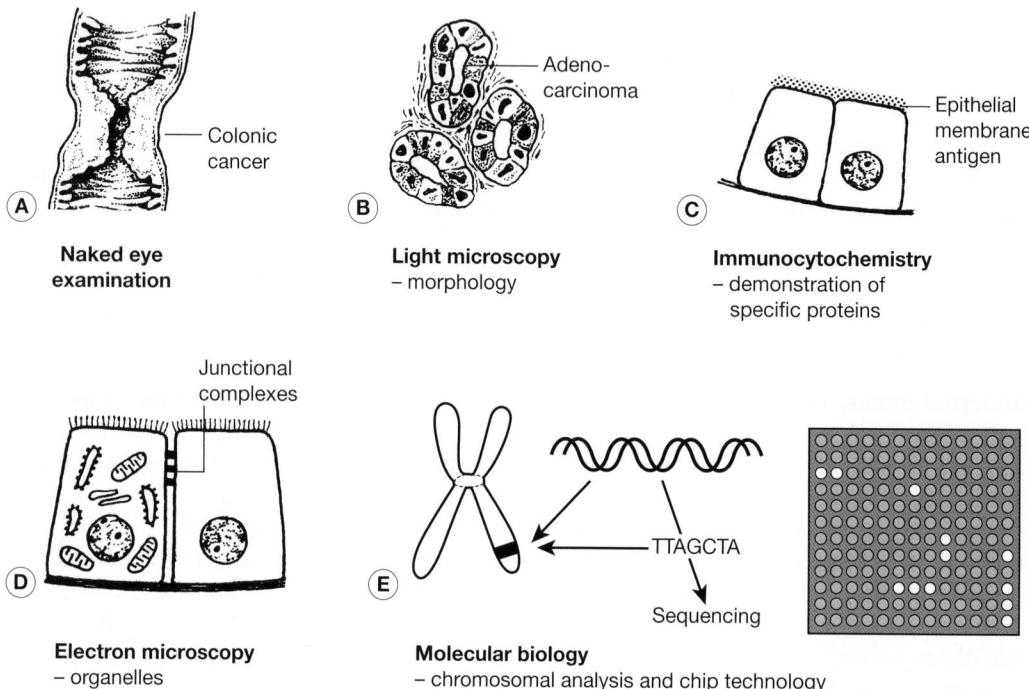

**A** Colonic cancer

**Naked eye examination**

**B** Adeno-carcinoma

**Light microscopy** – morphology

**C** Epithelial membrane antigen

**Immunocytochemistry** – demonstration of specific proteins

**D** Junctional complexes

**Electron microscopy** – organelles

**E** TTAGCTA Sequencing

**Molecular biology** – chromosomal analysis and chip technology

These increasingly sophisticated methods tend to influence the student to focus on detailed mechanisms at the molecular levels. It should not be forgotten that simple methods of gross examination and histological assessment are fundamental to the study of diseases. The following descriptions begin therefore with gross and microscopic pathology and proceed to the more detailed cellular changes when they are known. The student will find that such an approach is the basis of their learning in clinical practice.

# CELL AND TISSUE DAMAGE

## OBJECTIVES

1. To understand the control of cell numbers and how this differs in different tissues.
2. To understand the mechanisms of cell injury.
3. To define the differences between apoptosis and necrosis including morphological features and molecular mechanisms.
4. To describe the morphological features of coagulative, colliquative, gangrenous, caseous and fat necrosis.
5. To understand different types of intracellular and intercellular depositions and degenerations.
6. To define amyloidosis and its classification.

# CELLULAR PHYSIOLOGY AND PATHOLOGY

Understanding disease requires knowledge of cellular function and dysfunction.

Cellular physiology involves:

(a) Close relationships between cellular components and activities.
(b) Balancing control mechanisms to maintain constant conditions (homeostasis).
(c) Compensatory and repair mechanisms to minimise damage.

### PLASMA MEMBRANES

Main functions.

1. Maintain integrity of cell.
2. Contact with extracellular environment, e.g. cell surface receptors.

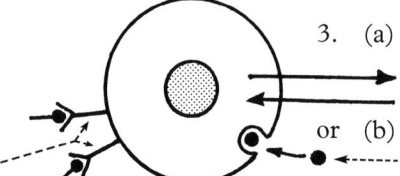

3. (a) Passage of ions through permeable channels, e.g. $Na^+$, $K^+$
   or (b) Passage of complex molecules by pinocytosis or phagocytosis.

Membrane damage may lead to cellular dysfunction or death.

### MITOCHONDRIA

These are the main sites of ENERGY production.

| Source | Production | Utilisation |
|---|---|---|
| | ADP $\rightarrow$ ATP | |

$O_2$ + glucose $\rightarrow$ (oxidative phosphorylation) $\rightarrow$ release of energy $\rightarrow$ for all cellular activities

Disorder of energy production affects all cellular functions.

### NUCLEUS

The nucleus controls all cellular activities through the action of at least 10 000 genes, each of which encodes a protein with structural, enzymatic or control functions.

Damage to DNA (e.g. by ionising radiation) is particularly likely in dividing cells. There are effective repair mechanisms but severe damage usually leads to cell death by apoptosis (see p. 6).

# CELLULAR PHYSIOLOGY AND PATHOLOGY

## Germ cell DNA damage

(i.e. to spermatogonia or oocytes)

1.  Severe damage to chromosomal structure ⟶ Prevention of conception
    Early abortion

2.  Less severe damage to groups ⟶ Developmental abnormalities
    of genes or single genes        Hereditary disease
                                     Susceptibility to diseases

## Somatic cell DNA damage

This is acquired during life. Damage to stem cells is especially important.

The development of cancer (p. 197) through activation of oncogenes or loss of tumour suppressor genes is the most important example.

## LYSOSOMES

These membrane bound organelles contain hydrolytic enzymes and are responsible for digestion and disposal of complex substances. ⟶ Disorder may lead to escape of enzymes or to accumulation of digestion products (e.g. storage disorders).

# CONTROL OF CELL NUMBER

In adult life the CELL NUMBER is fairly constant. Complex control mechanisms evenly balance new cell production with cell loss.

During SOMATIC GROWTH, cell proliferation outweighs cell loss.

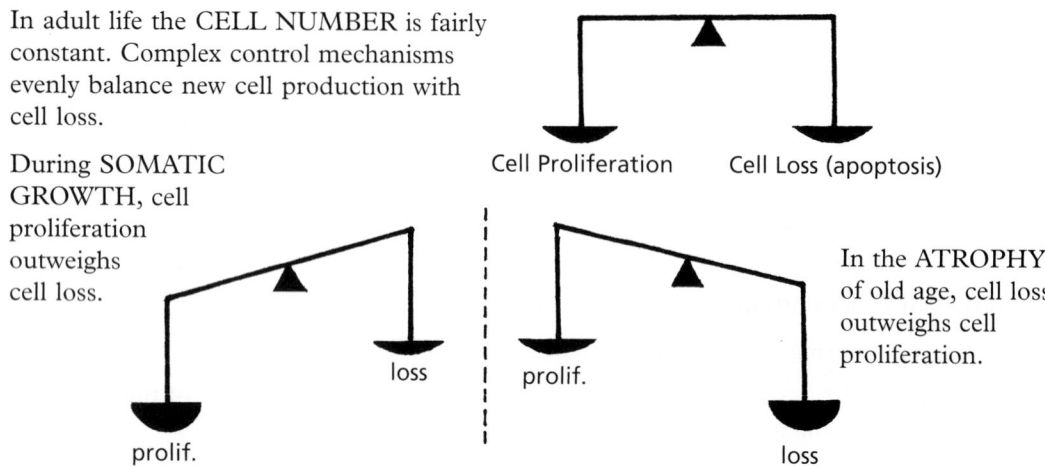

Cell Proliferation    Cell Loss (apoptosis)

In the ATROPHY of old age, cell loss outweighs cell proliferation.

loss    prolif.

prolif.    loss

In many diseases the balance is lost.

## CELL PROLIFERATION – THE CELL CYCLE

In adult life, cells can be classified into three groups according to their proliferation potential.

|  | PROLIFERATION POTENTIAL | EXAMPLES |
|---|---|---|
| 1. Labile cells | Rapid proliferation and cell turnover | Gut-lining epithelial cells |
| 2. Stable cells | Slow proliferation and cell turnover | Hepatocytes |
| 3. Permanent cells | NOT able to proliferate | Neurones |

In preparation for division, a cell passes through four consecutive phases ($G_1$, S, $G_2$, M) ending in *Mitosis* (M).

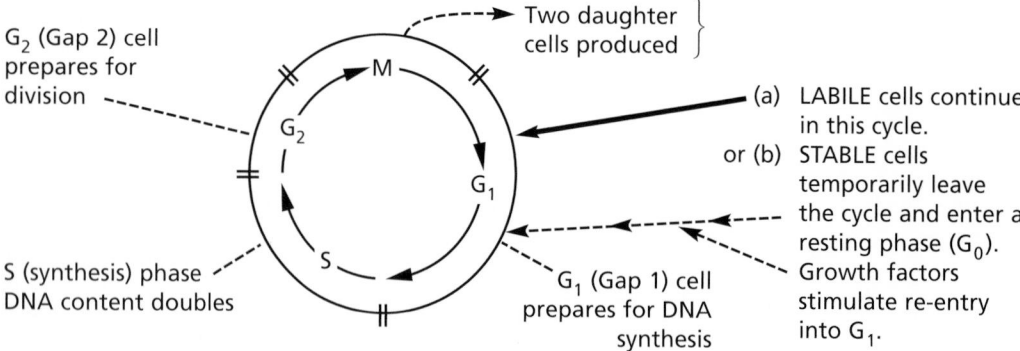

$G_2$ (Gap 2) cell prepares for division

Two daughter cells produced

(a) LABILE cells continue in this cycle.
or (b) STABLE cells temporarily leave the cycle and enter a resting phase ($G_0$). Growth factors stimulate re-entry into $G_1$.

S (synthesis) phase DNA content doubles

$G_1$ (Gap 1) cell prepares for DNA synthesis

A variety of growth promotors, inhibitors and drugs influence the cycle at various stages.

Knowledge of the cycle underlies the understanding of mechanisms involved in HEALING and REPAIR, and in CARCINOGENESIS.

# CELL INJURY

Cell injury results when cells are stressed so severely that they are no longer able to adapt, or when cells are exposed to inherently damaging agents.

A variety of noxious agents can damage cells. These include:

1. **Reduced oxygen supply** – respiratory disease, cardiovascular disease, anaemia.
2. **Physical agents** – mechanical trauma, excessive heat or cold, radiation.
3. **Chemical agents**.
4. **Toxins** – bacteria, plants, animals (e.g. snakes).
5. **Viruses**.
6. **Abnormal immunological reaction** – hypersensitivity states, glomerulonephritis.
7. **Nutritional deficiencies** – vitamin deficiency and malabsorption syndromes.
8. **Genetic abnormalities** – Down syndrome.

The severity of the injury determines the outcome:

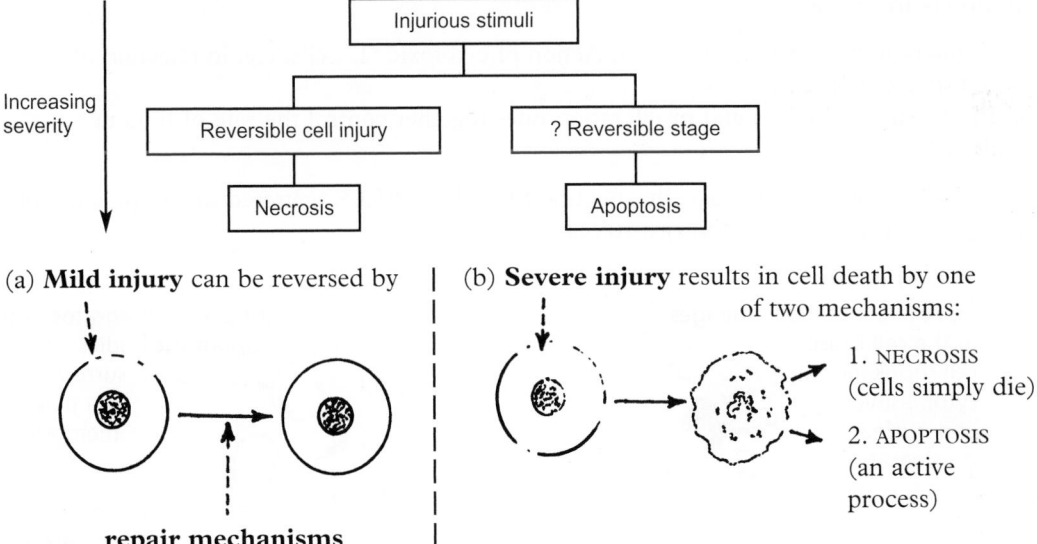

(a) **Mild injury** can be reversed by

**repair mechanisms**

(b) **Severe injury** results in cell death by one of two mechanisms:

1. NECROSIS (cells simply die)

2. APOPTOSIS (an active process)

# APOPTOSIS

Apoptosis (programmed cell death) (Greek: apoptosis = falling off, like leaves from a tree) is an important process in health and disease by which, unlike necrosis (p. 8), abnormal or unwanted cells are eliminated. It involves activation of a programmed series of events coordinated by a dedicated set of gene products. It is an active process. A few examples are:

### Apoptosis in health

In development and maintenance of steady cell populations:

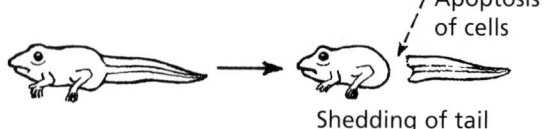

Apoptosis of cells

Shedding of tail

(i)   Metamorphosis of tadpole to frog or loss of webbing as hand develops.
(ii)  Hormone dependent involutions, e.g. menstrual breakdown of endometrium.
(iii) Cell deletion in proliferating populations, e.g. intestinal crypts or thymus.

### Apoptosis in disease

(i)   Irradiation, (ii) Viral infection, (iii) Action of cytotoxic 'T' cells, e.g. in rejection of transplanted organs.
(iv)  In tumours, apoptosis and proliferation rates together control the rate of tumour growth.

Apoptosis is a rapid process usually affecting SINGLE CELLS scattered in a population of healthy cells. It is considered in two stages:

Stage 1: **Cell death**

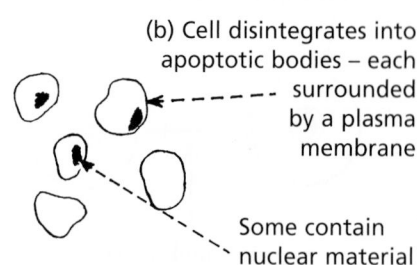

(a) Active metabolic changes in the cell cause – cell shrinkage, cytoplasmic and nuclear condensation

Plasma membrane intact

(b) Cell disintegrates into apoptotic bodies – each surrounded by a plasma membrane

Some contain nuclear material

Stage 2: **Cell elimination**

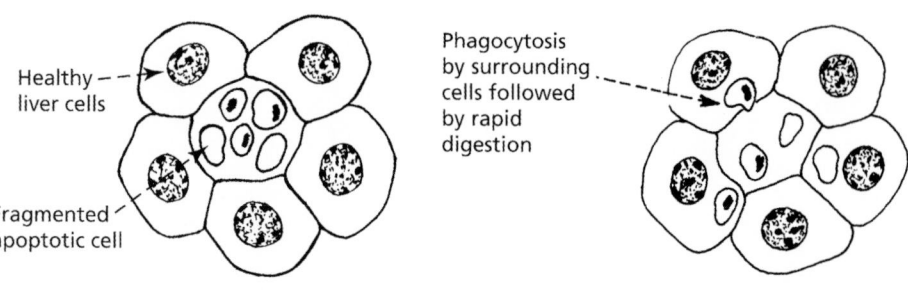

Healthy liver cells

Fragmented apoptotic cell

Phagocytosis by surrounding cells followed by rapid digestion

# APOPTOSIS

1. The surrounding cells move together to fill the vacant space, leaving virtually no evidence of the process.
2. The plasma membranes around the apoptotic bodies remain intact.
3. There is no inflammation.
4. Apoptosis is tightly regulated by many genes including *ced* and *bcl-2*.

## MECHANISMS OF APOPTOSIS

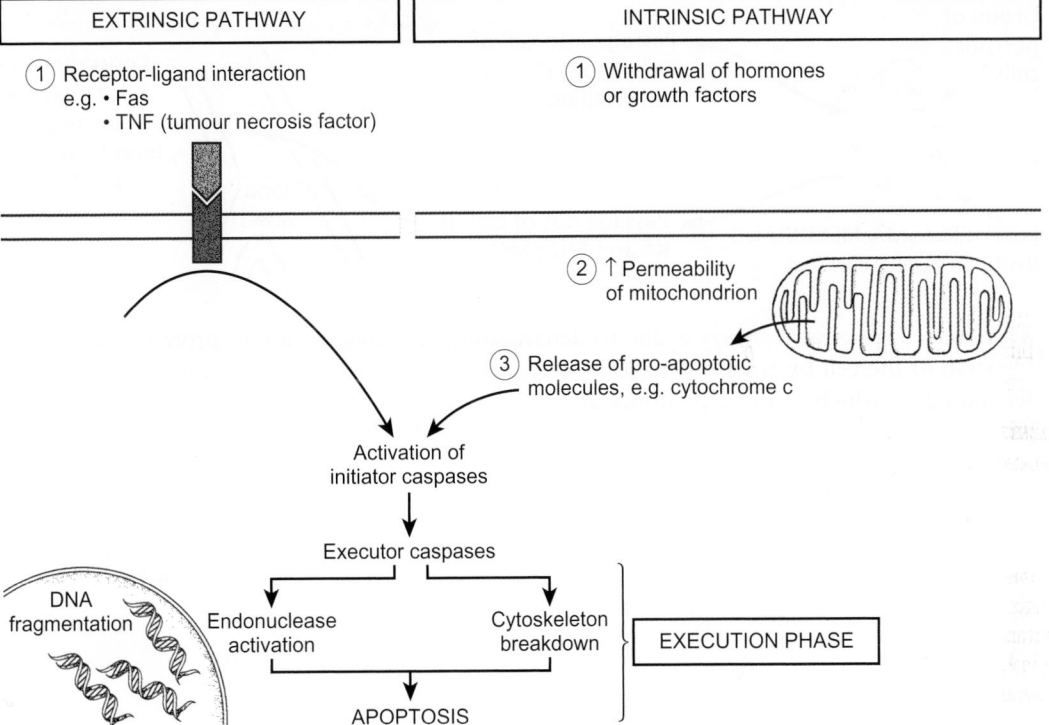

# APOPTOSIS

### NECROSIS

This term describes death of a cell or group of cells, typically following severe hypoxia, physical or chemical injury. Death of the cell is associated with rapid depletion of intracellular energy systems. Initially there are no morphologic changes, but within a few hours the cell membrane and intracellular organelles are disrupted. Electron microscopy demonstrates these changes earlier than light microscopy.

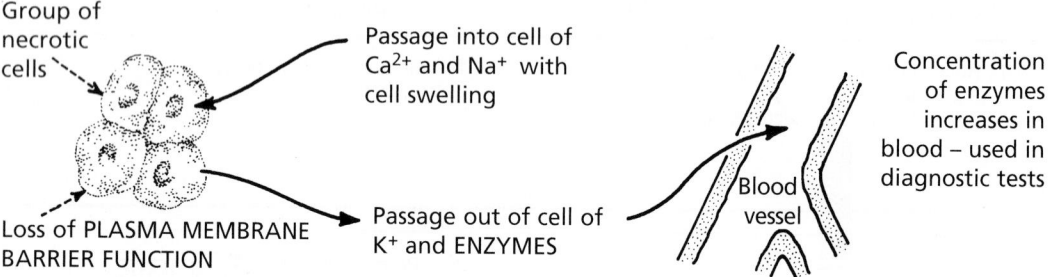

Group of necrotic cells

Passage into cell of $Ca^{2+}$ and $Na^+$ with cell swelling

Loss of PLASMA MEMBRANE BARRIER FUNCTION

Passage out of cell of $K^+$ and ENZYMES

Blood vessel

Concentration of enzymes increases in blood – used in diagnostic tests

What we recognise as necrosis is due to denaturation and coagulation of protein and/or digestion of the cell by released enzymes. There are several naked-eye appearances, depending on which of these predominates.

# NECROSIS

## COAGULATIVE NECROSIS

This type of necrosis is frequently caused by lack of blood supply, e.g. infarcts of the heart, spleen and kidney.

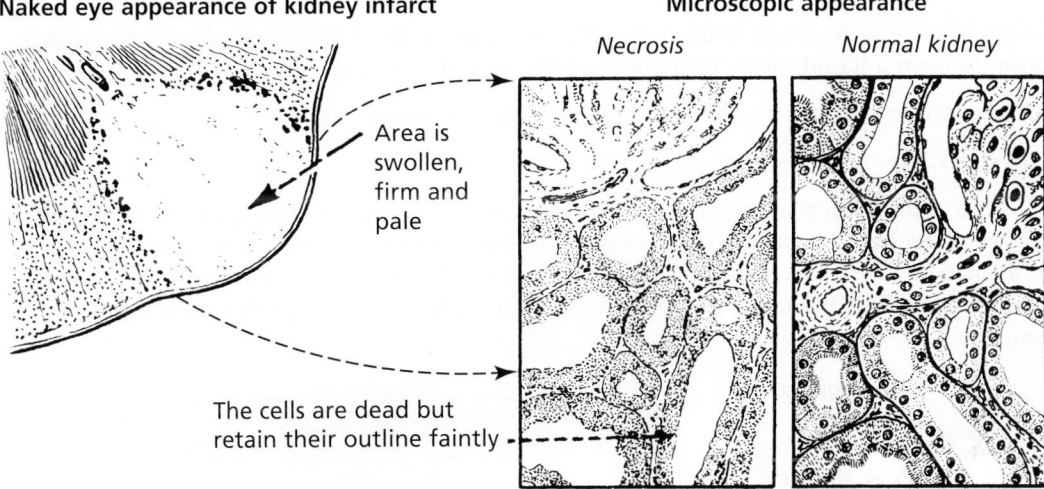

**Naked eye appearance of kidney infarct**

Area is swollen, firm and pale

The cells are dead but retain their outline faintly

**Microscopic appearance**

*Necrosis*    *Normal kidney*

The following changes are seen using the light microscope:

1. The nucleus shows one of three changes: (a) Karyolysis, (b) Karyorrhexis or (c) Pyknosis.
2. The cytoplasm becomes opaque and strongly eosinophilic (affinity for the red dye eosin).

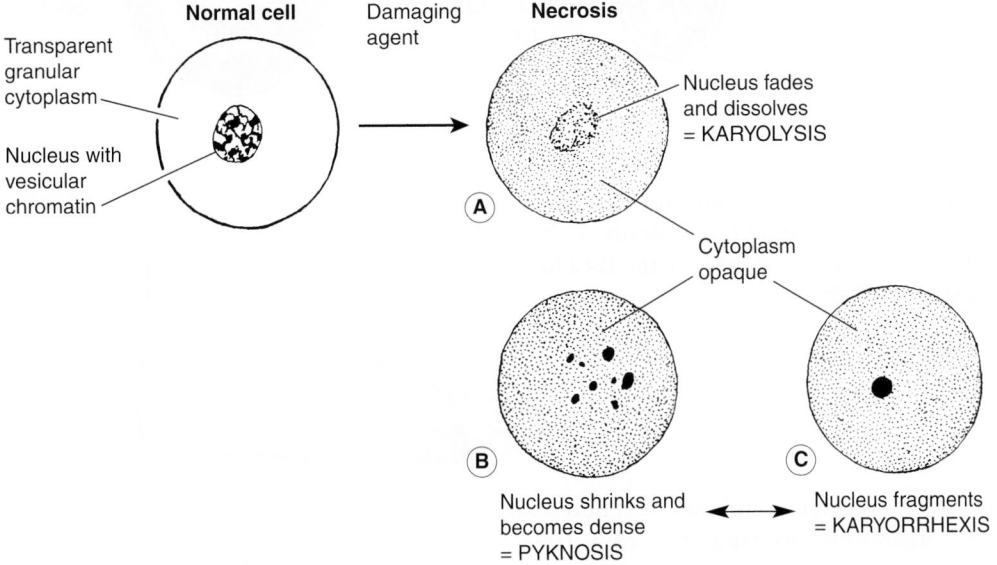

**Normal cell**    Damaging agent    **Necrosis**

Transparent granular cytoplasm

Nucleus with vesicular chromatin

Nucleus fades and dissolves = KARYOLYSIS

(A)

Cytoplasm opaque

(B)    (C)

Nucleus shrinks and becomes dense = PYKNOSIS

Nucleus fragments = KARYORRHEXIS

# NECROSIS

At *electron microscope* (E.M.) level, in addition to the above nuclear changes, disorganisation and disintegration of the cytoplasmic organelles and severe damage to the plasma membrane are seen with the formation of surface blebs.

### COLLIQUATIVE NECROSIS (LIQUEFACTIVE NECROSIS)

Death of cells in the brain result in liquefactive necrosis in which the dead cells are broken down to form a liquid mass. There is complete loss of structure (see p. 580).

An *abscess* (see p. 52) is another example of colliquative necrosis.

### GANGRENE

This is a complication of necrosis, which occurs when tissues are invaded by bacteria which release proteolytic enzymes. These enzymes degrade the necrotic tissue releasing foul-smelling gases. The tissue becomes green or black due to breakdown of haemoglobin. Obstruction of the blood supply to the bowel, for example, is almost inevitably followed by gangrene:

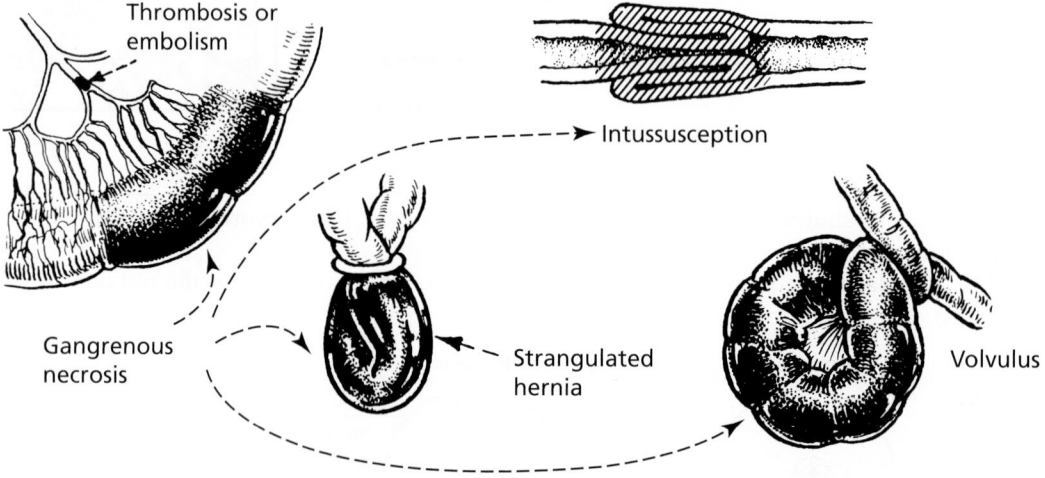

Thrombosis or embolism

Intussusception

Gangrenous necrosis

Strangulated hernia

Volvulus

Gangrene also occurs on the skin surface following arterial obstruction. It is particularly liable to affect the limbs, especially the toes in diseases such as diabetes.

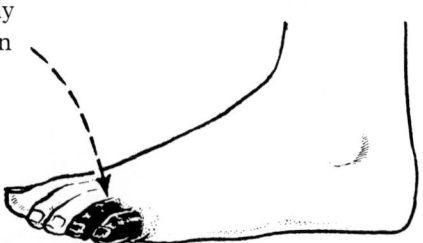

A special type of gangrene follows infection with clostridial organisms (gas gangrene; see p. 109).

# NECROSIS

## CASEOUS NECROSIS

This is commonly seen in tuberculosis (see p. 112). The necrotic tissue has a 'cream-cheesy' appearance.

## FAT NECROSIS

This is a descriptive term for a form of fat destruction seen, for example, in trauma and pancreatitis. The appearances are due to the action of lipases on triglycerides as follows:

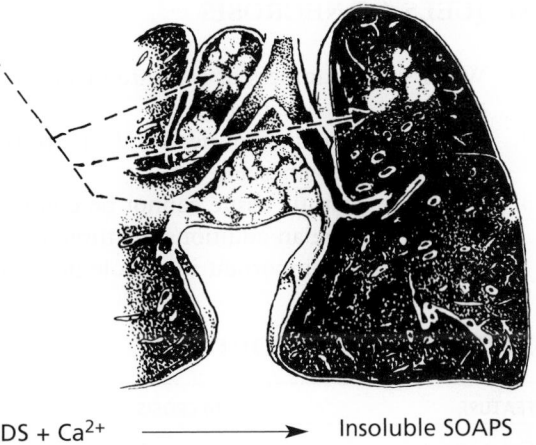

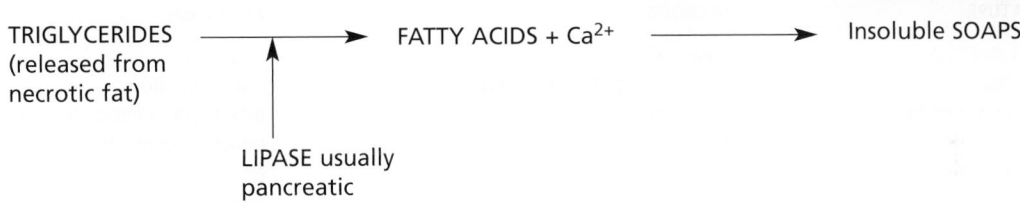

TRIGLYCERIDES (released from necrotic fat) $\longrightarrow$ FATTY ACIDS + $Ca^{2+}$ $\longrightarrow$ Insoluble SOAPS

LIPASE usually pancreatic

**Naked eye**

Fat

**Microscopic**

*Normal fatty tissue*          *Necrotic*

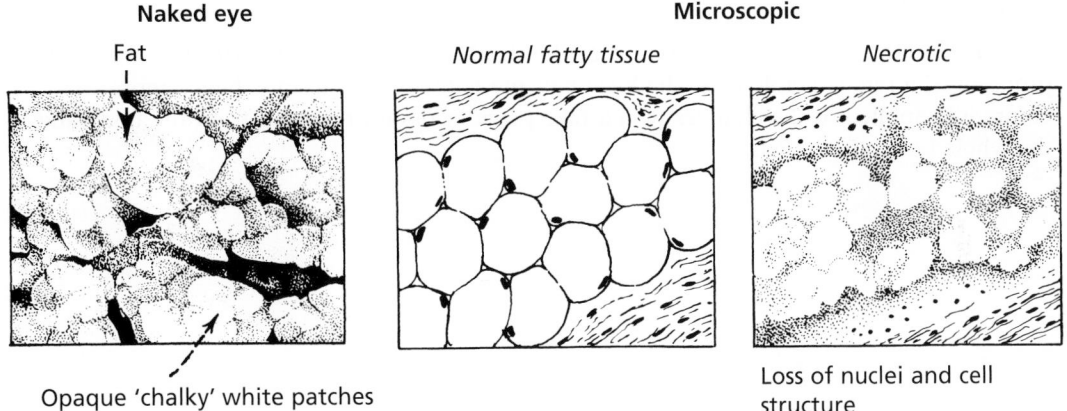

Opaque 'chalky' white patches

Loss of nuclei and cell structure

## FIBRINOID NECROSIS

This is a descriptive term in which connective tissues and especially arterial walls are infiltrated by a strongly eosinophilic hyaline material which shows some of the characteristics of fibrin.

# NECROSIS – AUTOLYSIS

### SEQUELS OF NECROSIS

1. When small numbers of cells are involved, the cellular debris is removed by PHAGOCYTOSIS (see p. 49).
2. With larger numbers of dead cells, there is an inflammatory response with organisation and fibrous repair (see p. 53).
3. When the necrotic tissue cannot be completely removed or organised, deposition of calcium may be an additional feature, for example in TUBERCULOUS CASEOUS NECROSIS. This feature is important in radiologic diagnosis. It is known as 'dystrophic calcification' (see p. 22).

### NECROSIS AND APOPTOSIS

| FEATURE | NECROSIS | APOPTOSIS |
|---|---|---|
| Cell size | Enlarged | Reduced |
| Nucleus | Karyolysis, pyknosis, karyorrhexis | Fragmentation |
| Plasma membrane | Disrupted | Intact with altered structure |
| Cellular contents | Enzymatic digestion, leakage | Intact apoptotic bodies |
| Inflammation | Frequent | No |
| Role | Pathological | Physiological or pathological |

### AUTOLYSIS

The process of 'self-digestion' begins after the death of the cell (as described above) and proceeds at a rate dependent on the local enzyme content. The term is hence more commonly applied to the changes which take place in tissues removed from the body and in the whole body after death.

# REVERSIBLE CELL DAMAGE

The various agents which can cause cell necrosis may also cause lesser cell damage which is reversible when the injurious agent is removed.

The appearances and effects are considered under these headings: (1) *hydropic swelling* and (2) *fatty change*.

## HYDROPIC SWELLING

Under the light microscope: E.M. appearances indicate the mechanisms:

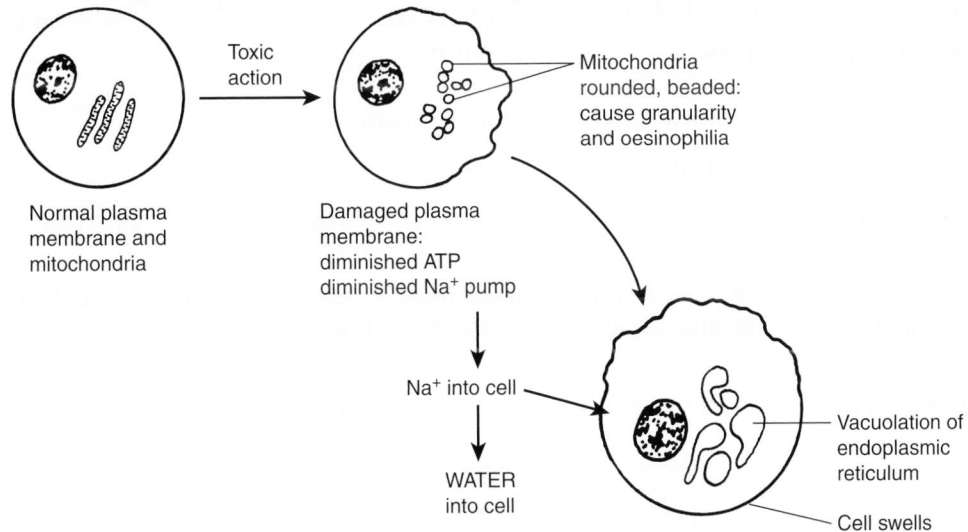

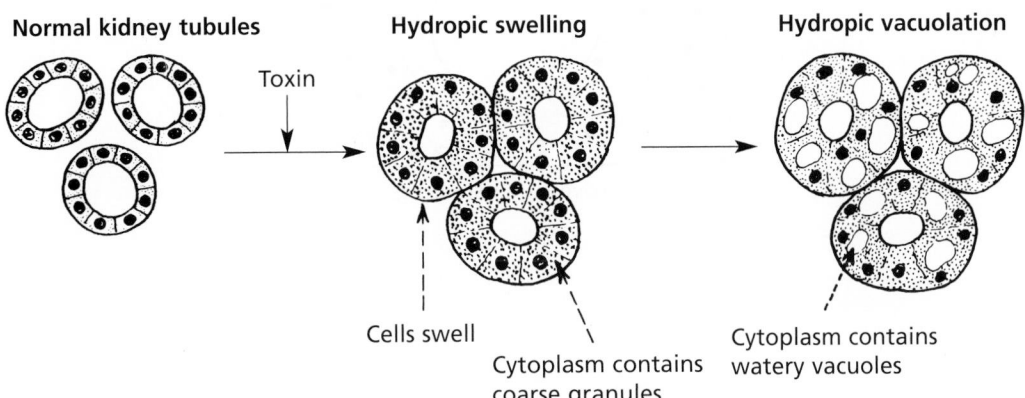

Naked eye: the damaged organs become swollen and are pale.

# REVERSIBLE CELL DAMAGE

### FATTY CHANGE

This is accumulation of fat in nonfatty tissues, e.g. skeletal muscles and the heart.

These tissues cannot metabolise the amount of lipid presented to them, resulting in its accumulation within the cells. Examples include:

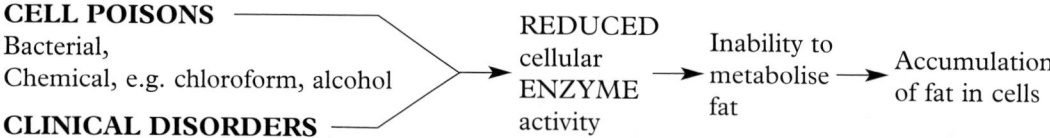

**CELL POISONS**
Bacterial,
Chemical, e.g. chloroform, alcohol

**CLINICAL DISORDERS**

REDUCED cellular ENZYME activity → Inability to metabolise fat → Accumulation of fat in cells

Anoxia due to anaemia, cardiac failure, respiratory disease.

Diabetes mellitus, chronic malnutrition.

In normal nonfatty tissues the intracellular fat is not visible by light microscopy using conventional fat stains.

In fatty change, the accumulated fat is visualised using frozen sections and fat-soluble dyes: e.g. Sudan, in routine paraffin sections the fat has been dissolved and is indicated by clear vacuoles.

For example, in the LIVER, the increase of deposited fat causes enlargement of the organ.

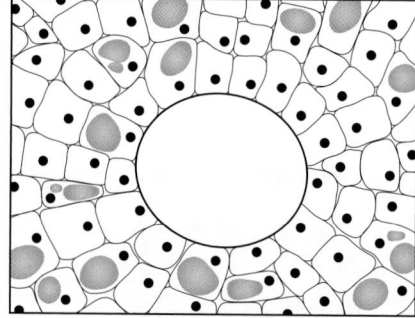

Macrovesicular steatosis

# REVERSIBLE CELL DAMAGE

## EFFECTS OF FATTY CHANGE

Impairment of cellular function is usually due to the pathologic process causing the fatty change (e.g. anoxia in severe anaemia) and not to the physical presence of fat within the cell. In the liver, for example, very large accumulations of fat do not impair basic liver functions.

A possible exception is the myocardium in certain circumstances.

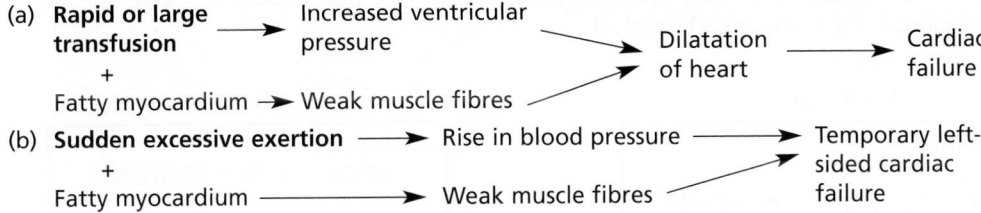

(a) **Rapid or large transfusion** + Fatty myocardium → Increased ventricular pressure / Weak muscle fibres → Dilatation of heart → Cardiac failure

(b) **Sudden excessive exertion** + Fatty myocardium → Rise in blood pressure / Weak muscle fibres → Temporary left-sided cardiac failure

# MECHANISMS OF CELL DAMAGE – FREE RADICALS

In addition to the depletion of ATP and mitochondrial damage, which results in alterations in the cell membrane with calcium influx, the formation of free radicals is an important contributory factor in many disease processes.

Free radicals are molecules with a single unpaired electron in an outer orbital position: they react with and modify a wide range of molecules, particularly lipids (of cell membranes), DNA and proteins.

A dot above the chemical symbol indicates the presence of a free radical: e.g. $OH^{\bullet}$ = hydroxyl radical, $O_2^{\bullet}$ = superoxide radical.

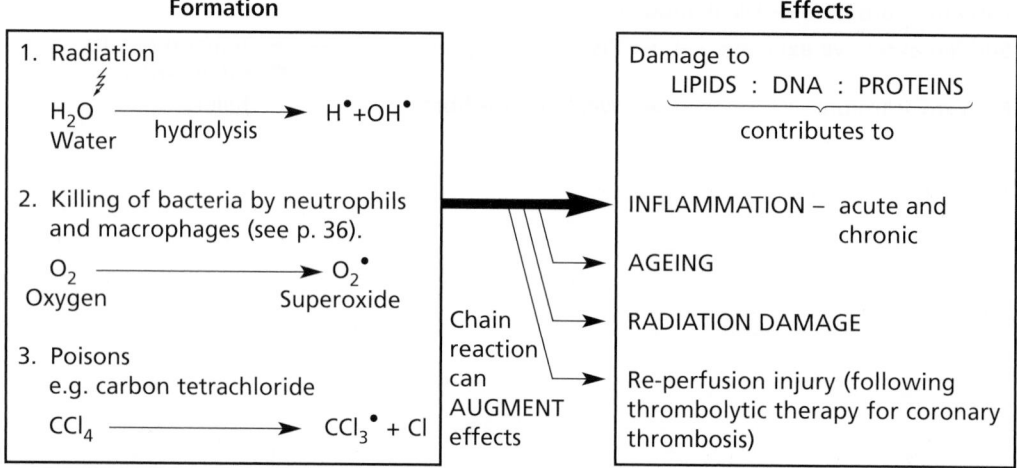

**Defence mechanisms to free radicals**

Some free radicals decay spontaneously (e.g. $O_2^{\bullet}$) but they can also be removed by ANTIOXIDANTS (e.g. vitamin E) and also by the action of enzymes such as superoxide dismutase and catalase.

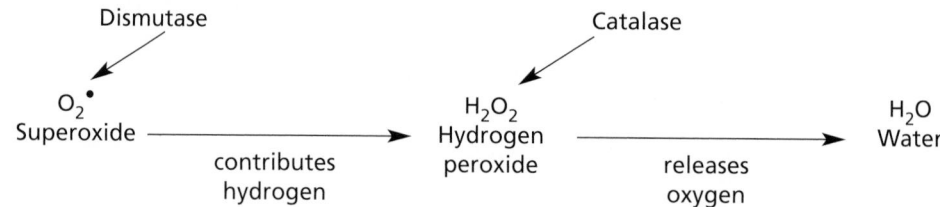

# ATROPHY

This is a simple decrease in cell size or number, resulting in shrinkage of affected tissues and organs. The most common example is atrophy of old age (see p. 18).

## CAUSES

1. **Gradual diminution in blood supply** ⟶ Reduction in oxygen supply and nutrients ⟶ Fall in cell activity and shrinkage, e.g. narrowing of coronary arteries → myocardial atrophy

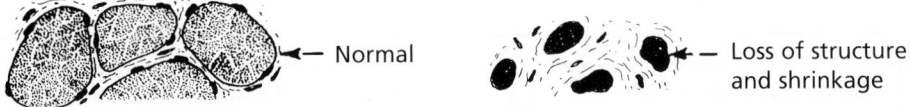

   Normal        Accumulation of lipofuscin around nucleus

2. **Reduced functional activity** (disuse atrophy) ⟶ Diminished demand for nutrition ⟶ Atrophy of cells

   *E.g.* Lack of exercise ⟶ Atrophy of skeletal muscle
   *E.g.* Obstruction of gland duct ⟶ Atrophy of gland (apoptosis is important here)

3. **Interrupted nerve supply** ⟶ Reduced reflex and metabolic activities, e.g. atrophy of skeletal muscles after destruction of motor nerves as in poliomyelitis.

   ◄— Normal      — Loss of structure and shrinkage

4. **Endocrine deficiency** ⟶ Loss of trophic mechanism ⟶ Reduced metabolic activity in dependent tissues

   *E.g.* Pituitary deficiency ⟶ Atrophy of ⟶ Thyroid
   ⟶ Adrenals
   ⟶ Gonads and genital organs

5. **Pressure** ⟶ Interruption of blood supply and interference with function, e.g. neoplasm pressing on surrounding tissues.

Atrophy is reversible provided the cause is eliminated or deficiencies restored.

# AGEING

The distinction between 'true' ageing and ageing complicated by disease processes may be difficult; as therapy can be directed at the latter, the distinction is important in clinical practice.

The changes associated with *true* ageing would be seen in a theoretical 'ideal' environment (minimal stress).

The following diagram is illustrative. The main controlling factors are *intrinsic*, i.e. genetic:
   ? associated with expression of ageing genes in mitochondria.
   ? loss of cells' ability to divide due to telomeric shortening (ends of chromosomes).

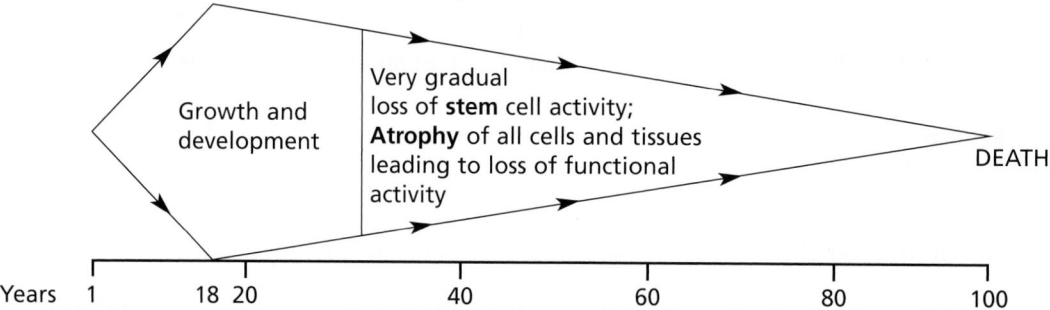

In the real environment this theoretical concept of ageing is accelerated and aggravated by two groups of *extrinsic* factors:

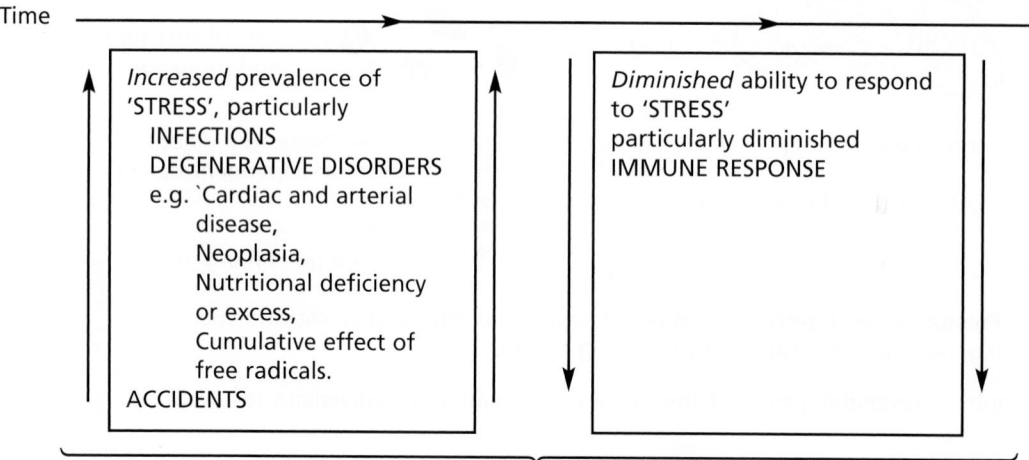

**Ageing accelerated and aggravated**

*Note*: Death is only very rarely, if ever, due to 'pure' ageing. It is the result of disease – either a single process or, with increasing age, more often several causes.

# DEPOSITIONS – AMYLOID

## AMYLOID

Amyloid is a waxy substance deposited in the extracellular tissues, particularly around blood vessels and in basement membranes. Various forms of amyloid are seen and they have varying effects. Amyloid is resistant to degradation and its deposition tends to progress relentlessly.

### Nature of amyloid

Chemical: amyloid fibrils are made up of:

(i) A major variable component >90%. This component is a protein related to acute phase reactive protein, which appears in the serum in many inflammatory conditions or is derived from fragments of immunoglobulin molecules (particularly lambda light chains).

(ii) A minor constant component, AMYLOID P PROTEIN – a glycoprotein normally found in serum.

Whatever its composition, amyloid fibrils are arranged in a β-pleated configuration; this accounts for its resistance to degradation and its staining properties.

### Detection

To the naked eye, the affected organs are pale, enlarged and have a firm, waxy texture.

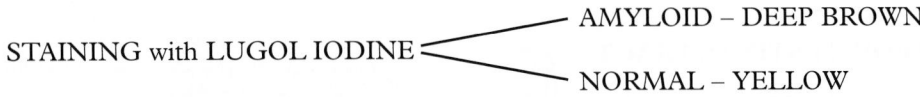

STAINING with LUGOL IODINE
— AMYLOID – DEEP BROWN
— NORMAL – YELLOW

### On light microscopy

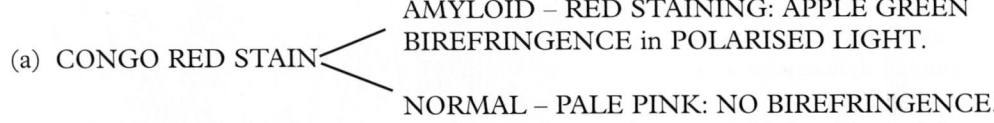

(a) CONGO RED STAIN
— AMYLOID – RED STAINING: APPLE GREEN BIREFRINGENCE in POLARISED LIGHT.
— NORMAL – PALE PINK: NO BIREFRINGENCE.

(b) IMMUNOSTAINING – for specific constituents (e.g. amyloid A or P protein).

**On electronmicroscopy** – closely packed interlacing fibrils 70–100 nm in diameter.

### Pathological effects

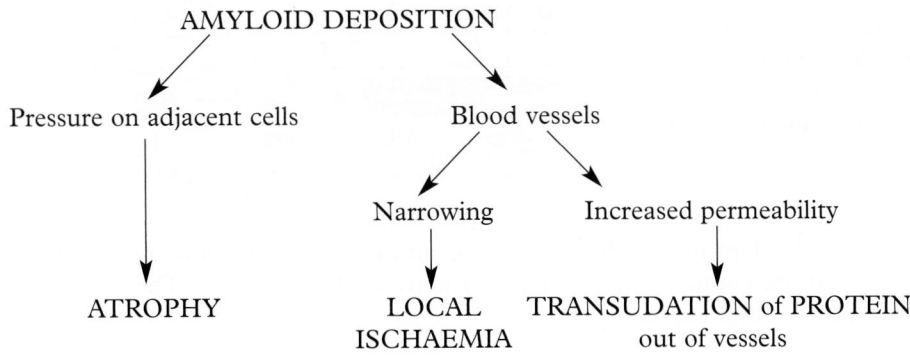

AMYLOID DEPOSITION

Pressure on adjacent cells → ATROPHY

Blood vessels
→ Narrowing → LOCAL ISCHAEMIA
→ Increased permeability → TRANSUDATION of PROTEIN out of vessels

# DEPOSITIONS – AMYLOID

Almost any tissue in the body may be affected by amyloid deposition, but the most important changes occur in the kidney, gastrointestinal tract and the heart. Other organs, such as the liver and spleen, may also be grossly affected without serious functional impairment.

### KIDNEY

In severe cases the kidneys are pale, firm and waxy, and with the iodine test the glomeruli stand out as brown dots to the naked eye.

Renal biopsy is useful in the diagnosis of amyloidosis.

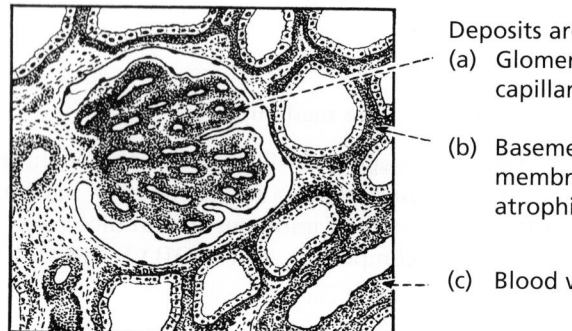

Deposits around:
(a) Glomerular capillaries

(b) Basement membranes of atrophic tubules

(c) Blood vessel

**Effects:**
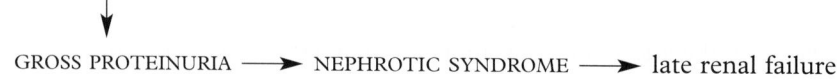

Glomerular capillary permeability altered

↓

GROSS PROTEINURIA ⟶ NEPHROTIC SYNDROME ⟶ late renal failure

### GASTROINTESTINAL TRACT

Due to altered permeability of the capillaries, the patient suffers from diarrhoea and protein loss. There may also be malabsorption, nutritional deficiencies and electrolyte imbalance.

Rectal biopsy is useful in the diagnosis of amyloidosis.

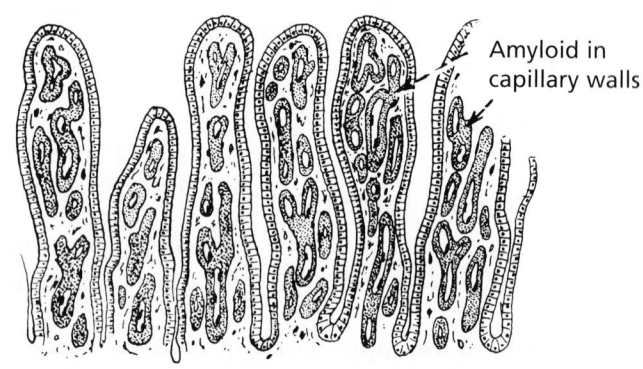

Amyloid in capillary walls

### HEART

Amyloid deposition occurs around the cardiac muscle fibres and the capillary basement membranes. The heart is enlarged with thick walls. Much of the thickness is due to amyloid deposition.

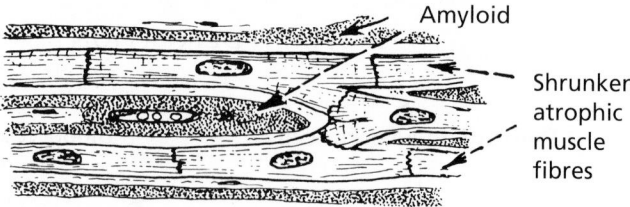

Amyloid

Shrunken atrophic muscle fibres

**Effects:**

Cardiac failure develops mainly due to the mechanical effect of amyloid, making the heart muscle stiff and preventing cardiac filling (restrictive cardiomyopathy). The blood supply to the muscle fibres is also impaired.

# AMYLOID CLASSIFICATION

## 1. SYSTEMIC AMYLOIDOSIS

(a) *Associated with monoclonal plasma cell proliferation*
(e.g. myeloma, monoclonal gammopathy, Waldenstrom macroglobulinaemia).

Increased production of:
Variable protein – AL (Amyloid Light chain derived) – from fragments of immunoglobulin, especially lambda light chains.

(b) *Associated with chronic inflammation*
(e.g. tuberculosis, osteomyelitis, rheumatoid arthritis, bronchiectasis and the genetically inherited familial Mediterranean fever).

Increased production of:
Variable protein – AA (Amyloid A protein) – derived from serum AA protein, an acute phase reactant in many inflammatory conditions.

### Summary of formation of amyloid

Abnormal (monoclonal) proliferation of plasma cells

↓

Abnormal immunoglobulins esp. lambda light chains

Proteolysis ⟶ ↓

'Major variable component'
AMYLOIDOGENIC PROTEIN >90%
(AL)
+ Amyloid P glycoprotein <10%

↓

SYSTEMIC AMYLOID (AL)

Long continued active inflammation

↓

Acute phase reactant protein

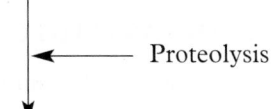 ↓ ⟵ Proteolysis

'Major variable component'
AMYLOIDOGENIC PROTEIN >90%
(AA)
+ Amyloid P glycoprotein <10%

↓

SYSTEMIC AMYLOID (AA)

## 2. LOCALISED AMYLOIDOSIS

In ENDOCRINE TUMOURS – amyloid derived from polypeptide hormones, e.g. medullary carcinoma of thyroid – calcitonin-derived amyloid.

In OLD AGE – the amyloidogenic protein is related to transthyretin (pre-albumin). Deposits of amyloid occur in the heart, brain and joints. In Alzheimer's disease (p. 588) local amyloid deposition in the brain is important. The amyloid is composed of peptide fragments of beta protein or A4 protein derived from a normal neuronal membrane protein (amyloid precursor protein).

# DEPOSITIONS – CALCIFICATION

Abnormal deposits of calcium occur in two circumstances: dystrophic calcification and metastatic calcification.

## 1. DYSTROPHIC CALCIFICATION

Local deposits of calcium may occur in:

(a) **Necrotic tissue** – old caseous lesions of tuberculosis, old infarcts, collections of pus, in fat necrosis associated with pancreatitis.

(b) **Tissues undergoing slow degeneration** – hyaline areas in benign tumours, e.g. fibroids (p. 545), in arteries due to atheromatous degeneration or in thrombi in old age; in diseased or abnormal heart valves.

The mechanism may be as follows:

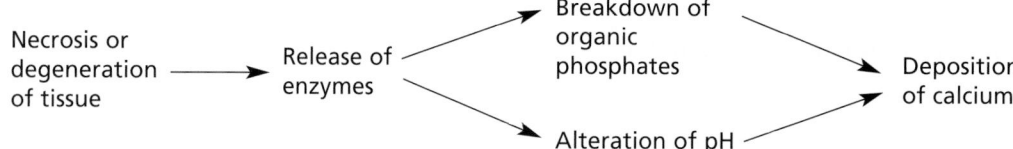

*Note*: $Ca^{2+}$ is radio-opaque and therefore can be seen on X-rays where it is of diagnostic use, for example in old healed disease (e.g. tuberculosis) and also in some tumours (e.g. breast cancer) where very small deposits of calcium may be present.

## 2. METASTATIC CALCIFICATION

In this case there is an increase in the calcium phosphate product in the blood (usually hypercalcaemia).

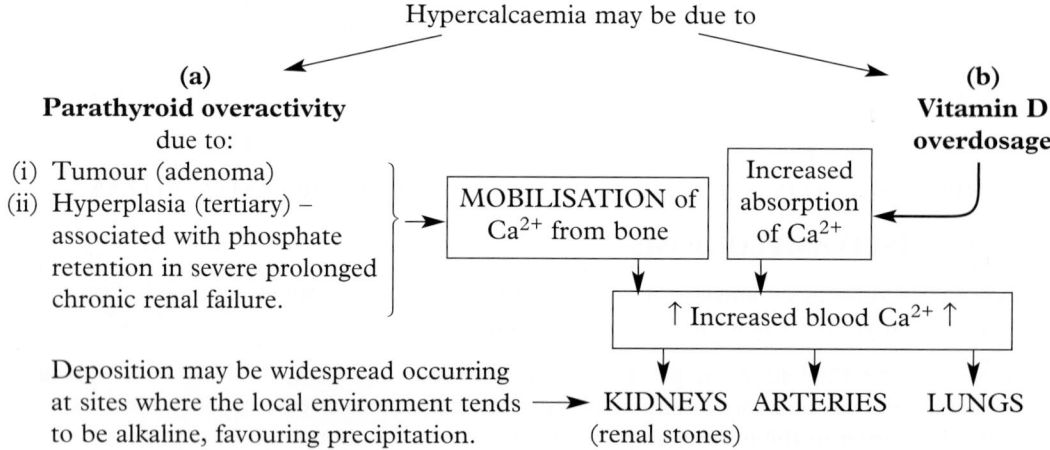

Some malignant tumours, e.g. breast and lung, are associated with hypercalcaemia and metastatic calcification.

The mechanisms are: (1) secretion by the tumour of a protein (parathyroid hormone-related peptide) which mimics the action of parathormone and (2) the local release of bone resorbing cytokines by tumour metastases in bones.

# ENDOGENOUS PIGMENTATION

## IRON-CONTAINING PIGMENT

Two main pigments are derived from the breakdown of red blood cells:

(1) HAEMOSIDERIN and (2) BILIRUBIN.

The detailed mechanism is described on page 372 in relation to JAUNDICE.

## HAEMOSIDERIN

The iron derived from red cell breakdown is held in the spleen, liver and bone marrow, combined with apoferritin. In the plasma it is transported by transferrin. The two mechanisms maintain an equilibrium between the iron contents in these three sites. When the amount of iron within the cells becomes excessive and overloads the ferritin system, it is deposited in a brown granular form – haemosiderin. This occurs in two situations:

### 1. Local breakdown of red cells in tissues, e.g. in a bruise

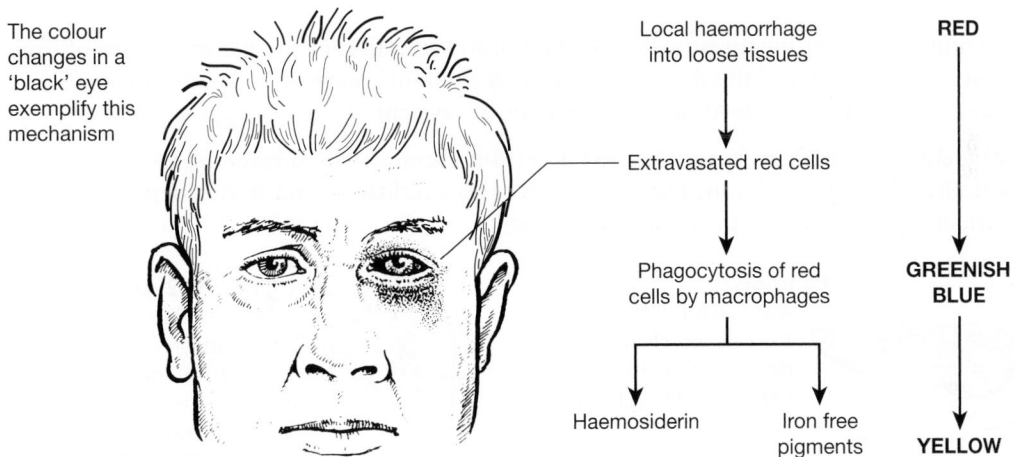

The colour changes in a 'black' eye exemplify this mechanism

Local haemorrhage into loose tissues → RED

↓

Extravasated red cells

↓

Phagocytosis of red cells by macrophages → GREENISH BLUE

↓

Haemosiderin    Iron free pigments → YELLOW

### 2. Iron overload in tissues

(a) *Haemosiderosis*

This is seen in the liver, spleen and sometimes the kidneys in cases of haemolytic anaemia, and in patients requiring repeated blood transfusion. The change is most dramatic in the liver, which becomes deep brown. Iron is found in the Kupffer cells first and, later, in liver cells. Perls stain highlights the iron deposits, which are stained blue. Iron deposits *per se* very rarely cause organ damage.

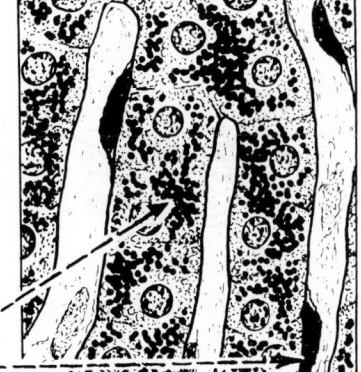

Granules of haemosiderin in liver cells in later stages

Kupffer cell

# ENDOGENOUS PIGMENTATION

(b) *Haemochromatosis (Bronzed diabetes)*

The absorption of iron from the intestine is controlled by the ferritin-transferrin mechanism.

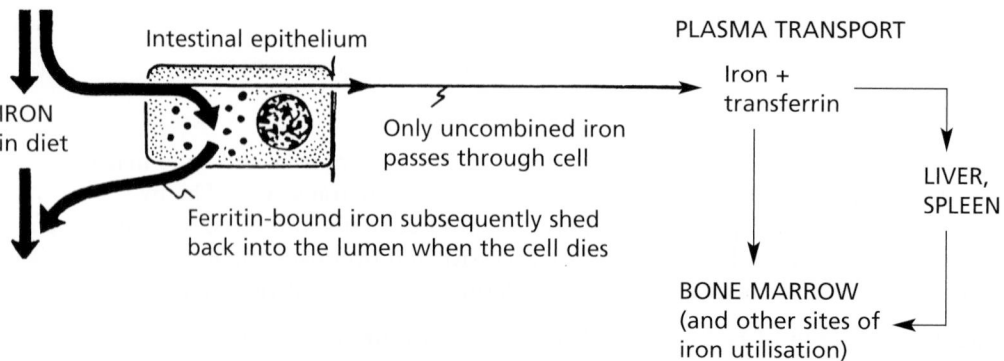

The ferritin content of the intestinal epithelium, iron saturation of the plasma, stores of iron in the liver and spleen and the demand for iron by the bone marrow form a balancing mechanism preventing overloading of any part of the system.

In haemochromatosis there is an inherited defect on chromosome 6 resulting in uncontrolled absorption of iron. The system becomes overloaded and iron is deposited as haemosiderin in many sites, the main ones being:

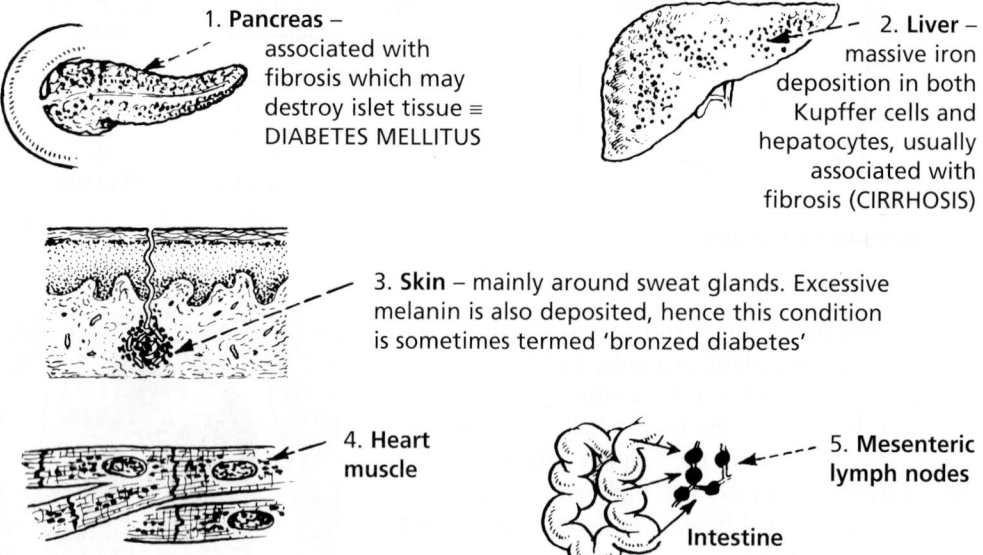

Haemosiderin may be found in almost any site in the body.

# ENDOGENOUS PIGMENTATION

## Haemoglobin

Intravascular haemolysis can result in haemoglobin appearing in the urine, giving it a dull red colour. In severe acute haemolysis (e.g. incompatible blood transfusion) acute renal tubular necrosis occurs. In chronic haemolysis (e.g. paroxysmal haemoglobinuria), some of the haemoglobin is reabsorbed and subsequently broken down so that iron, as haemosiderin, appears in the renal tubular epithelium.

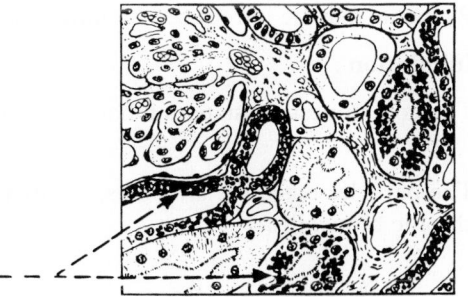

(Demonstrated by the Prussian blue reaction)

## Haematin (or haemazoin)

This is a brown pigment produced by malarial parasites from haemoglobin. It is taken up by the monocytes in the blood and subsequently deposited in the liver and spleen.

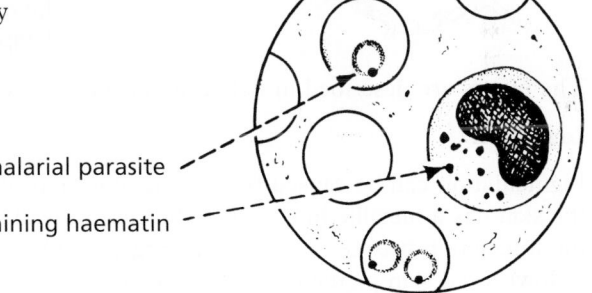

Red-cell – containing malarial parasite

Monocyte – containing haematin

## Lipofuscin

This is a yellowish brown pigment with a high lipid content, often found in the atrophied cells of old age – 'wear and tear' pigment. It is particularly common in the heart muscle, and the term 'brown atrophy' is often applied.

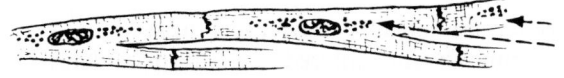

Thin myocardial fibre
Lipofuscin granules around nucleus

It is also found in liver cells, testes and nerve cells.

# EXOGENOUS PIGMENTATION

## EXOGENOUS PIGMENTATION

Pigments may be introduced by inhalation, ingestion or injection.

### Inhalation

The commonest substances inhaled are COAL DUST (carbon) – black, and STONE DUST (silica) – grey.

The particles reach the alveoli especially if the bronchial ciliary action is disturbed by chronic bronchitis.

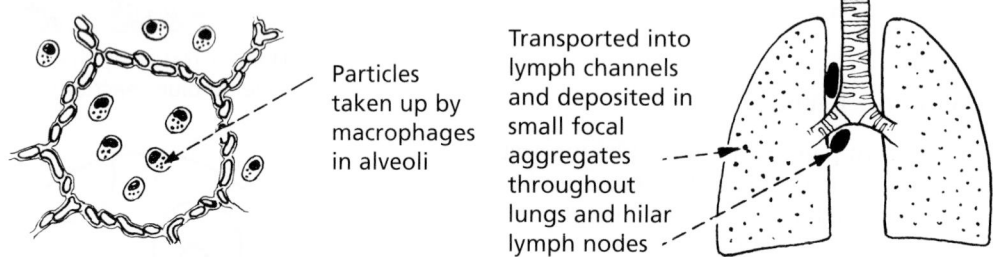

Particles taken up by macrophages in alveoli

Transported into lymph channels and deposited in small focal aggregates throughout lungs and hilar lymph nodes

The effects are described in detail under PNEUMOCONIOSIS.

### Ingestion

Pigmentation can be caused by chronic ingestion of metals such as silver or lead. In both, the skin has a metallic hue, and in the case of lead a blue line appears on the gums due to the interaction between lead and hydrogen sulphide. Excessive intake of carrots can lead to yellowish red skin pigmentation caused by carotene.

### Injection

Tattooing is the most striking example of pigmentation following injection.

## DEGENERATIONS

### 1. Hyaline

This is a descriptive term meaning a glossy, refractile appearance, seen in sections stained with haematoxylin and eosin. It is most commonly encountered in the form of dense collagen, particularly in benign tumours such as leiomyomas where the collagen has replaced muscle fibres, and in blood vessels in arteriosclerosis.

The term 'Mallory hyaline' refers to an *intra*cellular accumulation of cytoskeletal proteins, e.g. in alcoholic liver disease (p. 380).

### 2. Mucoid

This is a common change in epithelial tumours which secrete mucin. In these cases the epithelial cells undergo degeneration and appear to dissolve in the mucin.

Connective tissue may also accumulate mucin. Spaces filled with mucopolysaccharides (e.g. hyaluronic acid) appear between the fibres. The change is common in some tumours and the term 'myxomatous' may be used.

# GENETIC DISEASE

## OBJECTIVES

1. To understand the structure of DNA, gene expression and protein synthesis.
2. To state the differences between mitosis and meiosis.
3. To describe the common chromosomal abnormalities.
4. To understand single gene disorders and different types of inheritance.
5. To list the various common techniques available for the diagnosis of chromosomal and genetic abnormalities and their common applications.
6. To have an understanding of molecular biology in gene therapy and drug design.

# HEREDITY, GENES AND DISEASE

### CELL NUCLEUS AND CHROMOSOMES

The cell **NUCLEUS** contains CHROMOSOMES, which transmit hereditary traits from one generation to the next and also control the synthesis of all the proteins in the body.

The 46 chromosomes, which most human nuclei contain, are not identifiable in differentiated cells or cells in the non-proliferating phase of the cell cycle ($G_0$).

The different morphological appearances of nuclei in histological sections indicate the amount of nuclear activity.

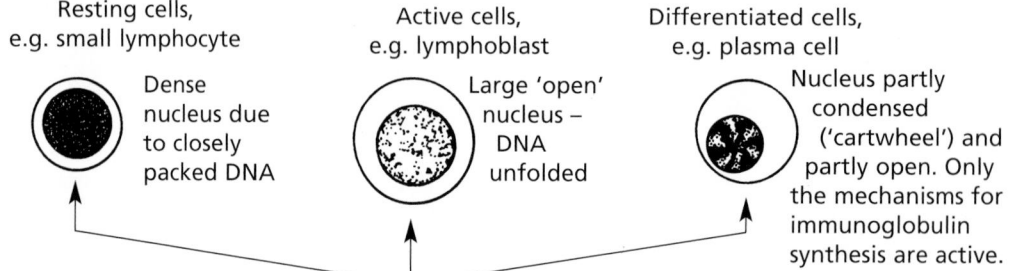

Resting cells, e.g. small lymphocyte — Dense nucleus due to closely packed DNA

Active cells, e.g. lymphoblast — Large 'open' nucleus – DNA unfolded

Differentiated cells, e.g. plasma cell — Nucleus partly condensed ('cartwheel') and partly open. Only the mechanisms for immunoglobulin synthesis are active.

Individual chromosomes NOT identifiable. (Can be demonstrated by molecular methods, e.g. fluorescent-in-situ hybridisation [FISH].)

# HEREDITY, GENES AND DISEASE

## Chromosomes

Chromosomes are packaged DNA within the cell nucleus. Each chromosome has a long arm designated the 'q arm' and a short arm designated the 'p arm'. Telomeres are present at the end of each chromosome. The DNA strand is wound around histones and packaged with other proteins into a compact structure.

Diagram of a typical chromosome 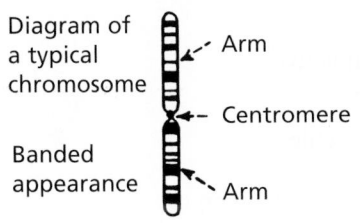 Arm

Centromere

Banded appearance

Arm

The following features are specific to each chromosome: (1) Overall length, (2) position of centromere (this dictates the length of each arm) and (3) the pattern of banding.

e.g. 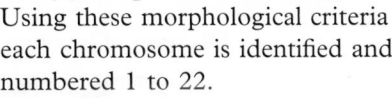 Using these morphological criteria each chromosome is identified and numbered 1 to 22.

The sex chromosomes are labelled 'X' large and 'Y' small

*Note:* This appearance represents a very condensed and coiled molecular arrangement, i.e. inactive.

A typical normal chromosome map (karyotype) shows 22 pairs of different but identifiable chromosomes...................................................... plus two sex chromosomes.

Each pair is called an AUTOSOME and consists of a PATERNAL and MATERNAL chromosome.

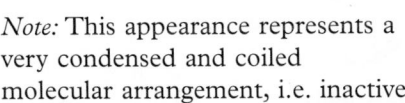 ×22

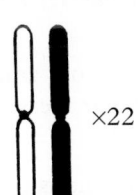

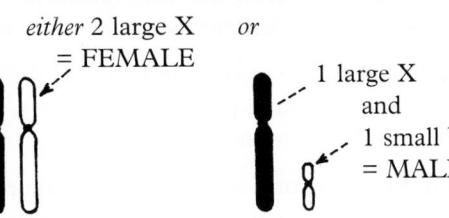

*either* 2 large X = FEMALE *or*

1 large X and 1 small Y = MALE

# DEOXYRIBONUCLEIC ACID (DNA)

Each chromosome is a very long single molecule of DNA, condensed during mitosis. The DNA molecule consists of a deoxyribose (sugar) and phosphate backbone with covalently bonded bases. It forms two strands, organised as a helix running in opposite directions, held together by hydrogen bonds. Adenine always pairs with thymine and guanine always pairs with cytosine.

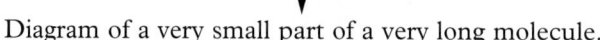

It is extended to its characteristic structure when active:

Diagram of a very small part of a very long molecule.

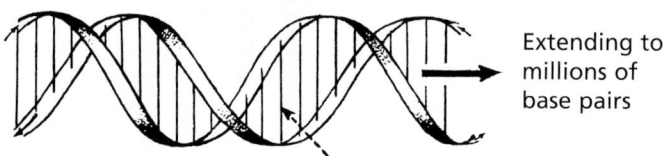

Extending to millions of base pairs

Joined by purine and pyrimidine base pairs

## The **DOUBLE HELIX**

Two long spirals of nucleotides (consisting of a deoxyribose [sugar] + phosphate) around a central axis, complementary but running in opposite directions.

The function is to initiate and control the synthesis of proteins from amino acids. All types of protein (structural proteins, hormones, receptors, intra-cellular messengers, etc.) are ENCODED along the molecule.

A **GENE** is the unit of the chromosome responsible for the synthesis of a single SPECIFIC PROTEIN. Genes vary in length but on average occupy about 20 000 base pairs of the molecule.

There are over 10 000 genes in all the human chromosomes, not all are active: some are repetitive: some form clusters subserving related activities (e.g. Major Histocompatibility Complex [Human Leukocyte Antigen] locus, see p. 131).

There is a complex REGULATION of gene activity involving stop and start signals, promotor and enhancer functions all within the DNA structure. The entire human genome has now been sequenced.

Every copy of the human genome contains multiple variations in sequence. These variations are described as polymorphisms. They do not always cause disease but they may predispose an individual to disease, e.g. HLA B27 and ankylosing spondylitis.

# DEOXYRIBONUCLEIC ACID (DNA)

## Gene expression and protein synthesis

A gene consists of coding regions (EXONS) interspersed with non-coding regions (INTRONS). In transcription the introns are eliminated and all the exons are transcribed to a ribonucleic acid form (mRNA) which is a copy of the DNA code sequencing the amino acids required for the production of a specific protein.

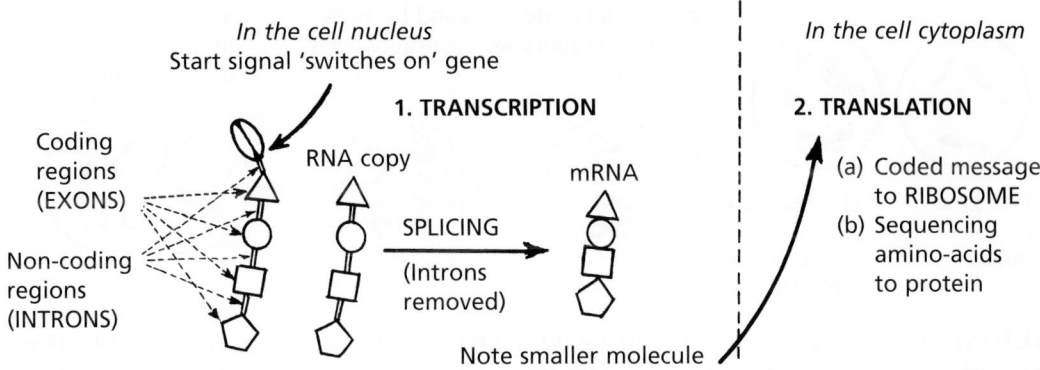

# MITOSIS AND MEIOSIS

**MITOSIS** is the process by which SOMATIC cells proliferate ensuring *exact replication of the daughter cells.* Following the stimulus to proliferate, the chromosomes condense and replicate exactly.

PROPHASE
All chromosomes
condense and replicate

METAPHASE
All chromosomes
are aligned along
equatorial plate:
nuclear membrane
'dissolves'.

ANAPHASE
Chromatids are
'pulled apart'
and become
chromosomes.

TELOPHASE
Two daughter cells
are about to form,
each containing
identical
chromosomes.

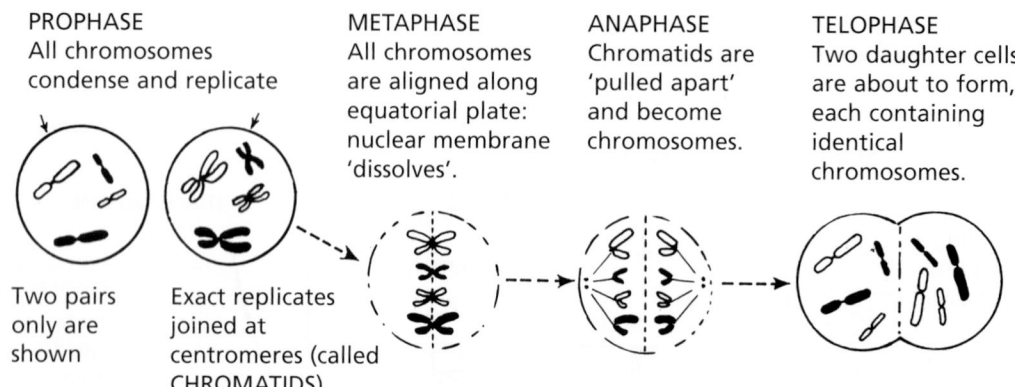

Two pairs
only are
shown

Exact replicates
joined at
centromeres (called
CHROMATIDS).

**MEIOSIS** is a complex process occurring during GAMETOGENESIS. It involves the reduction and division of chromosomes in such a way that: (1) a random mixture of both parental genes is present in the gamete and (2) the chances are equal for fertilisation to result in either sex. This simple diagram shows the important results of meiosis.

Primitive germ cell contains 46 chromosomes (i.e. 22 autosomes + XX or XY)

1. During MEIOSIS the chromosomes come close together and random segments are exchanged.
2. During MEIOSIS the sex chromosomes are similarly distributed.

# MITOSIS AND MEIOSIS

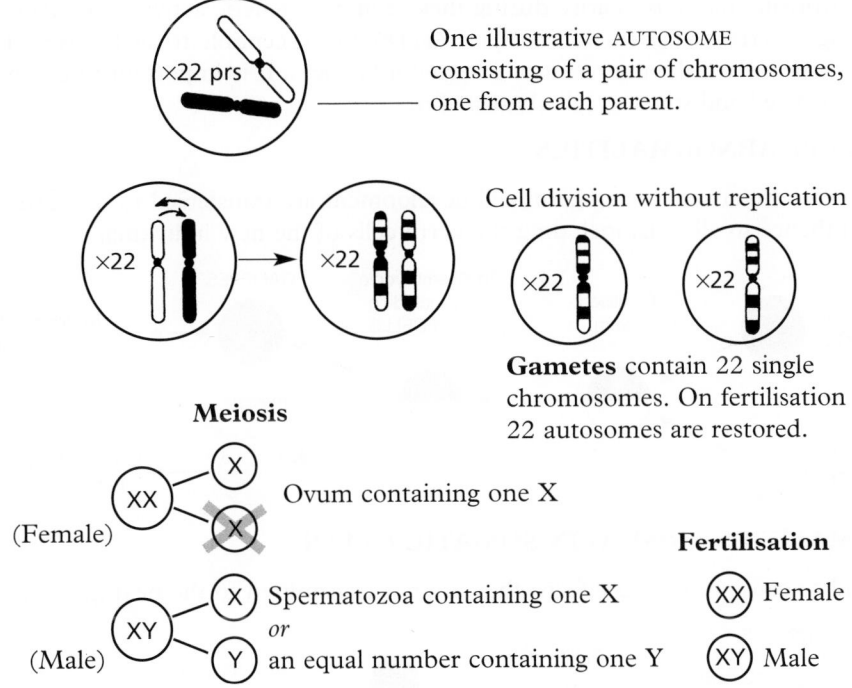

One illustrative AUTOSOME consisting of a pair of chromosomes, one from each parent.

Cell division without replication

**Gametes** contain 22 single chromosomes. On fertilisation 22 autosomes are restored.

**Meiosis**

Ovum containing one X

**Fertilisation**

(Female)

(Male)

Spermatozoa containing one X
*or*
an equal number containing one Y

XX Female

XY Male

*Note:* In this simplified diagram a preliminary replication before meiosis and mitotic divisions after meiosis are omitted. The chances of error are greatly increased.

# GENETIC ABNORMALITIES AND ASSOCIATED DISORDERS

It is not surprising that errors arise during these complex genetic activities. GERM CELLS and proliferating SOMATIC CELLS (including STEM CELLS) are susceptible to such errors. They may occur spontaneously or be the result of external influences. It is important to distinguish between germ cell and somatic cell abnormalities.

## GERM CELL ABNORMALITIES

Errors which have arisen during germ cell development are transferred to the fertilised ovum and thence to all cells, including the germ cells of the new individual.

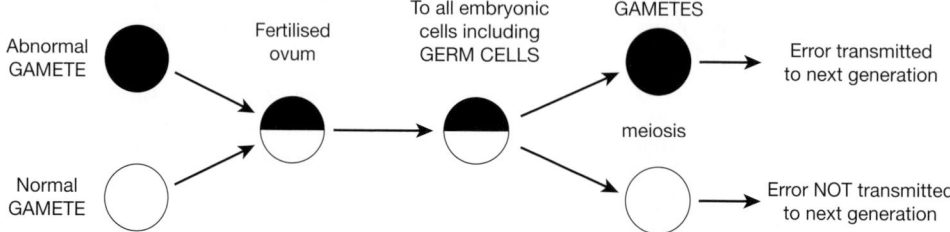

## ABNORMALITIES ARISING IN SOMATIC CELLS

These tend to cause restricted effects; they are not transmitted to the next generation.

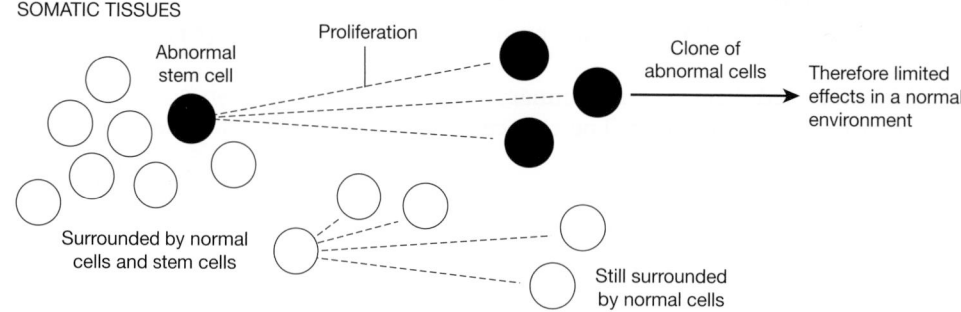

# TYPES OF GENETIC ABNORMALITIES

They range from large, involving whole chromosomes, through parts of chromosomes, to gene clusters and single genes.

## CHROMOSOMAL ABNORMALITIES

1. **Polyploidy** – when the chromosomal numbers are increased by an exact multiple of the normal (23), e.g. $23 \times 3 = 69$ chromosomes. Such nuclei are seen in hypertrophied muscle cells and ageing liver cells (i.e. somatic cell polyploidy). Such gross chromosomal abnormalities occurring during gametogenesis or at fertilisation are usually incompatible with life and a common cause of spontaneous abortion.

2. **Aneuploidy** – where the number of chromosomes is increased usually by one (TRISOMY) or decreased by one (MONOSOMY). Early spontaneous abortion is again common; survivors show mental retardation and varied physical abnormalities. Down syndrome is a good example of *autosomal trisomy* and is due to an extra chromosome (i.e. Trisomy 21 – karyotype 47XX + 21 or 47XY + 21). The abnormality occurs in utero after fertilisation of the ovum and is therefore autosomal. Increasing maternal age is a potentiating factor in Down syndrome and many other genetic defects.

3. **Structural abnormalities** – Despite the existence of efficient repair mechanisms, structural errors do arise when the long DNA molecules are accidentally broken during the physical changes occurring at replication. They include, for example, duplication and deletion of gene clusters and single genes, and translocation and inversion of fragments of DNA between chromosomes.

## SINGLE GENE DISORDERS

Factors regulating the production of the final specific protein are extremely complex.

1. *In the nucleus*                                                                   *In the cytoplasm*

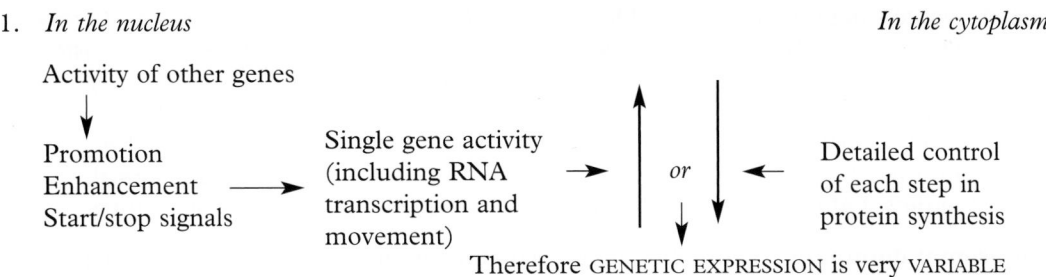

Therefore GENETIC EXPRESSION is very VARIABLE

# TYPES OF GENETIC ABNORMALITIES

2.  The corresponding genes on each parental chromosome exert important influences on each other. The inheritance of the Rhesus blood group D is a good example: there are two possibilities at the D locus on the chromosome – 'D' or 'd'. The three possible combinations give rise to the actual blood group (phenotype) as follows:

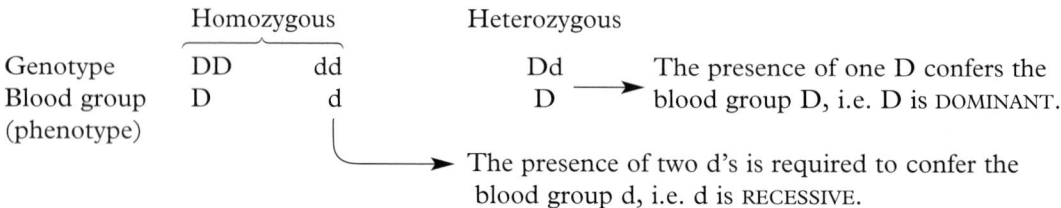

|  | Homozygous | | Heterozygous |
|---|---|---|---|
| Genotype | DD | dd | Dd |
| Blood group (phenotype) | D | d | D |

The presence of one D confers the blood group D, i.e. D is DOMINANT.

The presence of two d's is required to confer the blood group d, i.e. d is RECESSIVE.

This concept is important in *inherited single gene disorders.*

1.  In DOMINANT inheritance, any HETEROZYGOUS offspring bearing the abnormal trait will be affected: mating with a normal partner statistically produces 50% of normal offspring and 50% affected.
2.  In RECESSIVE inheritance, only HOMOZYGOTES for the trait are affected. Such cases usually arise from the mating of two heterozygous CARRIERS who, by definition, are themselves unaffected. The results of mating are as follows: (A = affected gene, N = normal gene)

NN = normal individual; NA = carrier; AA = affected individual.

The concept of dominant and recessive traits is useful in genetic counselling. Long lists of dominant and recessive disorders are available: only a few important examples are given.

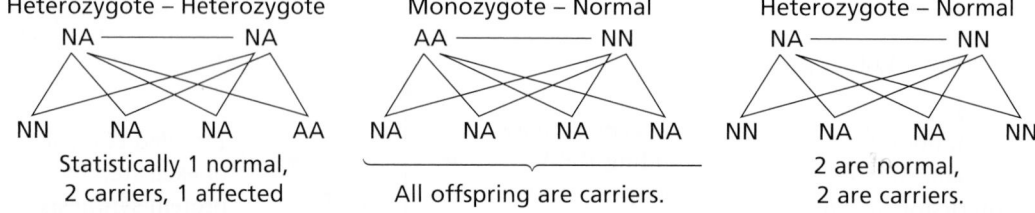

Heterozygote – Heterozygote
NA —— NA
NN  NA  NA  AA
Statistically 1 normal, 2 carriers, 1 affected

Monozygote – Normal
AA —— NN
NA  NA  NA  NA
All offspring are carriers.

Heterozygote – Normal
NA —— NN
NN  NA  NA  NN
2 are normal, 2 are carriers.

**Autosomal dominant** – neurofibromatosis, Huntington disease, polyposis coli, congenital spherocytosis.

**Autosomal recessive** – cystic fibrosis, congenital deafness, mucopolysaccharidoses.

**Sex-linked disorders** are usually recessive and are carried on the X chromosome: males are affected and females are carriers. Important disorders are haemophilia and muscular dystrophy.

# TYPES OF GENETIC ABNORMALITIES

## METABOLIC DISORDERS (INBORN ERRORS OF METABOLISM)

These are inherited disorders of single genes which code for the enzymes concerned in many metabolic pathways. The clinical effects show considerable variation in severity. Examples are disorders of carbohydrate (including glycogen storage), lipid and amino acid metabolism; lysosomal storage and membrane transport (including cystic fibrosis).

*Note*: Not all single gene abnormalities cause, by themselves, significant pathological effects. As indicated above, the controlling factors are complex and include the important effects of 'modifying genes'. It seems likely that abnormal recessive genes exist in the normal population but only present as clinical disorders in rare circumstances.

## MULTIFACTORIAL DISORDERS

Most human diseases have a genetic component but environmental factors usually play a very important part in the pathogenesis.

COMBINED ACTIVITY
of SEVERAL GENES       +    ENVIRONMENTAL    ⟶    DISEASE
(both normal and abnormal)        FACTORS

Examples are atopic (allergic) disorders, diabetes mellitus, hypertension, rheumatoid arthritis and various infections.

## SOMATIC CELL GENETIC DISORDERS

When mutation occurs after fertilisation of the ovum and at any stage throughout life the effects are limited to the disordered cell(s) and progeny. The clinical effects tend to be localised.

NEOPLASMS and hamartomas are examples of somatic cell genetic disorders (see Carcinogenesis).

*Note*: In the systematic section of this book significant genetic contribution to the pathogenesis of diseases will be recorded.

# DIAGNOSIS OF GENETIC ABNORMALITIES

The diagnosis of genetic disease requires examination of genetic material (i.e. chromosomes and genes) in various ways.

## CHROMOSOMAL ANALYSIS

The techniques include:

### 1. Karyotyping

During MITOSIS the chromosomes condense into specific morphological forms which are identifiable by light microscopy: when colchicine is added to a cell culture, mitosis is arrested at the metaphase: chromosomes are then separable and can be studied.

### 2. Comparative genomic hybridisation

Comparative genomic hybridisation is used to detect chromosomal imbalance, deletions and duplications by comparing sample DNA with control DNA.

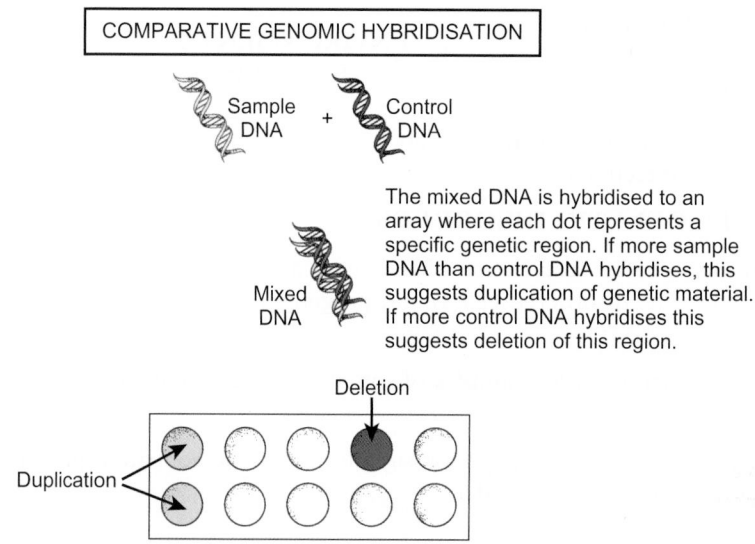

### 3. Fluorescence in situ hybridisation

Fluorescence in situ hybridisation (FISH) is a cytogenetic technique that uses fluorescent probes to bind to regions of chromosomes of interest. The principles are similar to immunohistochemistry except the target is DNA rather than protein.

FISH can be used for diagnosis of chromosomal translocations in soft tissue tumours and leukaemias and for assessment of Her2 copy number in breast cancer (see p. 565).

# DIAGNOSIS OF GENETIC ABNORMALITIES

## GENETIC ANALYSIS

### 1. Polymerase chain reaction

The polymerase chain reaction (PCR) is used to amplify a single copy or a few copies of a segment of DNA, generating thousands to millions of copies of a particular DNA sequence. The products of PCR are run on a gel.

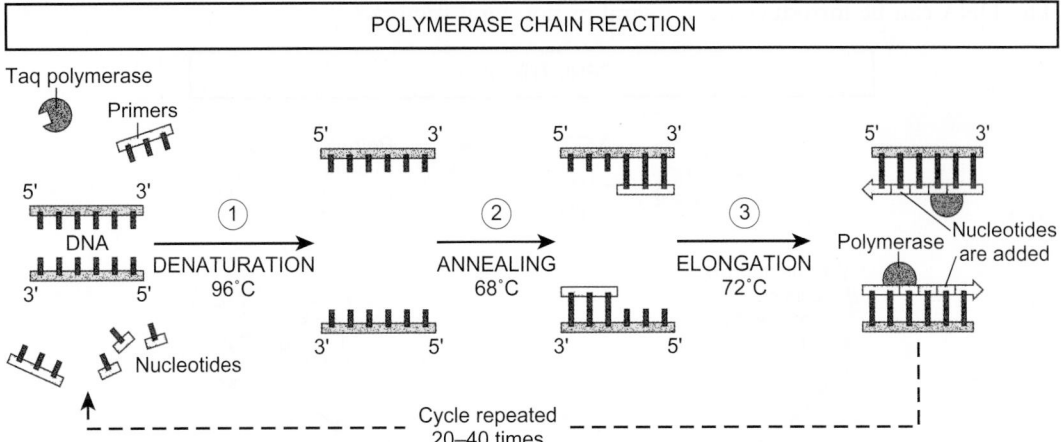

### 2. Sequencing

In conventional sequencing primers are added to DNA to be sequenced and one of the four nucleotides replaced with an altered nucleotide that binds and terminates the reaction. The four products are run on a gel. The gene is pieced together from the different products obtained. Conventional sequencing is slow and expensive.

Next generation sequencing sequences a large number of short DNA fragments in a single experiment. The extracted DNA is fragmented into small segments and these fragments are sequenced in parallel. The sequences are aligned to a reference gene.

The whole genome sequence is derived from the consensus of aligned reads.

## APPLICATIONS

These cytogenetic and molecular biology techniques have a wider remit than the diagnosis of genetic disease. They can be used for diagnosing infections (the HIV test is PCR based), tissue matching in transplantation and paternity testing to determine whether two individuals are biologically parent and child. These techniques are also important in forensic analysis with roles including victim identification and confirming suspects who may have inadvertently left DNA at the scene of a crime.

# GENE THERAPY

Gene therapy is the delivery of genetic material into a patient's cells with the aim of correcting a genetic abnormality. The aim is to fix a genetic problem at its source.

There are two main focuses:

1. To deliver DNA to correct damaged somatic cells.
2. To introduce functional genes into stem cells so the change is heritable.

The DNA can be introduced using viral or non-viral vectors.

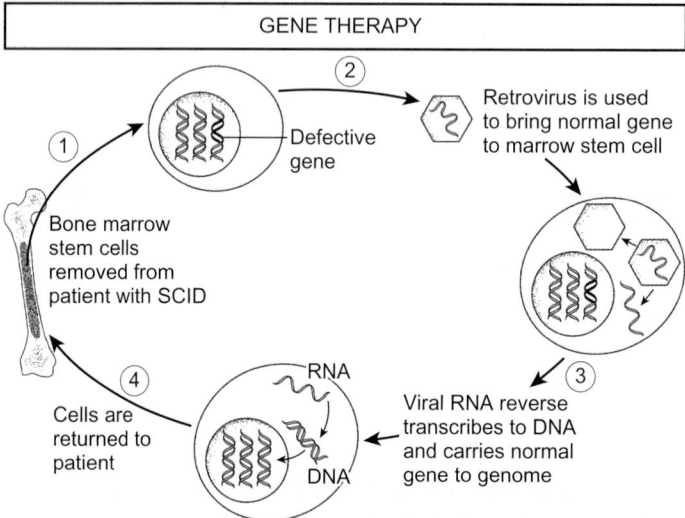

This is still very much experimental but is a potential treatment for single gene disorders such as haemophilia and cystic fibrosis. Severe combined immune deficiency (SCID) was one of the first genetic disorders treated with gene therapy. Problems have arisen with viral vectors which can trigger leukaemia.

# DRUG DESIGN

Advances in molecular biology have resulted in an explosion of targeted cancer therapies. These are drugs designed to target specific molecules that are involved in growth progression and spread of cancer. The use of these drugs usually requires confirmation of an abnormal gene (and therefore protein product) using molecular techniques such as PCR and FISH. Examples include tyrosine kinase inhibitors used in lung cancer in which there is a mutation in the epidermal growth factor receptor gene (p. 311)

# INFLAMMATION, HEALING AND REPAIR

## OBJECTIVES

**1.** To understand the causes and mechanisms of acute and chronic inflammation.
**2.** To understand the role of chemical mediators in inflammation.
**3.** To list the sequelae of acute inflammation.
**4.** To understand the formation and causes of granulomatous inflammation.
**5.** To describe the features and causes of ulcers, sinuses and fistulae.
**6.** To describe the mechanisms of wound healing at various sites.
**7.** To understand the factors that affect wound healing at various sites.

# INFLAMMATION

Inflammation is the dynamic process by which living tissues react to injury. It concerns vascular and connective tissues in particular.

**Causes:**

Various agents may kill or damage cells:

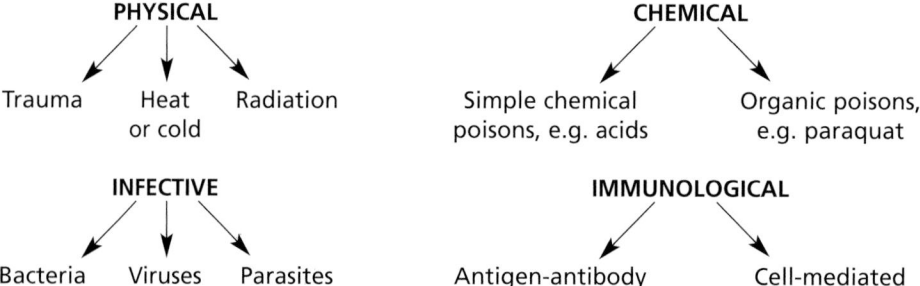

...and any other circumstance leading to tissue damage, e.g. VASCULAR or HORMONAL DISTURBANCE.

The inflammatory reaction takes place in the surviving adjacent vascular and connective tissues; the specialised parenchymal cells do not directly participate.

The initial stages are known as the **acute** inflammatory reaction. Where the process is prolonged the inflammation may be **subacute** or **chronic**.

# ACUTE INFLAMMATION

The classical signs are:

REDNESS (rubor)
HEAT (calor)
SWELLING (tumor)
PAIN (dolor)
LOSS OF FUNCTION (functio laesa)

*e.g.* boil

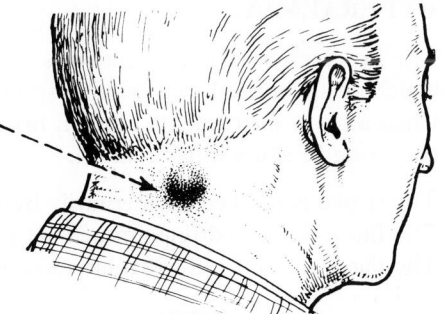

These gross signs are explained by changes occurring at microscopic level. Three essential features are:

1. **HYPERAEMIA**
2. **EXUDATION OF FLUID**
3. **EMIGRATION OF LEUCOCYTES**

# ACUTE INFLAMMATION

### HYPERAEMIA

The hyperaemia in inflammation is associated with the well-known microvascular changes which occur in the Lewis triple response – a FLUSH, a FLARE and a WEAL. It occurs when a blunt instrument is drawn firmly across the skin and illustrates the vascular changes occurring in acute inflammation.

The stroke is marked momentarily by a white line due to VASOCONSTRICTION.
The flush, a dull red line, immediately follows and is due to CAPILLARY DILATATION.
The flare, a bright red irregular surrounding zone, is due to ARTERIOLAR DILATATION.

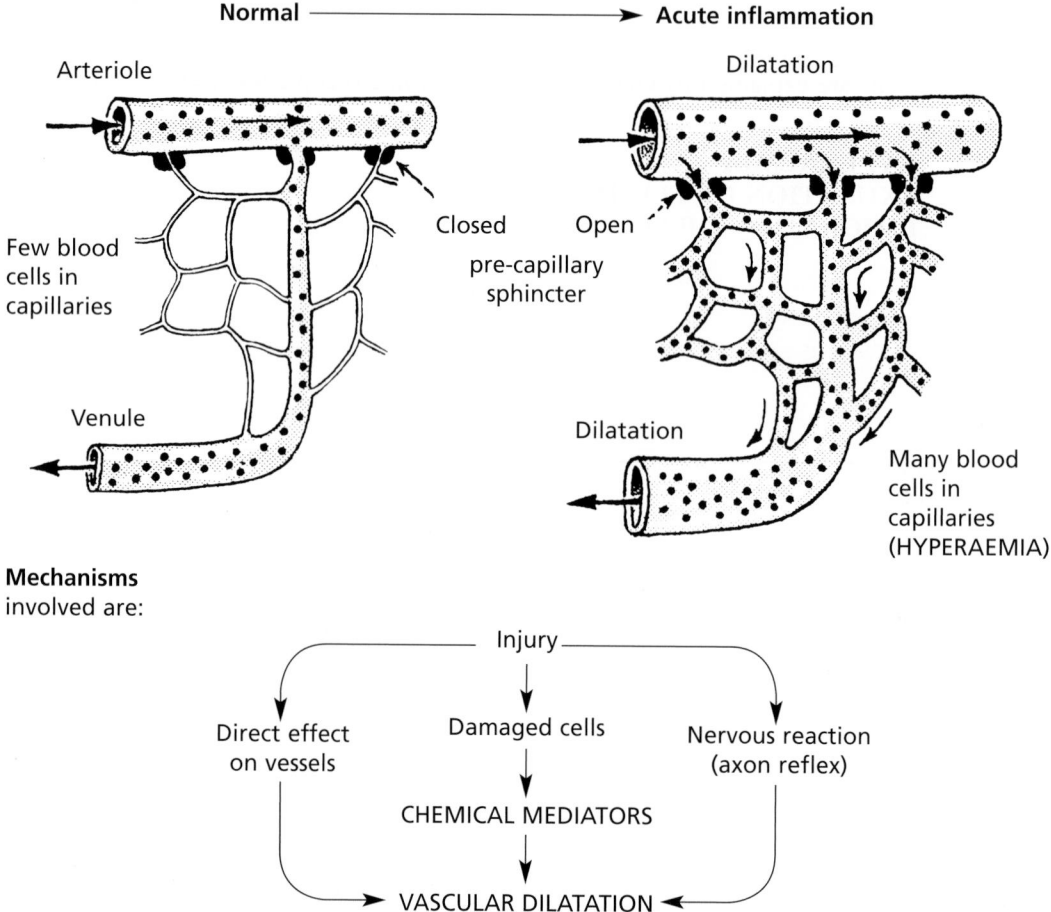

HYPERAEMIA explains the classical signs of REDNESS and HEAT.

# ACUTE INFLAMMATION

## EXUDATION

Exudation is the increased passage of protein-rich fluid through the vessel wall into the interstitial tissue. It explains the *weal* in the Lewis triple response.

**Advantageous results**

Fluid increase

↓

Dilution of toxins

**Contents of fluid**

(a) Globulins ➤ protective antibodies

(b) Fibrin deposition ➤ helps to limit spread of bacteria

(c) Various factors promoting subsequent healing

## Mechanism

1. *Protein passage*

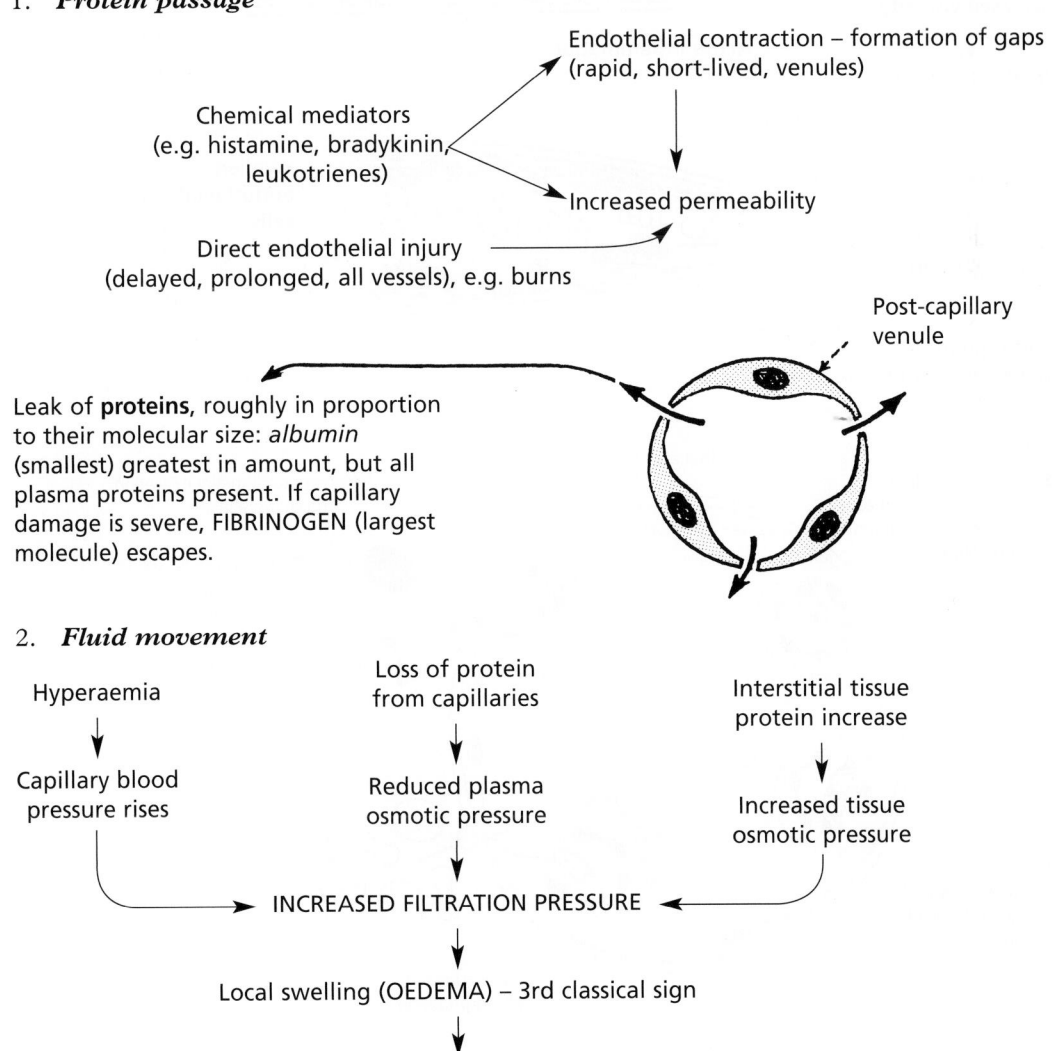

Chemical mediators
(e.g. histamine, bradykinin, leukotrienes)

Endothelial contraction – formation of gaps
(rapid, short-lived, venules)

↓

Increased permeability

Direct endothelial injury
(delayed, prolonged, all vessels), e.g. burns

Post-capillary venule

Leak of **proteins**, roughly in proportion to their molecular size: *albumin* (smallest) greatest in amount, but all plasma proteins present. If capillary damage is severe, FIBRINOGEN (largest molecule) escapes.

2. *Fluid movement*

| Hyperaemia | Loss of protein from capillaries | Interstitial tissue protein increase |
|---|---|---|
| ↓ | ↓ | ↓ |
| Capillary blood pressure rises | Reduced plasma osmotic pressure | Increased tissue osmotic pressure |

INCREASED FILTRATION PRESSURE

↓

Local swelling (OEDEMA) – 3rd classical sign

↓

Increased lymph flow from area

# ACUTE INFLAMMATION

## EMIGRATION OF LEUCOCYTES

Neutrophils and mononuclears pass between the endothelial cell junctions by amoeboid movement through the venule wall into the tissue spaces. In this process both neutrophils and endothelial cells are activated and both express cell adhesion molecules, initially SELECTINS and then INTEGRINS.

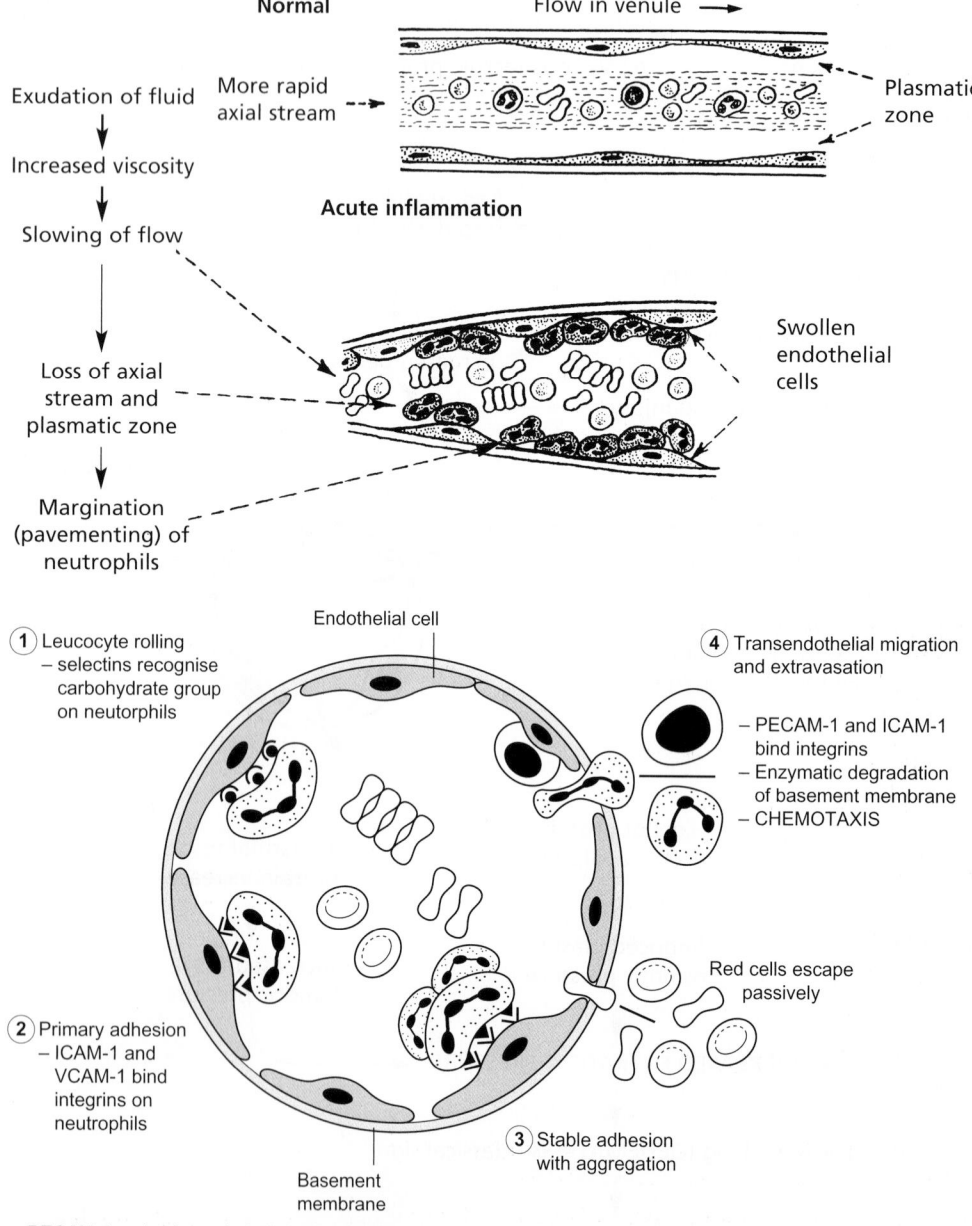

PECAM-1 – platelet endothelial cell adhesion molecule 1, ICAM-1 – intercellular adhesion molecule 1, VCAM-1 – vascular cell adhesion molecule 1.

# ACUTE INFLAMMATION

## CHEMOTAXIS

The initial margination of neutrophils and mononuclears is potentiated by slowing of blood flow and by increased 'stickiness' of the endothelial surface.

After penetration of the vessel wall, the subsequent movement of the leucocytes is controlled by CHEMOTAXIS. The cell moves in response to an increasing concentration gradient of the particular chemotactic agent, usually a protein or polypeptide.

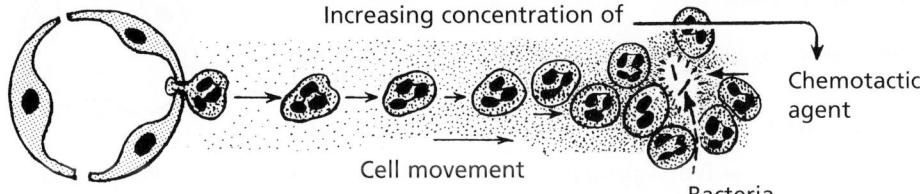

Important examples of chemotactic agents are:

Fractions of the COMPLEMENT SYSTEM (esp. C3a)
Factors derived from arachidonic acid by the neutrophils – LEUKOTRIENES (e.g. LTB4, leukotriene B4)
Factors derived from pathogenic BACTERIA
Factors derived from sensitised lymphocytes – CYTOKINES (e.g. IL-8, interleukin 8).

The leucocytes move by extension of an anterior pseudopod with attachment to extracellular matrix molecules such as fibronectin using cell adhesion molecules. The cell body is then pulled forward by actin and myosin filaments.

## PHAGOCYTOSIS

This is the process by which neutrophils and macrophages clear the injurious agent. It is an important defence mechanism in bacterial infections particularly.

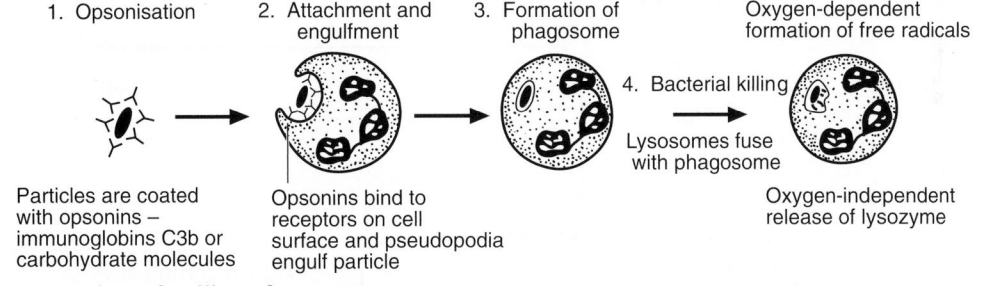

There are three families of OPSONIN:

1.  Immunoglobulin, especially IgG, immunoglobulin G
    – recognised by Fc receptors on neutrophil surface.
2.  Complement, especially C3b
    – recognised by C3b receptors on neutrophil surface.
3.  Secreted pattern recognition receptors, e.g. penetraxins, collectins, ficolins
    – bind sugar residues on bacterial cell walls.

The opsonic activity is enhanced when it is confined within a solid organ or rigid medium such as a fibrin network; where conditions are looser and more fluid, activity is diminished.

# ACUTE INFLAMMATION

### CHEMICAL MEDIATORS

Various chemical mediators have roles in the inflammatory process. They may be circulating in plasma and require activation or they may be secreted by inflammatory cells. Many of these mediators have overlapping actions.

Mediators derived from:

1.  Inflammatory cells.

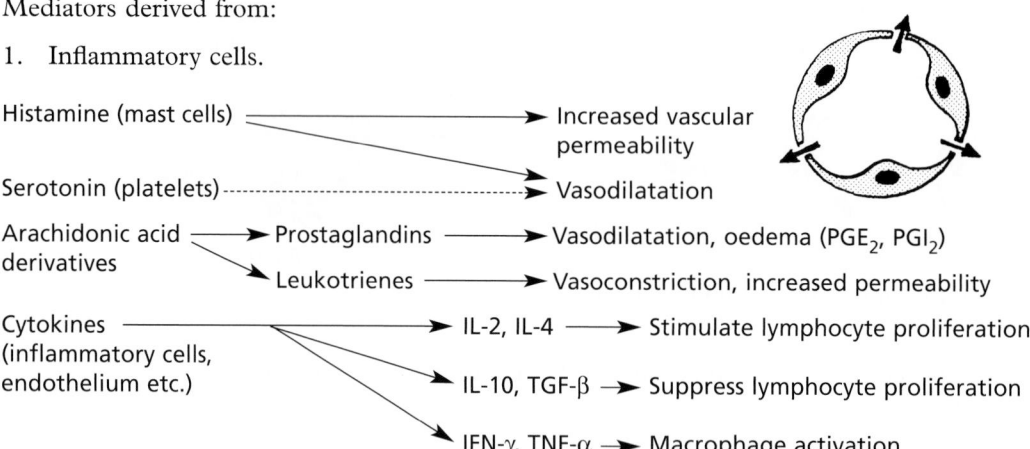

Histamine (mast cells) ⟶ Increased vascular permeability

Serotonin (platelets) ⟶ Vasodilatation

Arachidonic acid derivatives ⟶ Prostaglandins ⟶ Vasodilatation, oedema ($PGE_2$, $PGI_2$)

⟶ Leukotrienes ⟶ Vasoconstriction, increased permeability

Cytokines (inflammatory cells, endothelium etc.) ⟶ IL-2, IL-4 ⟶ Stimulate lymphocyte proliferation

⟶ IL-10, TGF-β ⟶ Suppress lymphocyte proliferation

⟶ IFN-γ, TNF-α ⟶ Macrophage activation

2.  Plasma. These pathways are all interrelated.

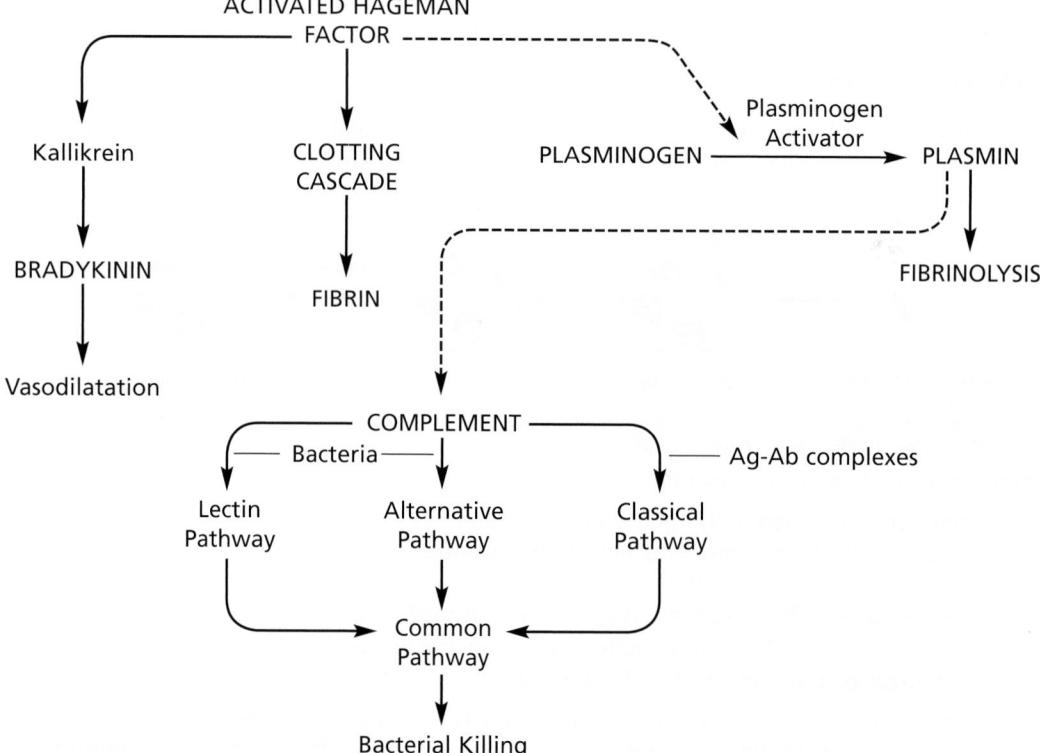

ACTIVATED HAGEMAN FACTOR

Kallikrein

BRADYKININ

Vasodilatation

CLOTTING CASCADE

FIBRIN

PLASMINOGEN ⟶ Plasminogen Activator ⟶ PLASMIN

FIBRINOLYSIS

COMPLEMENT

Bacteria — Ag-Ab complexes

Lectin Pathway

Alternative Pathway

Classical Pathway

Common Pathway

Bacterial Killing

# SEQUELS OF ACUTE INFLAMMATION

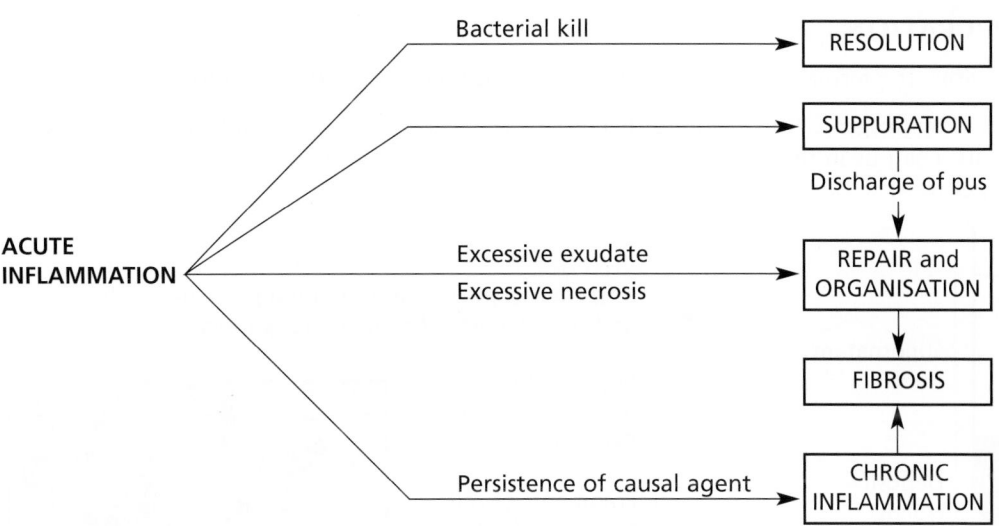

## RESOLUTION

This means the complete restoration of normal conditions after the acute inflammation. The three main features which potentiate this sequel are:

1. Minimal cell death and tissue damage.
2. Rapid elimination of the causal agent, e.g. bacteria.
3. Local conditions favouring removal of fluid and debris.

Resolution of lobar pneumonia (bacterial inflammation of lung alveoli) is a good example:

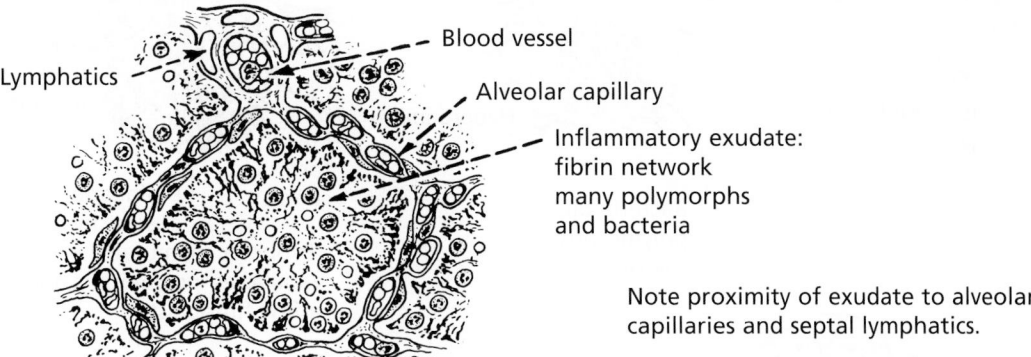

Note proximity of exudate to alveolar capillaries and septal lymphatics.

Following bacterial kill, the mechanism is as follows:

1. Solution of fibrin by enzyme action (polymorphs and fibrinolysin).
2. Removal of fluid by blood vessels and lymphatics.
3. Removal of all debris by phagocytes to hilar lymph nodes.
4. The capillary hyperaemia diminishes and restoration to normal is complete.

# SEQUELS OF ACUTE INFLAMMATION

### SUPPURATION

This means the formation of PUS; where pus accumulates an ABSCESS forms.

Infection by pyogenic (pus-forming) bacteria is the usual cause, e.g. staphylococcal abscess (or boil). The pus in this case is a thick, creamy yellow fluid which, on centrifugation, separates thus:

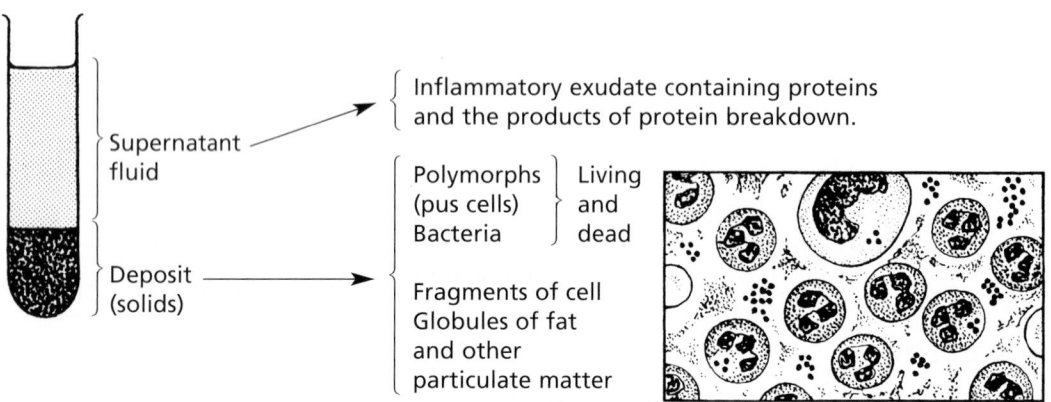

Supernatant fluid → { Inflammatory exudate containing proteins and the products of protein breakdown.

Deposit (solids) → {
Polymorphs (pus cells)  } Living and dead
Bacteria

Fragments of cell
Globules of fat
and other
particulate matter

### Evolution of an abscess

The usual evolution of an abscess is as follows:

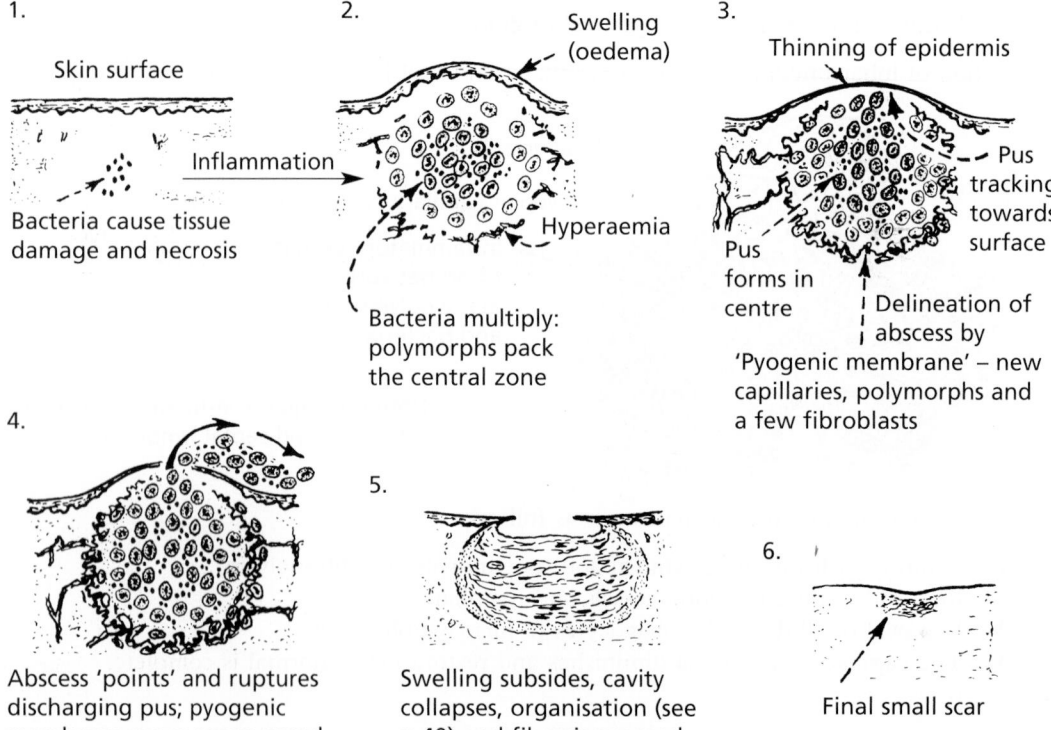

1. Skin surface

Bacteria cause tissue damage and necrosis

→ Inflammation →

2. Swelling (oedema)

Hyperaemia

Bacteria multiply: polymorphs pack the central zone

3. Thinning of epidermis

Pus tracking towards surface

Pus forms in centre

Delineation of abscess by 'Pyogenic membrane' – new capillaries, polymorphs and a few fibroblasts

4. Abscess 'points' and ruptures discharging pus; pyogenic membrane more pronounced

5. Swelling subsides, cavity collapses, organisation (see p.40) and fibrosis proceed

6. Final small scar

# SEQUELS OF ACUTE INFLAMMATION

When the abscess is deep seated, the process may be modified as follows:

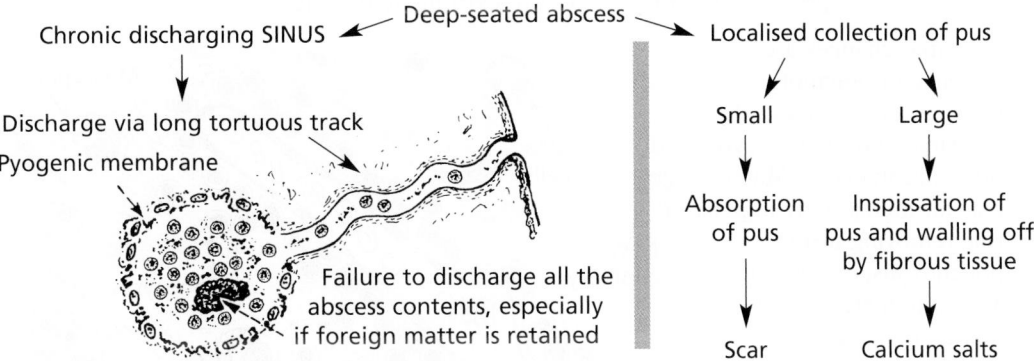

Chronic discharging SINUS ← Deep-seated abscess → Localised collection of pus

Discharge via long tortuous track

Pyogenic membrane

Failure to discharge all the abscess contents, especially if foreign matter is retained

Small → Absorption of pus → Scar

Large → Inspissation of pus and walling off by fibrous tissue → Calcium salts

## ORGANISATION AND FIBROSIS

Organisation occurs when, during the acute inflammatory process, (a) there is excessive exudation or necrosis or (b) when local conditions are unfavourable for the removal of exudate and debris. The term also applies to the local reaction to the presence of thrombus and also the necrosis associated with infarction.

The changes are similar to those described in wound healing – the growth of new capillaries into the inert material (exudate or thrombus), the migration of macrophages and the proliferation of fibroblasts resulting in FIBROSIS.

A good example of organisation following acute inflammation is seen in the pleura overlying pneumonia. The inflammation of the lung tissue proper usually resolves completely (p. 292); in contrast the pleural exudate is not easily removed and organisation takes place.

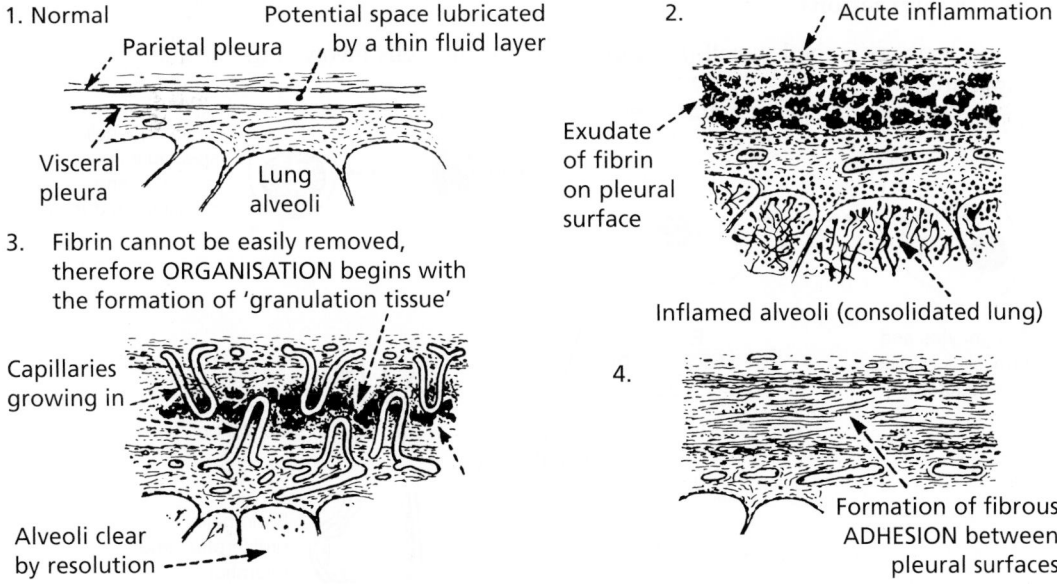

1. Normal
Potential space lubricated by a thin fluid layer
Parietal pleura
Visceral pleura
Lung alveoli

2. Acute inflammation
Exudate of fibrin on pleural surface
Inflamed alveoli (consolidated lung)

3. Fibrin cannot be easily removed, therefore ORGANISATION begins with the formation of 'granulation tissue'
Capillaries growing in
Alveoli clear by resolution

4. Formation of fibrous ADHESION between pleural surfaces

Other good examples of organisation are seen after infarction (p. 83).

# CHRONIC INFLAMMATION

**Chronic inflammation** may (a) follow acute inflammation if the causal agent is not removed or (b) be 'primary', i.e. there is no pre-existing acute stage.

The essential changes are:

1. Absence of polymorphs (natural life span of 1–3 days); the appearance of lymphocytes and often plasma cells. Macrophages play an increasingly important role removing dead polymorphs, presentation of antigenic material and granuloma formation.
2. Proliferation of vascular endothelium by 'budding' – formation of new capillaries (angiogenesis).
3. Proliferation of fibroblasts with collagen production leading to
4. Fibrosis.

Common causes of 'primary' chronic inflammation include:

(a) Persistent infections, e.g. tuberculosis, leprosy – where the organisms are resistant to neutrophil attack and bacteria survive within macrophages.
(b) Foreign material, e.g. silicates, including asbestos.
(c) Auto-immune diseases, e.g. auto-immune thyroiditis.
(d) Conditions of unknown aetiology, e.g. sarcoidosis: Crohn's disease.

**Cellular interactions**

The macrophage is the key cell that directs the various cells involved in chronic inflammation.

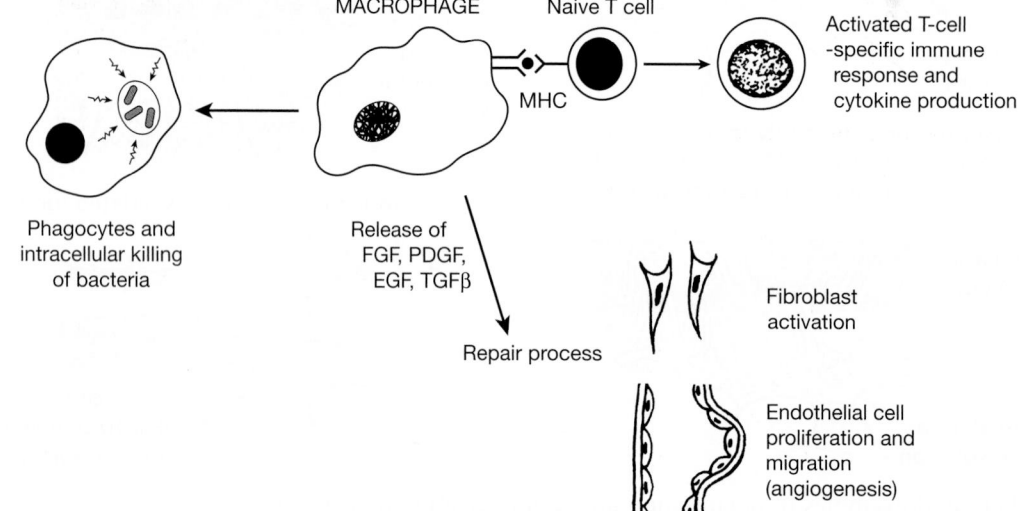

# CHRONIC INFLAMMATION

## GRANULOMATOUS INFLAMMATION

This is the term given to forms of chronic inflammation in which modified macrophages (epithelioid cells) accumulate in small clusters surrounded by lymphocytes. The small clusters are called GRANULOMAS. The basic lesion in TUBERCULOSIS is a good example.

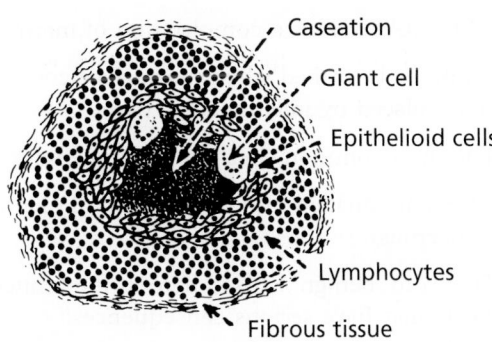

Caseation
Giant cell
Epithelioid cells
Lymphocytes
Fibrous tissue

Similar granulomas are seen in:

**Sarcoidosis** – a rare inflammatory disease of unknown aetiology affecting especially the lymph nodes and lungs, but also many other organs.

**'Talc' granuloma** – where particulate silicates introduced into the tissues evoke an inflammatory reaction after a latent period (usually years).

**Crohn's disease** – a chronic inflammatory disease affecting the terminal ileum and colon (p. 342).

**Lymph nodes** – draining ulcerated areas in which breakdown of lipid is occurring.

*Note:* In all of these granulomatous diseases the basic lesion may be identical, but CASEATION only occurs in tuberculosis.

The epithelioid cells of the granulomas are modified macrophages, and giant cells are derived from macrophages usually by cell fusion but occasionally by nuclear division without cytoplasmic separation.

The Langhans giant cell – seen in chronic granulomata, e.g. tuberculosis and sarcoidosis.

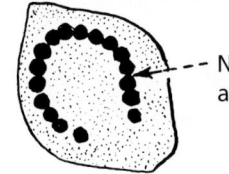

Nuclei in horse-shoe arrangement

The foreign body giant cell – seen in association with particulate insoluble material.

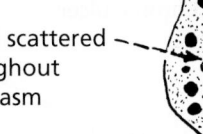

Nuclei scattered throughout cytoplasm

## Mechanism of granuloma formation

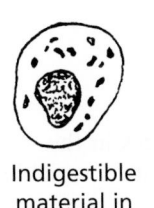

Indigestible material in MACROPHAGE

+

IMMUNE RESPONSE via ACTIVATED 'T' LYMPHOCYTE

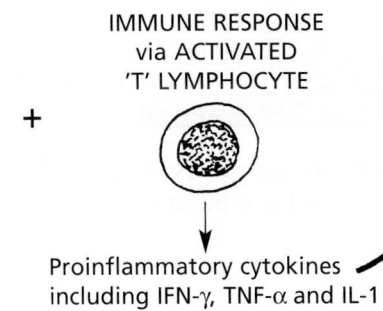

Proinflammatory cytokines including IFN-γ, TNF-α and IL-1

PROLIFERATION and ACTIVATION of MACROPHAGES

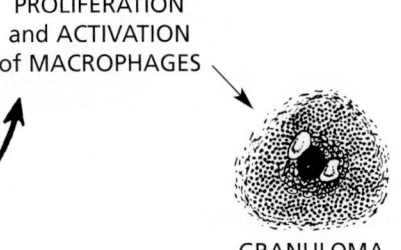

GRANULOMA FORMATION

# ULCERATION – BENIGN

ULCERATION is a complication of many disease processes.

An **ulcer** is formed when the surface covering of an organ or tissue is lost due to necrosis and replaced by inflammatory tissue.

The most common sites are the alimentary tract and the skin.

Ulcers are divided into two groups: (1) BENIGN (inflammatory) and (2) MALIGNANT (cancerous).

The word 'benign' is used here in the limited sense of contrasting with 'malignant': 'benign' ulcers may have serious consequences.

## EVOLUTION OF A BENIGN ULCER

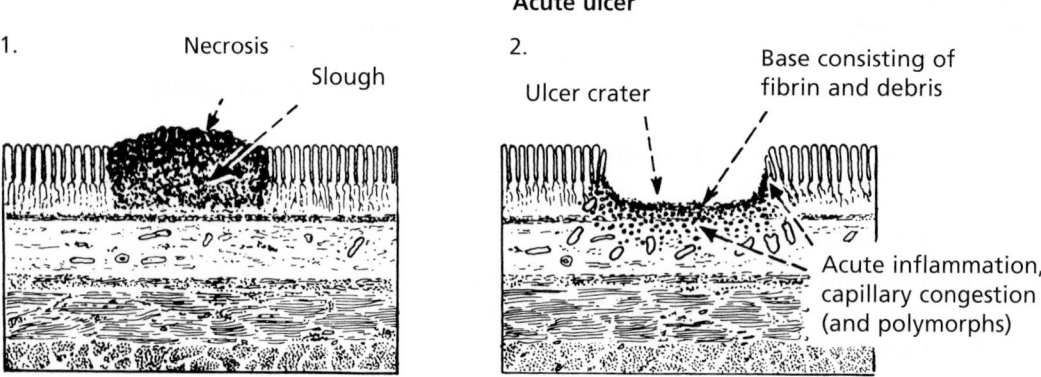

Healing can occur at this stage with restoration to normal, but if irritation (e.g. bacterial action, slight trauma, digestive juices and acid) continues, a CHRONIC ULCER forms.

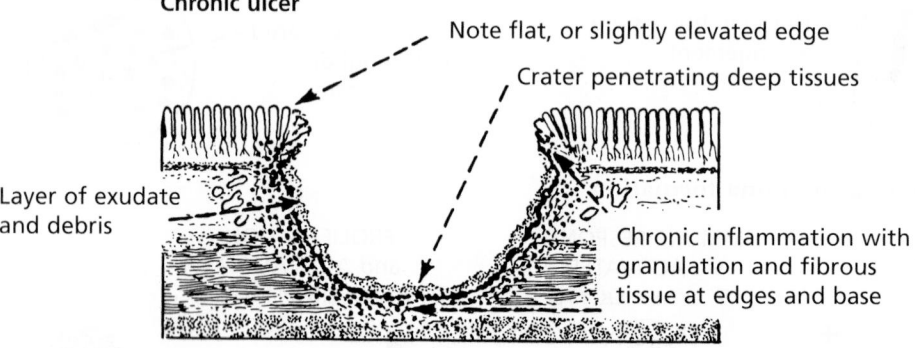

Healing of a chronic ulcer may be impeded by the secondary obliterative changes in the blood vessels due to the chronic inflammation, and it is inevitably associated with a variable amount of scarring.

# ULCERATION – MALIGNANT

## Evolution of a malignant ulcer (ulcerated tumour)

Such an ulcer is the result of the growth of a malignant tumour.

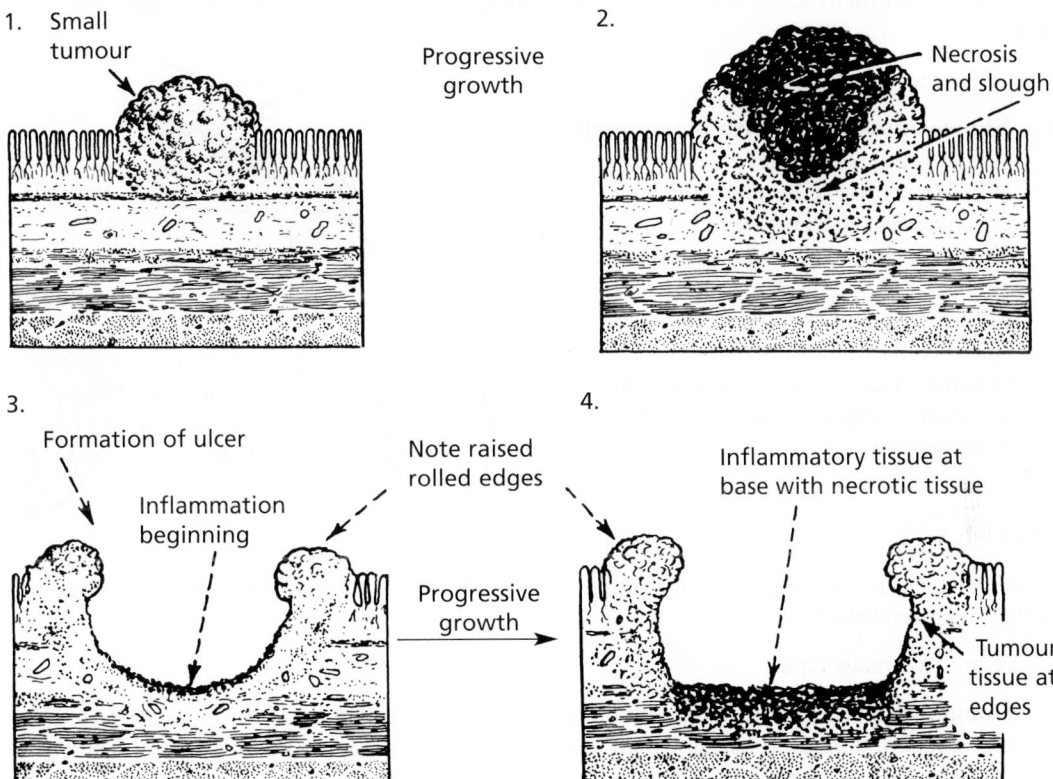

1. Small tumour

Progressive growth

2. Necrosis and slough

3. Formation of ulcer

Inflammation beginning

Note raised rolled edges

Progressive growth

4. Inflammatory tissue at base with necrotic tissue

Tumour tissue at edges

The differences between benign and malignant ulcers are most prominent at the edges from which a diagnostic biopsy should be taken. It is worth remembering that cancers often ulcerate but benign ulcers rarely undergo malignant change.

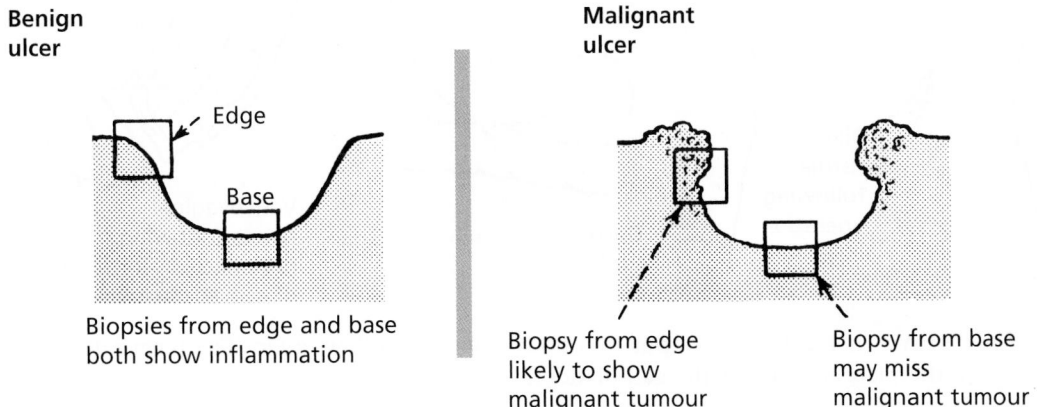

**Benign ulcer**

Edge

Base

Biopsies from edge and base both show inflammation

**Malignant ulcer**

Biopsy from edge likely to show malignant tumour

Biopsy from base may miss malignant tumour

# INFLAMMATION – ANATOMICAL VARIETIES

### SINUS

A sinus is a tract lined by granulation tissue leading from a chronically inflamed cavity to a surface. In many cases the cause is the continuing presence of 'foreign' or necrotic material.

Examples include:

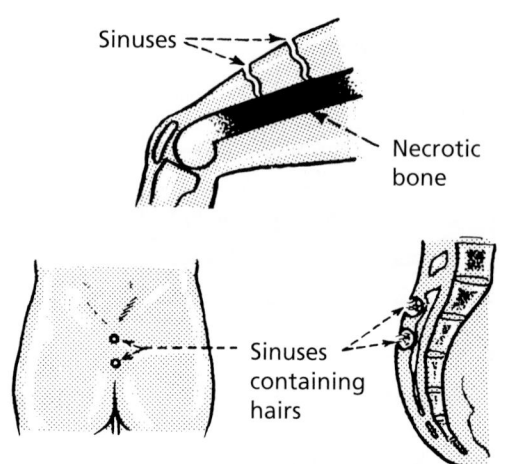

Sinuses

Necrotic bone

* **Sinuses associated with osteomyelitis** (inflammation of bone).
  Where necrosis of bone occurs, chronic sinuses form over it.
* **Pilonidal sinus** (pilonidal = nest of hairs).
  Seen in the mid-line over the sacrum (natal cleft) where hairs which have penetrated deeply under the skin are associated with chronic relapsing inflammation.

Sinuses containing hairs

### FISTULA

A fistula is a track open at both ends, through which abnormal communication between two surfaces is established.

There are two main types:

1.  **Congenital** – due to developmental abnormality: any inflammation is superimposed, e.g. tracheoesophageal fistula which can lead to choking and coughing during feeding in a newborn.
2.  **Acquired** – due to:

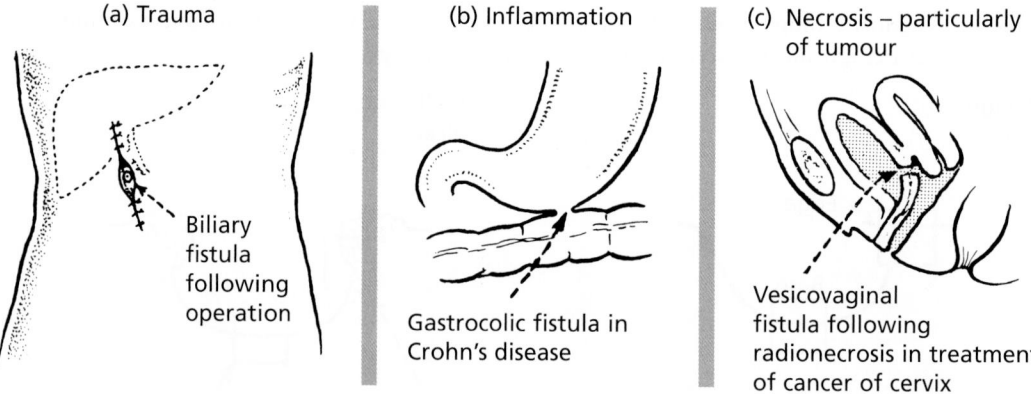

(a) Trauma

Biliary fistula following operation

(b) Inflammation

Gastrocolic fistula in Crohn's disease

(c) Necrosis – particularly of tumour

Vesicovaginal fistula following radionecrosis in treatment of cancer of cervix

An **EMPYEMA** is a collection of pus in a body cavity or hollow organ. The term refers usually to the pleural cavity or the gall bladder.

**CELLULITIS** occurs when inflammation spreads in the connective tissue planes.

# HEALING

Healing is the final stage of the response of tissue to injury.

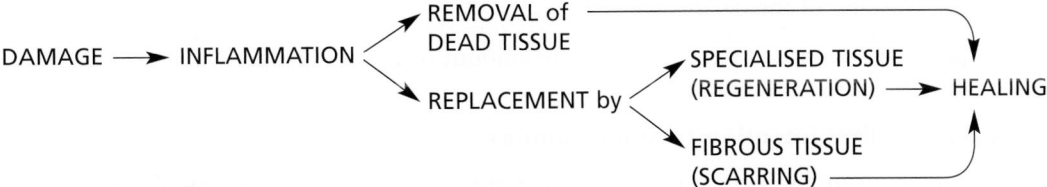

The capacity of a tissue for REGENERATION depends on its PROLIFERATIVE ABILITY and on the type and severity of the damage. In particular, regeneration is not possible if the STEM CELLS are destroyed.

Three broad GROUPS of cells are considered in the context of the cell cycle (p. 4).

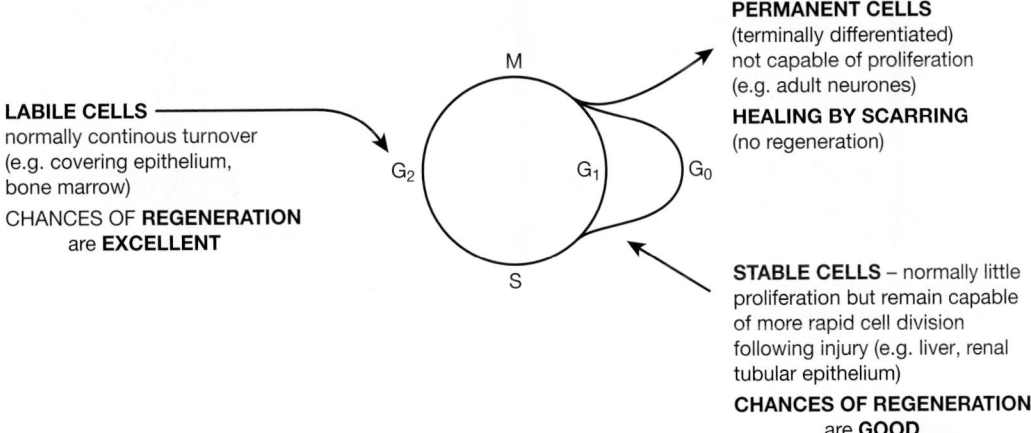

REGENERATION involves TWO PROCESSES:

1. PROLIFERATION of SURVIVING CELLS to replace lost tissue.
2. MIGRATION of SURVIVING CELLS into the vacant space.

**The FACTORS which CONTROL** healing and repair are complex: they include the production of a large variety of **growth factors**.

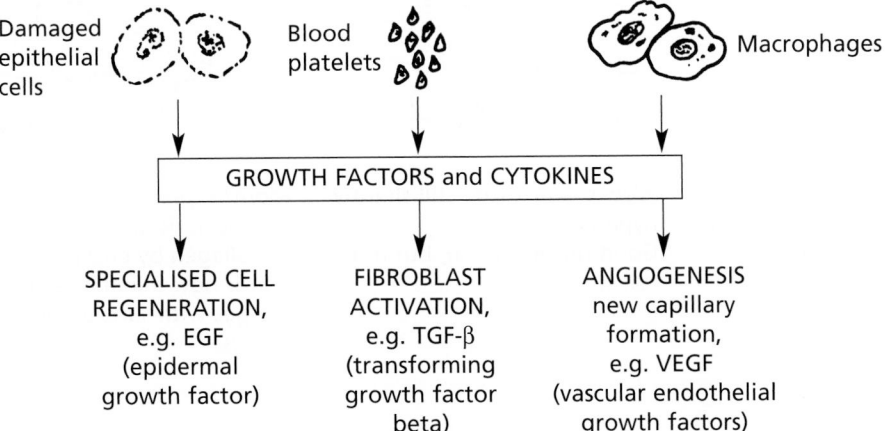

# WOUND HEALING

Healing of a wound shows both epithelial regeneration (healing of the epidermis) and repair by scarring (healing of the dermis).

Two patterns are described depending on the amount of tissue damage. These are the same process varying only in amount.

### 1. Healing by first intention (primary union)

This occurs in clean, incised wounds with good apposition of the edges – particularly planned surgical incisions.

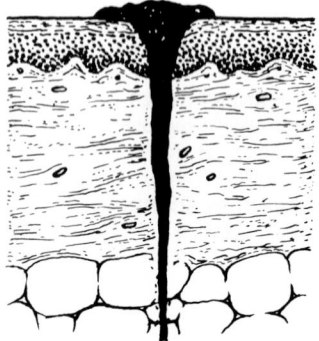

*Immediately:* Blood clot and debris fill the small cleft.

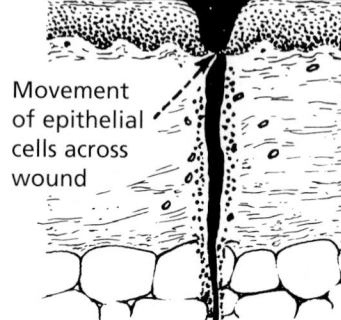

Movement of epithelial cells across wound

*2–3 hours:* Early inflammation close to edges. Mild hyperaemia and a few polymorphs.

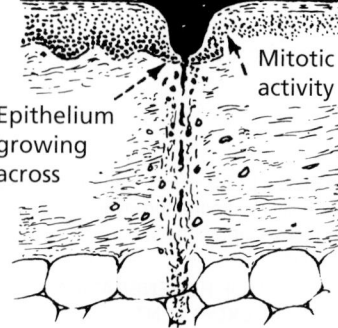

Mitotic activity

Epithelium growing across

*2–3 days:* Macrophage activity removing clot. Proliferation of blood vessels. Fibroblastic activity.

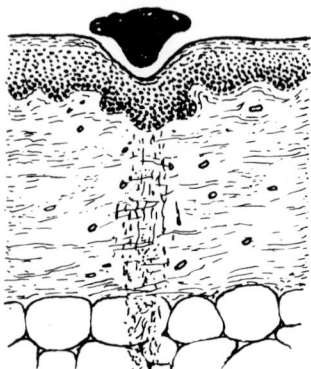

*10–14 days:* Scab loose and epithelial covering complete. Fibrous union of edges, but wound is still weak.

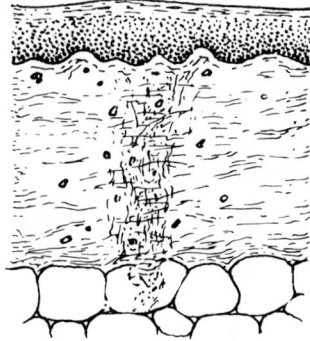

*Weeks:* Scar tissue still slightly hyperaemic. Good fibrous union, but not full strength.

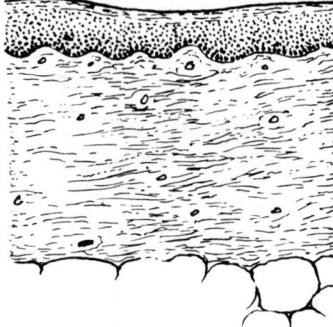

*Months–years:* Devascularisation. Remodelling of collagen by enzyme action. Scar is now minimal and merges with surrounding tissues.

# WOUND HEALING

## 2. Healing by second intention (secondary union)

This occurs in open wounds, particularly when there has been significant loss of tissue, necrosis or infection.

**Early**

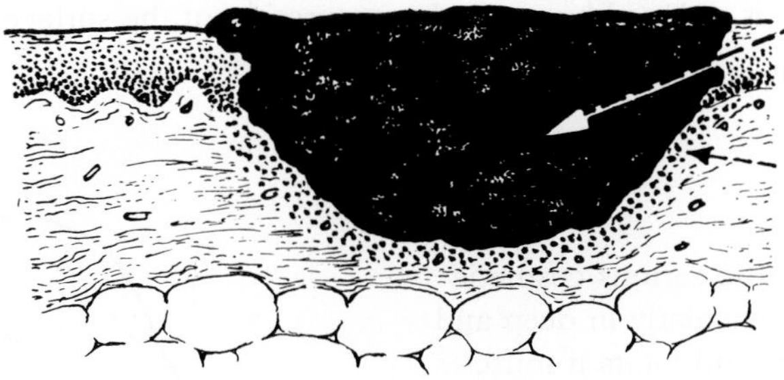

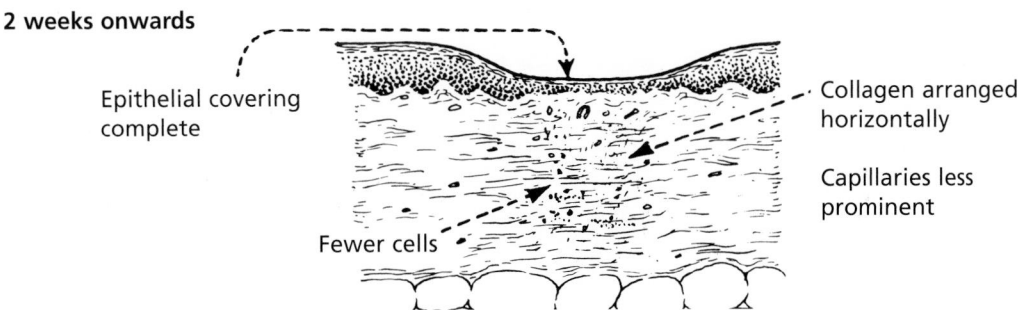

Cavity fills with blood and fibrin clot

Acute inflammation starts at junction of living tissue

**A few days**

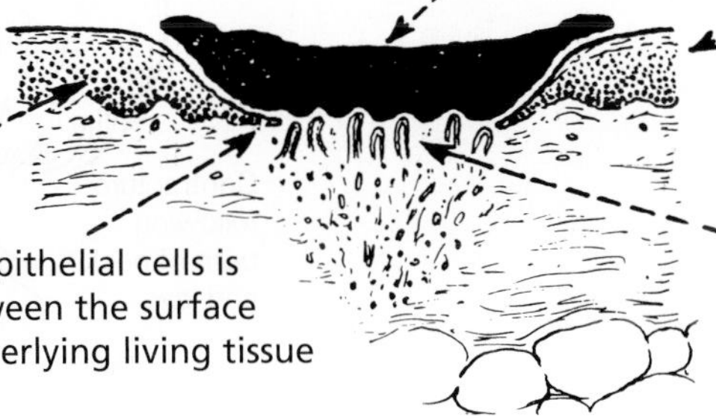

Scab dries out

Contraction of wound size due to action of myofibroblasts at edges

Mitotic activity in epithelium

A single sheet of epithelial cells is being pushed between the surface debris and the underlying living tissue

New capillary loops bring macrophages, neutrophils and fibroblasts

**1 week approximately**

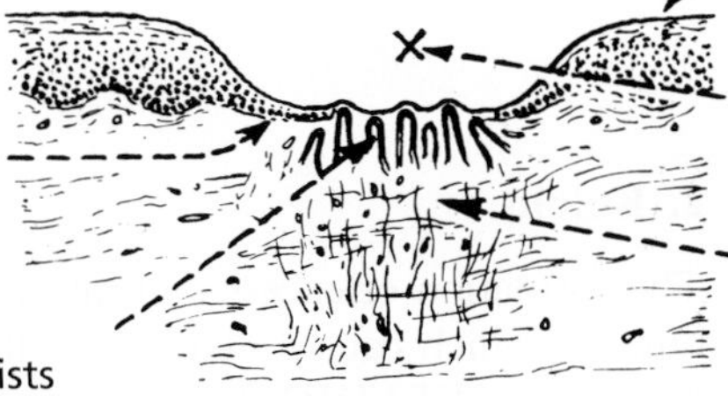

Contraction continuing

Surface debris has been shed

Epithelium continues to grow across

Loose connective tissue formed by fibroblasts

Granulation tissue is seen in the base of the wound. This tissue consists of newly formed capillaries with fibroblasts and macrophages and occurs in many circumstances in addition to wounds.

**2 weeks onwards**

Epithelial covering complete

Collagen arranged horizontally

Capillaries less prominent

Fewer cells

# WOUND HEALING

### Wound contraction

Wound contraction, which is beneficial and begins early, is due mainly to the young, specialised 'myofibroblasts' in the granulation tissue exerting a traction effect at the wound edges. The exposed surface is reduced by gradual regeneration of the surface epithelium.

The remodelling of the collagen continues for many months.

## COMPLICATIONS

### 1. Contracture

Later, CONTRACTURE may cause serious cosmetic and functional disability, particularly in deep and extensive skin burns and around joints if muscles are badly damaged.

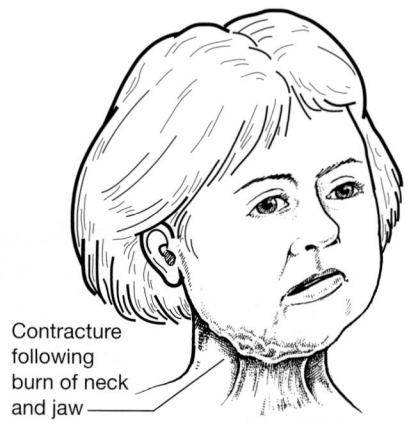

Contracture
following
burn of neck
and jaw

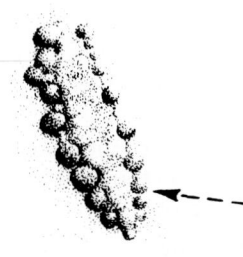

### 2. Keloid

The formation of excess collagen in the form of thick interlacing bundles which causes marked swelling at the site of the wound, is known as a KELOID. The essential cause is unknown. It is particularly common in black people.

# HEALING – FIBROSIS

FIBROSIS is the end result of WOUND HEALING, CHRONIC INFLAMMATION and ORGANISATION.

## Formation of fibrous tissue

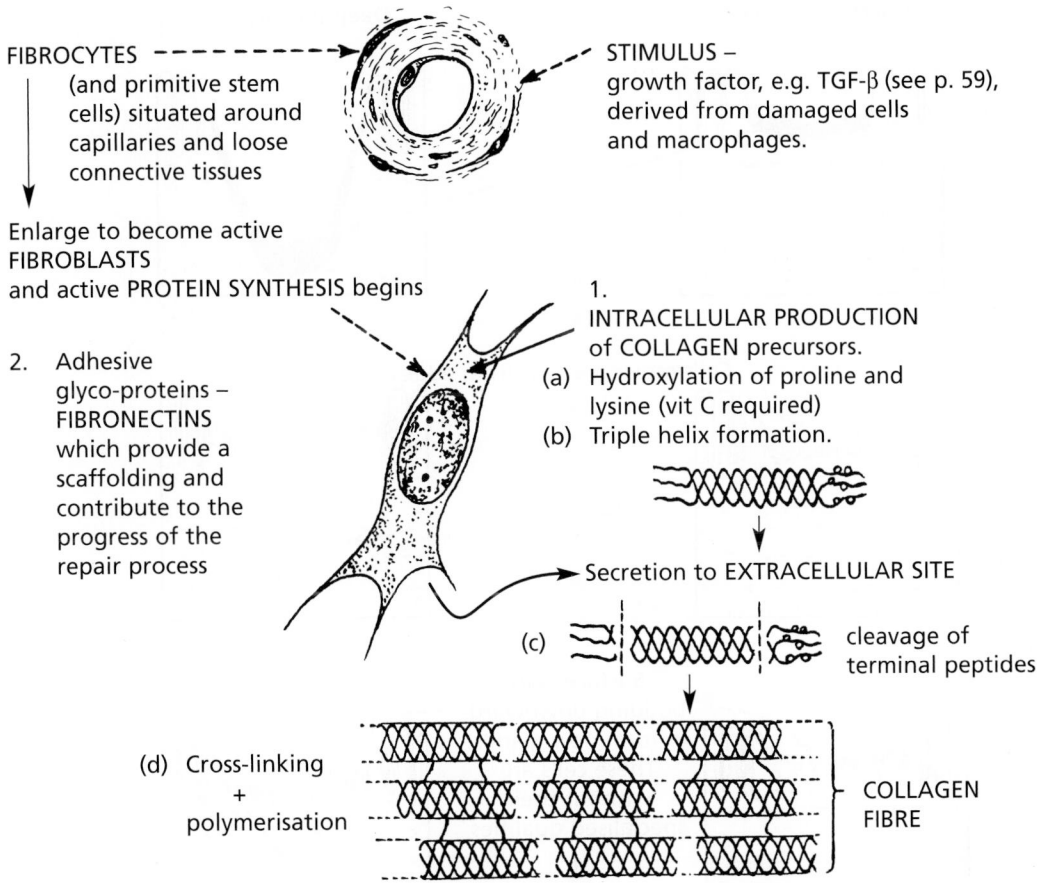

FIBROCYTES ---------→
(and primitive stem cells) situated around capillaries and loose connective tissues

STIMULUS –
growth factor, e.g. TGF-β (see p. 59), derived from damaged cells and macrophages.

Enlarge to become active
FIBROBLASTS
and active PROTEIN SYNTHESIS begins

2. Adhesive glyco-proteins – FIBRONECTINS which provide a scaffolding and contribute to the progress of the repair process

1.
INTRACELLULAR PRODUCTION of COLLAGEN precursors.
(a) Hydroxylation of proline and lysine (vit C required)
(b) Triple helix formation.

Secretion to EXTRACELLULAR SITE

(c)     cleavage of terminal peptides

(d) Cross-linking
+
polymerisation

COLLAGEN FIBRE

REMODELLING follows: Action of COLLAGENASE ──→ SCAR TISSUE
+ secretion of COLLAGEN

## Factors delaying healing

1. LOCAL
INFECTION, a POOR BLOOD SUPPLY, excessive movement and presence of foreign material DELAY HEALING.

2. GENERAL
DEFICIENCY of VITAMIN C
DEFICIENCY of AMINO ACIDS (in malnutrition)
DEFICIENCY of ZINC    } Failure of proper collagen synthesis with delayed healing and weak scars.
EXCESS of ADRENAL GLUCOCORTICOIDS
DEBILITATING CHRONIC DISEASE

# HEALING – SPECIAL SITUATIONS

### INTERNAL SURFACES

The epithelial lining of the gastrointestinal tract regenerates in a similar way to the skin.

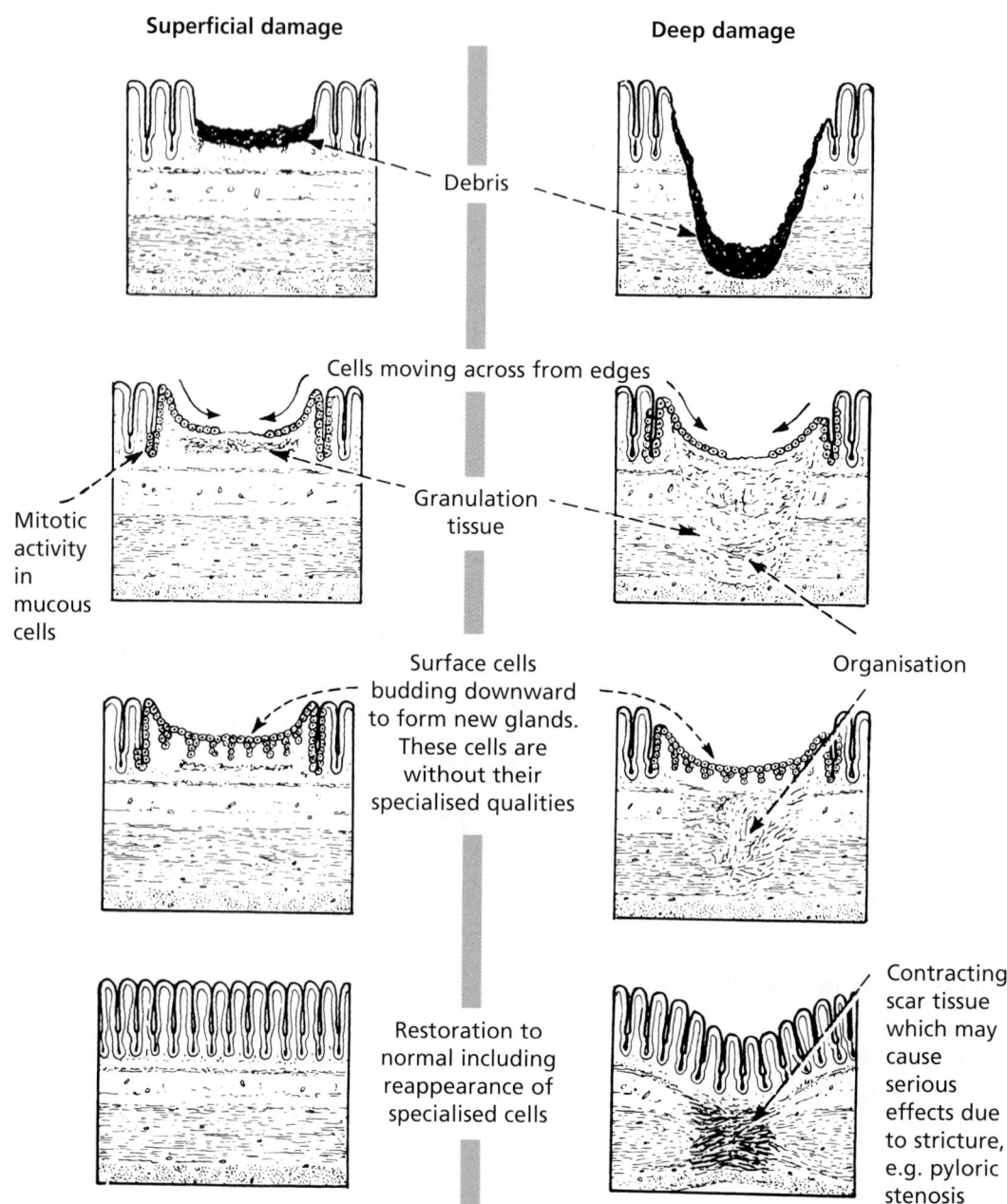

Superficial damage

Deep damage

Debris

Cells moving across from edges

Mitotic activity in mucous cells

Granulation tissue

Surface cells budding downward to form new glands. These cells are without their specialised qualities

Organisation

Restoration to normal including reappearance of specialised cells

Contracting scar tissue which may cause serious effects due to stricture, e.g. pyloric stenosis

# HEALING – SPECIAL SITUATIONS

## SOLID EPITHELIAL ORGANS

1. **Following gross tissue damage – including supporting tissue** (post-necrotic scarring)

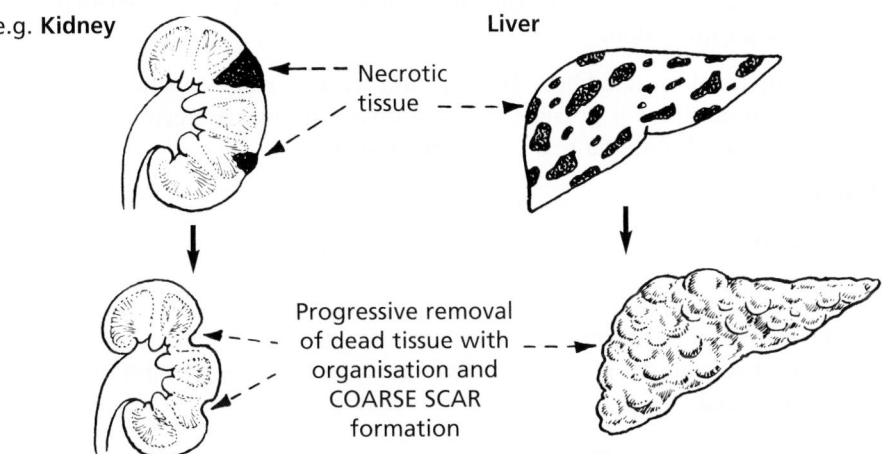

e.g. **Kidney**          **Liver**

Necrotic tissue

Progressive removal of dead tissue with organisation and COARSE SCAR formation

2. **Following cell damage with survival of the supporting (reticular) tissues**

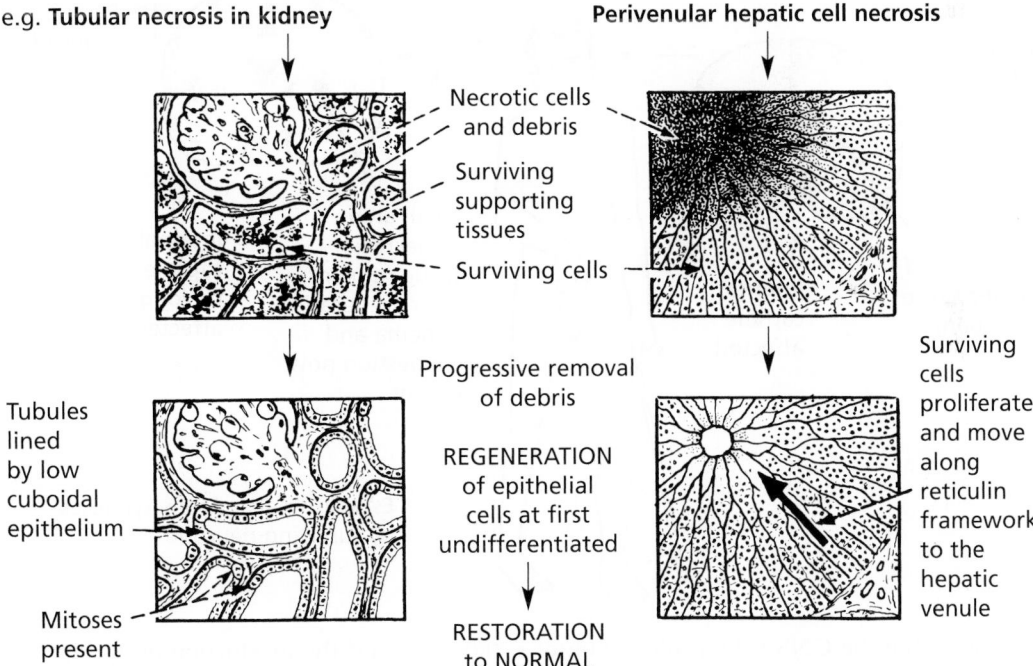

e.g. **Tubular necrosis in kidney**          **Perivenular hepatic cell necrosis**

Necrotic cells and debris

Surviving supporting tissues

Surviving cells

Tubules lined by low cuboidal epithelium

Mitoses present

Progressive removal of debris

REGENERATION of epithelial cells at first undifferentiated

↓

RESTORATION to NORMAL

Surviving cells proliferate and move along reticulin framework to the hepatic venule

# HEALING – SPECIAL SITUATIONS

### MUSCLE

Muscle fibres of all three types – skeletal, cardiac and smooth – have only limited capacity to regenerate.

When a MASS of muscle tissue is damaged, repair by SCARRING occurs. This is particularly important in the HEART after infarction.

If the damage affects individual muscle fibres diffusely and with varying severity, then regeneration of the specialised fibres is possible (e.g. the myocardium may recover completely from the effects of diphtheria toxin and virus infection).

### NERVOUS TISSUE

### Central nervous system

Regeneration does not occur when a neurone is lost.

In cases of acute damage the initial functional loss often exceeds the loss of actual nerve tissue because of the reactive changes in the surrounding tissue. As these changes diminish, some function may be restored.

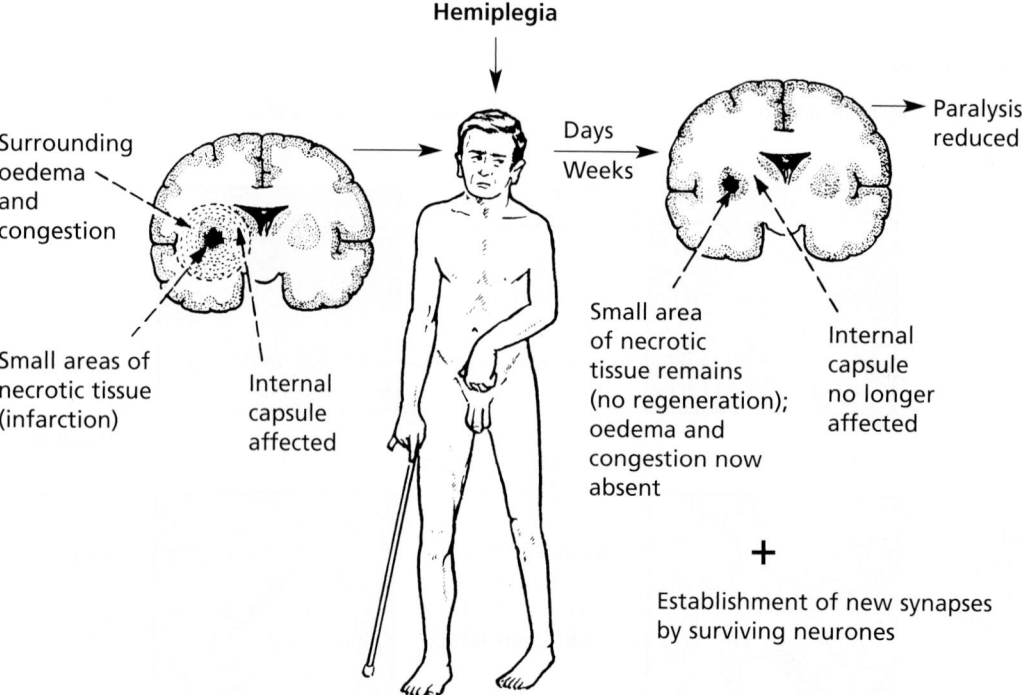

**Hemiplegia**

Surrounding oedema and congestion

Days
Weeks

Paralysis reduced

Small areas of necrotic tissue (infarction)

Internal capsule affected

Small area of necrotic tissue remains (no regeneration); oedema and congestion now absent

Internal capsule no longer affected

**+**

Establishment of new synapses by surviving neurones

Scarring within the CNS is by proliferation of ASTROCYTES and the production of fibrillary glial acidic protein – a process known as GLIOSIS.

# HEALING – SPECIAL SITUATIONS

## Peripheral nerves

When a peripheral nerve is damaged, the axon and its myelin sheath rapidly degenerate distally. The supporting tissues of the nerve (Schwann cells) degenerate slowly.

Regeneration can occur because the central neurone of which the axon is a peripheral extension is remote from the site of damage.

A spinal motor nerve is taken as an example.

## Normal spinal cord

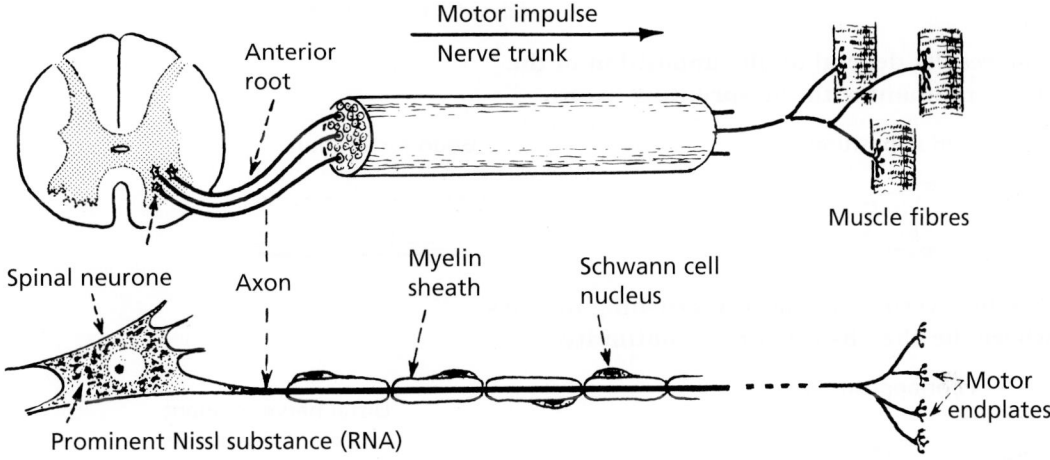

## Results of damage

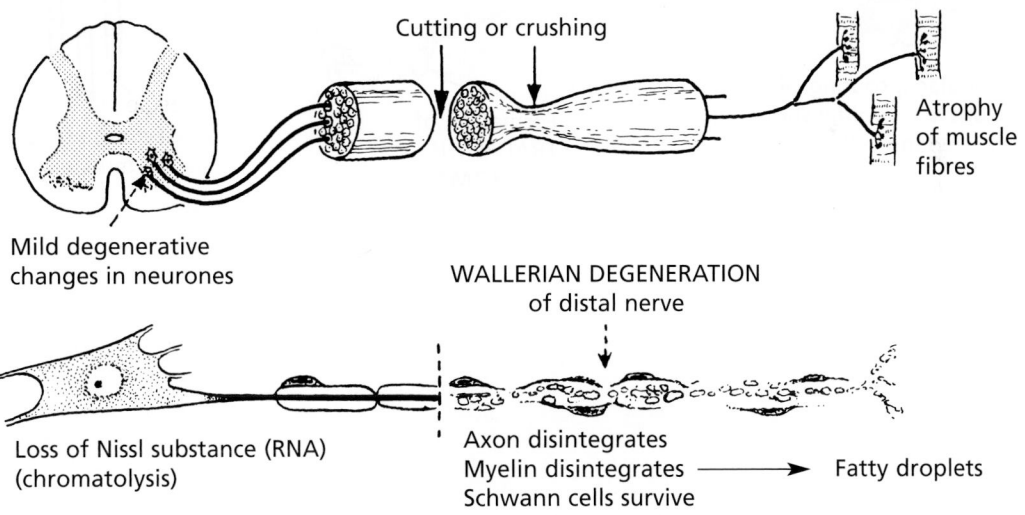

# HEALING – SPECIAL SITUATIONS

**Regeneration** takes the form of a sprouting of the cut ends of the axons.

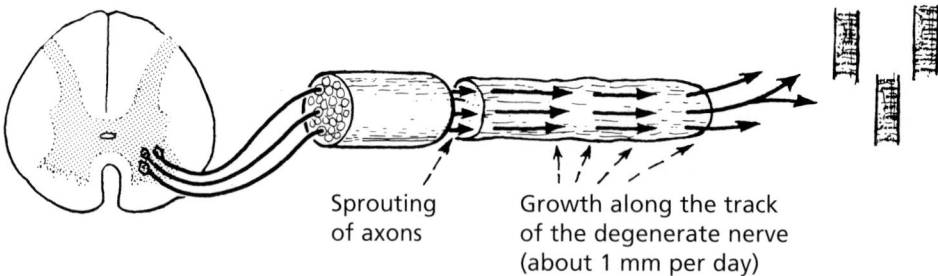

Sprouting of axons

Growth along the track of the degenerate nerve (about 1 mm per day)

**The results depend on the apposition of the distal remnant with the sprouting axons.**

**Good apposition**

**Good restoration**

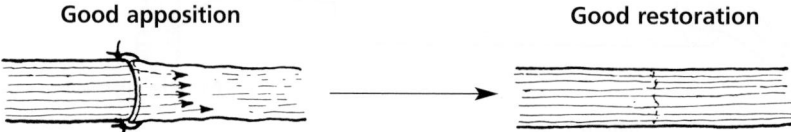

**The best results are seen in crushing injuries where the sheaths remain in continuity.**

**Poor apposition**

Distal nerve remnant disappears

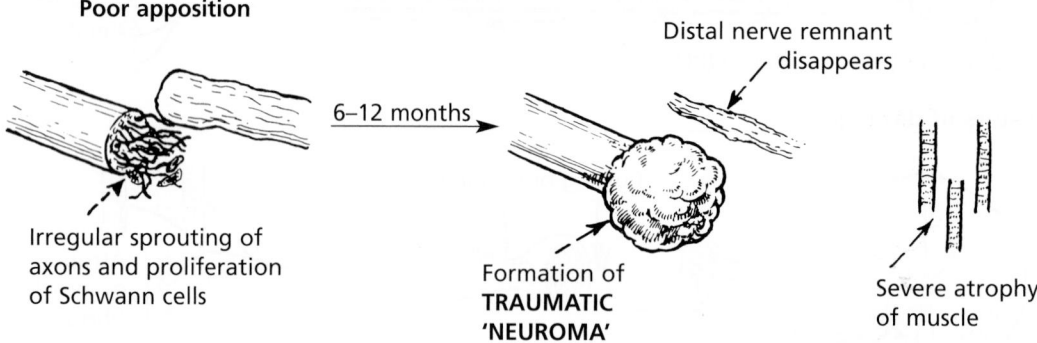

6–12 months

Irregular sprouting of axons and proliferation of Schwann cells

Formation of **TRAUMATIC 'NEUROMA'**

Severe atrophy of muscle

# FRACTURE HEALING

## BONE – FRACTURE HEALING

1. *Immediate effects*

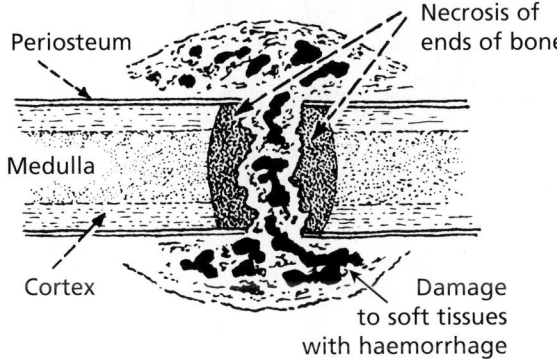

Periosteum

Medulla

Cortex

Necrosis of ends of bone

Damage to soft tissues with haemorrhage

2. *Early reaction-inflammatory*
   First 4–5 days

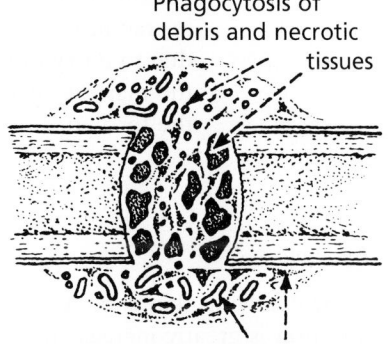

Phagocytosis of debris and necrotic tissues

Early organisation: capillaries and fibroblasts

3. *Formation of callus* (early bone regeneration) – after 1 week

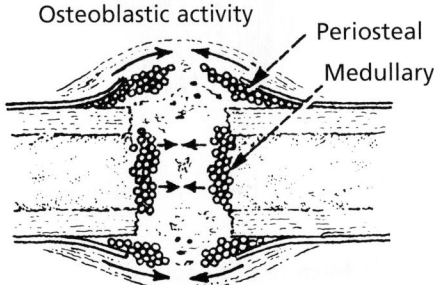

Osteoblastic activity

Periosteal

Medullary

**Provisional callus** bridges the gap – first, osteoid tissue (may include cartilage) then woven bone

4. *Mature callus* - from 3 weeks onwards

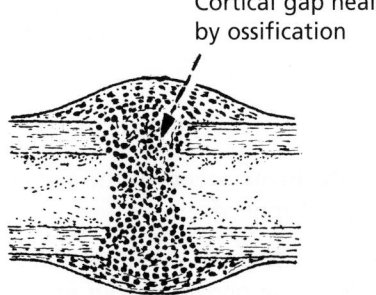

Cortical gap healed by ossification

Osteoblastic and osteoclastic activity proceeding

5. *Remodelling of callus*
   Definitive – weeks into months

Osteoblasts and osteoclasts active

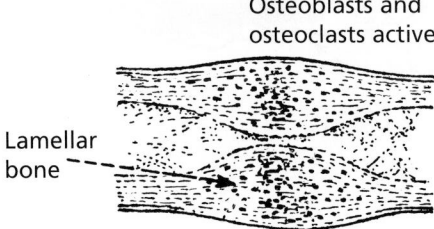

Lamellar bone

6. *Final reconstruction*

   Months later

Fracture site may be almost invisible

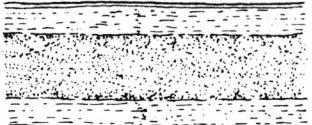

# FRACTURE HEALING

### Complications

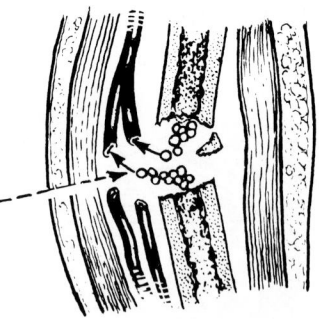

1. *Fat embolism* may occur in fracture of long bones due to entry of fat from the marrow cavity into the torn ends of veins.

2. *Infection*

If the overlying skin is breached in any way, i.e. the fracture is 'compound', the risk of infection is greatly increased; this is an important adverse factor in the healing process.

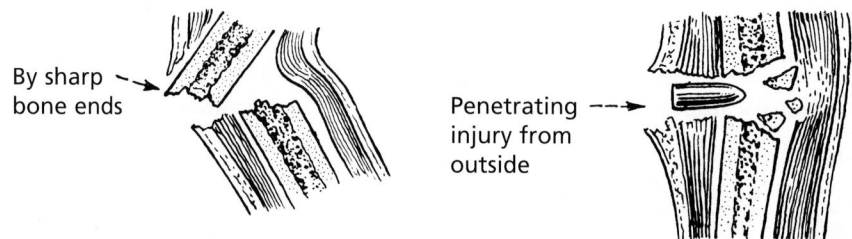

By sharp bone ends

Penetrating injury from outside

## PATHOLOGICAL FRACTURE

When the break occurs at the site of pre-existing disease of the bone, the term 'pathological fracture' is applied.

A common condition is a secondary tumour growing in and destroying the bone

Mixture of tumour and haematoma – healing inhibited

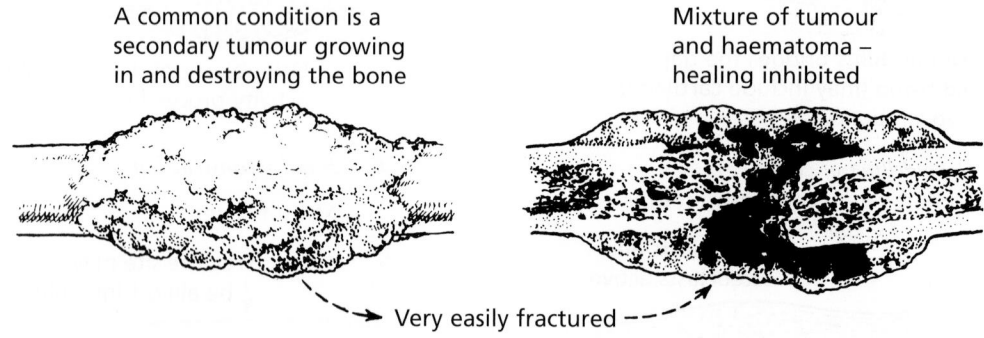

Very easily fractured

# FRACTURE HEALING

## FACTORS INFLUENCING HEALING OF FRACTURES

| ADVERSE | FAVOURABLE |

**1. Local factors**

(a) *Infore* ⎫ See previous
(b) *Pathological fracture* ⎭ page

(a) *Infection* ⎫ See previous
(b) *Pathological fracture* ⎭ page

(c) *Poor apposition and alignment* . . . . . . . . . . . . . . . . . . *Good apposition*

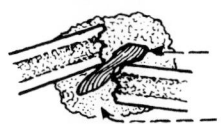

There may be interposition
of soft tissue, e.g. muscle

Large irregular callus:
slow repair, permanent deformity of bone

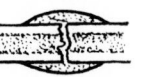

Small callus,
quick repair

(d) *Continuing movement of bone ends* . . . . . . . . . . . . . *Good immobilisation*

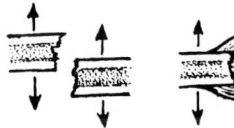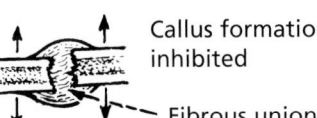

Callus formation
inhibited

Fibrous union

In extreme cases, a rudimentary joint
(pseudoarthrosis)
may form

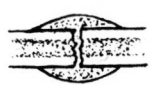

Small callus, good
bone formation

(e) *Poor blood supply* . . . . . . . . . . . . . . . . . . . . . . . *Good blood supply*

This is largely influenced by the anatomical site
of the fracture, for example:
(a) Nutrient artery entering remote from the
    fracture or damaged by fracture
    (e.g. scaphoid, femoral head)
(b) Fracture through area devoid of periosteum
    (e.g. neck of femur)
(c) Minimal adjacent soft tissue (e.g. tibia).

In favourable conditions
blood supply is derived
from:
(a) periosteal arteries
(b) nutrient artery
(c) adjacent soft tissues.

**2. General factors**

(a) *Old age* . . . . . . . . . . . . . . . . . . . . . . . *Youth*
(b) *Poor nutrition* – e.g. famine, . . . . . . . . . . . . . . . . . . . *Good nutrition* – especially
    malabsorption leading to lack of          protein, calcium, vit D and vit C.
    protein, calcium, vit D and vit C.

# HAEMODYNAMIC DISORDERS, THROMBOSIS AND SHOCK

## OBJECTIVES

**1.** To list the three main factors leading to thrombosis and know examples of each.
**2.** To understand the consequences of thrombosis in the brain and heart.
**3.** To define embolism and to understand the main types of embolism and resulting pathological consequences.
**4.** To define shock, list the causes and understand the main consequences.
**5.** To understand the circulatory changes that take place in both early and late shock.
**6.** To understand the pathological changes of established shock on end organs.

# GENERAL CONSIDERATIONS

Conditions resulting from thrombo-embolic phenomena are a major cause of morbidity and mortality in the Western world. The main forms are:

1. **Myocardial infarction** 2. **Cerebrovascular infarction** 3. **Pulmonary embolism**

Thrombosis usually precedes embolism leading to infarction, but embolism may have antecedent causes other than thrombosis.

## THROMBOSIS

A thrombus is a mass formed from blood constituents within a vessel or the heart during life. Blood clotting is a physiological protective mechanism but thrombosis is a pathological process with serious consequences. Thrombosis should be distinguished from 'clot', which is blood that coagulates outside of the vascular system (or within the vascular system after death).

# GENERAL CONSIDERATIONS

## MECHANISM OF FORMATION

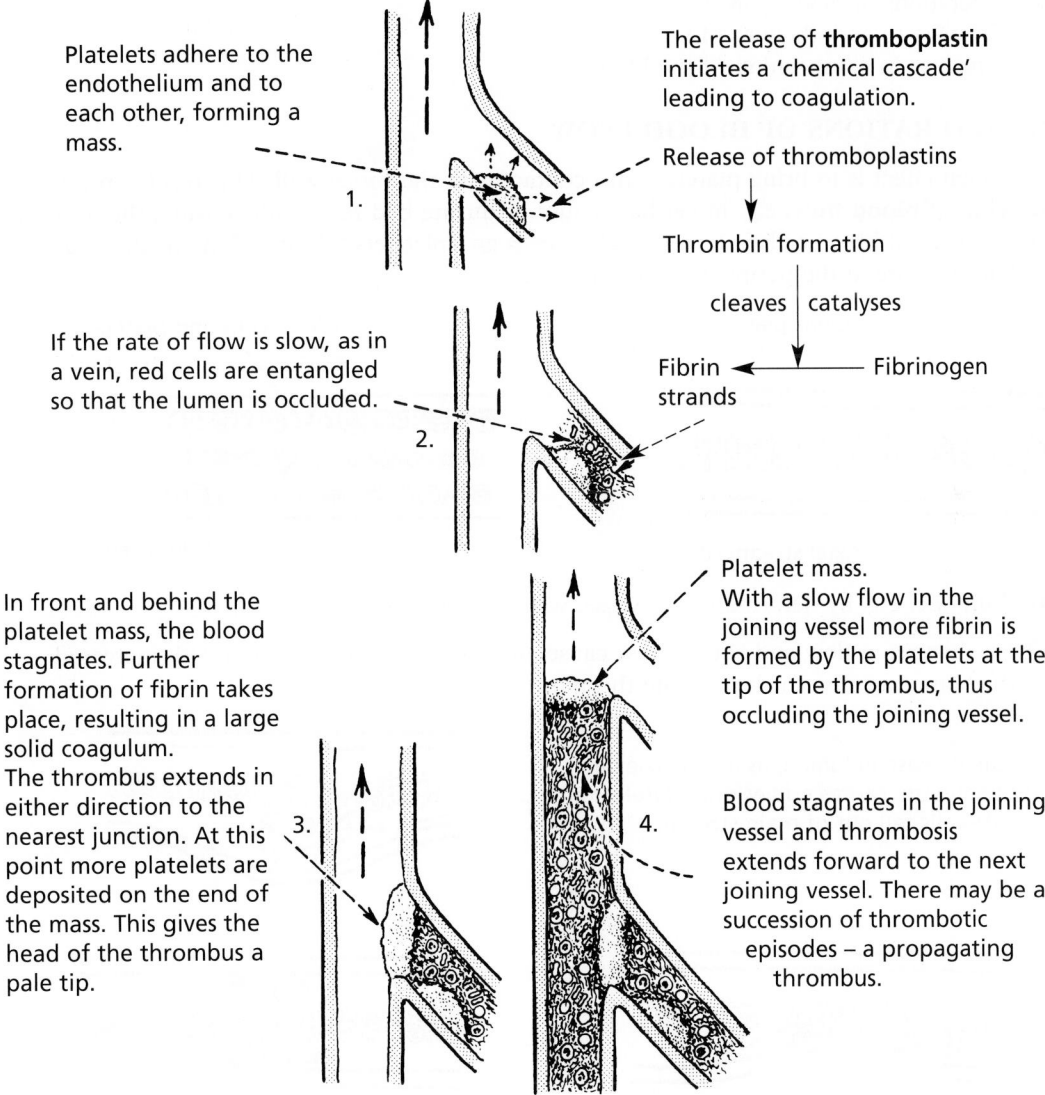

Platelets adhere to the endothelium and to each other, forming a mass.

1.

The release of **thromboplastin** initiates a 'chemical cascade' leading to coagulation.

Release of thromboplastins

Thrombin formation

cleaves | catalyses

Fibrin strands ← Fibrinogen

If the rate of flow is slow, as in a vein, red cells are entangled so that the lumen is occluded.

2.

In front and behind the platelet mass, the blood stagnates. Further formation of fibrin takes place, resulting in a large solid coagulum.
The thrombus extends in either direction to the nearest junction. At this point more platelets are deposited on the end of the mass. This gives the head of the thrombus a pale tip.

3.

Platelet mass.
With a slow flow in the joining vessel more fibrin is formed by the platelets at the tip of the thrombus, thus occluding the joining vessel.

Blood stagnates in the joining vessel and thrombosis extends forward to the next joining vessel. There may be a succession of thrombotic episodes – a propagating thrombus.

4.

# FACTORS LEADING TO THROMBOSIS

The three MAIN factors leading to thrombosis are known as the Virchow triad:

1. Alterations of blood flow.
2. Damage to endothelium of vessel.
3. Changes in composition of the blood.

## 1. ALTERATIONS OF BLOOD FLOW

The main effect is to bring platelets into contact with the vessel wall. This results from: **slowing of blood flow**, e.g. in cardiac failure or during bed rest. With slowing, the normal axial stream of blood cells is lost and white cells and platelets fall out of the main stream and accumulate in the peripheral plasma zone.

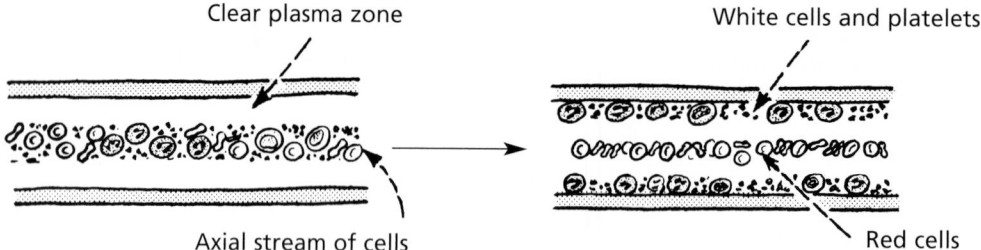

Clear plasma zone

White cells and platelets

Axial stream of cells

Red cells

**Turbulence**, e.g. by deformation of vessel wall or around venous valves.

These changes in flow and shear stress cause altered endothelial function with increased production of agents which promote thrombosis (p. 77).

Local increase in lumen, as in varicose veins or aneurysm, causes eddies and platelets and white cells fall out of main stream.

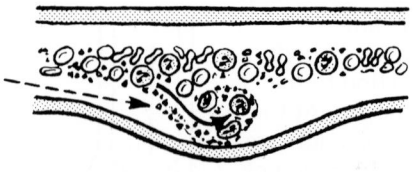

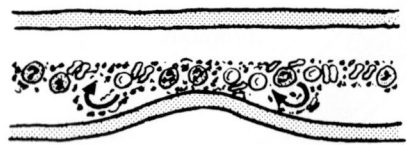

Swelling or compression of vessel wall by disease. Eddies form in front and behind obstruction.

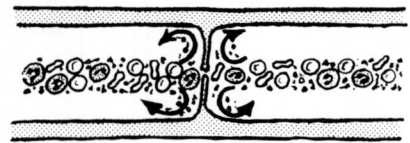

Eddies form around valves if flow slows.

# FACTORS LEADING TO THROMBOSIS

## 2. DAMAGE TO ENDOTHELIUM OF VESSEL

This leads to platelet adhesion and aggregation. Common causes are:

(a) Disease in vessel wall, e.g. atheroma.

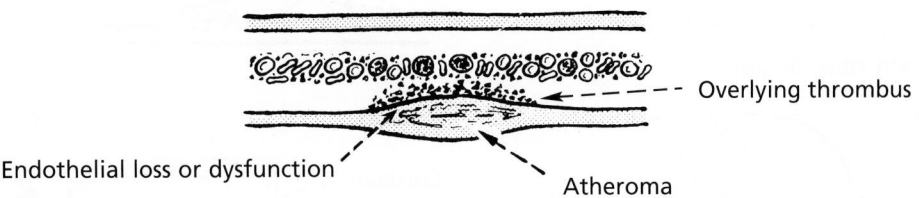

Overlying thrombus

Endothelial loss or dysfunction

Atheroma

(b) Toxins from nearby inflammatory processes.
(c) Local compression of vessels (e.g. during operations).

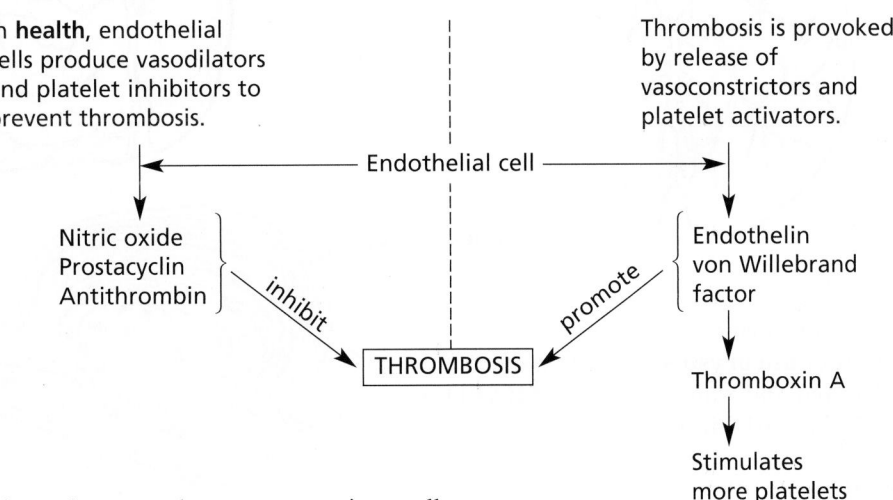

In **health**, endothelial cells produce vasodilators and platelet inhibitors to prevent thrombosis.

Thrombosis is provoked by release of vasoconstrictors and platelet activators.

Endothelial cell

Nitric oxide
Prostacyclin
Antithrombin

*inhibit*

THROMBOSIS

*promote*

Endothelin
von Willebrand factor

Thromboxin A

Stimulates more platelets

The balance between these processes is usually AGAINST THROMBOSIS.

## 3. CHANGES IN COMPOSITION OF THE BLOOD

(a) INCREASE in platelets, fibrinogen and prothrombin after operations and childbirth: usually after 5–10 days.
(b) INCREASE in platelet adhesiveness – again after surgery.
(c) Rare inherited abnormalities of thrombosis inhibitors – e.g. antithrombin III deficiency, protein C deficiency.
(d) Miscellaneous factors – e.g. oral contraceptives, smoking, some cancers.

# COMMON SITES AND TYPES OF THROMBUS

### ARTERIAL

Thrombi are common in arteries as a
complication of **atheroma** (p. 216). Forming
in a rapid circulation, the thrombus consists
mainly of PLATELETS (WHITE thrombus).

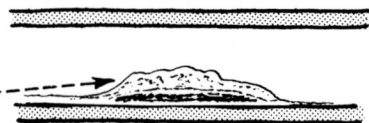

Common sites include:

BRAIN

HEART

Middle
cerebral
arteries

Coronary
arteries

Thrombus

Thrombus

Thrombus formation is common in
the walls of **aneurysms**, consisting of
layers of red and white thrombus (MIXED
or LAMINATED thrombus).

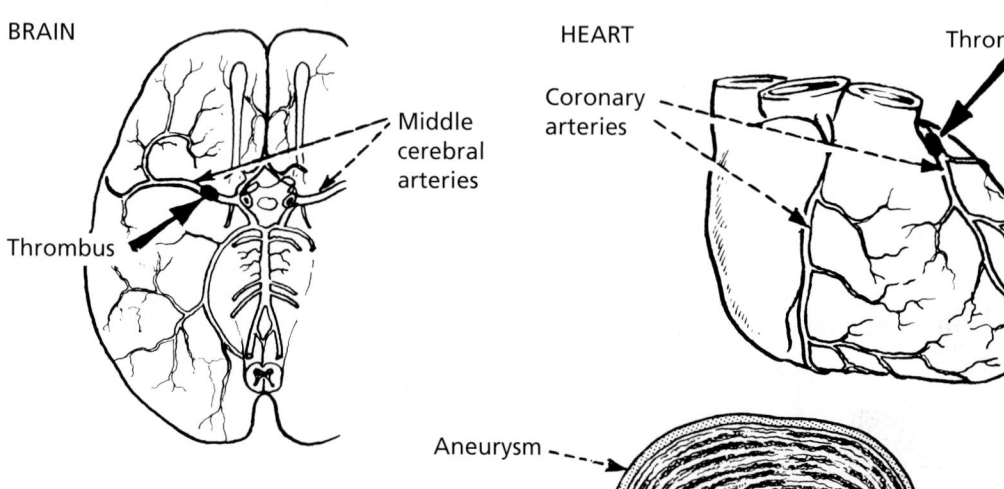

Aneurysm

### VENOUS

**Systemic** venous thrombosis is common
because of the slow blood flow and lower
pressure. It consists
of red cells, platelets
and fibrin
(RED thrombus).

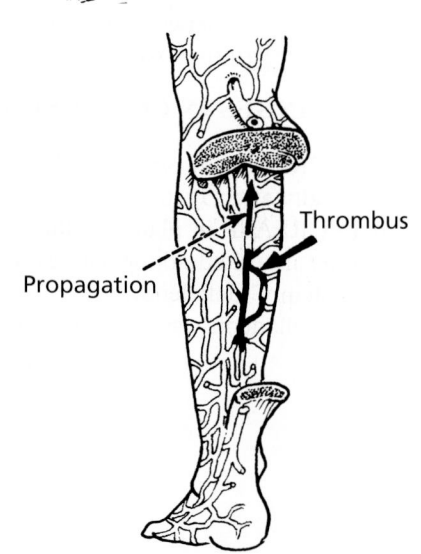

Thrombus

Propagation

It is most common in the deep veins of the calf and
frequently propagates in the femoral and iliac veins
– from where it may embolise to the lungs (p. 81).

Bed rest, operations and cardiac disease are
predisposing conditions.

**Portal** thrombosis is a rare complication of
abdominal disease, e.g. hepatic cirrhosis.

# COMMON SITES AND TYPES OF THROMBUS

## CAPILLARY

Thrombi, composed mainly of fused red cells, form when capillaries are damaged, usually in acute inflammatory processes.

Capillaries are occluded by fibrin thrombi in cases of disseminated intravascular coagulation (DIC, disseminated intravascular coagulation – see p. 451).

## CARDIAC

Thrombi may be seen in the ATRIA (especially in the auricles in ATRIAL FIBRILLATION); in the VENTRICLES and on the heart VALVES.

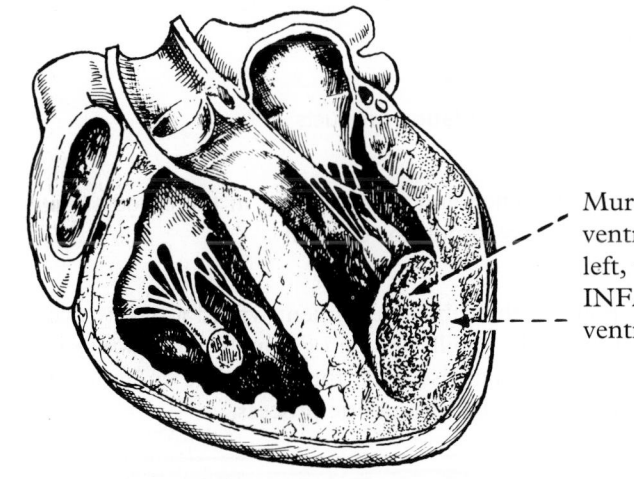

Mural thrombi occur in ventricles, especially the left, usually secondary to INFARCTION of the ventricular wall.

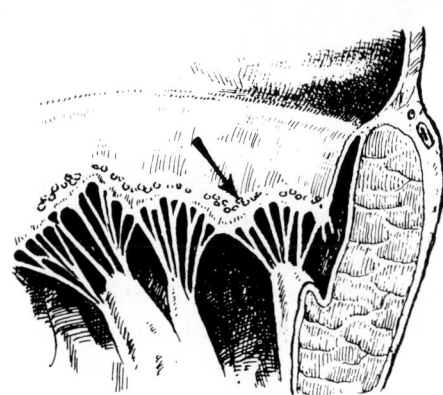

Thrombi can occur on the heart valves in rheumatic endocarditis.

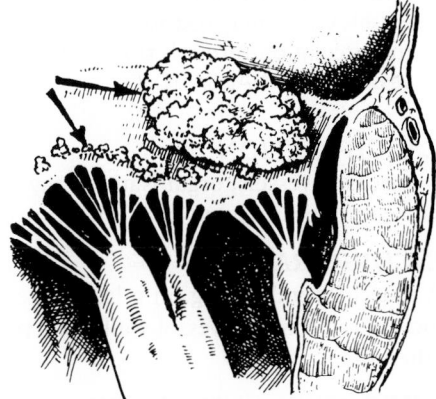

In infective endocarditis thrombi form on the valves. They are larger, mixed, friable and contain masses of micro-organisms.

# SEQUELS OF THROMBOSIS

1.  **FIBRINOLYSIS**

    Many small thrombi are completely removed by the fibrinolytic system which exists to limit thrombosis.

    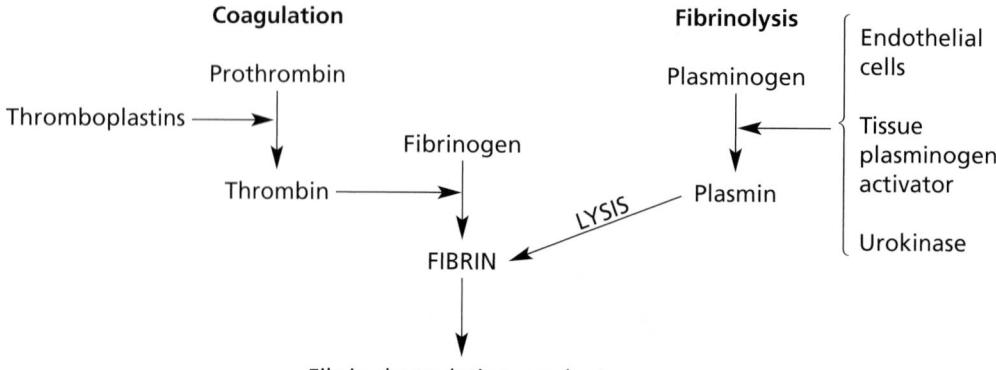

2.  **EMBOLISM**

    Part of the thrombus may be detached and carried along in the blood stream to impact in a distant vessel. This is extremely important clinically.

3.  **ORGANISATION**

    Capillaries grow into the point of thrombus attachment within a day or two. Fibroblasts and phagocytic cells accompany the capillaries, and gradually the thrombus material is dissolved and replaced by fibrovascular tissue. At the same time endothelium covers the ends of the thrombus, thus limiting the thrombotic process.

    Ultimately, the branching capillaries may be converted into one or two larger vessels which may restore the circulation through the vessel – RECANALISATION.

    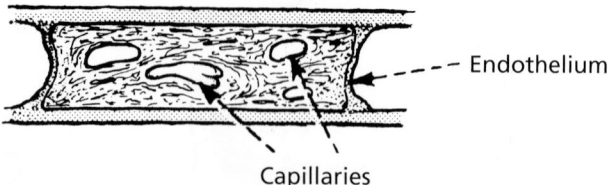

4.  **CALCIFICATION**

    In diseased vessels, organisation may not take place. The thrombus shrinks, calcium salts are deposited and convert it into a phlebolith – seen in X-rays.

5.  **INCORPORATION**

    A mural thrombus, e.g. in a large artery, may be covered by endothelium and incorporated in the vessel wall. This process may be important in the formation of atheroma.

**PROPHYLAXIS** and **THERAPY** of thrombosis aims at:

1.  Reducing coagulability utilising (a) anticoagulants aimed at specific sites in the coagulation cascade, e.g. warfarin derivatives, heparin (see p. 450) and (b) inhibiting specific prostaglandin synthesis, e.g. aspirin.
2.  Encouraging fibrinolysis, using fibrinolysins.

# EMBOLISM

An embolus is any abnormal mass of matter carried in the blood stream large enough to **occlude some vessel.**

The commonest emboli are derived from material generated within the vascular system, e.g. fragments of thrombus or material from atheromatous plaques.

1.  **Pulmonary thrombo-embolism**
    **Emboli from the systemic veins** (especially deep venous thrombosis, e.g. in the calf) pass through the right side of the heart to the pulmonary circulation. The consequences depend on the size of the embolus and the patient's previous health.
    (a) **Massive** embolus → blocks main pulmonary artery trunk → acute total circulatory block → SUDDEN DEATH.
    (b) **Moderate** embolus
        As the lungs have a double blood supply (pulmonary and bronchial arteries), and a vast anastomosis, obstruction of a pulmonary artery branch does not necessarily cause infarction. If, however, there is pre-existing cardiac failure, infarction may occur as the bronchial arterial blood flow is sluggish.

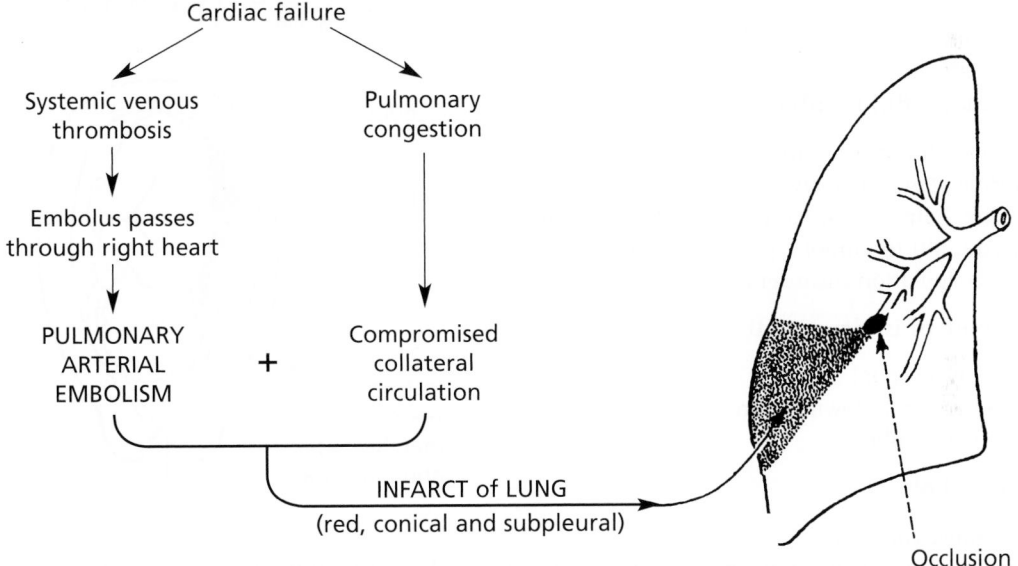

Cardiac failure

Systemic venous thrombosis → Pulmonary congestion

Embolus passes through right heart

PULMONARY ARTERIAL EMBOLISM + Compromised collateral circulation

INFARCT of LUNG
(red, conical and subpleural)

Occlusion

    (c) **Small** emboli
        Many are removed by the fibrinolytic system and are asymptomatic. However, repeated minor emboli may result in pulmonary hypertension and right heart failure. Repeated small emboli → blockage of peripheral pulmonary arterial branches → **pulmonary hypertension.**

2.  **Emboli of the arterial system** are derived from the heart or the larger arteries which have become atheromatous. The results of arterial obstruction are very important.

# EMBOLISM

### EMBOLISM – OTHER FORMS

Matter entering the vascular system may be:

(a) *Solid* – tumour cells, bacterial clumps, fat, parasites
(b) *Gaseous* – air
(c) *Liquid* – amniotic fluid with fetal derived matter

### Fat embolism

This may occur when a long bone is fractured, usually 24–72 hours later. Fat globules enter torn veins and pass to the lungs; obstruction of pulmonary blood flow may be sufficient to cause *anoxia*. Cerebral symptoms are common due to anoxia but also due to the fat globules which have passed through the lung capillaries.

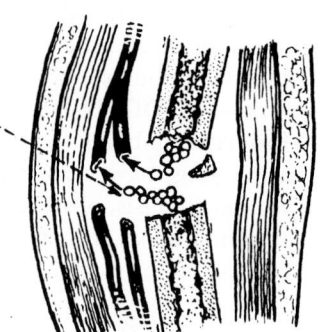

### Amniotic fluid embolism

During childbirth, amniotic fluid may enter a uterine vein, especially after manipulations. Vernix, hairs and squames enter the circulation. In addition to embolic phenomena, there are also coagulation disorders (p. 451).

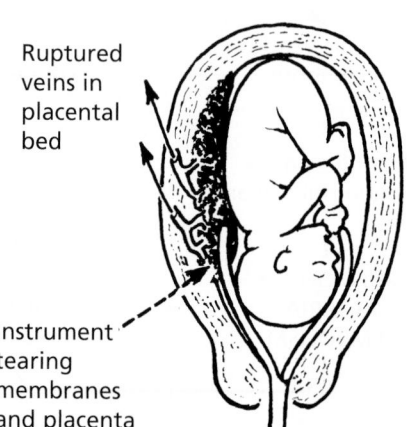

Ruptured veins in placental bed

Instrument tearing membranes and placenta

### Embolism in drug addicts

Foreign material (e.g. talc) may enter the bloodstream following intravenous injection and form emboli.

### Air embolism

(a) *Single embolism*
    Atmospheric air may enter the blood when a neck or intracranial vein is incised. Inspiration induces a suction effect by causing a negative pressure in the veins. As a result of frothing in the right ventricle, cardiac function is seriously impaired.
(b) *Multiple embolism*, in 'caisson disease'.

    This occurs in people working in barometric pressures of several atmospheres, e.g. diving to great depths. The atmospheric gases go into solution in high concentration in the blood and tissues. If decompression occurs too quickly, these gases 'boil' off and appear as bubbles in the circulation. The oxygen is taken up by the tissues but insoluble gases cause widespread 'embolism', especially in the nervous system and bone.

# ARTERIAL OBSTRUCTION

Arterial obstruction is usually due to thrombosis or embolism and may be (a) partial or complete, (b) acute or slowly progressive.

The effects depend on the local anatomy, particularly on the presence of an anastomotic collateral circulation.

### Occlusion of end arteries

These may have    (a) no collaterals (e.g. splenic artery)

                        (b) capillary anastomoses (e.g. renal and coronary arteries)

                        (c) arterial anastomoses which are too small to maintain circulation (e.g. superior mesenteric artery)

### Result:

Obstruction → anoxia of tissues → necrosis

### INFARCTS

An infarct is an area of necrosis due to ischaemia. It is often found at the periphery of an organ, e.g. the kidney.

Blocked
artery

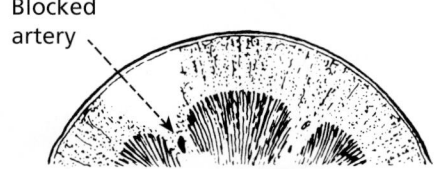 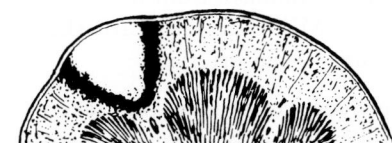

*After 12 hours:* area is pale. Degenerative changes already seen with electron microscope.

*After 36 hours*: area shows pallor and swelling due to coagulative necrosis. The surrounding tissues are congested.

### Healing

This takes place slowly. Capillaries and fibroblasts replace the necrotic tissue. Collagen is formed, the fibroblasts contract and this results in a depressed scar.

# IMPORTANT SITES OF INFARCTION

The HEART, the LUNGS and the BRAIN are the most common sites. Less common are the SMALL INTESTINES kidney and spleen.

### HEART (p. 226)

Infarction is almost always due to coronary arterial thrombosis complicating atheroma.

Cardiac function is immediately compromised, eddies form, the endocardium may be damaged and a thrombus forms on the inner surface of the infarcted area. The damage may extend to the external surface causing pericarditis.

If the patient survives, the infarct heals by fibrosis.

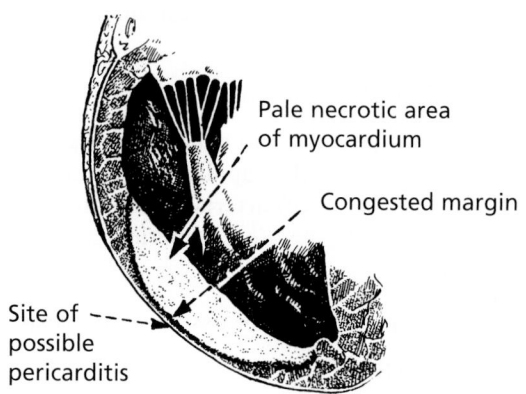

Pale necrotic area of myocardium

Congested margin

Site of possible pericarditis

### BRAIN (p. 578)

Infarcts are commonly due to thrombosis of diseased vessels or to embolism from the left heart or carotid arteries, e.g. MIDDLE CEREBRAL, posterior cerebral and basilar arteries.

The usual changes of infarction take place, but the necrosis is colliquative – **cerebral softening**.

Infarction may occur without arterial occlusion in severe, prolonged hypotension (shock). Parts of the brain at the junction of arterial territories are affected (boundary zone or watershed infarcts) (see p. 579).

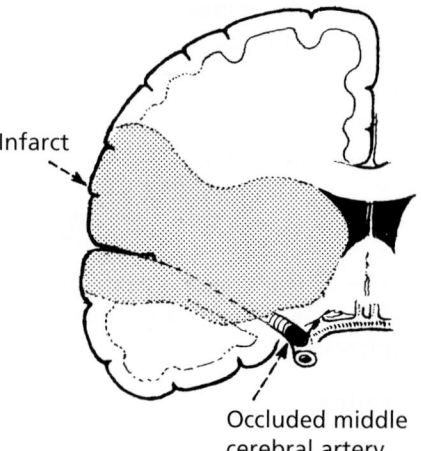

Infarct

Occluded middle cerebral artery

# IMPORTANT SITES OF INFARCTION

## INTESTINE

Infarction may follow thrombosis of or embolisation to the mesenteric arteries. The sequence of changes usually seen in solid organs is altered by the effects of anastomoses and, in the later stages, by **bacterial invasion** (gangrenous necrosis).

Occlusion ⟶ Ischaemia ⟶ Collateral congestion ⟶ CONGESTION and HAEMORRHAGE

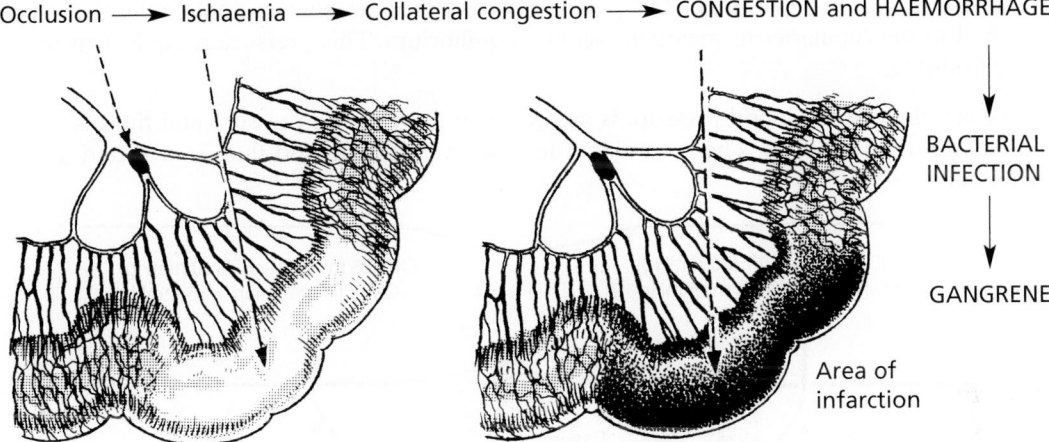

BACTERIAL INFECTION

GANGRENE

Area of infarction

# NORMAL TISSUE FLUID CIRCULATION

There is continuous interchange of fluid between blood and tissues. Some fluid enters the lymphatics before eventually returning to the blood stream. Two main forces operate pressure gradients controlling the fluid movement.

1. **Hydrostatic pressure**, i.e. capillary blood pressure (BP) encouraging the passage of fluid through the capillary wall, = 35 mm mercury (mmHg).
2. **Protein osmotic pressure** (OP), i.e. the plasma proteins encourage the retention of fluid in the capillaries to maintain osmotic equilibrium. This pressure is equivalent to 25 mmHg.

At the arterial end the blood pressure is greater than the osmotic pressure and fluid is forced out of the capillary. The reverse is true at the venous end and fluid is attracted into the vessel.

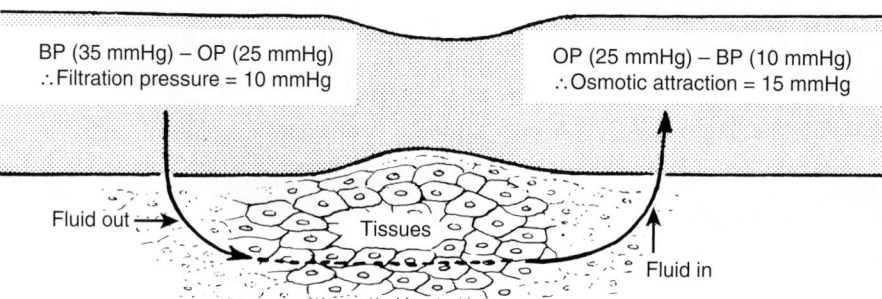

BP (35 mmHg) − OP (25 mmHg)
∴Filtration pressure = 10 mmHg

OP (25 mmHg) − BP (10 mmHg)
∴Osmotic attraction = 15 mmHg

Fluid out →

Tissues

Fluid in

A small amount of fluid enters lymphatics. This is partly the result of tissue pressure and partly due to osmotic attraction of proteins in the lymphatic system.

In addition to those forces operating at capillary level, there are other mechanisms which influence the movement of fluid within the body.

1. **Fluid intake**
   Intake via the gut or parenterally may exceed the ability of the kidneys to eliminate water.
2. **Integrity of the kidneys**
   Damage to the kidney may diminish the elimination of fluid.
3. **Hormone activity**

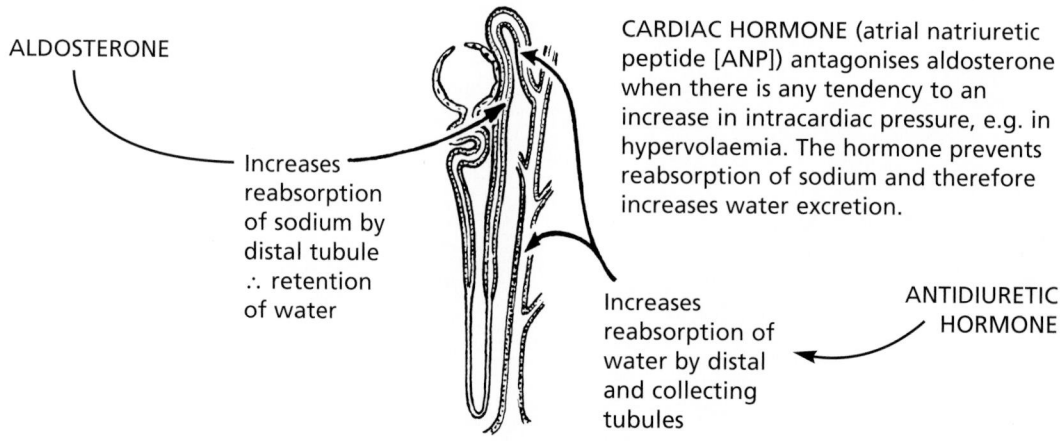

ALDOSTERONE

Increases reabsorption of sodium by distal tubule ∴ retention of water

CARDIAC HORMONE (atrial natriuretic peptide [ANP]) antagonises aldosterone when there is any tendency to an increase in intracardiac pressure, e.g. in hypervolaemia. The hormone prevents reabsorption of sodium and therefore increases water excretion.

Increases reabsorption of water by distal and collecting tubules

ANTIDIURETIC HORMONE

# OEDEMA

Oedema is an accumulation of excess fluid in the extravascular tissues. It can be local or generalised. There are a wide variety of causes.

DECREASE in blood osmotic pressure (usually due to HYPOALBUMINAEMIA)

*Common causes:*
Liver disease – deficient synthesis.
**Renal disease** – protein loss.
Starvation.

INCREASE in venous pressure (hydrostatic pressure ↑)

*Common causes:*
**Cardiac failure**
Venous obstruction in lower limbs.

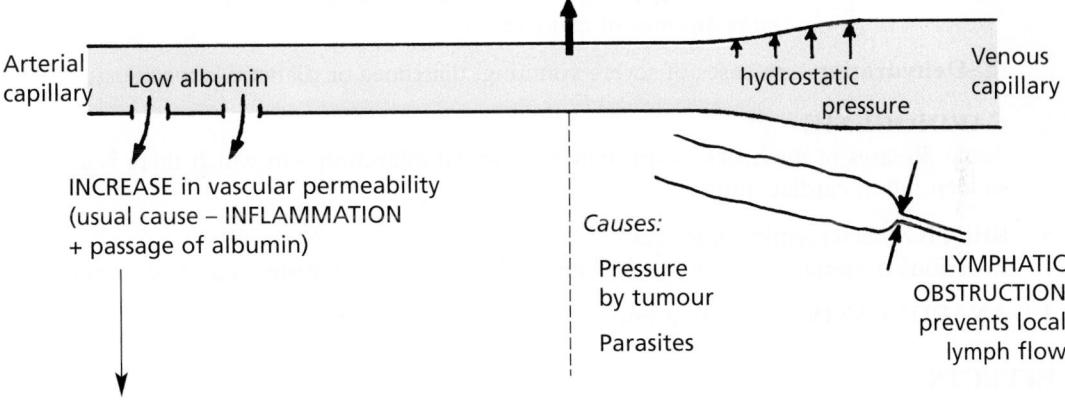

NET INCREASE
in FLOW from CAPILLARY

Arterial capillary
Low albumin
hydrostatic pressure
Venous capillary

INCREASE in vascular permeability
(usual cause – INFLAMMATION
+ passage of albumin)

*Causes:*

Pressure
by tumour

Parasites

LYMPHATIC
OBSTRUCTION
prevents local
lymph flow

Loss of osmotic pressure

More than one factor may apply:

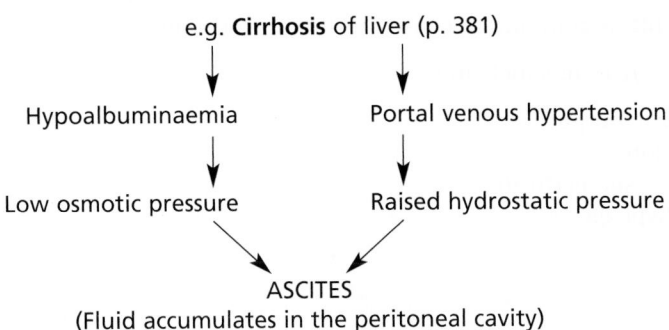

e.g. **Cirrhosis** of liver (p. 381)

Hypoalbuminaemia

Low osmotic pressure

Portal venous hypertension

Raised hydrostatic pressure

ASCITES
(Fluid accumulates in the peritoneal cavity)

Cerebral (p. 575) and pulmonary (p. 210) oedema are life threatening and are dealt with separately.

# SHOCK

Shock is a condition in which there is reduced perfusion of the vital organs due to a severe and acute reduction in cardiac output and effective circulating blood volume. There is progressive cardiovascular collapse characterised by hypotension, hyperventilation and clouding of consciousness.

## CAUSES

1. **HYPOVOLAEMIC (i.e. diminished blood volume)**
   Associated with:

   (a) **Trauma**
   - (i) Severe haemorrhage – external or internal
   - (ii) Severe injury – especially fractures of bones and crushing of tissues
   - (iii) Burns – especially where extensive surface damage allows loss of a large amount of exudate.

   (b) **Dehydration** – in cases of severe vomiting, diarrhoea or diabetic ketoacidosis.

2. **CARDIOGENIC**
   Acute diseases of the heart – especially myocardial infarction – in which there is a sudden fall in cardiac output.

3. **SEPTIC** (bacteraemic, endotoxic)
   In serious bacterial infections (especially Gram-negative organisms, e.g. *Escherichia coli*).

4. **ANAPHYLAXIS** – a severe immune hypersensitivity reaction (p. 143).

## EFFECTS

The loss of effective circulating blood causes tissue and cell damage. At the same time, there are reactive changes in the circulation.

These two mechanisms combine to cause the shock syndrome.

The main consequences of shock are:

1. Low cardiac output
2. Hypotension
3. Impaired tissue perfusion
4. Cellular hypoxia

# SHOCK

## REACTIVE CIRCULATORY CHANGES – EARLY STAGE

These changes are concerned with the maintenance of an adequate cerebral and coronary circulation and are effected by redistribution of the blood in the body as a whole.

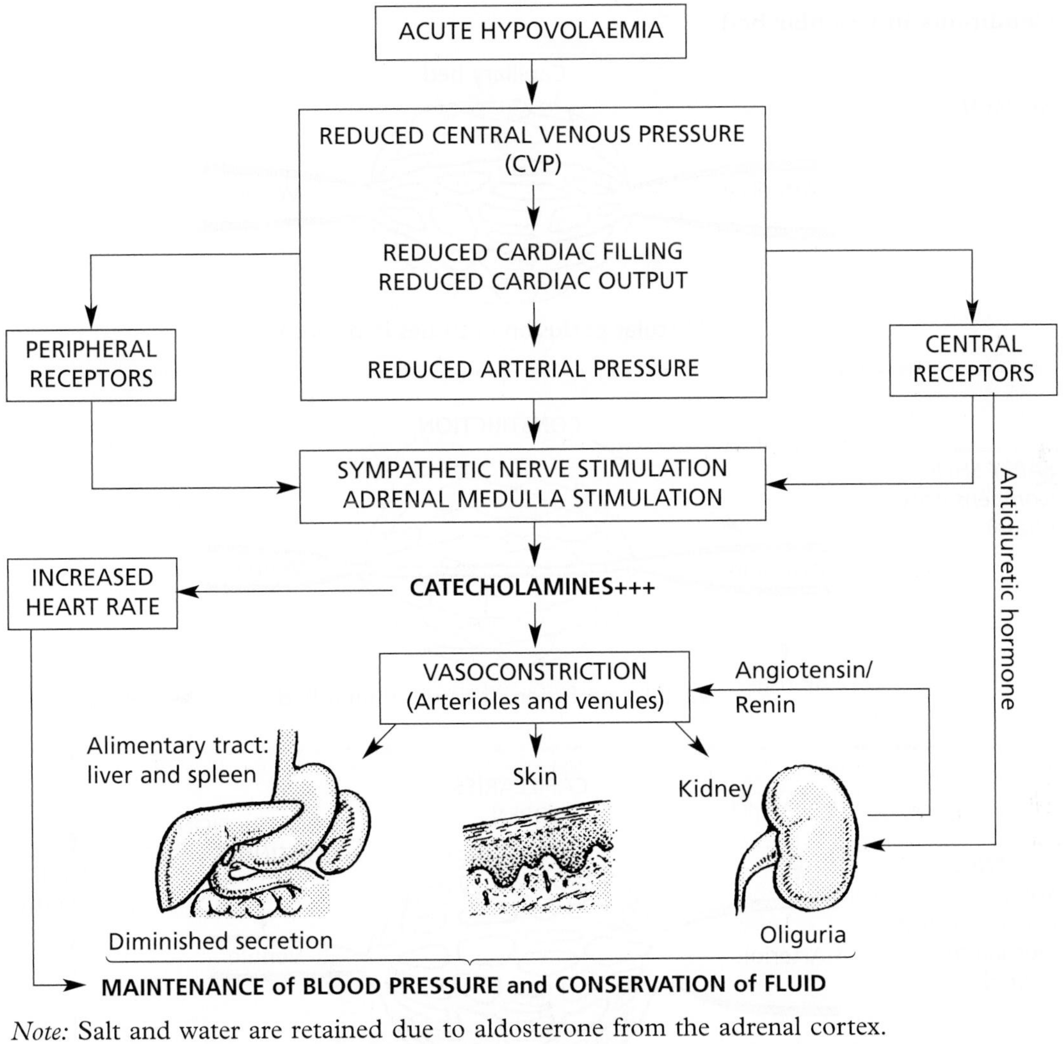

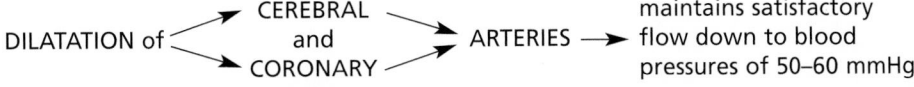

**MAINTENANCE of BLOOD PRESSURE and CONSERVATION of FLUID**

*Note:* Salt and water are retained due to aldosterone from the adrenal cortex.

At the same time, the circulations in the brain and heart are protected by autoregulatory mechanisms. They are not subject to the generalised vasoconstriction.

Instead:

DILATATION of CEREBRAL and CORONARY ARTERIES maintains satisfactory flow down to blood pressures of 50–60 mmHg

If the loss of circulating fluid volume is great, the limits of the compensatory mechanism are exceeded and the patient develops severe shock.

89

# SHOCK

### DECOMPENSATION – ADVANCED STAGE

The patient is now listless, pale and cold, the face is pinched and the lips blue. The pulse is rapid and weak and the blood pressure is low.

**Conditions in vascular bed**

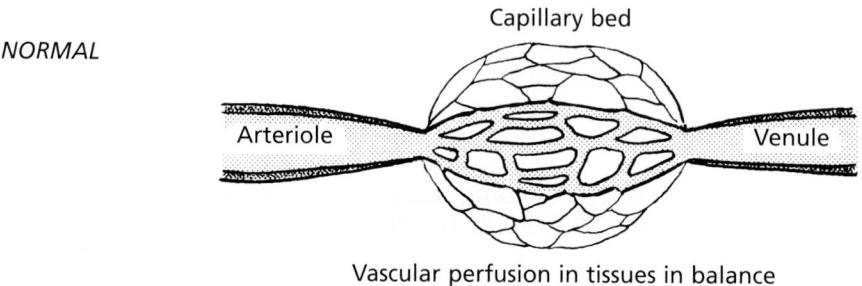

*NORMAL*

Capillary bed

Arteriole

Venule

Vascular perfusion in tissues in balance

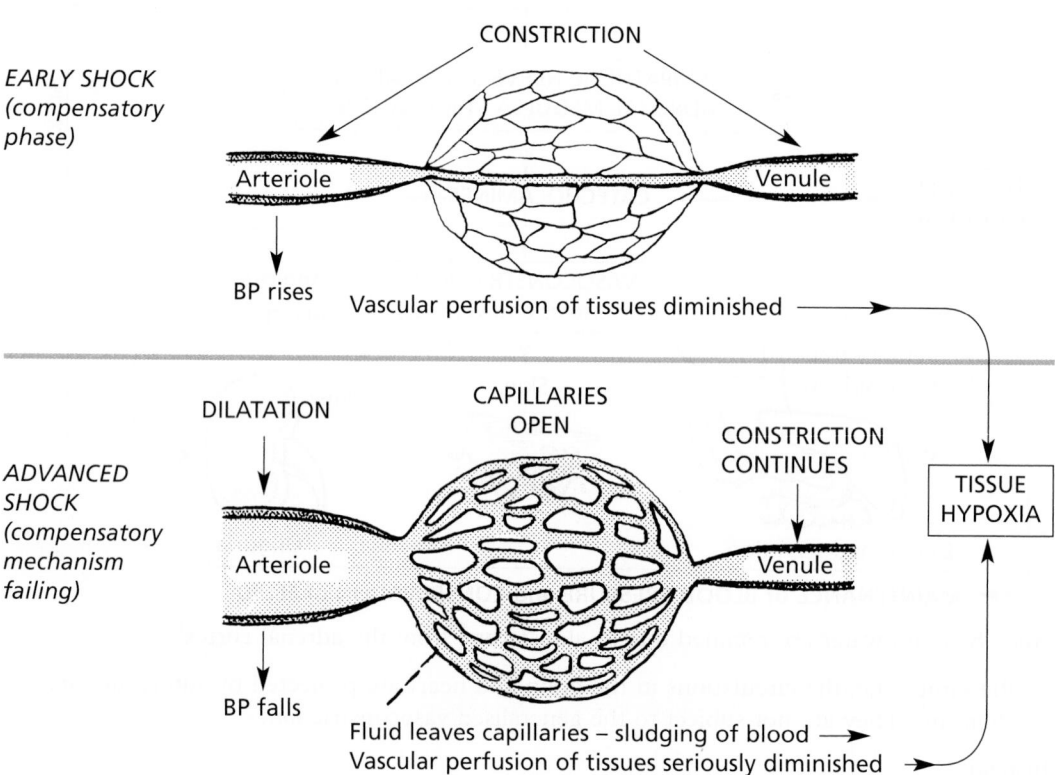

*EARLY SHOCK (compensatory phase)*

CONSTRICTION

Arteriole

Venule

BP rises

Vascular perfusion of tissues diminished

*ADVANCED SHOCK (compensatory mechanism failing)*

DILATATION

CAPILLARIES OPEN

CONSTRICTION CONTINUES

TISSUE HYPOXIA

Arteriole

Venule

BP falls

Fluid leaves capillaries – sludging of blood ⟶
Vascular perfusion of tissues seriously diminished ⟶

# SHOCK

Thus from the beginning of the shock process, all the body tissues, with the exception of the brain and the heart, suffer from hypoxia. This sets up vicious circles which aggravate the condition:

1.

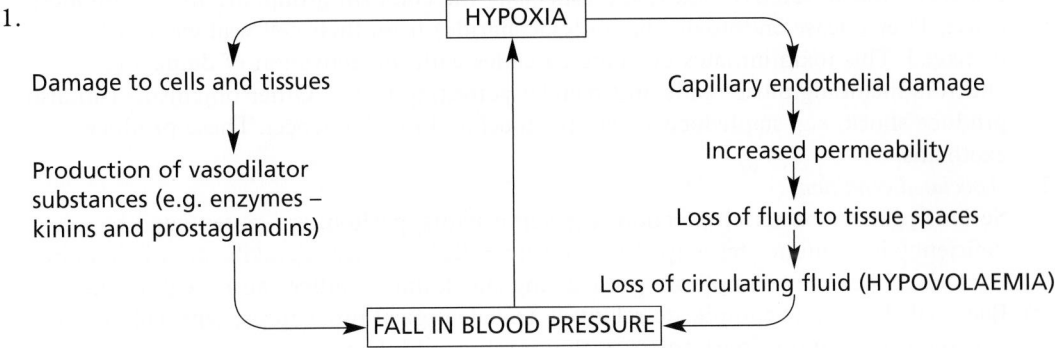

2. When the blood pressure falls below 50–60 mmHg, the autoregulatory control of the cerebral and coronary circulation fails. Serious damage to the brain and heart may occur.

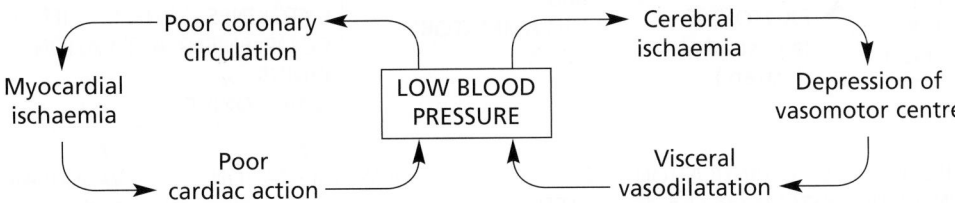

## CHANGES IN THE BLOOD AND CELL METABOLISM

As well as these basic circulatory disturbances, important changes in the blood and cellular metabolism occur in shock.

**Blood coagulation system**

Acute hypoxia → Damaged endothelium → Coagulation cascade triggered → May proceed to formation of FIBRIN → Disseminated intravascular coagulation (DIC) syndrome

**Cellular metabolism**

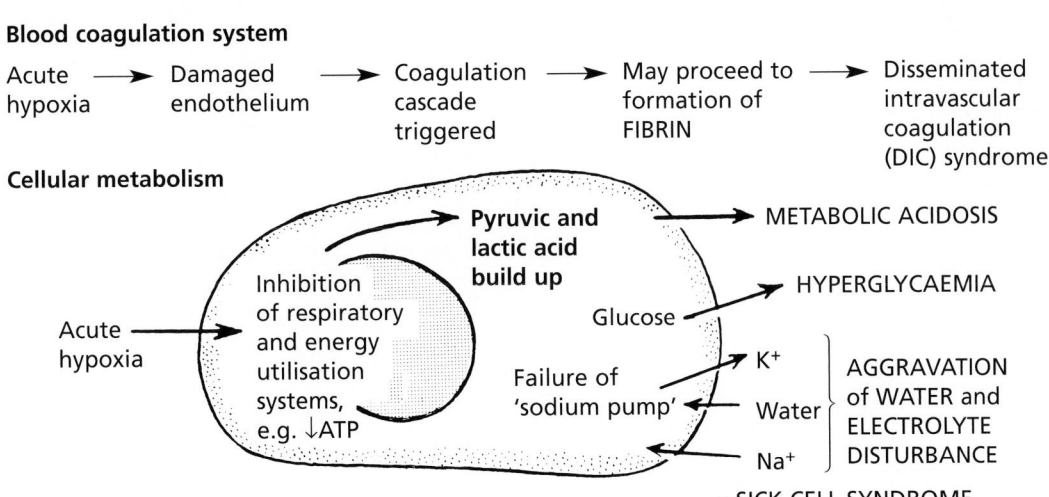

# SHOCK

### SEPTIC SHOCK (ENDOTOXIC)

### Causes

1. *Bacteria* – GRAM-NEGATIVE BACTERIA, especially the coliform group, are the commonest cause. They release endotoxin (lipopolysaccharide) from their cell wall when it is damaged. This toxin initiates cytokine cascades with the activation of damaging effectors including nitric oxide and platelet-activating factor. Other organisms can also produce shock, e.g. staphylococci, streptococci and meningococci. These produce exotoxins.

2. *Associated conditions*

(a) Serious primary bacterial infection, e.g. septicaemia, peritonitis – potentiated by deficiency in immune status (p. 146) and liver disease where detoxification is impaired.

(b) Bacterial shock may complicate pre-existing shock due to other causes, e.g. burns.

(c) Bacterial shock may complicate relatively trivial surgical procedures, especially in the gastrointestinal and urinary tracts in the presence of infection.

### Mechanism

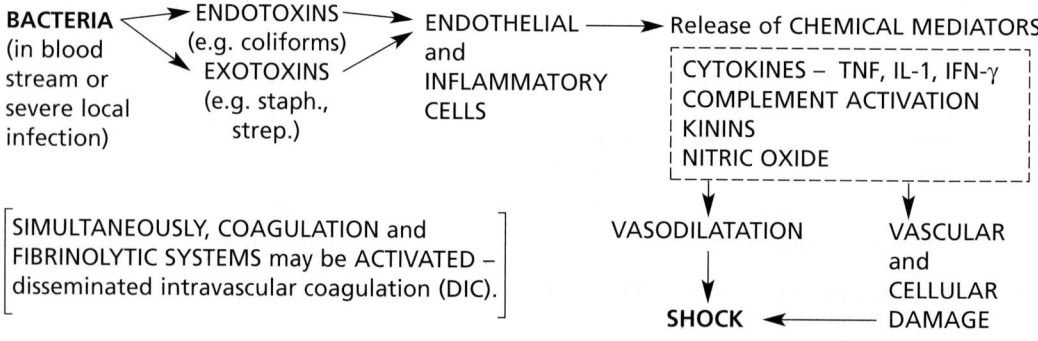

# SHOCK

## SHOCK IN BURNS AND SCALDS

### Mechanism

1. There is stimulation of afferent nerves, followed by:
2. An INFLAMMATORY RESPONSE evoked by the burned tissues.

> Massive exudation and
> loss of PROTEIN-RICH fluid ⟶ HYPOVOLAEMIA ⟶ SHOCK
> (sludging of blood in capillaries)

The mechanism explains why the SEVERITY of the shock is roughly proportional to the exuding SURFACE AREA and not to the depth of the burn.

Other factors are chemical mediators derived from the burned tissues.

3. Complications which aggravate the shock:

> (a) Infection: Burned ⟶ Susceptible to infection ⟶ SEPTIC
> tissues   esp. *Staph. aureus*,   SHOCK
>    *Strep. pyogenes*, Gram-neg.   may be superimposed
>    bacilli (e.g. *Pseudomonas*)
>
> (b) Anaemia: Haemolysis of red cells at burned
>    site and later if sludging is severe ⟶ ANAEMIA

# SHOCK – INDIVIDUAL ORGANS

### HEART

There are two ways in which heart failure may be associated with shock.

1. In hypovolaemic and bacteraemic shock, heart failure is a *COMPLICATION*.
2. In cardiogenic shock, acute heart failure is the *CAUSE* of shock.

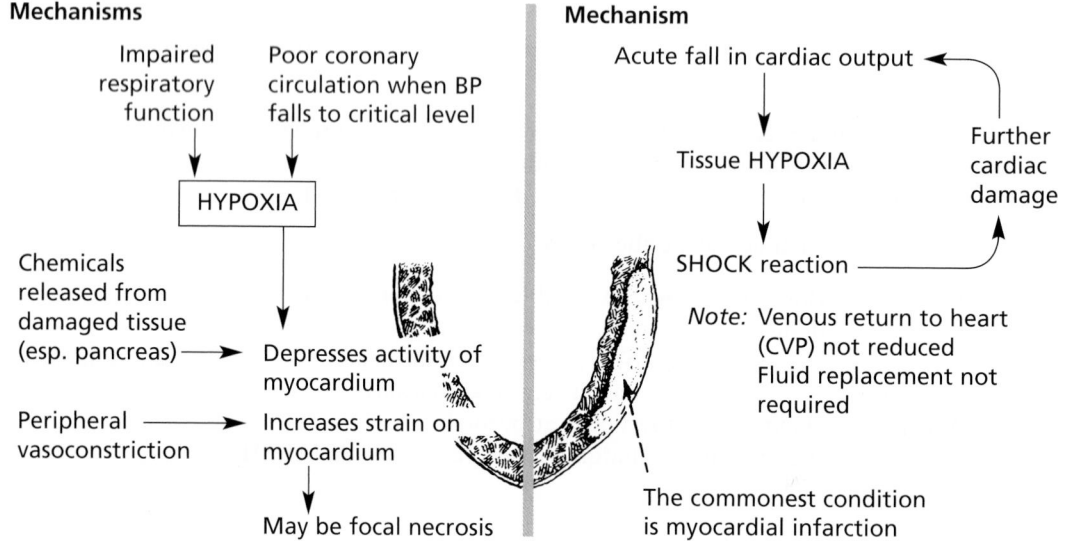

**Mechanisms**

Impaired respiratory function · Poor coronary circulation when BP falls to critical level → HYPOXIA

Chemicals released from damaged tissue (esp. pancreas) → Depresses activity of myocardium

Peripheral vasoconstriction → Increases strain on myocardium

May be focal necrosis

**Mechanism**

Acute fall in cardiac output → Tissue HYPOXIA → SHOCK reaction → Further cardiac damage

*Note:* Venous return to heart (CVP) not reduced. Fluid replacement not required

The commonest condition is myocardial infarction

### LUNGS

Respiratory function is disturbed in two ways:

**Circulatory changes in the lung** (especially in septic/traumatic shock). These occur when compensatory mechanisms are failing. There is congestion and oedema, with the formation of hyaline membranes. At autopsy the lungs are heavy and wet. This condition is called 'shock lung' or acute respiratory distress syndrome (ARDS). The pathological term is diffuse alveolar damage (DAD).

**Early** patchy changes throughout the lungs:

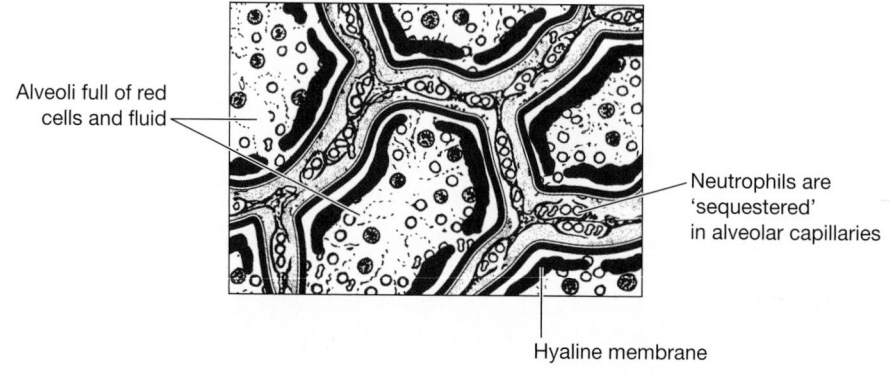

Alveoli full of red cells and fluid

Neutrophils are 'sequestered' in alveolar capillaries

Hyaline membrane

# SHOCK – INDIVIDUAL ORGANS

## KIDNEYS

The excretory function of the kidneys is always disturbed in shock. This is due to the general circulatory collapse and hypotension, but it may be aggravated by the secretion of renin and angiotensin by the kidney, aldosterone by the adrenal and antidiuretic hormone by the posterior pituitary. These hormones are secreted in an attempt to retain fluid and restore the blood volume, but by inducing vasoconstriction they will tend to increase renal damage.

### Mechanism

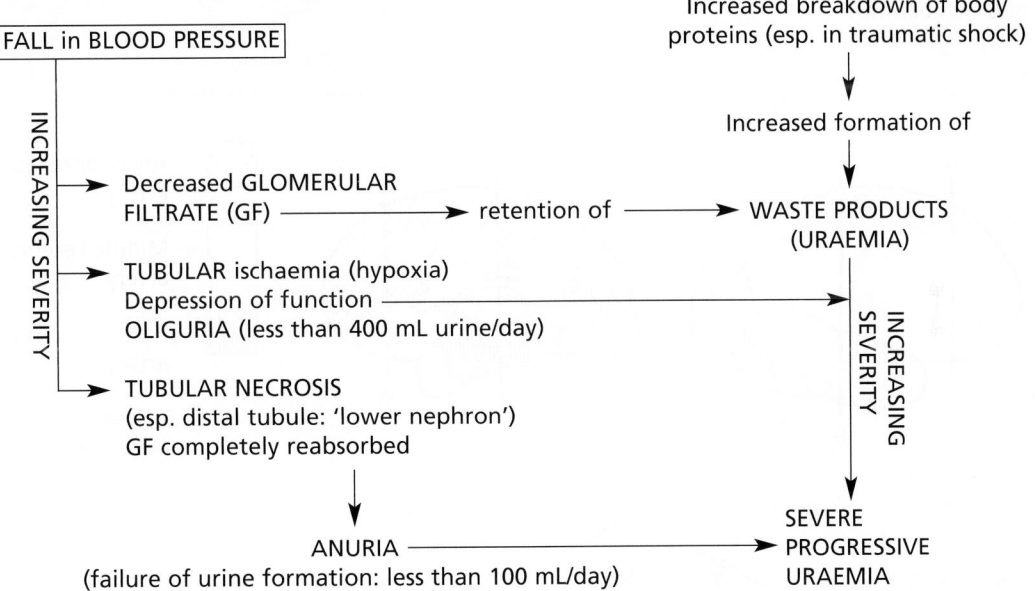

FALL in BLOOD PRESSURE

INCREASING SEVERITY

Increased breakdown of body proteins (esp. in traumatic shock)

Increased formation of

Decreased GLOMERULAR FILTRATE (GF) → retention of → WASTE PRODUCTS (URAEMIA)

TUBULAR ischaemia (hypoxia)
Depression of function
OLIGURIA (less than 400 mL urine/day)

INCREASING SEVERITY

TUBULAR NECROSIS
(esp. distal tubule: 'lower nephron')
GF completely reabsorbed

ANURIA
(failure of urine formation: less than 100 mL/day)

SEVERE PROGRESSIVE URAEMIA

In such cases, at post mortem the kidneys are pale and swollen and the architectural markings are blurred

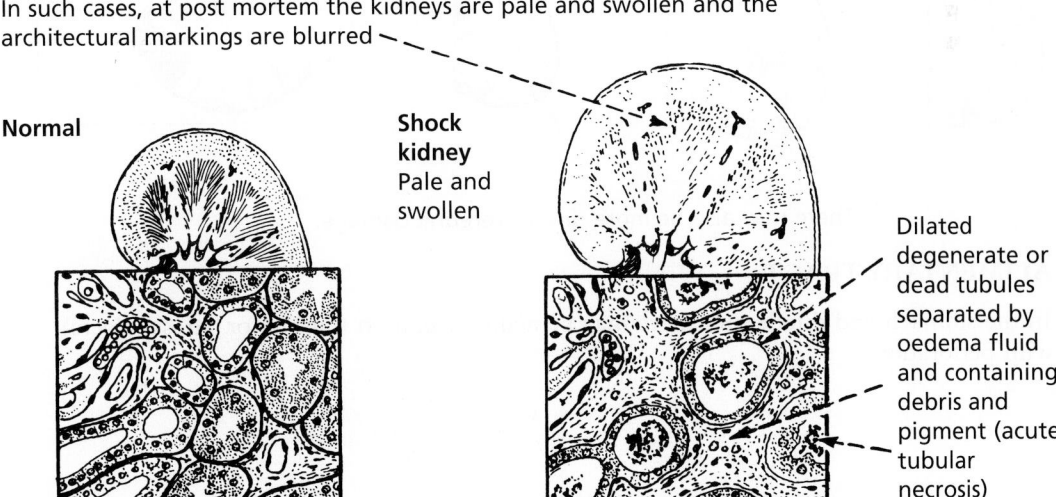

Normal

Shock kidney
Pale and swollen

Dilated degenerate or dead tubules separated by oedema fluid and containing debris and pigment (acute tubular necrosis)

In even more severe shock the entire cortex may become necrotic (acute cortical necrosis).

# SHOCK – INDIVIDUAL ORGANS

### BRAIN

During the compensated phase of shock, relatively mild cerebral ischaemia is associated with changes in the state of consciousness. When the blood pressure falls to below 50–60 mmHg, the brain suffers serious ischaemic damage with infarction in the 'boundary zones' of the cerebral cortex and cerebellum.

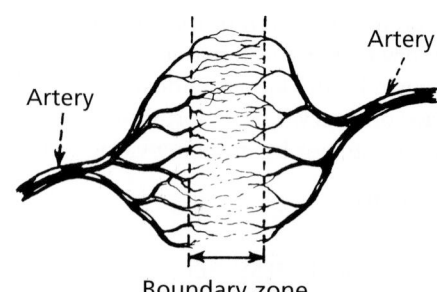

Boundary zone
(Sluggish circulation)

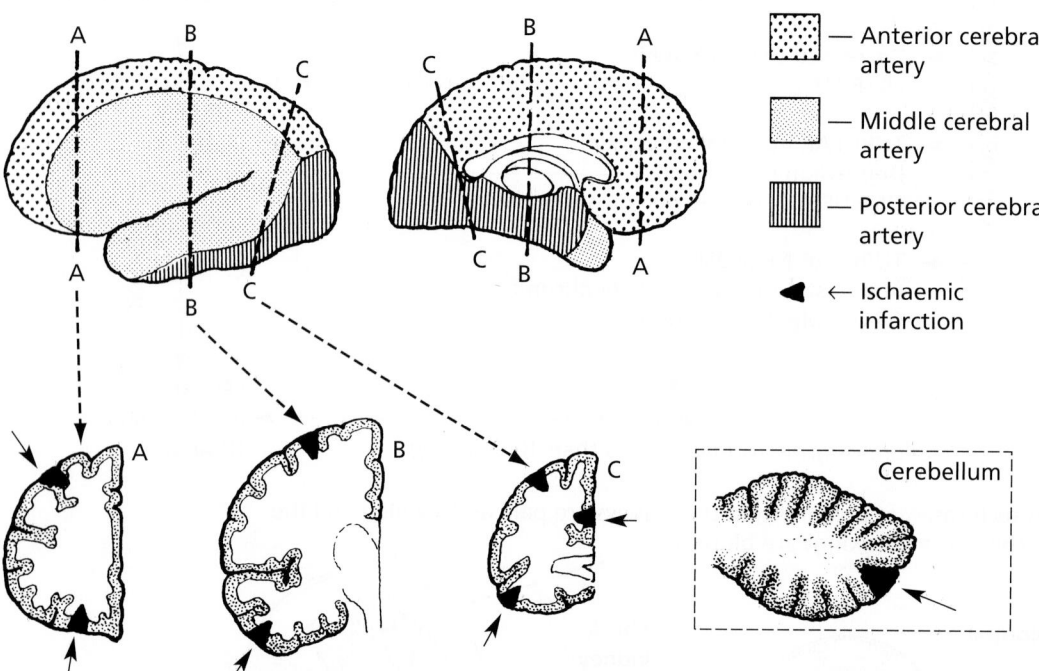

There may also be more diffuse cerebral damage.

### ALIMENTARY TRACT

In the stomach and duodenum there may be acute ulceration (curling or 'stress' ulcers) with perforation.

# SHOCK – INDIVIDUAL ORGANS: OUTCOME

## LIVER

The liver acinus is supplied by portal venous blood and hepatic arterial blood: in shock, Zone 3 of the hepatic acinus is vulnerable to anoxia.

Shock ⟶ reduced arterial blood supply ⟶ ANOXIA

May proceed to Zone 3 necrosis.

## THE OUTCOME OF SHOCK

There are three possibilities, depending on several factors:

1. RECOVERY after convalescence, which may be long.
2. SURVIVAL with permanent damage to various organs.
3. DEATH.

| FACTORS FAVOURING RECOVERY | FACTORS FAVOURING PROGRESSION OF SHOCK |
|---|---|
| 1. AVAILABILITY of EARLY TREATMENT of:<br>(a) the INITIATING CAUSE<br>(b) the HYPOVOLAEMIA<br>2. Youth<br>3. Good general health | 1. DELAY in TREATMENT<br>2. FAILURE to REMOVE the INITIATING CAUSE<br>3. Old age<br>4. Poor general health<br>5. Pre-existing cardiovascular and lung disease<br>6. Onset of complications, esp. infection and organ damage |

## LIVER

The liver is supplied by partial venous blood and large arterial blood reserve.
Zone 3 of the hepatic acinus is vulnerable to hypoxia.

Muscle, skin and used arterial blood supply.

## THE OUTCOME OF SHOCK

There are three possibilities, depending on several factors:

1. RECOVERY – most cases survive, which may be rapid
2. SURVIVAL with permanent damage to various organs
3. DEATH

| FACTORS FAVOURING RECOVERY | FACTORS AVOIDING PROGRESSION OF SHOCK |
|---|---|
| a. AVAILABILITY of EARLY TREATMENT of: | 1. DELAY in TREATMENT |
| (a) the precipitating cause | 2. FAILURE to REMOVE the INITIATING CAUSE |
| (b) the HYPOVOLAEMIA | 3. TISSUE |
| 2. YOUTH | 4. Circulating toxin |
| 4. Good general health | 5. Pre-existing cardiovascular and lung disease |
| | 6. Onset of complications e.g. infection and organ damage |

# INFECTION AND IMMUNITY

## OBJECTIVES

1. To define infection, colonisation, pathogen, commensals, pathogenicity and virulence.
2. To outline the categories of infectious agents, their key features and main differences.
3. To describe the host response to infections of varying type.
4. To describe the inflammatory response to infection.
5. To define the key components, cell types and molecular mediators of the innate and adaptive immune response.
6. To describe the four types of hypersensitivity reaction.
7. To understand the causes of primary and secondary immunodeficiency including HIV.
8. To understand immune tolerance and the pattern of common auto-immune disorders.

# INFECTION

There are many infections: this chapter will deal only with principles and a few examples.

| TYPE OF INFECTING AGENT | EXAMPLE | EXAMPLE OF DISEASE |
|---|---|---|
| Bacteria (a very wide range) | *Staphylococcus* | Abscess |
| Viruses (a wide range) | Herpes zoster | Chickenpox and shingles |
| Fungi (a limited range) | *Candida* | Buccal and vaginal thrush |
| Protozoa | *Plasmodium* | Malaria |
| Infestation with parasites, worms and flukes | *Echinococcus granulosis* | Hydatid disease |

### COLONISATION AND COMMENSAL GROWTH

Vast numbers of bacteria normally colonise the external body surfaces (skin, alimentary and upper respiratory tracts). These **commensal** inhabitants usually do not harm the host. Organisms that injure the host are said to be **pathogenic**. If the host defences are damaged a commensal organism may cause an **opportunistic infection**.

### INFECTION AND INFECTIOUS DISEASE

INFECTION occurs when microorganisms invade the sterile internal body tissues. (Multiplication usually follows invasion.)

An INFECTIOUS DISEASE occurs when infection is associated with clinically manifest tissue damage.

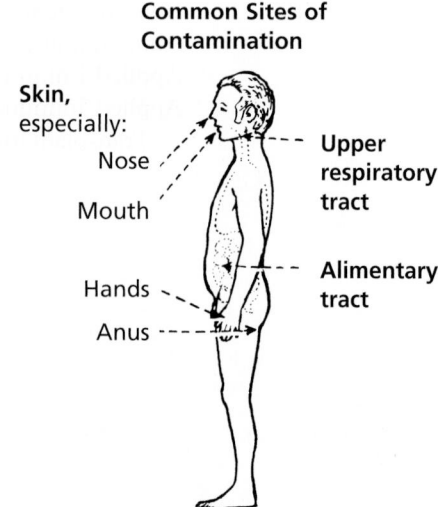

**Common Sites of Contamination**

Skin, especially:
- Nose
- Mouth
- Hands
- Anus

Upper respiratory tract

Alimentary tract

# INFECTION

## Routes of entry of infecting organisms

1.  Through the *skin* or *mucous membranes*
    (a)  By direct close contact, e.g. venereal disease, HIV.
    (b)  By contamination of abrasions and wounds, e.g. wound infections, rabies.
    (c)  By inoculation, e.g. insect bite – yellow fever, syringe – hepatitis B and C, AIDS.
2.  By *ingestion*
    Contaminated food and water, e.g. enteric fever, hepatitis A, poliomyelitis, cholera.
3.  By *inhalation*
    Dust and droplets, e.g. influenza, tuberculosis.

## Factors influencing the establishment of infection

1.  *In the HOST*

In addition to a good state of general health and nutrition, the following mechanisms operate in preventing and limiting infection.

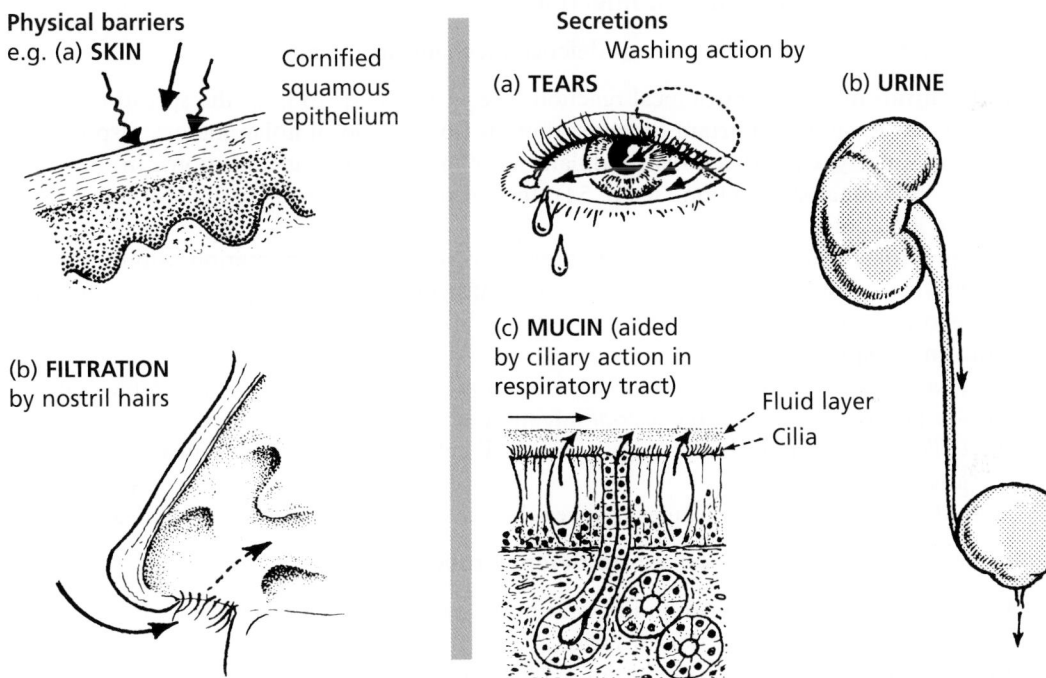

**Physical barriers**
e.g. (a) **SKIN**
Cornified squamous epithelium

(b) **FILTRATION** by nostril hairs

**Secretions**
Washing action by
(a) **TEARS**
(b) **URINE**

(c) **MUCIN** (aided by ciliary action in respiratory tract)
Fluid layer
Cilia

## Chemical action

(a)  Acid secretion in stomach and urinary tract.
(b)  Lysozymes – enzymes capable of dissolving bacterial capsules, e.g. in tears and saliva.
(c)  Immunoglobulin A (IgA) – a specialised immunoglobulin (see p. 137) – tears, intestinal secretions.
(d)  Nonspecific inhibitory substances – urine, sweat, sebum.

# INFECTION

### Innate immune response

(a) Natural Killer (NK) cells and macrophages with pattern recognition receptors.
(b) Plasma proteins including the complement system.

2. *In the MICRO-ORGANISM*

Factors potentiating invasive capacity include:

(a) **Quantity of dose** – the larger the dose the more likely that the defences are penetrated.
(b) **Virulence** – describes the degree of pathogenicity, including:
  (i) Capacity to resist phagocytosis and enzyme attack.
  (ii) Adhesive properties.
  (iii) Production of exoenzymes which act on host tissues, e.g. hyaluronidase (streptococci), coagulase (staphylococci) and of toxins, e.g. leucocidins, enterotoxins.

### Factors influencing the course of infection

Once infection has occurred, important defence mechanisms operate:

1. **Inflammation** in the **acute** local reaction (see p. 44) tends to limit the spread of organisms. In some important diseases, there is no acute local inflammatory response at the site of entry, e.g. brucellosis (undulant fever) and many virus infections. In the *chronic* inflammatory reaction (see p. 54), the formation of fibrous tissue also helps to localise infection.
2. **Phagocytosis** (see p. 49). *Note*: some organisms may survive or multiply within phagocytes – usually associated with chronic infection. Good examples are tuberculosis, brucellosis, leprosy.
3. **Immune response**
  (a) *Humoral antibody* reactions, e.g. agglutination, opsonisation, lysis via complement – especially important in *bacterial* infections.
  (b) *Cellular immunity* reactions, e.g. cytotoxic T cells, especially important in viral infections.
4. **Cytokines** – signalling molecules that regulate the immune response to pathogens.

### Examples of failure of protective and defence mechanisms

1. **In skin** – direct breach by wounding and burns; softening of the surface by exposure to water and sweat, or due to skin disorders.
2. **In the respiratory tract** – inhibition of ciliary movement by nicotine in smokers potentiates infection.
3. **In the stomach** – in achlorhydria (no hydrochloric acid) organisms flourish in the stomach.
4. **When secretions are prevented from flowing freely** by narrowing of natural passages, bacterial growth in the 'stagnant' fluid is potentiated (e.g. enlarged prostate urethral obstruction, urinary infection).
5. **When commensal growth is impaired** by antibiotic treatment, pathogenic bacteria may colonise the 'vacant site'.

# INFECTION

6. **Deficiency of the immunological system**
   (a) Natural deficiency due to hereditary defect, e.g. X-linked agammaglobulinaemia.
   (b) Acquired due to administration of drugs in treatment of disease, e.g. steroids, cytotoxic drugs or specific virus infection, e.g. HIV causing AIDS.
7. **Deficiency of phagocytosis** – especially polymorphs (either low numbers or deficient function – see p. 49).
8. **In debilitating diseases** such as diabetes, chronic failure and nutritional deficiency.
9. **Genetic susceptibility** – may be a factor in some infections.

## Mechanisms by which disease is produced

The local reaction to infections is usually INFLAMMATORY and is evoked by cellular damage and death. The detailed mechanisms are different in bacteria and viruses.

## BACTERIA

1. **Production of toxins (poisons)**

| EXOTOXINS | ENDOTOXINS |
|---|---|
| Secreted by living bacteria | Integral part of bacterial cell wall<br>Released on death of organism (usually Gram-negative) |
| Simple proteins | Lipid polysaccharide (LPS) complexes<br>TSST1 – superantigen produced by *Staphylococcus aureus* causing toxic shock syndrome |
| Neutralised by specific antibody (antitoxin) | Do not stimulate antibody production |
| Many actions<br>　–Enzymes, e.g. *S. aureus* protease<br>　–Action on intracellular signalling, e.g. *Vibrio cholerae*<br>　–Neurotoxins, e.g. *Clostridium botulinum*<br>　–Superantigens, e.g. *Streptococcus pyogenes* | Beneficial effects: In low dose, stimulates protective immunity<br>Harmful effects: In high dose, ENDOTOXIC SHOCK – due to massive release of cytokines with activation of coagulation, fibrinolytic and complement cascades<br>LPS binds cell surface receptor CD14 and is delivered to the pattern recognition receptor TLR4 – Toll-like receptor 4. This starts intracellular signalling cascade |

2. **Hypersensitivity reaction causing tissue injury**
   This is a form of the immune response in which reaction between the bacterial protein and sensitised lymphocytes initiates the inflammatory reaction (see p. 143).
3. **Tissue invasion: lymphatic spread and invasion of blood stream**

# SEPSIS

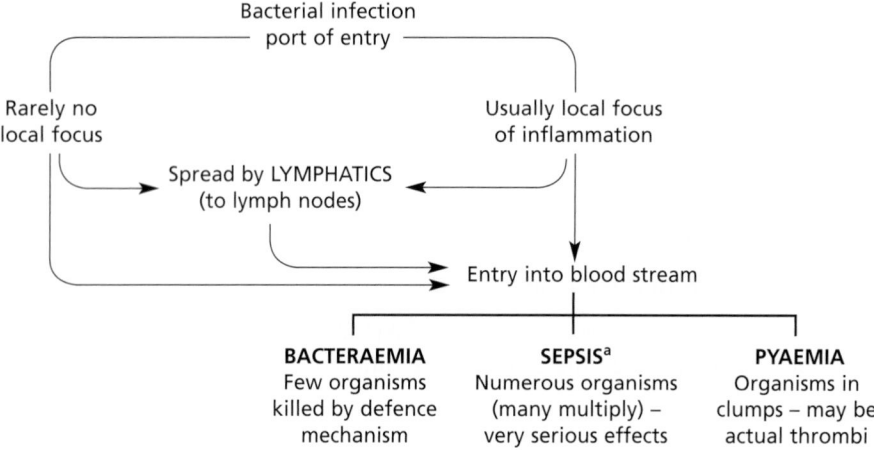

<sup>a</sup>Sepsis is a very serious condition in which there is a whole-body inflammatory state (systemic inflammatory response syndrome) in the presence of infection.

Mortality is between 20% and 50%, even with modern medical treatment. It commonly occurs in response to LPS in the wall of Gram-negative bacteria.

**Mechanisms**

LPS triggers innate immunity via TLR4. With infection disseminated via the bloodstream there is widespread activation of phagocytes.

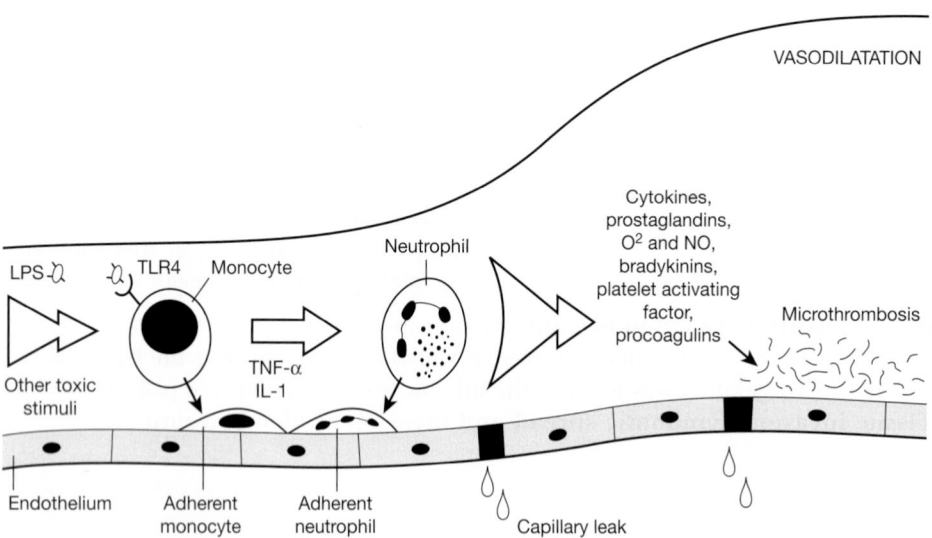

The initial stimulus triggers production of proinflammatory cytokines, and monocytes and neutrophils adhere to endothelium. Activated macrophages, neutrophils and endothelial cells release secondary inflammatory mediators. This release of proinflammatory cytokines is known as a CYTOKINE STORM. Procoagulants produced by endothelial cells may trigger microthrombosis and if widespread this is known as DISSEMINATED INTRAVASCULAR COAGULATION.

# BACTERAEMIA

(a) Occurs commonly: usually of no serious significance.
(b) An integral part of some infections, e.g. typhoid fever.

**Important special cases**

1. *Dental extraction*

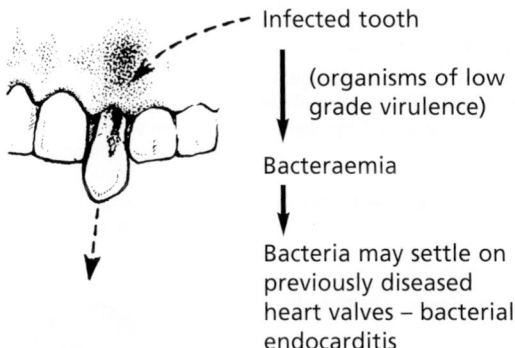

Infected tooth

↓ (organisms of low grade virulence)

Bacteraemia

↓

Bacteria may settle on previously diseased heart valves – bacterial endocarditis

2. *Established bacterial endocarditis*

Mitral valve

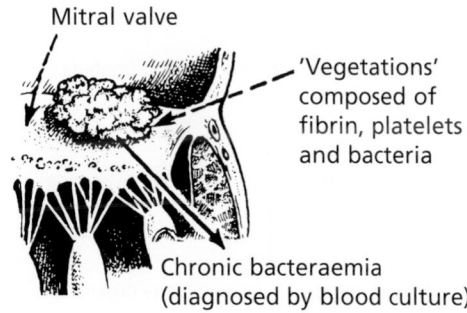

'Vegetations' composed of fibrin, platelets and bacteria

Chronic bacteraemia (diagnosed by blood culture)

# PYAEMIA

Pyaemia occurs when pathogenic organisms escape into the bloodstream in the form of small aggregates – micro-emboli. This results in either:

| **PYAEMIC ABSCESSES** | **SEPTIC INFARCTION** |
|---|---|

Septic focus – usually staphylococcal

↓

Thrombosis of venules incorporating bacteria

↓

Showers of micro-emboli

↓

Multiple micro-absesses in many organs

The lesions are larger and less numerous than pyaemic absesses

They are associated with

(a) Septic thrombosis of larger veins (suppurative thrombophlebitis)
e.g. Leg veins → Embolism → Infarction with suppuration in lungs

Portal vein → Embolism → Infarction with suppuration in lungs

(b) Acute infective endocarditis

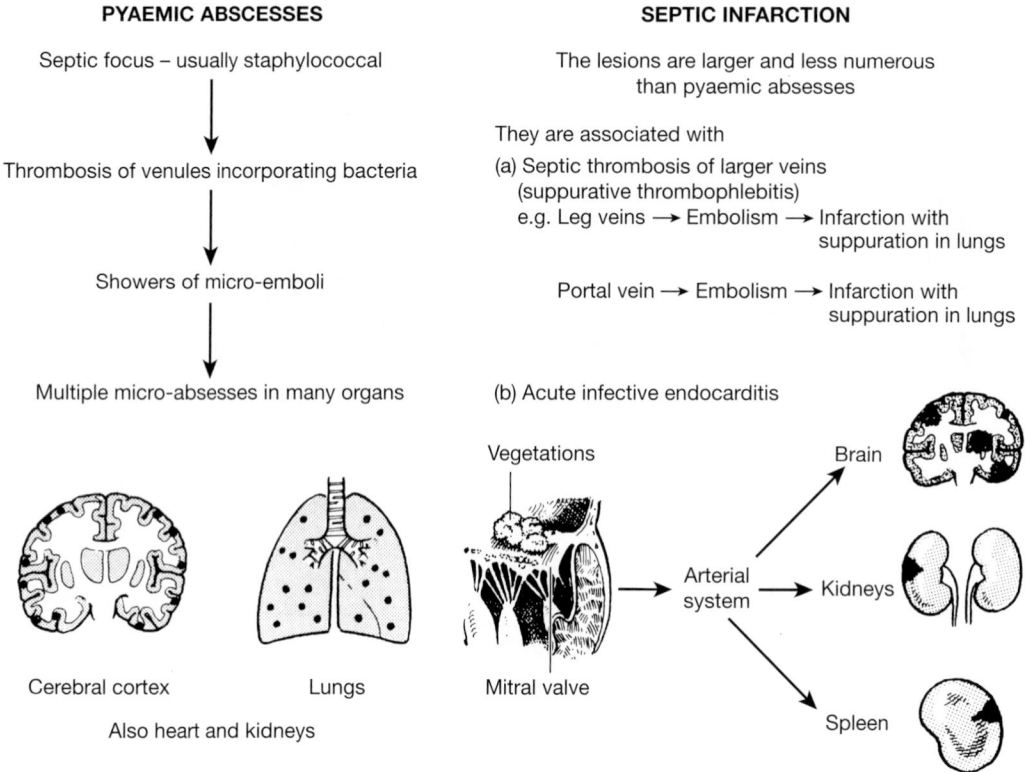

Cerebral cortex          Lungs

Also heart and kidneys

Vegetations

Mitral valve

Arterial system

Brain

Kidneys

Spleen

# ACUTE BACTERIAL INFECTION

## PYOGENIC BACTERIA

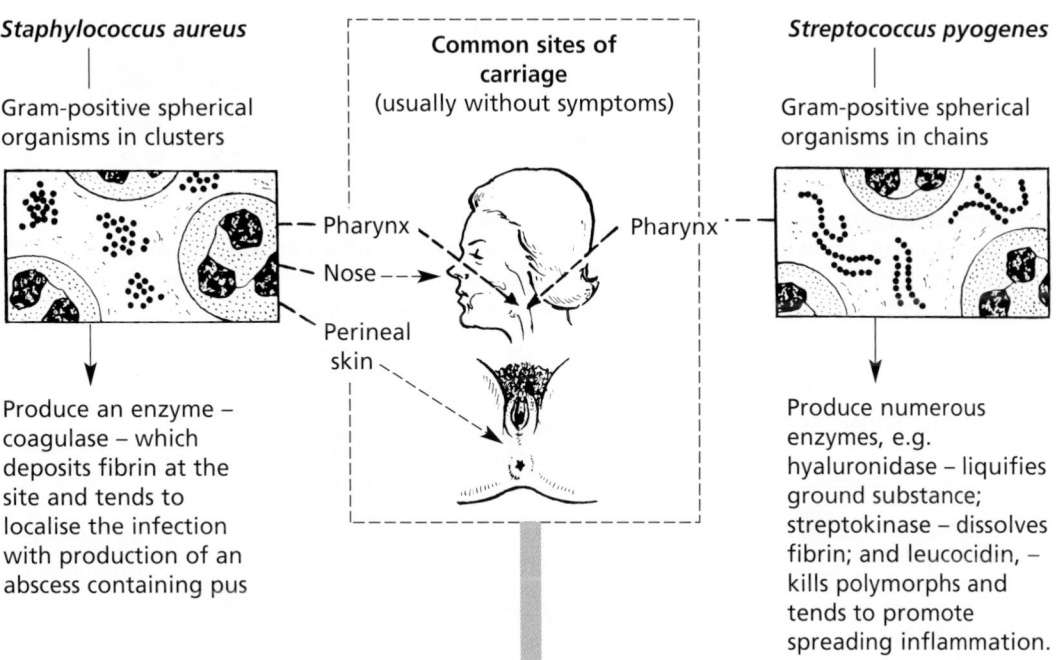

*Staphylococcus aureus*

Gram-positive spherical organisms in clusters

Produce an enzyme – coagulase – which deposits fibrin at the site and tends to localise the infection with production of an abscess containing pus

**Common sites of carriage**
(usually without symptoms)

– Pharynx

– Nose

Perineal skin

Pharynx

*Streptococcus pyogenes*

Gram-positive spherical organisms in chains

Produce numerous enzymes, e.g. hyaluronidase – liquifies ground substance; streptokinase – dissolves fibrin; and leucocidin, – kills polymorphs and tends to promote spreading inflammation.

*Note:* In hospitals staphylococci are becoming increasingly resistant to multiple antibiotics (MRSA = methicillin resistant *Staphylococcus aureus*).

---

### Lesions produced

*Skin infections* – pustules, oils, carbuncles
*Wound infection*
*Staphylococcal broncho-pneumonia* may be a serious complication in epidemic influenza
Exotoxin production → food poisoning: toxic shock syndrome

*Skin infections* – impetigo, erysipelas, cellulitis
*Wound infection*
*TONSILLITIS* and pharyngitis
Exotoxin production
↓
The skin rash of scarlet fever

---

### GENERAL BLOOD SPREAD

*PYAEMIA*
OSTEOMYELITIS – acute inflammation of long bones – particularly in children

*SEPSIS*

*Note*: Rheumatic fever and acute glomerulonephritis are complications of streptococcal infection in which the heart and kidneys are damaged. This is caused by disturbance in the immune mechanisms (Type III hypersensitivity reaction) and is not due to the actual presence of streptococci in the heart and kidneys.

# ACUTE BACTERIAL INFECTION

**Neisseria**

**Meningococcus**          **Gonococcus**

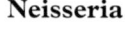

Both are **Gram-negative intracellular** diplococci

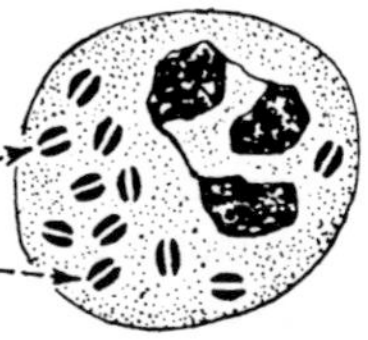

*Carried* in nasopharynx.
*Causes* **purulent** *meningitis*
and, in children, occasionally
a fatal septicaemia.

Skin rash          Massive adrenal
                   haemorrhage

(Waterhouse-Friderichsen syndrome)

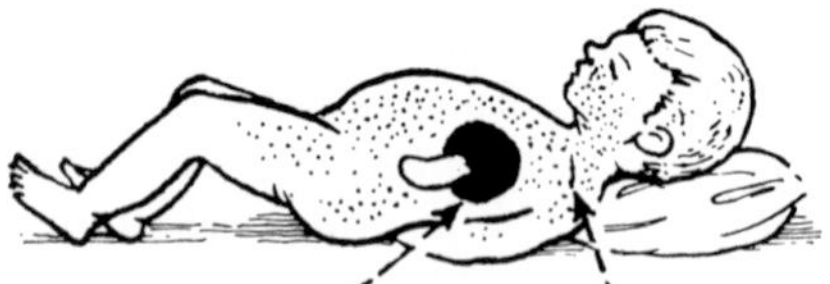

Massive adrenal          Purpuric
haemorrhage              skin rash

*Carried* in genital mucous membrane.
*Causes* purulent inflammation of urethra in
male and of uterine cervix in the female with
spread to adjacent organs.

**Male**

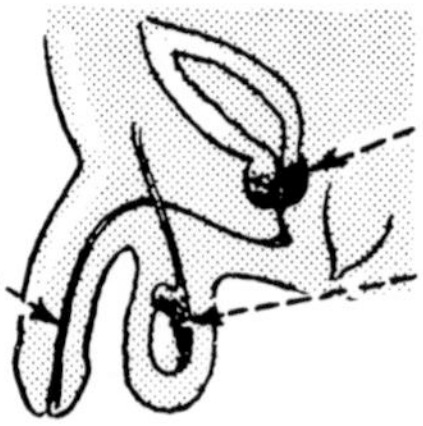

Anterior
urethritis

Prostatitis

Epididymitis

**Female**

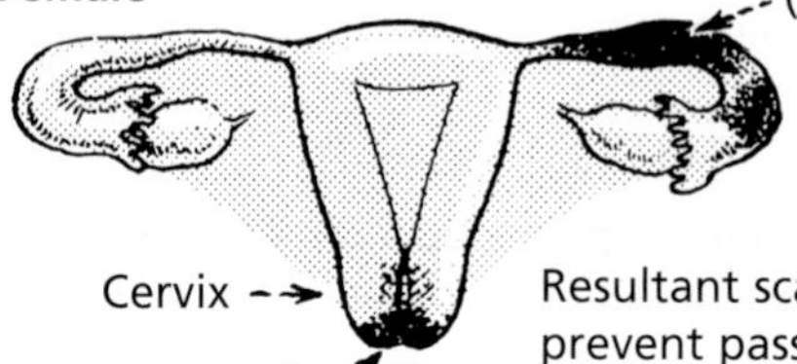

Acute salpingitis
(inflammation
of fallopian
tubes)

Cervix

Gonococcal
infection

Resultant scarring may
prevent passage of ovum
to uterus → sterility

## Gram-negative bacilli

These are usually commensals in the alimentary tract and include facultative and obligatory anaerobes.

'Coliform' organisms can cause local inflammation in the alimentary tract, the urinary tract and wound infections.

In addition, ENDOTOXINS liberated in the blood stream cause severe sepsis with SHOCK (p. 104).

### FOOD POISONING

*Escherichia coli 0157*, a commensal in cattle, is a human pathogen – production of a powerful *verocytotoxin* is associated with *haemolytic uraemic syndrome* (see p. 512) and may cause death in the very young and elderly.

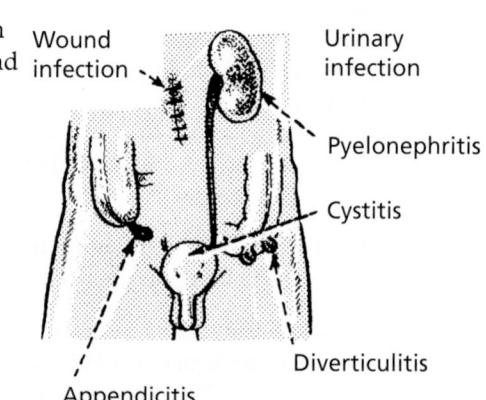

Wound
infection

Urinary
infection

Pyelonephritis

Cystitis

Appendicitis

Diverticulitis

## ACUTE BACTERIAL INFECTION

### GANGRENE

Gangrene is a complication of NECROSIS in which bacterial infection is superimposed. There are three main types:

1. **Dry gangrene**

   This occurs in the toes and feet of elderly people or diabetics suffering from gradual arterial occlusion. The putrefactive process spreads slowly until it reaches the part where the blood supply is adequate. Small numbers of organisms are present.

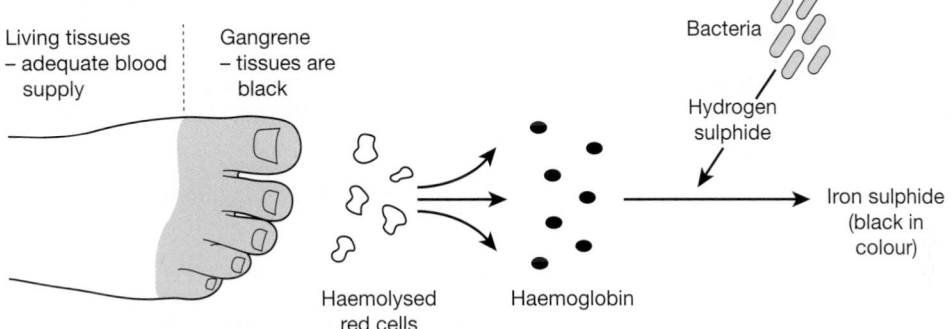

Living tissues – adequate blood supply

Gangrene – tissues are black

Bacteria

Hydrogen sulphide

Iron sulphide (black in colour)

Haemolysed red cells

Haemoglobin

2. **Wet gangrene**

   The tissues are moist at the start of the process due to venous congestion or oedema, e.g. strangulation of viscera. The disease spreads rapidly and may be associated with sepsis. Tissue discolouration occurs by the same mechanism as dry gangrene.

3. **Gas gangrene**

   Dry and wet gangrene are associated with mixed bacterial infection. Gas gangrene is caused by exotoxin-producing bacteria of the CLOSTRIDIA group – ANAEROBIC sporulating Gram-positive bacilli (*Clostridium perfringens* most common). These organisms, found in soil, can enter a wound and proliferate in necrotic tissue with formation of gas bubbles. Spread is rapid with sepsis syndrome. Historically it was a serious complication of war wounds.

### Special types of gangrene

Necrotising fasciitis – this infection spreads along fascial planes within subcutaneous tissue. The infection may be polymicrobial or due to a single organism, commonly group A streptococcus or, in hospitals, MRSA.

Fournier gangrene – this is a form of necrotising fasciitis affecting the male genitals particularly in diabetics.

# ACUTE BACTERIAL INFECTION

### TETANUS

This organism itself does not cause local tissue damage. The effects are due to a powerful ENDOTOXIN secreted by the organism. This is in contrast to the usual bacterial diseases where tissue damage is important and is due to the local bacterial action.

The infecting organism, *Clostridium tetani*, a STRICT ANAEROBE, is a Gram-positive rod. Often the presence of a terminal spore gives a characteristic drumstick appearance. The highly resistant spores are widespread in the environment due to contamination by animal faeces.

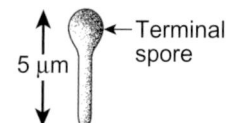

### Method of infection

Contamination of wounds in which there are anaerobic conditions, e.g. deep-penetrating wounds and wounds with severe soft tissue damage (road traffic accidents and battle casualties), and only very occasionally trivial thorn punctures.

In developing communities the umbilical stump of the newborn may be infected by faecal material.

### Effects

The exotoxin is highly potent and causes paroxysmal muscular spasm, which becomes progressively more severe and was fatal in many cases; modern therapy including muscle relaxation and ventilation has improved the prognosis dramatically.

### Course

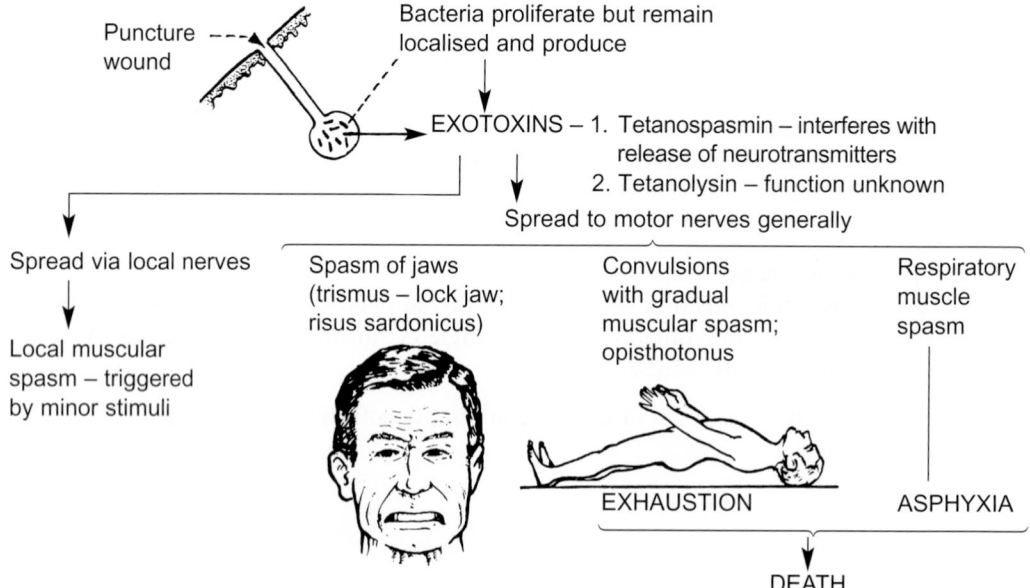

# ACUTE BACTERIAL INFECTION

## Immunity

- Active immunisation by **TOXOID** – prophylactic.
- Passive immunisation by **ANTITOXIN** – therapeutic (only effective before toxin is fixed to nerve tissues).

Other important bacteria-producing toxins are *C. botulinum* (botulism), *V. cholerae* (cholera), *Corynebacterium diphtheriae* (diphtheria).

# CHRONIC BACTERIAL INFECTION (GRANULOMAS)

In these infections chronic inflammation is the basic mechanism (see p. 54). The detailed evolution of the inflammatory reaction is modified by several factors of which the immune response of the host is important (see p. 129).

## TUBERCULOSIS

Tuberculosis is caused by the *Mycobacterium tuberculosis* (tubercle bacillus, TB), an organism which has a resistant waxy component in its structure and is acid and alcohol-fast (i.e. resists bleaching with strong acid and alcohol after being stained red with fuchsin). The highest incidence of tuberculosis is in Southern Asia and sub-Saharan Africa. The disease rapidly declined in Western Europe and North America after World War II due to (a) improved nutrition and hygiene, (b) *BCG (Bacillus Calmette Guérin)* immunisation and (c) chemotherapy (*note*: drug resistance is becoming an increasing problem). At risk groups include the elderly, the immunosuppressed (esp. HIV infection) and alcoholics. The disease remains prevalent in developing countries.

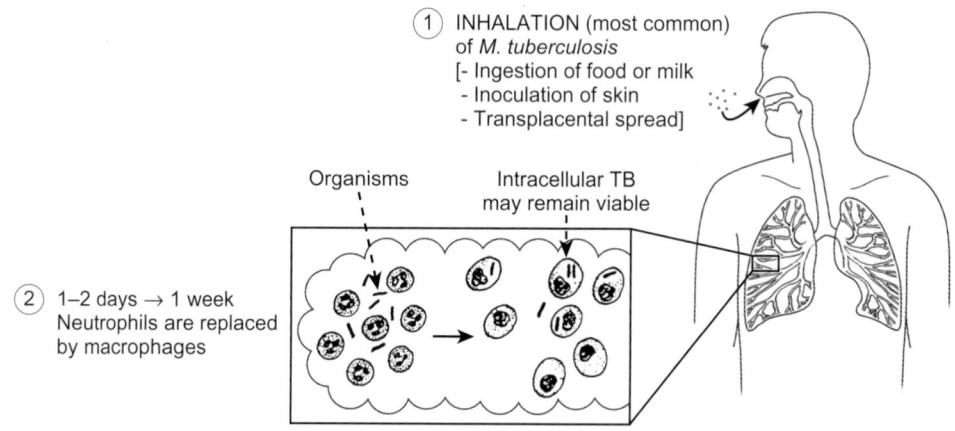

① INHALATION (most common) of *M. tuberculosis* [- Ingestion of food or milk - Inoculation of skin - Transplacental spread]

Organisms

Intracellular TB may remain viable

② 1–2 days → 1 week Neutrophils are replaced by macrophages

③ 2–3 weeks
Cellular immune response (Type IV hypersensitivity p. 145) to tuberculous cell wall constituents

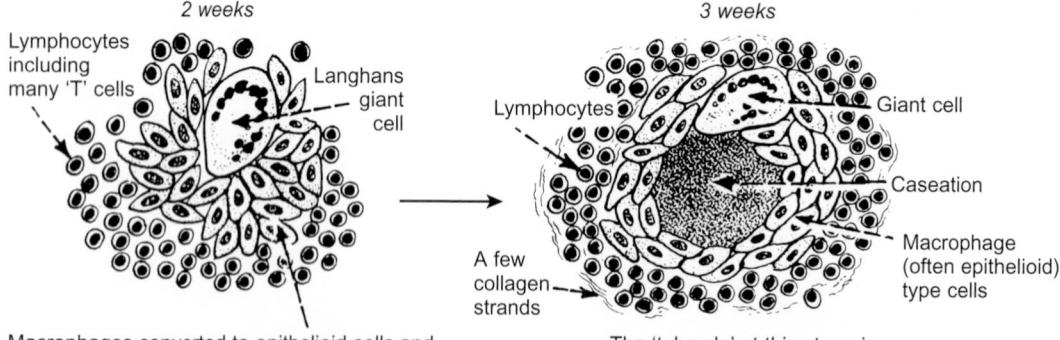

*2 weeks*

Lymphocytes including many 'T' cells

Langhans giant cell

*3 weeks*

Lymphocytes

Giant cell

Caseation

Macrophage (often epithelioid) type cells

A few collagen strands

Macrophages converted to epithelioid cells and arranged around central focus. KILLING of TB begins.

The 'tubercle' at this stage is just visible to the naked eye.

④ Spread and confluence of these proliferative granulomatous lesions are the basic mechanism in active progressive disease.

# CHRONIC BACTERIAL INFECTION (GRANULOMAS)

## OTHER MYCOBACTERIAL INFECTIONS

Mycobacteria other than tubercle sometimes infect humans. They are commonly present in soil and water and are less virulent than *M. tuberculosis*. Most exposures do not produce disease unless there is a defect in local or systemic host defences.

*M. avium* and *M. intracellulare* – these are closely related and are often grouped together as *M. avium-intracellulare* (MAI) – they may cause pneumonia, lymphadenitis or disseminated disease in immunosuppressed patients.

*M. kansasii* – this may cause a chronic cervical lymphadenitis with cutaneous fistulas and scarring in children.

*M. marinum* – this can cause a cutaneous granulomatous ulcerating lesion which can be contracted from contaminated swimming pools or from cleaning an aquarium (swimming pool granuloma).

## ACTINOMYCOSIS

Actinomycosis is a localised but gradually spreading chronic suppuration affecting the lower jaw, the ileocaecal region of the bowel, the female genital tract and occasionally the lung.

The organism – *Actinomyces israelii* – widespread in nature, is a Gram-positive, branching, filamentous anaerobe found around the teeth and in the pharyngeal crypts. In the tissues, it forms yellow, densely felted together spherical colonies just visible to the naked eye; the pus is seen to contain 'sulphur granules'.

**Sites of infection**

**Abscess formation**

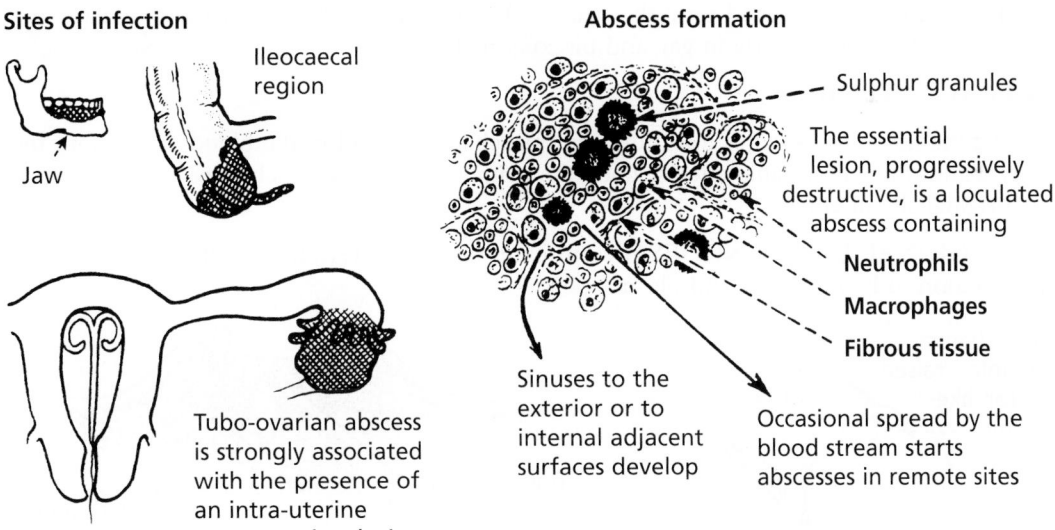

Ileocaecal region

Jaw

Tubo-ovarian abscess is strongly associated with the presence of an intra-uterine contraceptive device

Sinuses to the exterior or to internal adjacent surfaces develop

Sulphur granules

The essential lesion, progressively destructive, is a loculated abscess containing

**Neutrophils**

**Macrophages**

**Fibrous tissue**

Occasional spread by the blood stream starts abscesses in remote sites

# CHRONIC BACTERIAL INFECTION (GRANULOMAS)

### LEPROSY

This slowly progressive disease which causes serious effects by damage to peripheral nerves is still widespread in the tropics and subtropics. The infection is acquired by close, prolonged contact and is due to *M. leprae*, a slender acid and alcohol-fast bacillus. The disease presents in two contrasting extreme forms and with cases of intermediate type.

1. **Lepromatous leprosy**
   Disfiguring nodularity of the skin – 'leonine facies'.
   Peripheral nerves affected late.
   The lesions contain lymphocytes, plasma cells and macrophages – filled with organisms.
   Organisms + + + in tissues.

2. **Tuberculoid leprosy**
   Focal areas of skin pallor and anaesthesia due to early involvement of nerves.
   Basic lesion is a follicular granuloma (tubercle) not unlike the true tubercle follicle.
   Organisms are scanty.

These differences are due in the main to differences in the immune reaction of the host.

A defective Th1 response or dominant Th2 response.

A predominant Th1 response with IL-2 and IFN-γ production.

### SYPHILIS

This is a sexually transmitted disease caused by a spirochaete (*Treponema pallidum*). It has a close set spiral structure that can be demonstrated by dark ground illumination, silver staining of immunofluorescence and immunohistochemistry in tissue sections. The incidence of syphilis declined until the late 1990s but there has been a marked increase in cases since 2001 particularly in gay and bisexual males.

### PRIMARY SYPHILIS

During the first 3 weeks after infection, the spirochaetes spread in the blood throughout the body without any noticeable effects. Then the primary lesion – hard chancre – appears at the original site of entry.

The INGUINAL LYMPH NODES present clinically as painless, firm swellings due to proliferation of lymphocytes and plasma cells.

Hard chancre – a painless raised button-like nodule

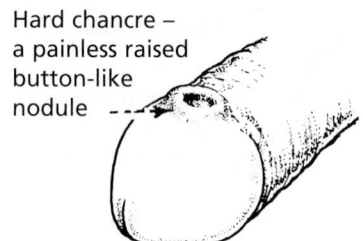

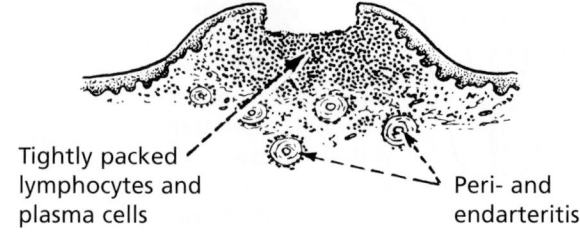

Tightly packed lymphocytes and plasma cells

Peri- and endarteritis

Diagnosis is by examination under dark ground illumination of serum taken from ulcer.

*Note:* No neutrophils – this is not an abscess. There is minimal tissue destruction and healing occurs without scarring.

# CHRONIC BACTERIAL INFECTION (GRANULOMAS)

## SECONDARY SYPHILIS

During the next 2 or 3 months, the spread of the organisms throughout the body causes secondary stage effects. These are a widespread rash (pox) of varying appearance, ulceration of mucous membranes, generalised lymphadenopathy and damage to various individual organs and tissues. There are constitutional effects – particularly fever and anaemia.

The essential pathology is the presence of very numerous spirochaetes accompanied by focal infiltration of lymphocytes, plasma cells and macrophages with mild arteritis. Infectivity is very high. Tissue destruction is minimal and healing occurs without scarring. A latent stage of long duration is followed in 35% of cases by tertiary syphilis.

## TERTIARY (LATE) SYPHILIS

The lesions, which may occur at any time for many years after the healing of the secondary phase, offer striking contrasts. This stage is characterised mainly by local destructive lesions, the result of cellular immunity (T cells) causing necrosis of tissue. The main forms are:

1. **Gumma**
   This is a localised area of necrosis which may affect large parts of any organ or tissue but particularly bones, testis and liver.
2. **Syphilitic aortitis**
   The arch and thoracic aorta is damaged with weakening of the media: this leads to ANEURYSM formation (see p. 256), which causes serious local pressure effects and may also rupture with severe haemorrhage.
3. **Neurological syphilis**
   (a) **Meningovascular** – mainly affects the meningeal blood vessels and causes neurological impairment secondarily.
   (b) **Parenchymatous**

(i) General paralysis of the insane – severe destruction of cerebral tissue

(ii) Tabes dorsalis – the damage specifically affecting the posterior roots and columns of spinal cord – is associated with characteristic clinical symptoms due to loss of proprioceptive sensation in the legs

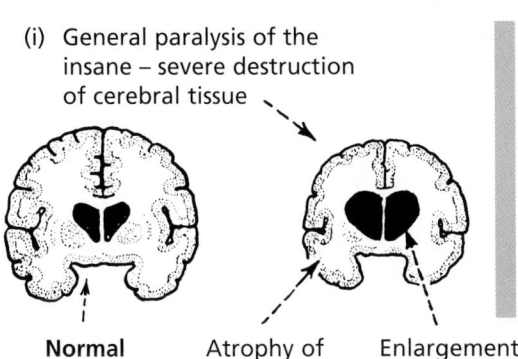

**Normal**  Atrophy of convolutions  Enlargement of ventricles

# CHRONIC BACTERIAL INFECTION (GRANULOMAS)

## CONGENITAL SYPHILIS

Transplacental infection of the fetus occurs with the following possible consequences:

(a) Abortion or stillbirth – many organs damaged.
(b) Birth of marasmic infant – organ and tissue damage at birth and in later childhood.

## DIAGNOSIS OF SYPHILIS

1. **Demonstration of organisms**
   In primary syphilis and early secondary syphilis, organisms may be detected in smears from lesions by dark-ground microscopy or in tissue sections using immunohistochemical staining with appropriate antibodies.
2. **Serological tests**
   (a) *Non-treponemal tests*
       These tests detect antibodies that react to a cardiolipin-cholesterol-lecithin antigen in the serum of infected patients. False positives occur in 1–2%. The outdated Venereal Diseases Reference Laboratory (VDRL) has been replaced by the rapid plasma reagin (RPR) test. Results are quantitative and can be negative with latent infection.
   (b) *Treponemal tests*
       Specific anti-treponemal antibodies are detected to treponemal antigens. These tests include *Treponema pallidum* enzyme immunoassay (EIA), *T. pallidum* particle agglutination (TPPA), *T. pallidum* haemagglutination assay (TPHA) and *T. pallidum* IgG or IgM immunoblot. EIA and TPPA are most commonly used. The results remain positive even after treatment.

## OTHER SPIROCHAETE INFECTIONS

*Borrelia burgdorferi* is transmitted to humans by deer tick bites and causes Lyme disease – symptoms include a rash, arthralgia and occasionally meningitis.

# VIRUS INFECTIONS

## VIRUS INFECTIONS

Viruses are obligate intracellular pathogens that can replicate only by utilising the resources of the infected cell. The virus particle, or *virion*, consists of a central core of genetic material, either ribonucleic acid (RNA) or DNA, surrounded by a protein coat (*capsid*). Retroviruses are an important subgroup of RNA viruses. In addition, there may be a membranous *envelope* containing host and viral lipids.

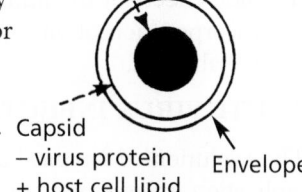

Central core DNA or RNA

Capsid
– virus protein
+ host cell lipid

Envelope

The diagram shows how viruses use the host cell for replication, at the same time causing cell death.

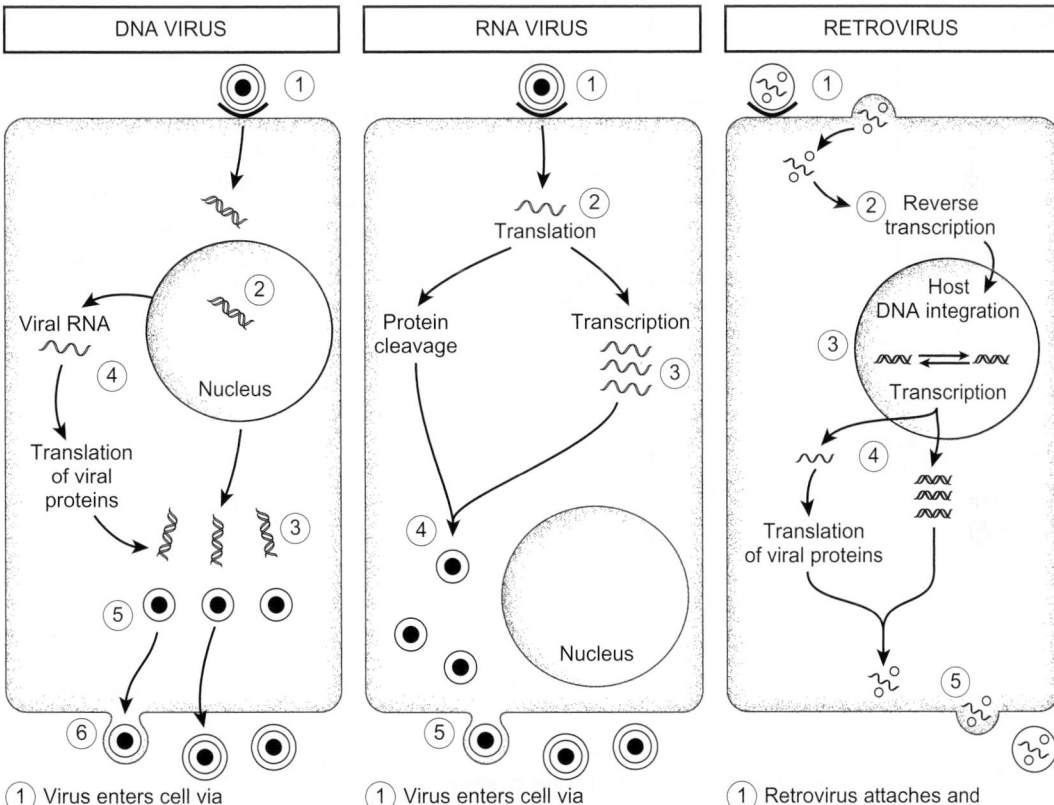

| DNA VIRUS | RNA VIRUS | RETROVIRUS |
|---|---|---|

① Virus enters cell via surface receptor

② Viral DNA enters nucleus

③ Multiple copies of viral DNA produced

④ Viral RNA translated to viral proteins

⑤ Viral DNA packaged with viral proteins to form virus particles

⑥ Virus particles released by budding from cell membrane

① Virus enters cell via surface receptor

② Viral RNA translated to viral proteins

③ Transcription of viral RNA to produce multiple copies

④ Viral RNA packaged with viral proteins to form virus particles

⑤ Virus particles released by budding from cell membrane

① Retrovirus attaches and penetrates cell membrane

② Retrovirus uncoated and reverse transcription of viral RNA to produce dsDNA

③ Viral DNA integrated into host DNA in nucleus - provirus

④ Transcription of provirus to produce RNA for retrovirus genome and viral protein

⑤ Retrovirus leaves cell acquiring envelope on exit

# VIRUS INFECTIONS

In addition to this direct cytopathic effect of the virus, damage to host may be caused by:

(i)   Side effects of the immune response.
(ii)  Incorporation of virus into the cell genome severely affecting the intracellular metabolism.

### ACUTE VIRUS INFECTION

The evolution of a typical acute virus infection can be understood in terms of virus replication, release and spread within the body, and of the host's reaction.

### Typical evolution

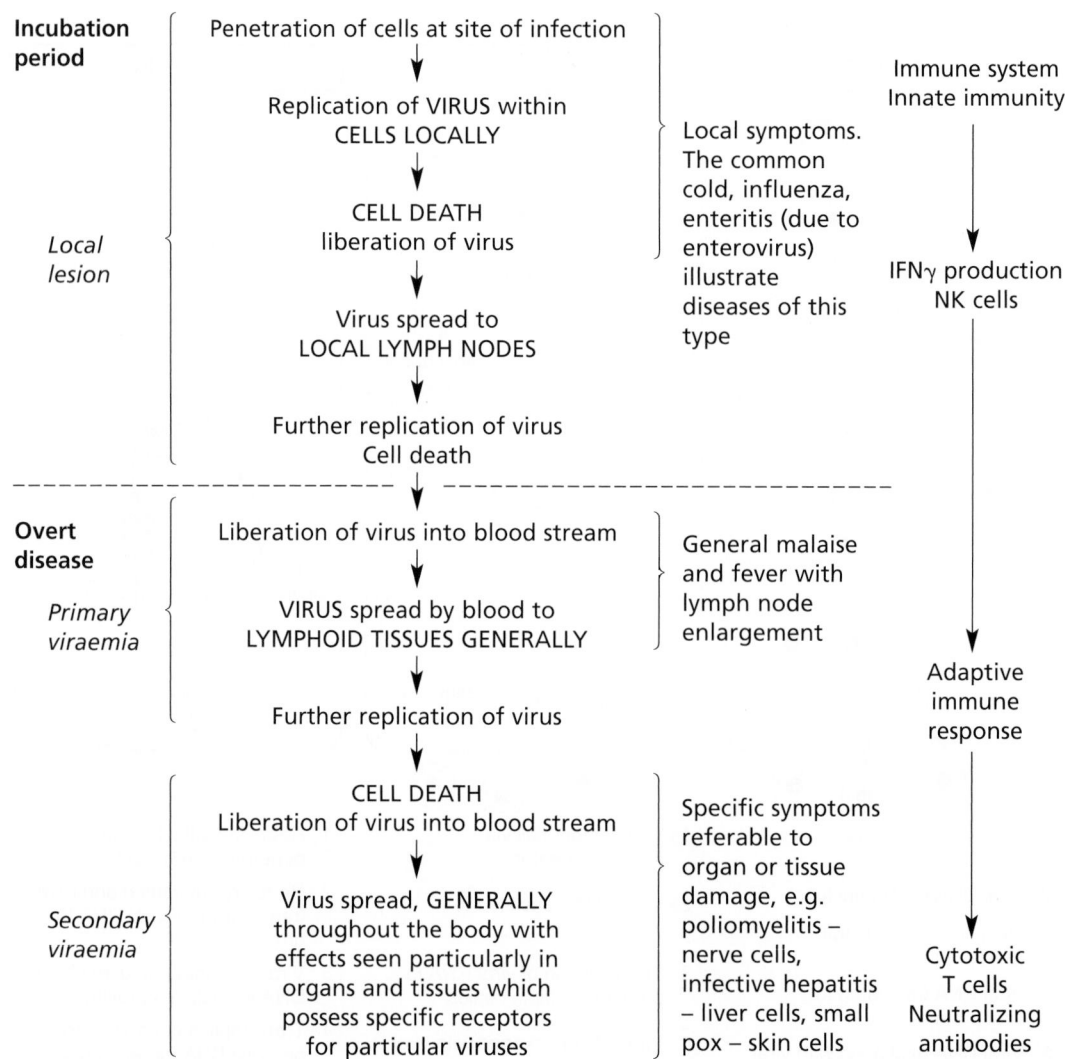

# VIRUS INFECTIONS

This typical evolution is produced by successive waves of virus. However, the great majority of virus infections are clinically latent or mild because virus replication and spread are prevented by the body's defence mechanisms. Severe overt disease occurs when there is an especially virulent virus or when the body's resistance is inadequate, especially in a primary infection.

Not all virus infections cause disease in this way; two important variations are:

1. LATENT and     2. ONCOGENIC

**LATENT VIRUS INFECTION**

A good example is the common 'cold sore' of the lips and face caused by the **Herpes simplex** virus (an enveloped DNA virus).

Initial infection                                                           Reactivation

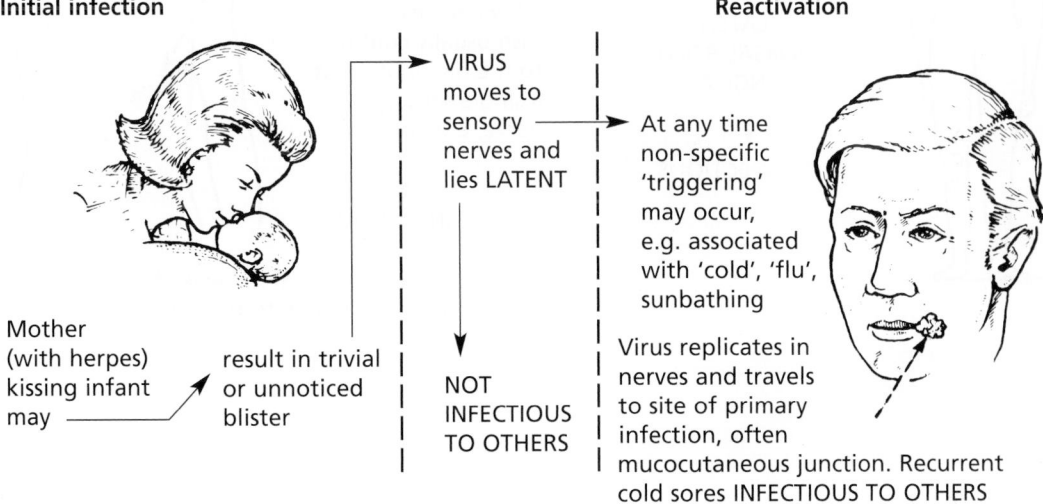

VIRUS moves to sensory nerves and lies LATENT

At any time non-specific 'triggering' may occur, e.g. associated with 'cold', 'flu', sunbathing

Mother (with herpes) kissing infant may → result in trivial or unnoticed blister

NOT INFECTIOUS TO OTHERS

Virus replicates in nerves and travels to site of primary infection, often mucocutaneous junction. Recurrent cold sores INFECTIOUS TO OTHERS

# VIRUS INFECTIONS

Another example is **Herpes zoster (shingles).**

This is a painful affection of segmental sensory nerves and root ganglia due to infection by CHICKEN POX VIRUS **Varicella.**

**Initial infection in childhood**

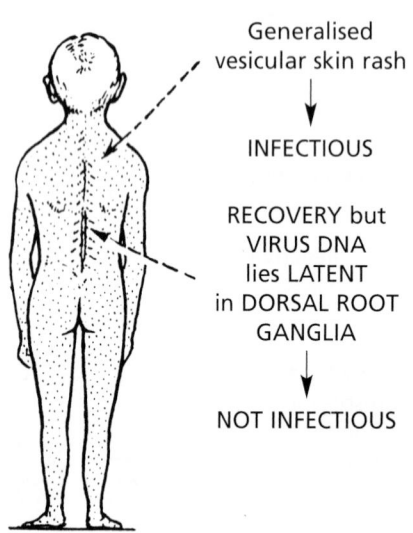

Generalised
vesicular skin rash

↓

INFECTIOUS

RECOVERY but
VIRUS DNA
lies LATENT
in DORSAL ROOT
GANGLIA

↓

NOT INFECTIOUS

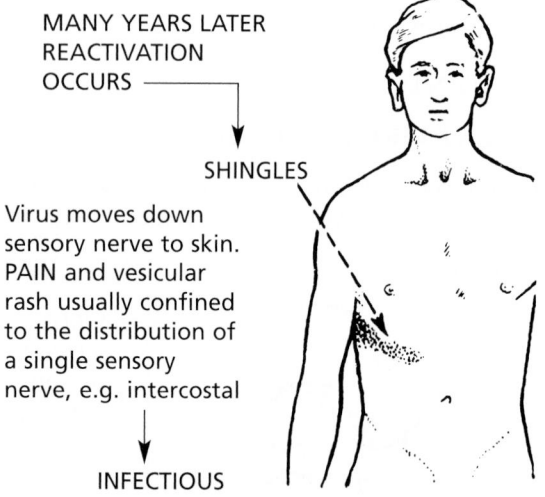

MANY YEARS LATER
REACTIVATION
OCCURS

SHINGLES

Virus moves down
sensory nerve to skin.
PAIN and vesicular
rash usually confined
to the distribution of
a single sensory
nerve, e.g. intercostal

↓

INFECTIOUS

If the trigeminal nerve is affected
serious damage to the eye may result.

# VIRUS INFECTIONS

## ONCOGENIC VIRUS INFECTION

Several DNA viruses and retroviruses of the RNA family can give rise to tumours (see also p. 195).

Examples include the following:

(a) Human papilloma virus (HPV) – HPV-16 and 18, strains of the common wart virus, are the primary cause of cervical carcinoma. Young girls are now vaccinated against HPV to reduce the incidence of cervical cancer.

(b) Hepatitis virus – both hepatitis B and C viruses are firmly associated with hepatocellular carcinoma, whether sufferers develop cirrhosis or not.

(c) Epstein–Barr virus – a member of the herpes group causes glandular fever (infectious mononucleosis – a non-malignant condition) in young adults in Western societies. This virus is also closely associated with Burkitt lymphoma (a malignant tumour) found in young Africans living in malarial areas, with nasopharyngeal carcinoma, particularly in the Far East, with Hodgkin disease and with post-transplant lymphoma.

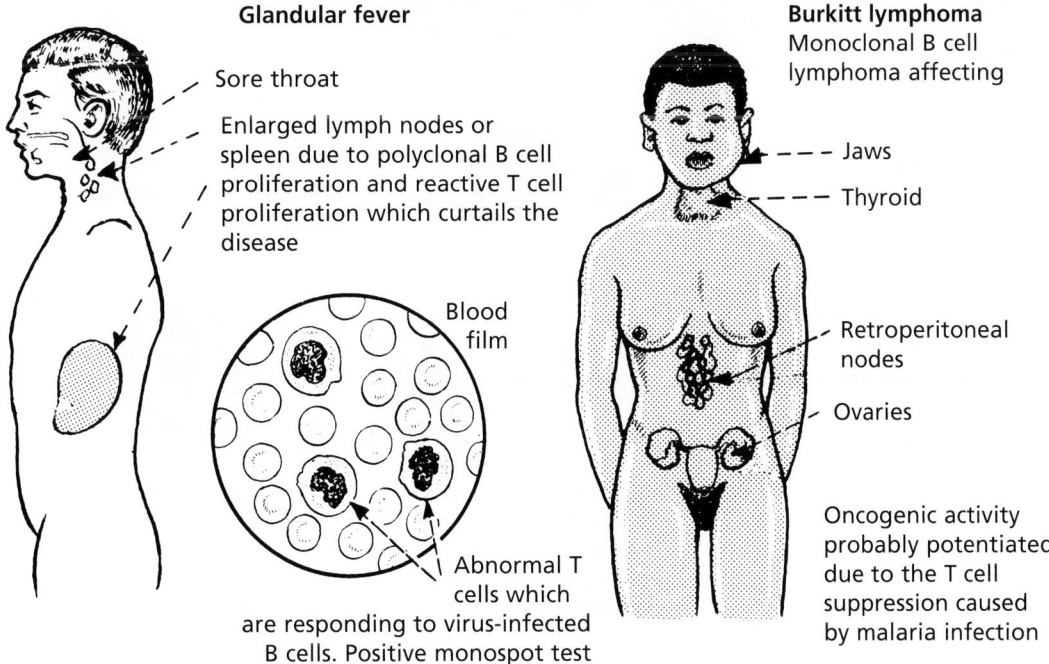

**Glandular fever**

Sore throat

Enlarged lymph nodes or spleen due to polyclonal B cell proliferation and reactive T cell proliferation which curtails the disease

Blood film

Abnormal T cells which are responding to virus-infected B cells. Positive monospot test

**Burkitt lymphoma**
Monoclonal B cell lymphoma affecting

Jaws

Thyroid

Retroperitoneal nodes

Ovaries

Oncogenic activity probably potentiated due to the T cell suppression caused by malaria infection

(d) Retroviruses – T cell leukaemias are caused by specific retroviruses, i.e. human T cell leukaemia-lymphoma virus (HTLV). HTLV-1 is endemic in Japan, the West Indies and central belts of Africa.

The mechanisms by which viruses cause tumours are illustrated on page 195.

# HOST/VIRUS INTERACTION

**The reactions occurring in the host** are important.

1. **Changes in the infected cells**

(a) Cell degeneration (with loss of function) leading to cell death.

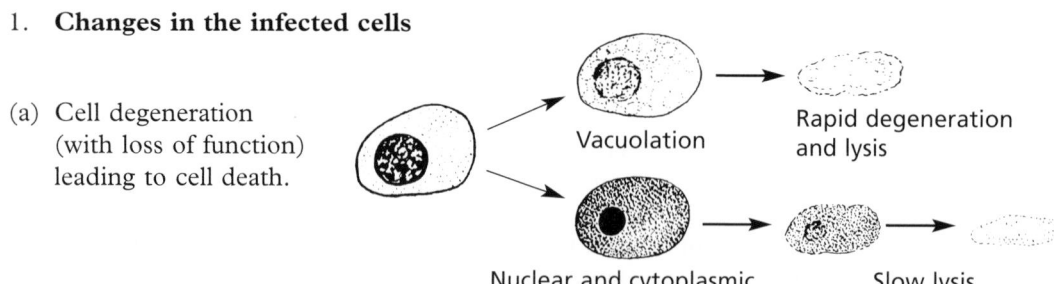

Vacuolation

Rapid degeneration and lysis

Nuclear and cytoplasmic condensation

Slow lysis

(b) Fusion of adjacent infected cells – giant cell formation, e.g. the Warthin-Finkeldy cell of measles.

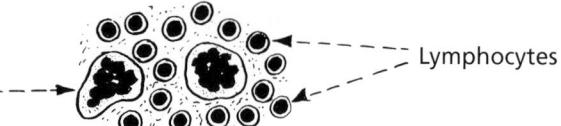

Lymphocytes

(c) Cell proliferation, e.g. common wart of HPV infection.

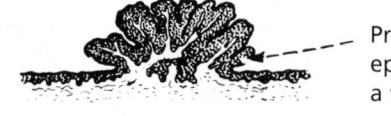

Proliferation of skin epithelial cells causing a warty growth

(d) Formation of 'inclusion' bodies within cytoplasm or nucleus: they consist of aggregates of virus and/or products of cell degeneration.

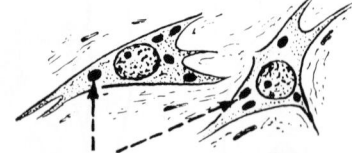

Diagnostic eosinophilic intracytoplasmic Negri bodies in nerve cells of the hippocampus in **RABIES**

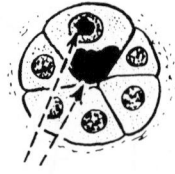

Nuclear and cytoplasmic inclusion in cytomegalic virus infection of salivary ducts

(e) No apparent change in cell but virus remains latent – reactivation later with continuous and slow release associated with gradually progressive disease.

(f) No apparent change but later malignant proliferation occurs, i.e. oncogenic infection.

# HOST/VIRUS INTERACTION

2. **Interferon production** by the infected cells and specifically activated T lymphocytes. Interferons are a group of protein molecules – not antibodies. They represent the first and very important line of defence by interfering with the synthesis of viral protein and thus protect healthy cells. Interferons also stimulate production of MHC (major histocompatibility complex) class I molecules and special proteins that enhance the ability of virally infected cells to present viral peptides to T cells. They also activate NK cells.

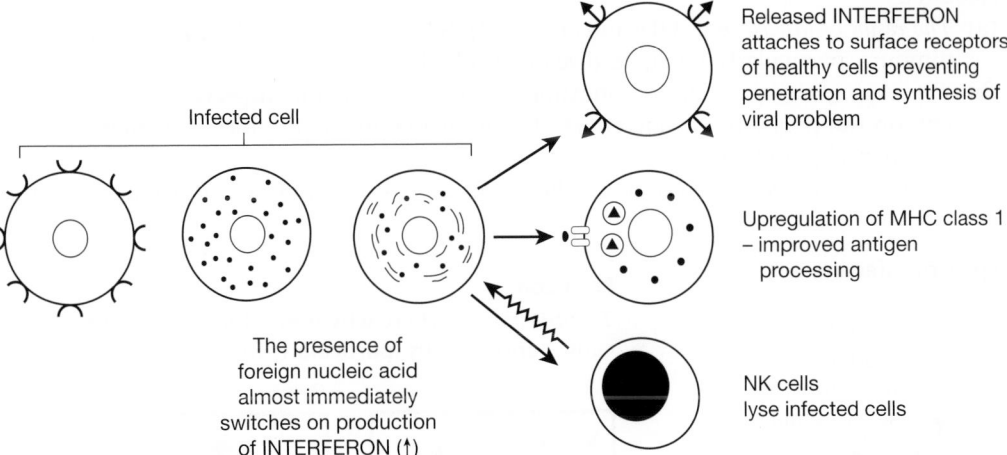

Infected cell

Released INTERFERON attaches to surface receptors of healthy cells preventing penetration and synthesis of viral problem

Upregulation of MHC class 1 – improved antigen processing

The presence of foreign nucleic acid almost immediately switches on production of INTERFERON (↑)

NK cells lyse infected cells

3. **The adaptive immune response** (see p. 129) begins 4–7 days after initial infection.

   (a) Antibodies to virus } limit initial infection via antibody-dependent cell-
   (b) Cellular immunity } mediated cytotoxicity (ADCC) but are very important in protecting against RE-INFECTION.

   (c) Occasionally virus antibody complexes cause special types of reaction in the host, e.g. inflammatory necrosis of arteries (arteritis), some forms of kidney damage and the skin rashes of childhood viral infections.

4. **The inflammatory response**

   The vascular and exudative elements follow the usual pattern; **neutrophils** are **not** a feature unless there is considerable tissue necrosis or secondary bacterial infection. However, **macrophage** phagocytic activity is important in the defence against viral infection. There is often a relative **lymphocytosis**.

# OPPORTUNISTIC INFECTIONS

This term is used for infections caused by organisms which are often non-pathogenic or of low grade virulence, occurring in individuals whose resistance to infection is impaired. They are occurring more frequently in modern medical practice because of the increasing use of powerful immunosuppressive drugs.

## CAUSES OF LOWERED RESISTANCE

1. Congenital immunological deficiencies (rare).
2. Acquired
   (a) *The result of disease*, e.g. HIV infection (AIDS); uraemia; liver disease; malignant tumours, particularly Hodgkin disease and leukaemias.
   (b) *The result of therapy*, e.g. immunosuppression in transplant surgery; immunosuppression – a side effect of tumour therapy; antibiotics – changing commensal populations.
   (c) *Introduction of foreign material*, e.g. heart valve prostheses; intravenous long lines in intensive care; tracheostomy.

### Examples of infecting organisms

**Bacteria** → *Acinetobacter* wound infections: septicaemia

*Staph. epidermidis* on heart valves; low grade septicaemia

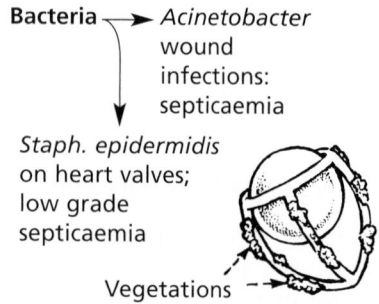

Vegetations on artificial heart valve

### Protozoa

*Toxoplasma gondii* reactivation of latent infection causes encephalitis (particularly in AIDS patients)

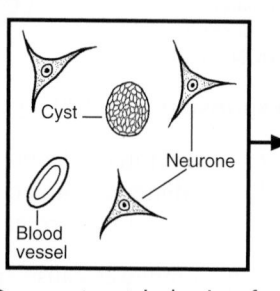

Dormant cyst in brain of immuno-competent person

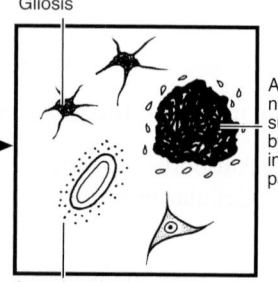

Reactivation of this cyst in immuno-suppressed patient leads to encephalitis

### Virus

Cytomegalovirus pneumonia

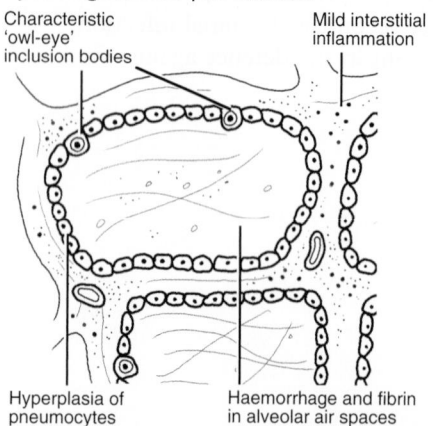

### Fungi

*Pneumocystis jiroveci* (previously known as *carinii*) a severe pneumonia (seen in AIDS cases particularly)

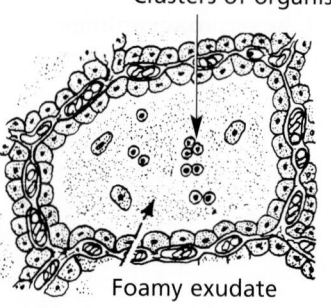

Clusters of organisms

Foamy exudate

# INFECTION – GENERAL EFFECTS

The more general body reactions in infection are: FEVER and CHANGES IN METABOLISM.

## FEVER (PYREXIA)

The body temperature rises above normal initially due partly to an imbalance between heat production and loss, but mainly due to a resetting at a higher level of the 'thermostat' mechanism in the hypothalamus. This results in:

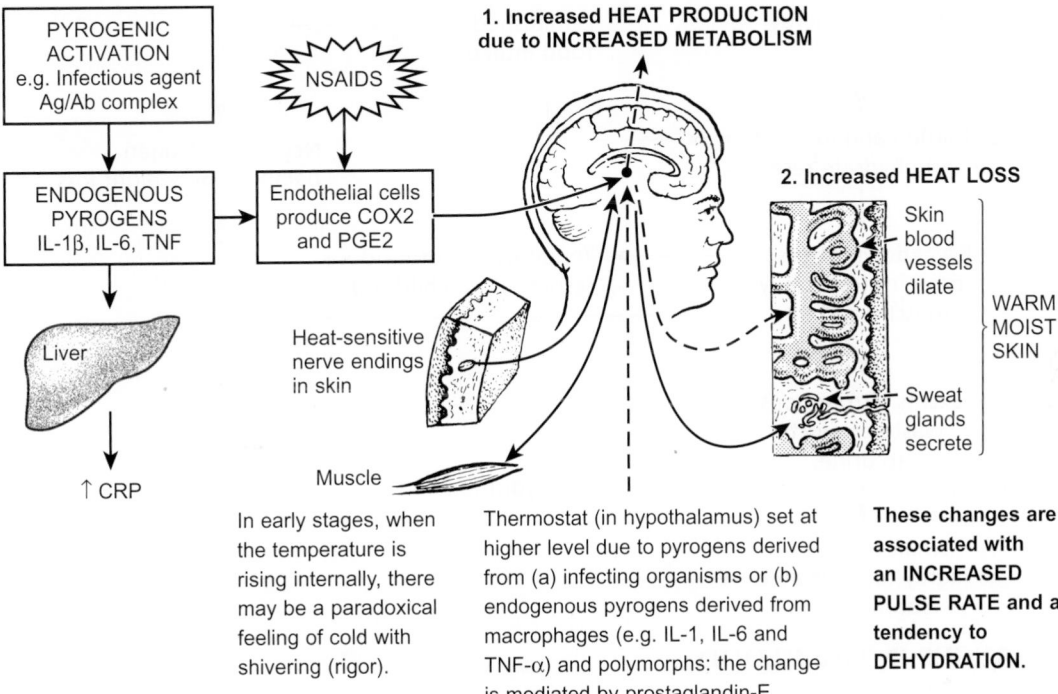

In early stages, when the temperature is rising internally, there may be a paradoxical feeling of cold with shivering (rigor).

Thermostat (in hypothalamus) set at higher level due to pyrogens derived from (a) infecting organisms or (b) endogenous pyrogens derived from macrophages (e.g. IL-1, IL-6 and TNF-α) and polymorphs: the change is mediated by prostaglandin-E.

These changes are associated with an INCREASED PULSE RATE and a tendency to DEHYDRATION.

**Pyrexia** also occurs when there is:

(a) Considerable tissue necrosis, e.g. infarction and tumours.
(b) Cerebral disease – especially in the region of the pons.
(c) Heat-stroke – where the environmental temperature and humidity are high and there is excessive water and salt loss.

**Hyperpyrexia** (when the temperature exceeds 41 °C [106 °F]) is extremely dangerous because of damage to the nerve cells in the brain.

# INFECTION – GENERAL EFFECTS

### CHANGES IN METABOLISM

Tissue breakdown is greatly increased, and in some infectious fevers there is a marked loss of body weight.

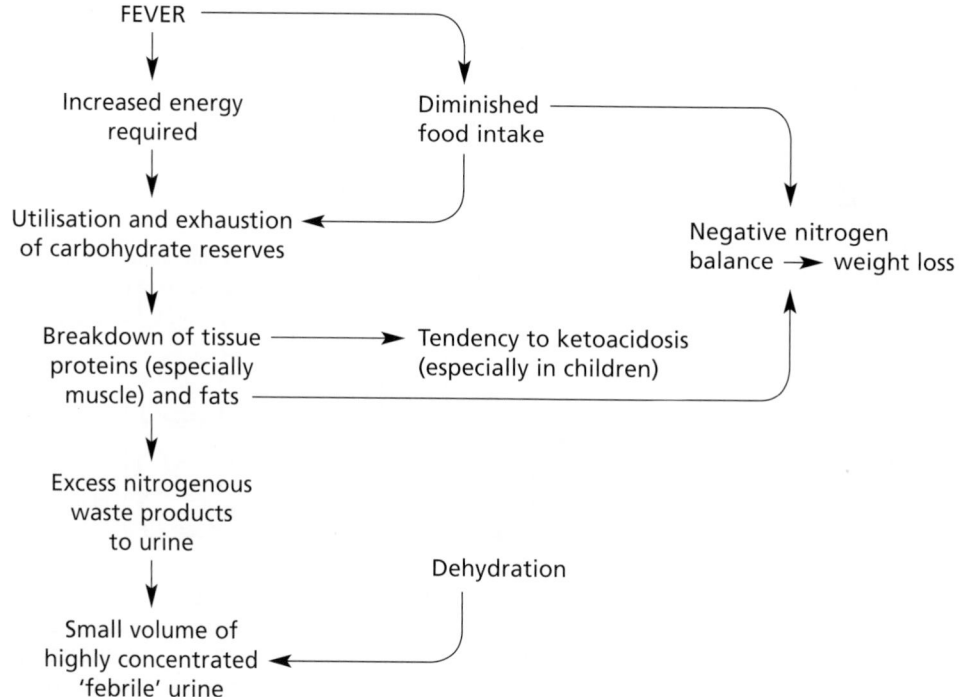

### CHANGES IN THE BLOOD

(a) **Celllular changes**
   (i) **Neutrophil leukocytosis** – in acute bacterial infections.
   (ii) **Lymphocytosis** – often in viral infections.
   (iii) **Lymphopenia** – in typhoid fever and chronic debilitating infections.

(b) **Biochemical changes**
   (i) **Non-specific** changes in plasma proteins → cause a rise in the **Erythrocyte Sedimentation Rate (ESR)**.
   (ii) **Specific antibodies** are present in both bacterial and viral infections (see next chapter).
   (iii) **Acute phase proteins** – a group of serum proteins which rise in response to inflammation: examples are C-reactive protein (used in diagnosis): complement components: mannin-binding lectin (MBL) and serum amyloid A protein: in long-standing chronic inflammation AMYLOIDOSIS may be a complication (see p. 19).
   (iv) Other chemical changes are listed on page 49.

# IMMUNITY

The immune system protects us from invading pathogenic microorganisms and cancer. Immunity – the state of protection from infectious disease – has both a less specific or INNATE and a more specific or ADAPTIVE component.

## INNATE IMMUNITY

This provides the first line of defence against infection. It is a rapid response (minutes); it is not specific to a particular pathogen. It has no memory and does not confer long-lasting immunity to the host. It has four main components and is found in all classes of plant and animal life.

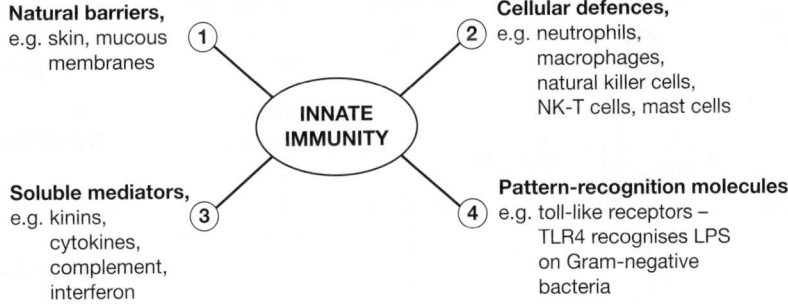

**Natural barriers,** e.g. skin, mucous membranes ①

② **Cellular defences,** e.g. neutrophils, macrophages, natural killer cells, NK-T cells, mast cells

INNATE IMMUNITY

**Soluble mediators,** e.g. kinins, cytokines, complement, interferon ③

④ **Pattern-recognition molecules,** e.g. toll-like receptors – TLR4 recognises LPS on Gram-negative bacteria

## ADAPTIVE IMMUNITY

This provides a specific immune response directed at an invading pathogen. Following exposure to a foreign organism there is an initial EFFECTOR RESPONSE that eliminates or neutralises a pathogen. Later re-exposure to the same foreign organism induces a MEMORY RESPONSE with a more rapid immune reaction that eliminates the pathogen and prevents disease. This response is found only in vertebrates.

It has been known from historical times that a person who has recovered from an infectious disease, e.g. smallpox, is most unlikely to suffer from it again – even when exposed maximally – although he would remain susceptible to other infections.

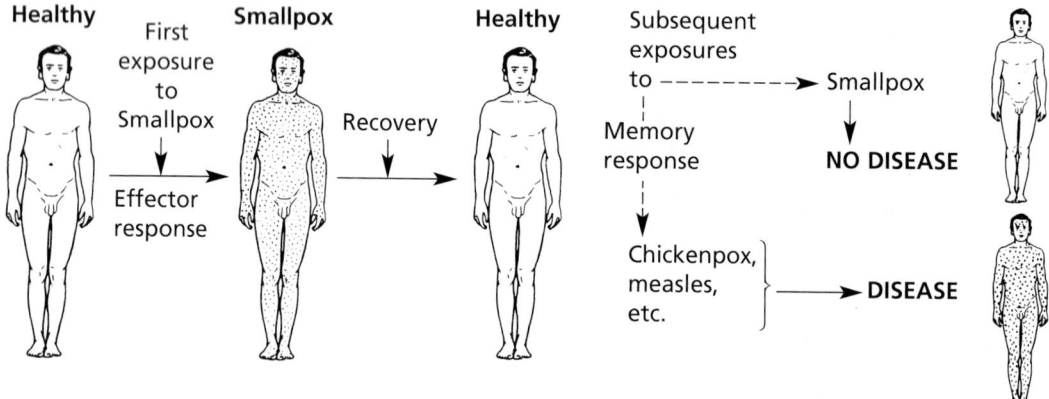

That is, during the recovery period he has ACQUIRED SPECIFIC IMMUNITY to smallpox but not to other unrelated infections.

*Note*: This immunity may extend to related infections: the use of the immunity against smallpox conferred by worldwide vaccination with cowpox (pioneered by Jenner in the 18th century) has completely eliminated smallpox throughout the world.

# THE ADAPTIVE IMMUNE RESPONSE

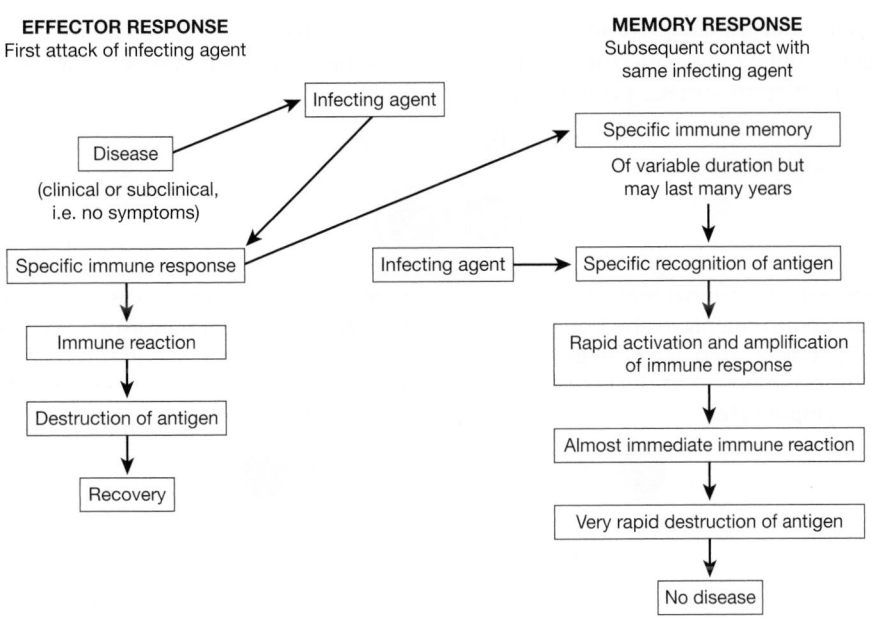

**EFFECTOR RESPONSE**
First attack of infecting agent

Infecting agent

Disease

(clinical or subclinical,
i.e. no symptoms)

Specific immune response

Immune reaction

Destruction of antigen

Recovery

**MEMORY RESPONSE**
Subsequent contact with
same infecting agent

Specific immune memory

Of variable duration but
may last many years

Infecting agent

Specific recognition of antigen

Rapid activation and amplification
of immune response

Almost immediate immune reaction

Very rapid destruction of antigen

No disease

## ADAPTIVE IMMUNE RESPONSE

**ANTIGENS** are substances that can be recognised by the immunoglobulin receptor of B cells or the T-cell receptor when complexed with MHC. They are usually part of infectious agents such as bacteria and some viruses, although other foreign materials are also antigenic. Most antigens are proteins but some large carbohydrate molecules such as lipopolysaccharides will induce antibody formation.

**EPITOPES** are the immunologically active regions of an antigen that bind to specific membrane receptors on lymphocytes or to secreted antibodies. B and T cells recognise different epitopes on the same antigenic molecule. B cells usually recognise soluble antigen (exogenous). Epitopes recognised by T cells are often internal peptides that are exposed by processing with antigen-presenting cells (endogenous).

## INTER-RELATIONSHIP OF INNATE & ADAPTIVE IMMUNITY

**INNATE IMMUNITY**

Natural barriers

**Cellular defenses**
PMN, macrophages,
NK cells

Soluble mediators

Cytokines
Antibodies

Cytokines

B cells

T cells

**ADAPTIVE IMMUNITY**

# CELLULAR BASIS OF THE ADAPTIVE IMMUNE RESPONSE

The main cells of the adaptive immune response are the lymphocytes. They are indistinguishable by light microscopy using conventional stains but can be separated by the presence of different surface proteins on T and B cells.

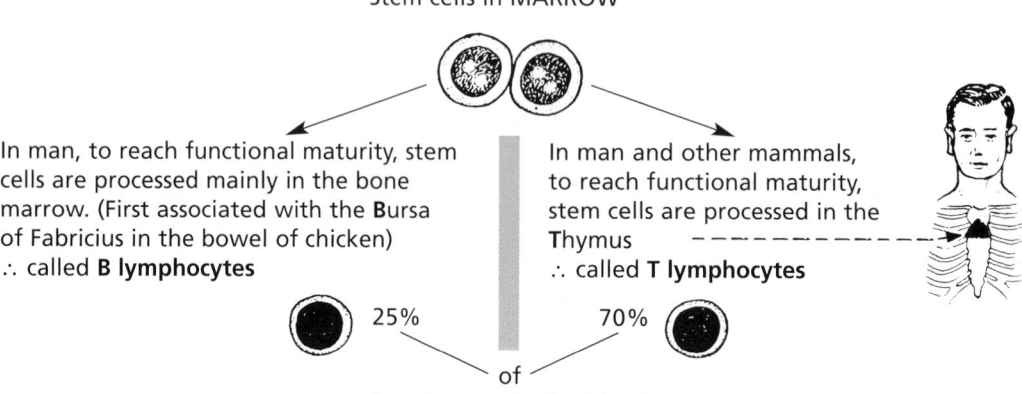

Stem cells in MARROW

In man, to reach functional maturity, stem cells are processed mainly in the bone marrow. (First associated with the **B**ursa of Fabricius in the bowel of chicken)
∴ called **B lymphocytes**

In man and other mammals, to reach functional maturity, stem cells are processed in the **Thymus**
∴ called **T lymphocytes**

25%          70%

of lymphocytes in the blood

The introduction of an antigen results in activation and proliferation of these two lymphocyte populations. This activity takes place in the lymphoid tissues.

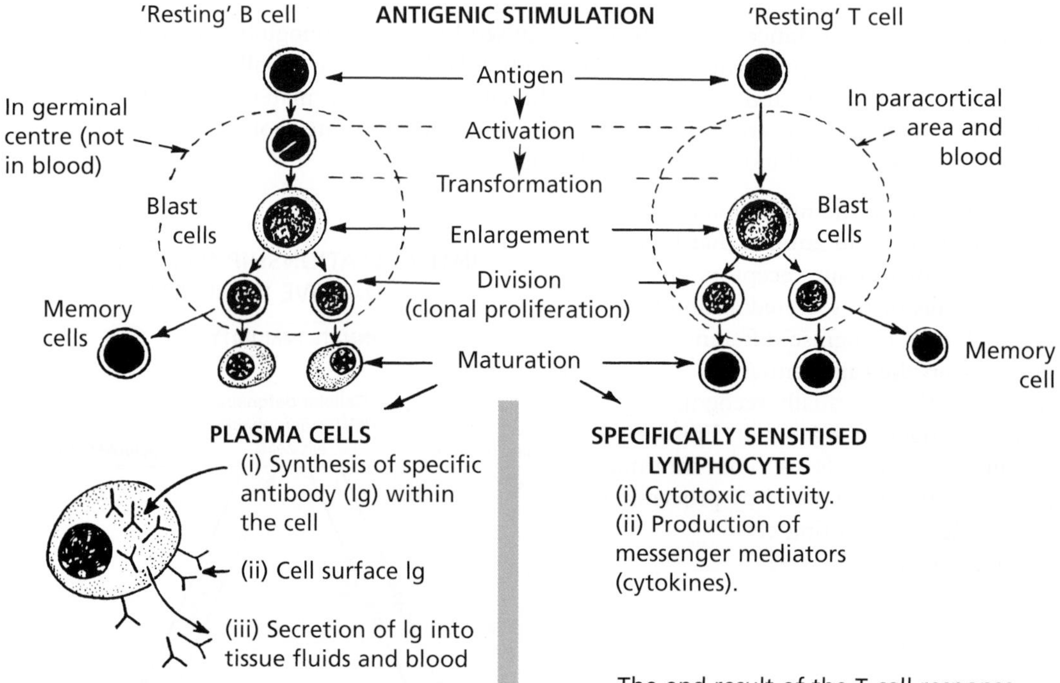

'Resting' B cell          **ANTIGENIC STIMULATION**          'Resting' T cell

In germinal centre (not in blood)

Antigen

Activation

Transformation

In paracortical area and blood

Blast cells

Enlargement

Blast cells

Memory cells

Division (clonal proliferation)

Maturation

Memory cell

**PLASMA CELLS**
(i) Synthesis of specific antibody (Ig) within the cell

(ii) Cell surface Ig

(iii) Secretion of Ig into tissue fluids and blood

The end result of the B-cell response is the formation of humoral antibodies or **HUMORAL IMMUNITY**
– protection against extracellular infection.

**SPECIFICALLY SENSITISED LYMPHOCYTES**
(i) Cytotoxic activity.
(ii) Production of messenger mediators (cytokines).

The end result of the T-cell response is the formation of **CELLULAR IMMUNITY**
– protection against intracellular organisms, e.g. viruses and some bacteria (e.g. TB).

# GENETIC INFLUENCES ON THE IMMUNE RESPONSE

The MAJOR HISTOCOMPATIBILITY complex, also known as the human leucocyte antigen (HLA), has an important role in the IMMUNE RESPONSE and DISEASE.

The genes controlling the system are in two major groups (Class I and Class II) on CHROMOSOME 6: each group has three genes which are highly polymorphic (i.e. show great variation within individual members of the same animal species). The multiple alleles of each gene encode for surface membrane glycoproteins.

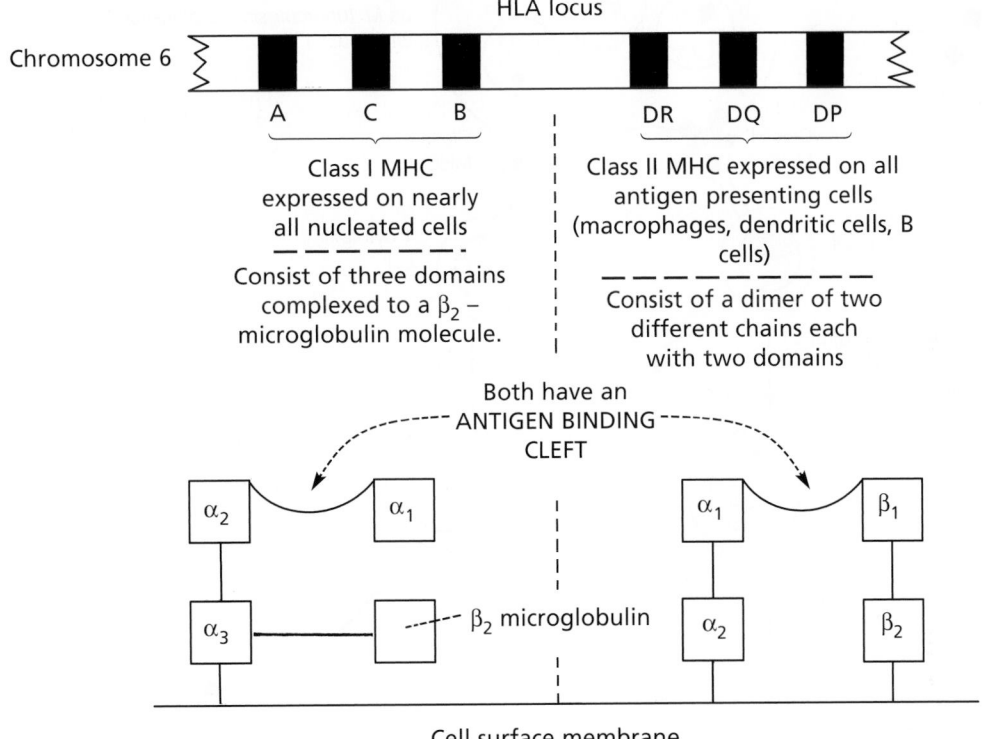

## The important roles of HLA are:

(i)   Presentation of peptides from foreign antigens to T lymphocytes
        Class I antigens to cytotoxic T cells (normally CD8 +ve)
        Class II antigens to helper T cells (normally CD4 +ve).
(ii)  They are the main stimulus to **graft rejection** in incompatible hosts. (The better the HLA match, the better the chance of graft survival.)
(iii) There is a strong association with diseases – especially **auto-immune** disorders (p. 159).
        The most striking example is **ankylosing spondylitis** where >90% of patients carry the allele HLA B27.
(iv)  They control individual resistance/susceptibility to certain infections, e.g. HLA B52 is associated with resistance to HIV infection.

# CELLULAR IMMUNITY

Activation of T cells requires the involvement of ANTIGEN PRESENTING CELLS (APC). Within these cells, foreign antigen is proteolytically digested to short peptides and then presented with HLA molecules to the T cell which possesses a specific receptor for that antigen.

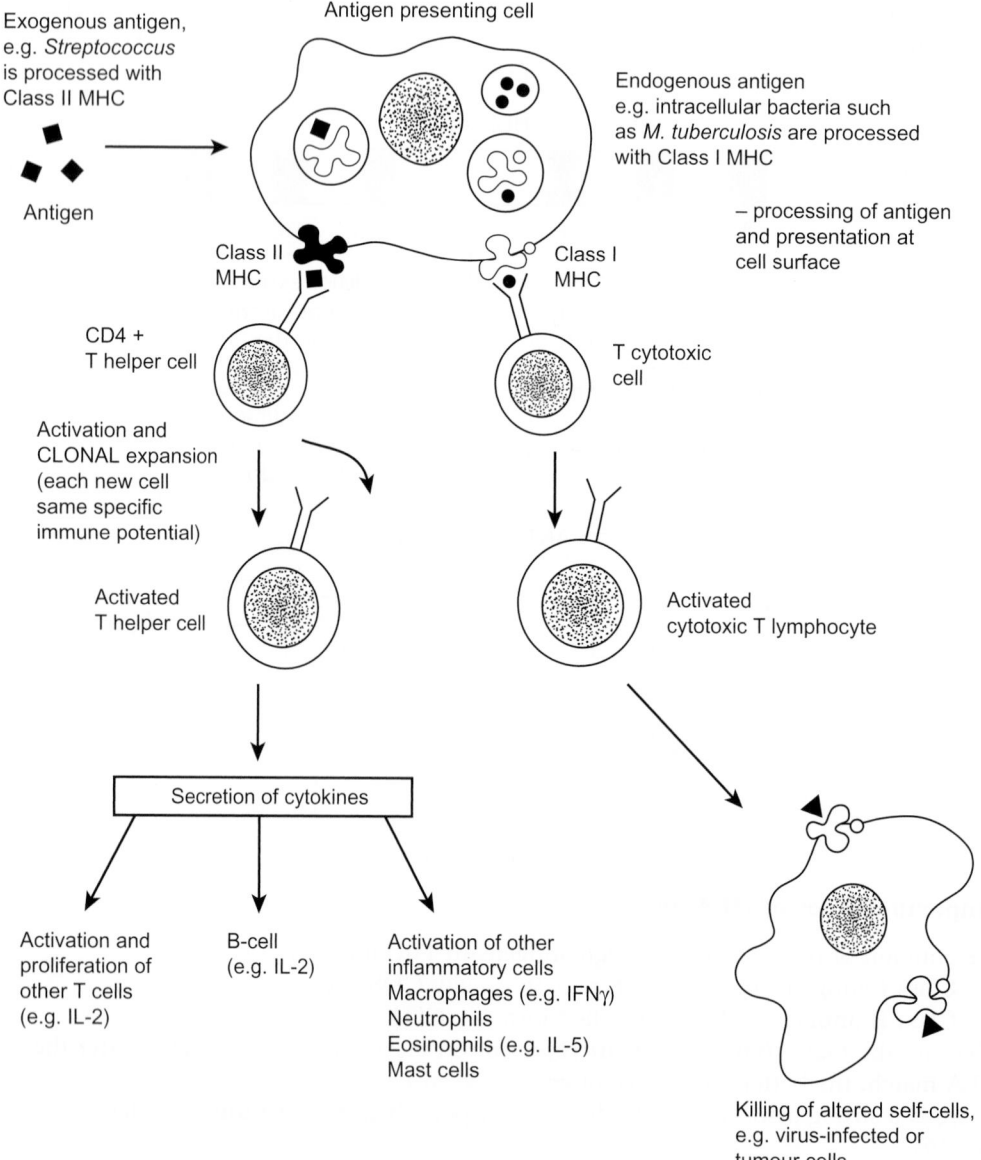

Exogenous antigen, e.g. *Streptococcus* is processed with Class II MHC

Antigen presenting cell

Antigen

Endogenous antigen e.g. intracellular bacteria such as *M. tuberculosis* are processed with Class I MHC

– processing of antigen and presentation at cell surface

Class II MHC

Class I MHC

CD4 + T helper cell

T cytotoxic cell

Activation and CLONAL expansion (each new cell same specific immune potential)

Activated T helper cell

Activated cytotoxic T lymphocyte

Secretion of cytokines

Activation and proliferation of other T cells (e.g. IL-2)

B-cell (e.g. IL-2)

Activation of other inflammatory cells Macrophages (e.g. IFNγ) Neutrophils Eosinophils (e.g. IL-5) Mast cells

Killing of altered self-cells, e.g. virus-infected or tumour cells

# CYTOKINES

The chemical messengers of the immune system are known as CYTOKINES. These small proteins are produced by virtually all cells of the innate and adaptive immune system, particularly CD4+ lymphocytes. The quantity and type of cytokine can positively and negatively regulate cells and cytokine effect is in turn controlled by expression or down-regulation of cytokine receptors on the cell surface.

## CYTOKINES INVOLVED IN INNATE IMMUNITY

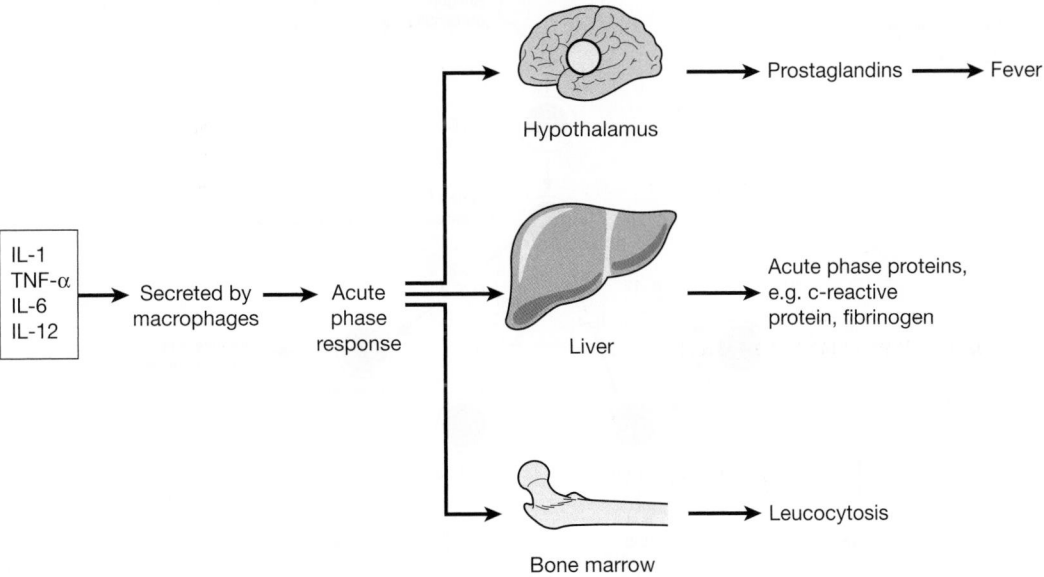

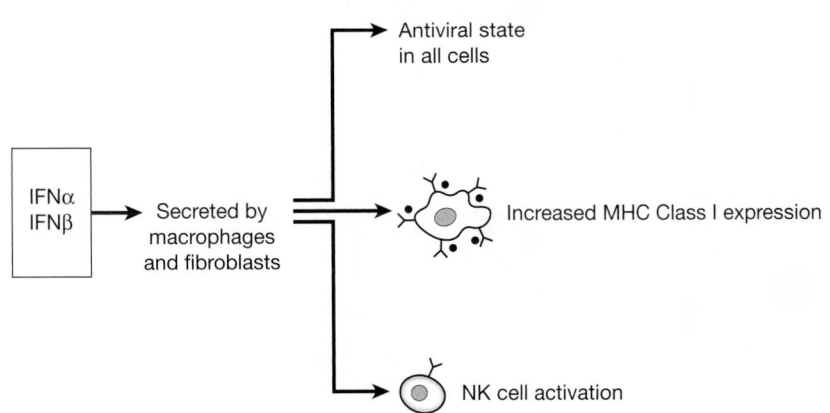

# CYTOKINES INVOLVED IN ADAPTIVE IMMUNITY

The immune response to a particular pathogen must induce an appropriate set of effector functions that can eliminate the pathogen from the host. Differences in cytokine secretion patterns among T helper cells are determinants of the type of immune response made to a particular antigenic challenge. Accordingly the cytokines secreting T helper cells are currently divided into four subsets:

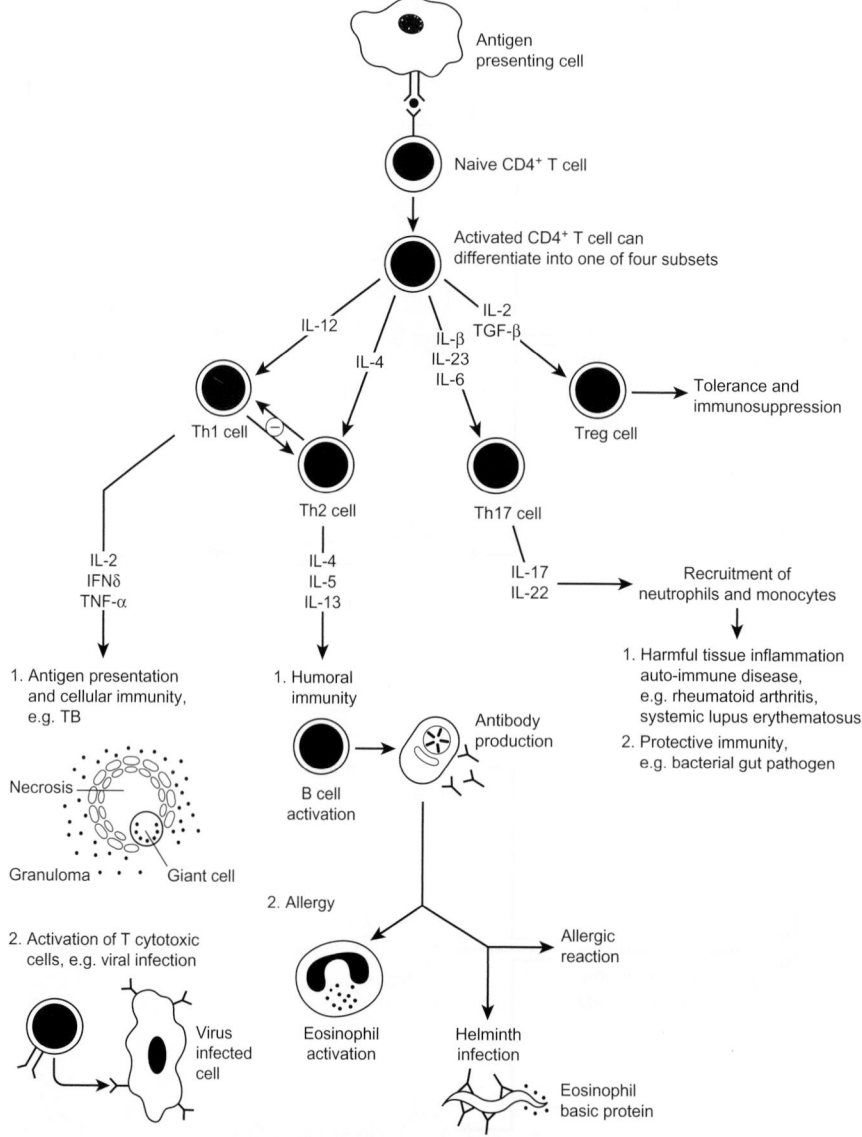

The balance between the two main subsets determines disease outcome, e.g. tuberculoid leprosy is characterised by a Th1 response (destructive granulomas, few parasites). In lepromatous leprosy there is a Th2 response (disseminated disease, many parasites).

# HUMORAL IMMUNITY

## BASIC STRUCTURE OF IMMUNOGLOBULIN

The basic immunoglobulin is a protein molecule consisting of two identical LIGHT chains and two identical HEAVY chains. Each light chain is bound to a heavy chain by a disulphide bond. Similarly disulphide bridges link the two heavy and light chain combinations to form the basic four-chain structure.

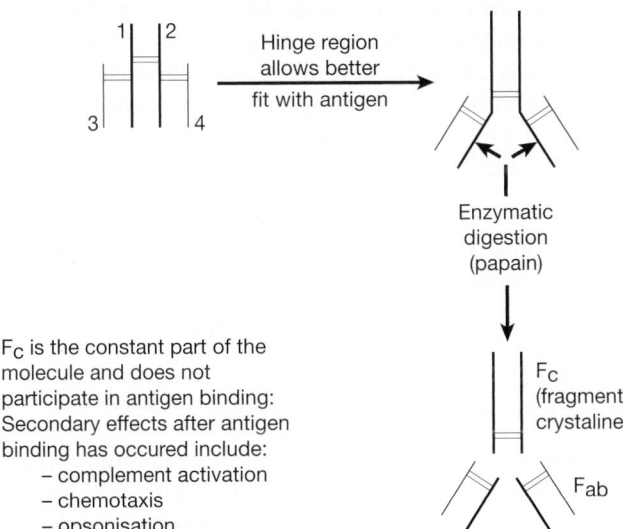

Hinge region allows better fit with antigen

Enzymatic digestion (papain)

$F_C$ (fragment crystaline)

$F_{ab}$

1 and 2 are heavy chains. Differences in structure allow separation of five main Ig classes – IgG; A; M; D; E.

3 and 4 are light chains. They exist in two forms – Kappa ($\kappa$) and Lambda ($\lambda$). In any one molecule both chains are either $\kappa$ or $\lambda$.

$F_{ab}$ are the variable parts of the molecule and are the site of antigen binding, the variation in amino acid content allowing a wide range of specific activity.

$F_C$ is the constant part of the molecule and does not participate in antigen binding: Secondary effects after antigen binding has occured include:
– complement activation
– chemotaxis
– opsonisation.

## ANTIBODY MEDIATED EFFECTOR FUNCTIONS

1. **Opsonisation**
   Fc receptors on macrophages and neutrophils can bind the Fc of Ig molecules, resulting in phagocytosis of the antigen-antibody complex.
2. **Complement activation**
   IgM and IgG subclasses can activate the complement system.
3. **ADCC**
   The linking of antibody bound to target cells (e.g. virus infected cells) with the Fc receptors of NK cells enables the NK cell to recognise and kill the target cell.
4. **Crossing of epithelium (transcytosis)**
   The delivery of antibody to the mucosal surfaces of the eyes, nose, mouth, bronchi and gut, as well as transport to breast milk, requires the movement of immunoglobulin across epithelium, a process called transcytosis.
5. **Activation of mast cells, eosinophils, basophils**
   This is unique to IgE (see p. 143).

# IMMUNOGLOBULINS

### ANTIBODY CLASSES AND ACTIVITIES

These groups are named according to the composition of the heavy chains.

IgM

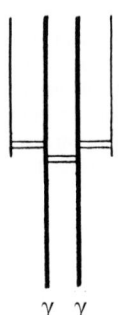

**IgM** (heavy chain = μ) is a polymer, joined by J chains, of five identical Ig molecules, therefore called macroglobulin.

Although in low concentration in the blood, 0.5–2 mg/mL, it is the main Ig on the surface of B lymphocytes (before conversion to plasma cells). It is the first immunoglobulin class produced and is active in the primary response. It neutralises viruses. In combination with complement, it is actively bactericidal and is especially effective in bacteraemia.

*Note*: The numerous (10) antigen-binding sites increase its efficiency.

The natural blood group antibodies, anti-A and anti-B are M globulins.

IgG

**IgG** (heavy chain = γ) is a single molecule with two antigen binding sites.

This is the most abundant class of immunoglobulin, with a concentration in blood of 8–16 mg/mL. There are four subclasses IgG1, IgG2, IgG3 and IgG4. Of its several activities the important ones are:

1.  Passive transfer of IgG (IgG1, IgG3 and IgG4) from mother to baby occurs via the placenta and colostrum. The immunity only lasts a few months.

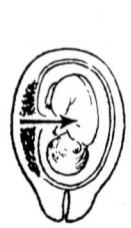

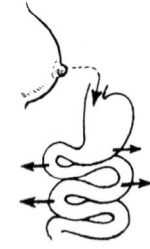

Transplacental passage of IgG

Colostrum, rich in IgG, absorbed from alimentary tract into the blood stream of the neonate

2.  Neutralisation of virus and toxins.

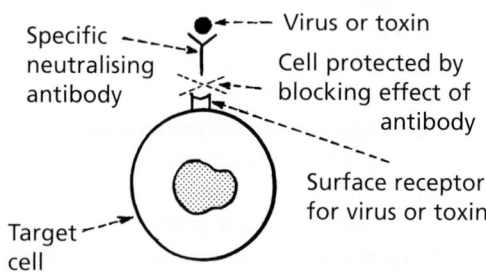

3.  Opsonisation (IgG1 and IgG3). See page 49.
4.  Complement Activation (IgG3, IgG1 and IgG2). See page 139.

# IMMUNOGLOBULINS

IgA

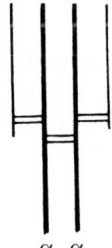

**IgA** (heavy chain = α) occurs in the blood (1.5–4 mg/mL), where its function is unknown.

It is the predominant immunoglobulin in secretions of eyes, nose, mouth, bronchi and gut. Its function is to protect mucous surfaces from antigenic attack and prevent access of foreign substances to the circulation and general immune system. It may neutralise toxins and prevent binding to mucous surfaces. IgA is a single molecule in the serum.

The diagram illustrates the local production of IgA in the gut.

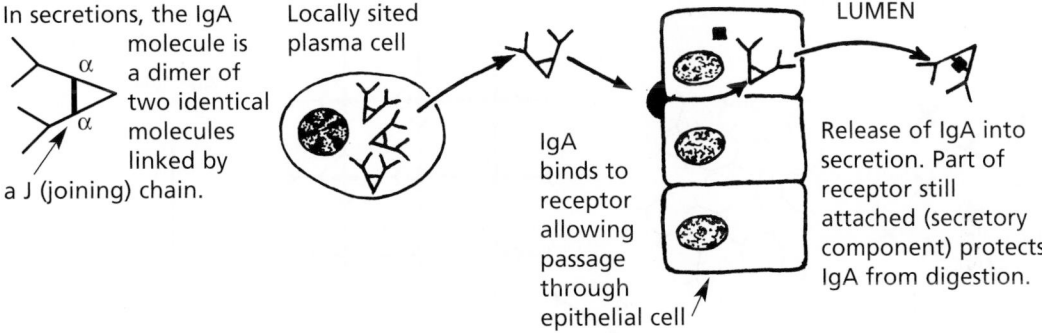

In secretions, the IgA molecule is a dimer of two identical molecules linked by a J (joining) chain.

Locally sited plasma cell

IgA binds to receptor allowing passage through epithelial cell

LUMEN

Release of IgA into secretion. Part of receptor still attached (secretory component) protects IgA from digestion.

**IgD** (heavy chain Δ) of uncertain function: concentration in blood very low probably because it is not secreted by plasma cells. Like IgM it is present on the surface of B lymphocytes prior to transformation.

**IgE** (heavy chain ε) – a single molecule similar to IgG and IgA. It is sometimes called REAGIN: concentration in blood is low (20–500 ng/mL). The serum level is raised in worm infestation and is probably protective. Its main activity is mediated by MAST CELLS (or BASOPHILS); it is the principal mediator of atopic and anaphylactic disease.

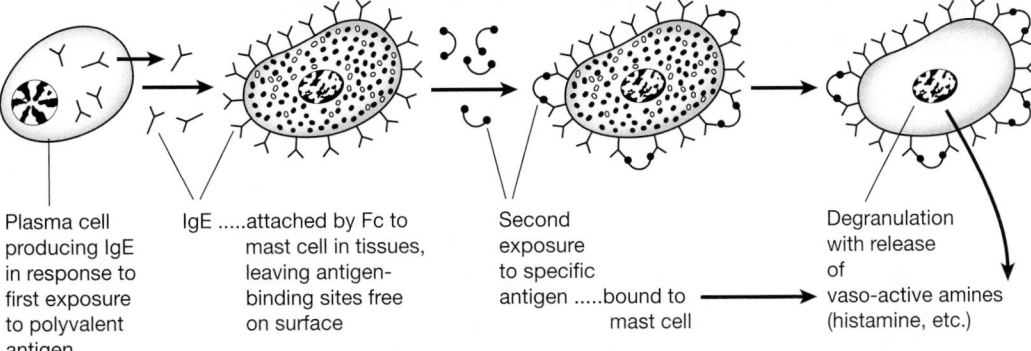

Plasma cell producing IgE in response to first exposure to polyvalent antigen

IgE .....attached by Fc to mast cell in tissues, leaving antigen-binding sites free on surface

Second exposure to specific antigen .....bound to mast cell

Degranulation with release of vaso-active amines (histamine, etc.)

The range of antibodies is immense. B cells produce this vast number by rearranging the genes from the immunoglobulin light and heavy chains. The appropriate clone of plasma cells is stimulated by binding of antigen to the cell surface receptor (so-called 'clonal selection').

# IMMUNE REACTIONS

### ANTIGEN-ANTIBODY INTERACTIONS

When an antigen (Ag) binds with an antibody (Ab) an Ag/Ab complex is formed. This reaction is reversible in varying degrees and depends on the **affinity** of the antibody for an individual antigen and the **avidity** (strength when multiple epitopes on an antigen interact with multiple binding sites).

The consequences of Ag/Ab interaction include:

### 1. PRECIPITATION

A soluble antigen is rendered insoluble by aggregation of the Ag/Ab complexes into a lattice.

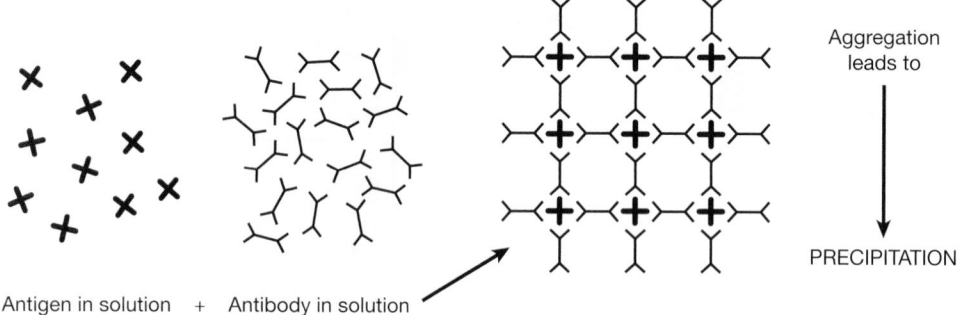

Antigen in solution    +    Antibody in solution

Aggregation leads to

PRECIPITATION

This reaction is the basis of immunoelectrophoresis, used e.g. to identify a monoclonal band in myeloma.

### 2. AGGLUTINATION

Particulate antigens, e.g. bacteria and red blood cells, are aggregated in the same way as in the precipitation reaction and the process is called AGGLUTINATION. Agglutination reactions are routinely performed to type red cells (ABO typing).

### 3. CROSS-REACTIVITY

In some cases antibody elicited by one antigen can cross-react with an unrelated antigen usually because they share a similar epitope, e.g. *S. pyogenes*.

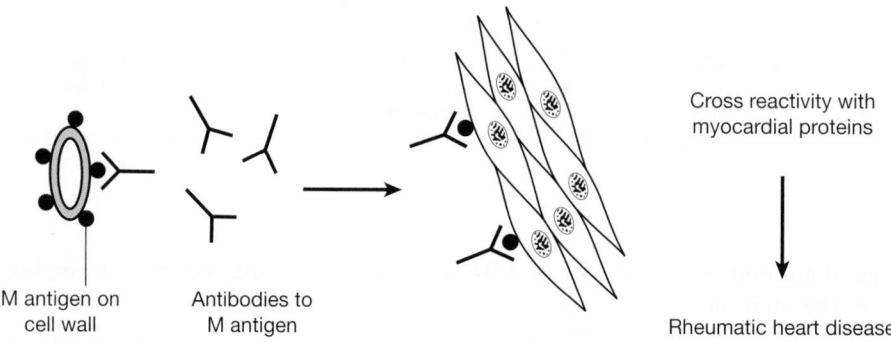

M antigen on cell wall

Antibodies to M antigen

Cross reactivity with myocardial proteins

Rheumatic heart disease

# IMMUNE REACTIONS

## COMPLEMENT SYSTEM

Complement consists of nine main protein components present in inactive form in the blood. There are three pathways of complement activation. Activation results in the formation of multi-molecular enzymes that activate further components in a cascade, ultimately generating a membrane attack complex that is capable of causing cell lysis.

The Mannose-binding lectin (MBL) and alternative pathways do not require antibody for activation and are therefore a component of the **innate** immune system.

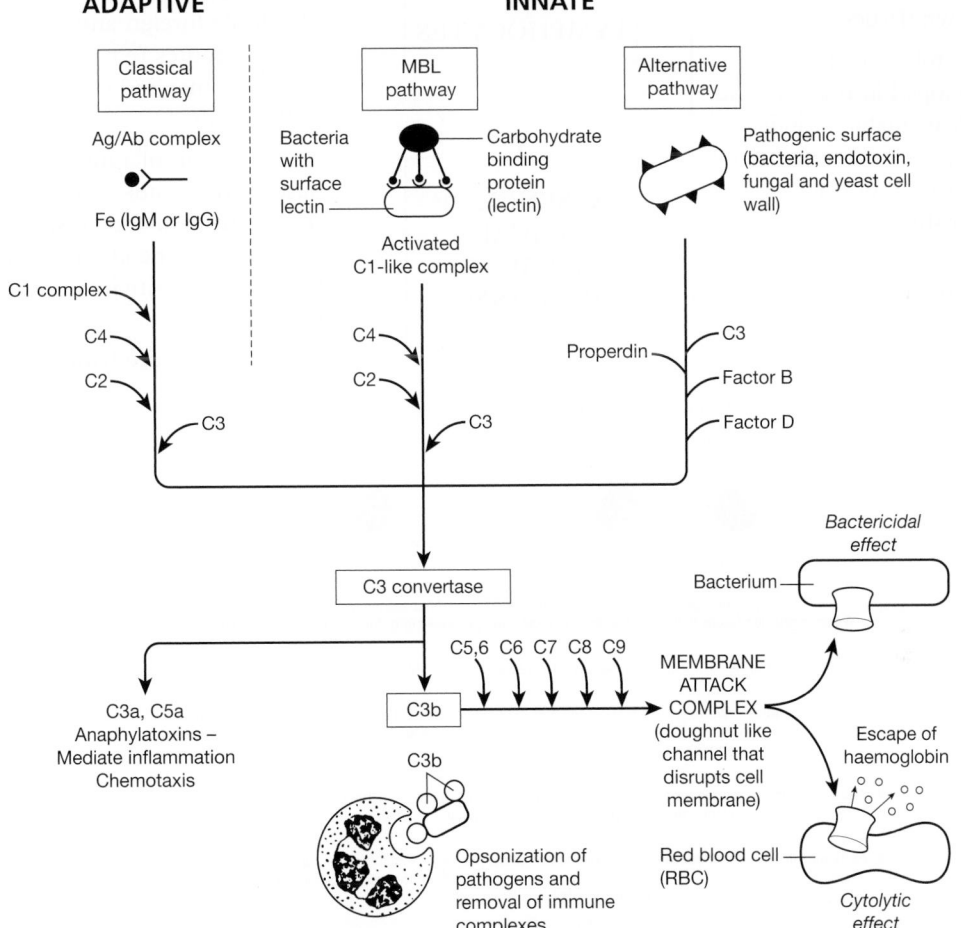

Activation of complement by Ag/Ab complex is called **fixation**. Using red cells as markers, this fixation can detect the presence of antigen or antibody in serum.

E.g.    Test serum + antigen + complement.
        If serum contains antibody, complement is fixed, otherwise it remains free.
        Add sensitised RBC (coated with Ab).
        Lysis of RBC = complement still free ∴ no Ab in original serum.
        No lysis = complement was fixed by Ab in test serum.

# TOLERANCE

Humoral and cell-mediated immunity are specific active immune responses with a protective function.

In certain circumstances an antigen does not evoke these active responses. This is because the lymphocytes, although recognising the antigen, do not react – this is TOLERANCE.

**Natural 'self' tolerance**
(Central Tolerance)

The immune system recognises and tolerates its own tissues.

This tolerance is developed in the fetal and early neonatal periods, and prevents autoimmune diseases in normal individuals.

Occurs in bone marrow and thymus.

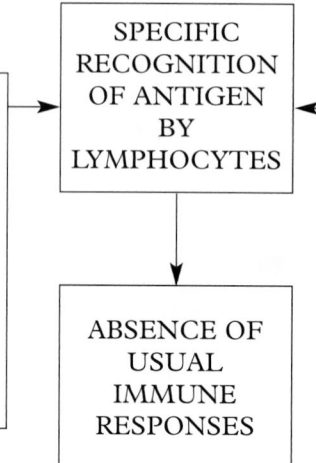

SPECIFIC RECOGNITION OF ANTIGEN BY LYMPHOCYTES

↓

ABSENCE OF USUAL IMMUNE RESPONSES

**Acquired tolerance**
(Peripheral Tolerance)

After the neonatal period and throughout adult life, injections of soluble foreign antigens by selected routes (e.g. intravenous, mucosal) may induce tolerance in the adult.

This form of tolerance is the basis of desensitisation treatment in allergic disease and explains the absence of, e.g. food hypersensitivity in normal individuals.

Occurs in mature lymphocytes.

① **Anergy** – Both B and T cells require two signals for activation. Lack of the second signal switches the cell off.

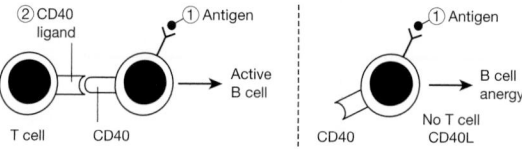

For T cells the signals are ① MHC peptide and ② costimulatory molecule B7.2 on APC
A third signal for T cells that provides direction has been proposed (e.g. for Th1, IL-12 and for Th2, IL-4)

② **Deletion** – In fetal life all T and B lymphocytes that recognise 'self' antigens are eliminated by apoptosis.

③ **Clonal ignorance** – Autoreactive lymphocytes may remain unactivated because they have a weak affinity for the 'self' antigen. They have the potential to be activated under certain circumstances and therefore pose a threat to the host.

④ **Receptor editing** – In this process there is secondary rearrangement of an immunoglobin variable region altering receptor specificity and averting autoimmunity.

⑤ **Activation-induced cell death** – Fas-mediated apoptosis plays a critical role in the removal of mature autoreactive B and T lymphocytes. Fas-mediated apoptosis plays an important role in immune privileged sites (e.g. brain, eye).

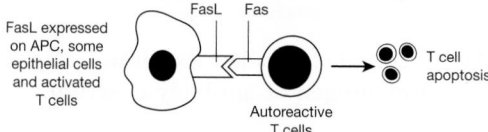

⑥ **Suppression by regulatory T cells** – A specialised population of T cells that suppress the response of other lymphocytes. These cells express CD25, one of the chains of the IL-2 receptor. They also express FOXP3 at transcription factor and mutations in this gene can result in auto-immune disease.

Tolerance is an important protective mechanism. When it breaks down, the serious effects give rise to **auto-immune disease** (see p. 150).

# IMMUNOPATHOLOGY

The complicated and delicately balanced immune mechanisms clearly have been developed to protect against antigens, particularly infections. When these immune reactions are upset, the protective mechanism can itself be a source of disease states.

There are three main categories: (1) hypersensitivity states, (2) immune deficiency states and (3) auto-immune diseases.

## HYPERSENSITIVITY REACTIONS

These consist of an inappropriate response by an individual to an antigen, following a previous exposure. They differ from the protective immune response in that they are exaggerated, inappropriate or damaging to the host. Depending on the main type of immune response concerned, these are classified as follows:

(a) Those associated with *HUMORAL ANTIBODIES* ∴ immediate – Types I, II, III.
(b) Those associated with *CELLULAR IMMUNITY* ∴ delayed (24–72 hours) – Type IV.

This classification is to some extent artificial. Hypersensitivity may start as an immediate humoral reaction but end in a mixed state with both humoral and cellular activities. In the 1960s, Coombs and Gell divided hypersensitivity reactions into four types that are still used today.

### Type I immediate

This occurs within 20–60 minutes of exposure to antigen and is often referred to as 'immediate type hypersensitivity'.

All three terms have been used for this reaction. The basic mechanism is as follows:

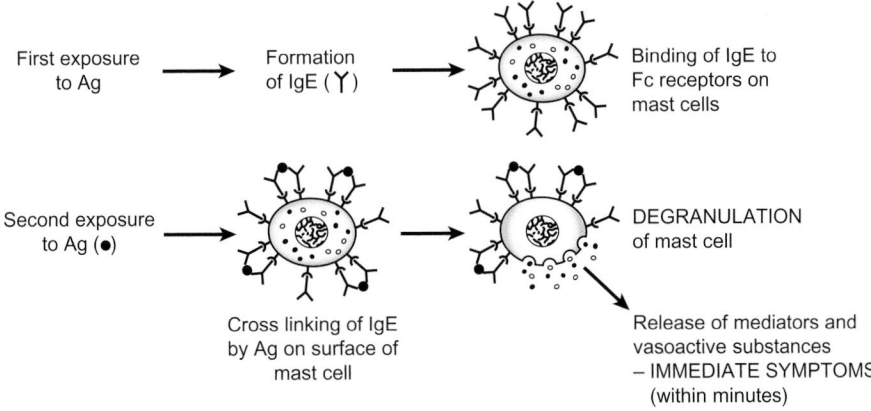

# IMMUNOPATHOLOGY

### Antigens and 'allergens'

The most potent allergens are usually large molecules with molecular weights up to 40 000. Examples of common 'allergens' are pollen, house mite dust, cat fur and penicillin. Food allergy, e.g. to peanuts and milk, is uncommon.

### Antibody

This is IgE. Plasma cells forming IgE are not normally found in the internal secretory surfaces of the body – tonsils, bronchi, gastrointestinal tract – but are present in large numbers in cases of allergy (and in defence against parasitic infections).

### Mast cells

These have a wide distribution but are prominent in the same areas as the IgE-producing plasma cells, plus skin, bladder and synovial membranes. This explains the frequently used term 'target organs' when discussing hypersensitivity.

# HYPERSENSITIVITY STATES

## Clinical examples of Type I reaction

### ANAPHYLACTIC SHOCK

*1st injection* of antigen, e.g. penicillin or a bee sting → general sensitisation

------------------------------------

*2nd injection* of above → acute collapse: bronchial constriction; vomiting; diarrhoea; perhaps a skin rash. May be fatal. Note that the antigens are injected – enter blood stream → basophils affected → widespread reaction

### HAY FEVER

*1st contact* with grass pollen → local sensitisation of conjunctiva and nasal passages

------------------------------------

*2nd contact* with above → irritation or swelling of conjunctiva with nasal excessive watery secretion

### ASTHMA

*1st contact* with house mite dust or animal dander → local sensitisation of bronchi

------------------------------------

*2nd contact* with above → bronchial constriction and secretion of thick mucus cause dyspnoea (difficult breathing)

Chronic asthma may involve cellular immunity with tissue destruction.

**Eosinophils** are a common finding in the tissues of patients with allergies, attracted by eosinophil chemotactic factor released by mast cells. Allergic conditions are often familial with a genetic basis. Several candidate loci have been proposed including loci linked to cytokine genes and a gene for the IgE receptor on mast cells.

## Type II – antibody mediated

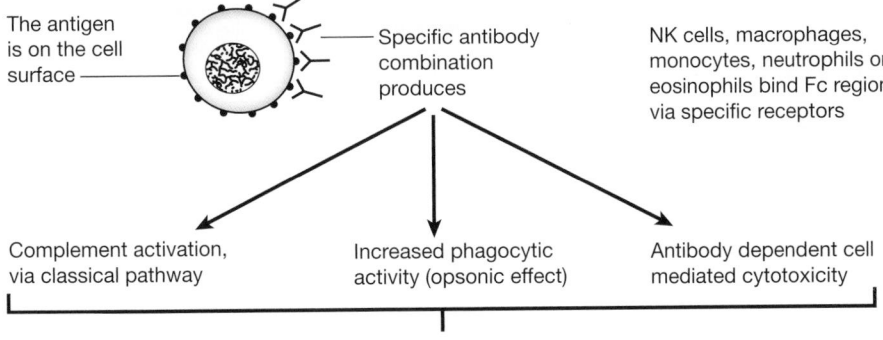

The antigen is on the cell surface — Specific antibody combination produces

NK cells, macrophages, monocytes, neutrophils or eosinophils bind Fc region via specific receptors

Complement activation, via classical pathway

Increased phagocytic activity (opsonic effect)

Antibody dependent cell mediated cytotoxicity

DESTRUCTION OF CELL

This antibody mediated reaction causes some forms of haemolytic anaemia (HA) (e.g. auto-immune HA [p. 432], Rhesus incompatibility [p. 430]) and some blood transfusion reactions. Certain drugs (e.g. penicillins) can also cause auto-immune HA by acting as a *hapten*. This is a small molecule that only becomes immunogenic when combined with a host protein carrier.

In some auto-immune disorders antibodies of this type are directed against specialised cell surface receptors, e.g. Grave disease or myasthenia gravis (see p. 152).

## Type III – immune complex

The reaction is due to the consequences of specific direct antigen/antibody combination. These immune complexes form in the circulation and may deposit in blood vessels leading to complement activation (p. 139), platelet aggregation and acute inflammation. The antibodies involved are IgG or IgM.

# HYPERSENSITIVITY STATES

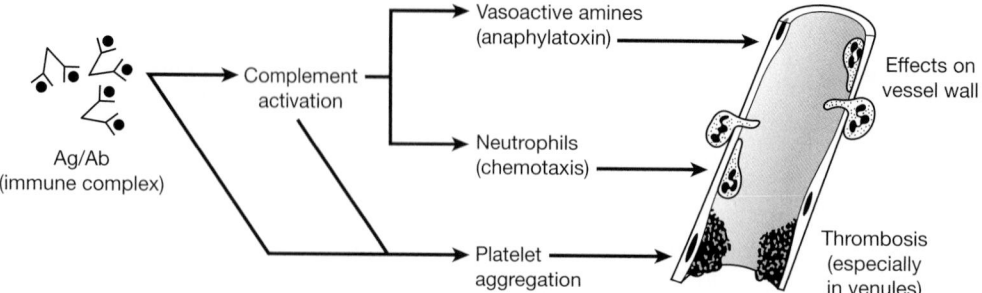

Ag/Ab
(immune complex)

Complement
activation

Vasoactive amines
(anaphylatoxin)

Neutrophils
(chemotaxis)

Platelet
aggregation

Effects on
vessel wall

Thrombosis
(especially
in venules)

Type III hypersensitivity may be systemic or localised.

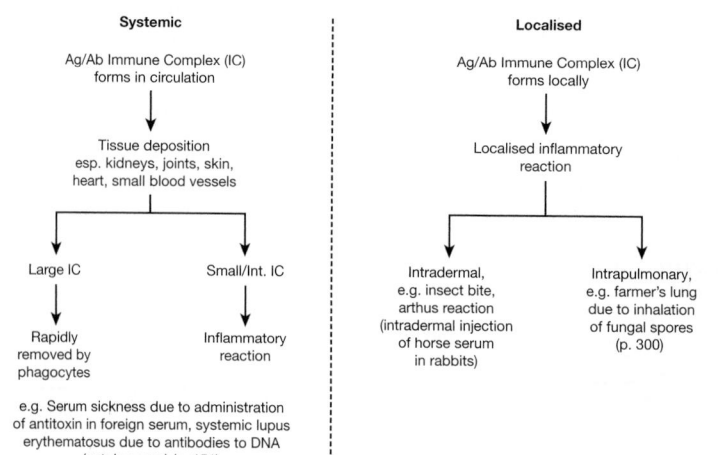

**Systemic**

Ag/Ab Immune Complex (IC)
forms in circulation

↓

Tissue deposition
esp. kidneys, joints, skin,
heart, small blood vessels

Large IC

↓

Rapidly
removed by
phagocytes

Small/Int. IC

↓

Inflammatory
reaction

e.g. Serum sickness due to administration
of antitoxin in foreign serum, systemic lupus
erythematosus due to antibodies to DNA
(autoimmune) (p. 151)

**Localised**

Ag/Ab Immune Complex (IC)
forms locally

↓

Localised inflammatory
reaction

Intradermal,
e.g. insect bite,
arthus reaction
(intradermal injection
of horse serum
in rabbits)

Intrapulmonary,
e.g. farmer's lung
due to inhalation
of fungal spores
(p. 300)

# HYPERSENSITIVITY STATES

## Type IV – T cell-mediated

This reaction is an antigen-elicited cellular immune response which produces tissue injury independently of the presence of antibody. The reaction is usually delayed, taking 24–72 hours to develop (previously known as delayed type hypersensitivity). Classic examples include the tubercle follicle, graft rejection and contact dermatitis.

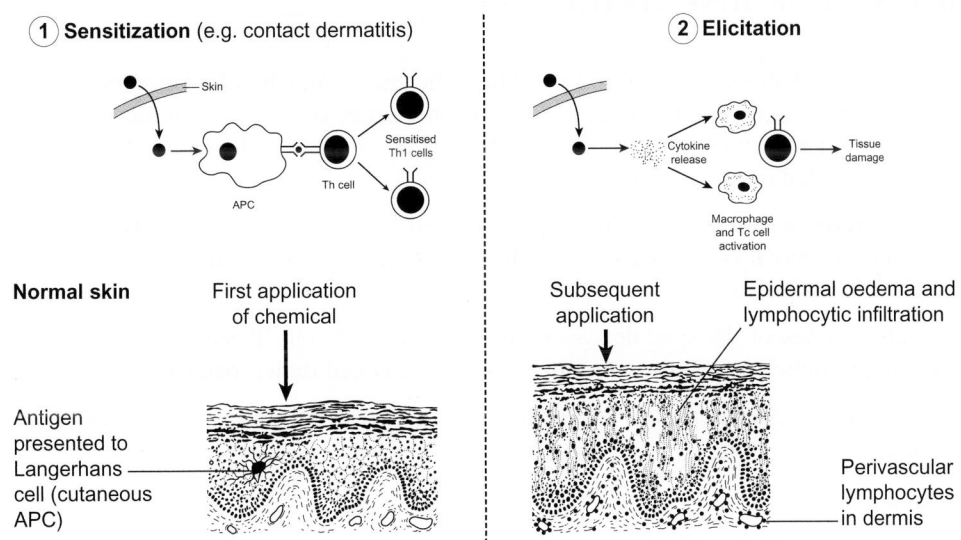

① **Sensitization** (e.g. contact dermatitis)

Skin
Sensitised Th1 cells
Th cell
APC

② **Elicitation**

Cytokine release
Tissue damage
Macrophage and Tc cell activation

**Normal skin**

First application of chemical

Antigen presented to Langerhans cell (cutaneous APC)

Subsequent application

Epidermal oedema and lymphocytic infiltration

Perivascular lymphocytes in dermis

# IMMUNE DEFICIENCY STATES

The systems involved are:

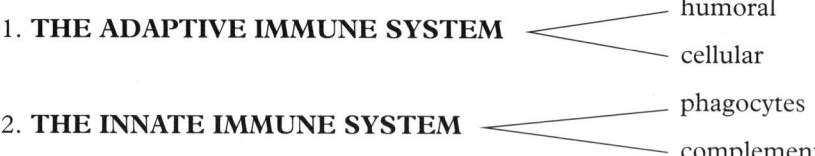

1. **THE ADAPTIVE IMMUNE SYSTEM** — humoral
— cellular

2. **THE INNATE IMMUNE SYSTEM** — phagocytes
— complement

Failure in any one alters the immune response. The deficiencies may be of a primary nature, commonly genetic in origin, or secondary to some other disease or circumstance. Equally, the alteration in any system may be quantitative or qualitative. In many of these deficiencies there is a failure in more than one system.

**Primary (inherited) deficiencies** of the specific system are rare. They include B cell, T cell, and combined B and T cell deficits. B cell deficiency leads to infection by pyogenic bacteria. T cell deficits lead to infection by viruses, fungi and intracellular bacteria.

**Secondary deficiencies** of the specific system are common. Usually T cell activity is affected, resulting in deficient cellular immunity and, later, B cell deficit occurs.

AIDS is now a major worldwide public health problem. Other predisposing conditions and diseases include:

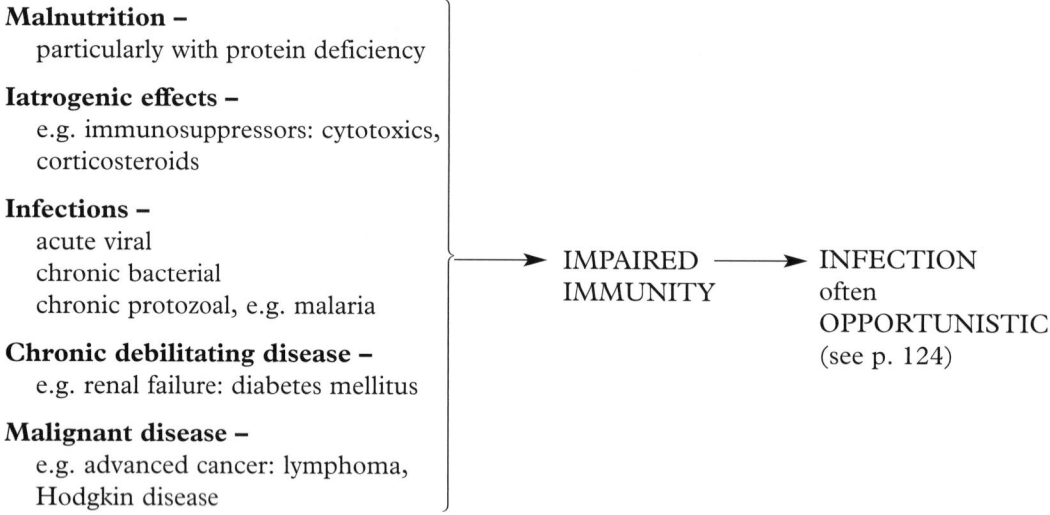

**Malnutrition –**
    particularly with protein deficiency

**Iatrogenic effects –**
    e.g. immunosuppressors: cytotoxics, corticosteroids

**Infections –**
    acute viral
    chronic bacterial
    chronic protozoal, e.g. malaria

**Chronic debilitating disease –**
    e.g. renal failure: diabetes mellitus

**Malignant disease –**
    e.g. advanced cancer: lymphoma, Hodgkin disease

IMPAIRED IMMUNITY → INFECTION often OPPORTUNISTIC (see p. 124)

Deficiencies of the innate immune system are rare. The disorders of neutrophil function are described on page 445.

# IMMUNE DEFICIENCY STATES – AIDS

AIDS is a worldwide epidemic with large numbers of cases in sub-Saharan Africa and South-East Asia. Globally, an estimated 40 million people are infected with the virus.

The virus (HIV) is of the retrovirus group: it infects and destroys CD4 T lymphocytes (macrophages, monocytes and dendritic cells are also infected). There are two strains of HIV: HIV1, which is more virulent, and HIV2, which predominates in West Africa.

The disease is slowly progressive and untreated is usually ultimately fatal. Recently highly active antiretroviral therapy (HAART), usually a combination of drugs such as nucleoside analogues and proteases, has been shown to reduce viral load to undetectable levels and has decreased the incidence of opportunistic infections and the death rate in the United States. However, these drugs are expensive and have significant side effects.

| Infection | Latent period | AIDS |
|---|---|---|
| CD4 $> 500 \times 10^6$ | CD4 $- 200$–$500 \times 10^6$ | CD4 $< 200 \times 10^6$ |
| Asymptomatic or a short febrile illness. Although the patient's cells contain HIV, tests for antibodies may be negative for up to several months. | Virus present in lymphocytes: may be persistent lymph node enlargement and fever. | Infections and tumours<br><br>Infection — opportunistic / others<br><br>Tumours — Kaposi sarcoma / lymphomas |

The whole range of opportunistic infection (see p. 124), including disseminated virus infection (e.g. herpes simplex and cytomegalovirus), occurs.

The diagram shows the more common AIDS-associated diseases and sites:

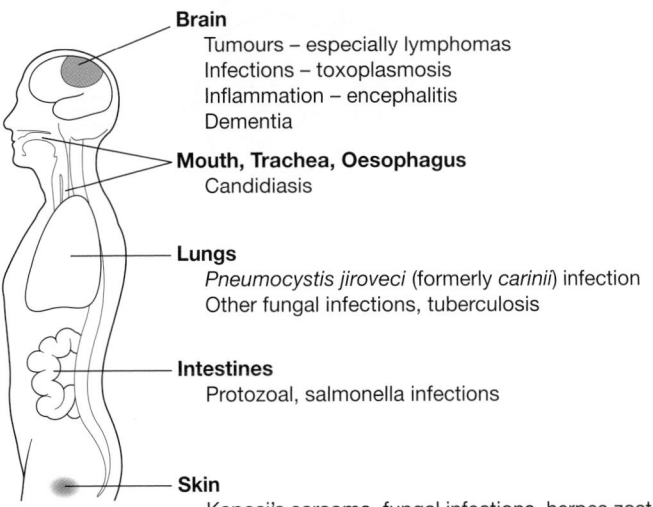

**Brain**
Tumours – especially lymphomas
Infections – toxoplasmosis
Inflammation – encephalitis
Dementia

**Mouth, Trachea, Oesophagus**
Candidiasis

**Lungs**
*Pneumocystis jiroveci* (formerly *carinii*) infection
Other fungal infections, tuberculosis

**Intestines**
Protozoal, salmonella infections

**Skin**
Kaposi's sarcoma, fungal infections, herpes zoster

## Blood changes

*Antibodies* – Specific antibodies appear up to 6 months after infection and form the basis of the diagnostic test for HIV. The antibody titre may fall greatly late in the disease.
*Immunoglobulins* are usually elevated in the early stages.
*CD4 lymphocytes* may be severely reduced, producing a lymphopenia (see above).

# IMMUNE DEFICIENCY STATES – AIDS

### EPIDEMIOLOGY AND TRANSMISSION

Although the virus may be present in many body fluids and secretions, transmission is by the parenteral route, usually by (1) **sexual contact**, (2) **infected blood** or (3) **from mother to infant**.

Transmission does not occur with normal social contact and there is a very low risk to medical or nursing personnel using normal procedures.

1.  **Sexual contact**: HIV is present in semen and vaginal fluid. Transmission may occur by homosexual intercourse. The risk of transmission is increased where there is genital ulceration or abrasion.
2.  **Infected blood**: the risk from blood transfusion and blood products has now been virtually eliminated by screening and sterilisation procedures (in the past many haemophiliacs were infected). The communal use of contaminated syringes and needles is important among drug addicts.
3.  **Mother to infant**: around half a million infants become infected with HIV each year. The majority of these infections result from transmission of virus from HIV-infected mothers during childbirth or by transfer of virus in milk during breastfeeding. Maternal antiretroviral therapy can reduce the incidence of transmission.

### CELLULAR MECHANISMS

1.  **Viral structure**

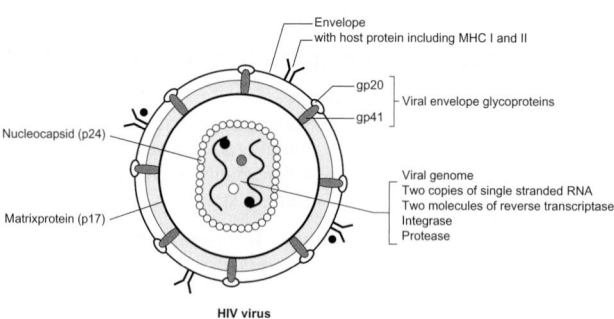

HIV virus

# IMMUNE DEFICIENCY STATES – AIDS

## 2. Infection and Replication

### (A) Infection of cells

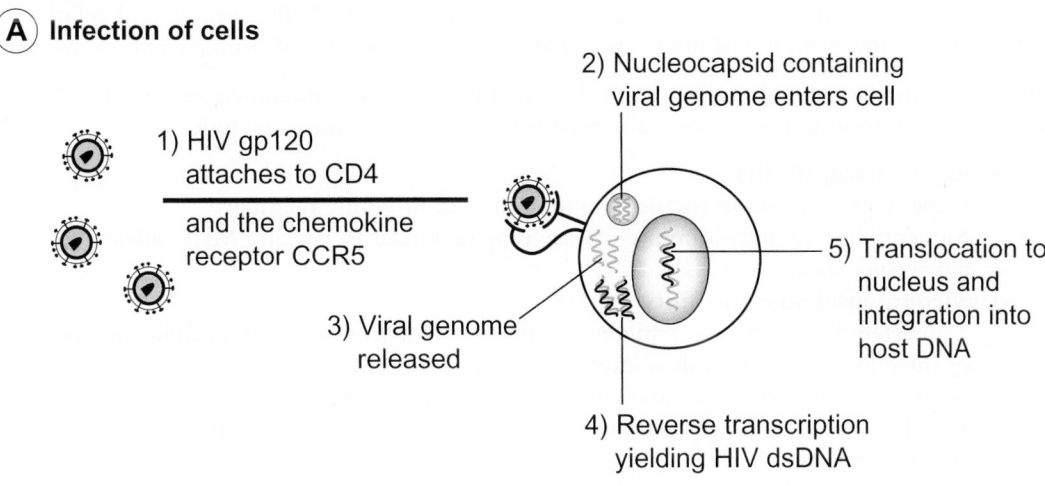

1) HIV gp120 attaches to CD4

and the chemokine receptor CCR5

2) Nucleocapsid containing viral genome enters cell

3) Viral genome released

4) Reverse transcription yielding HIV dsDNA

5) Translocation to nucleus and integration into host DNA

### (B) Effects

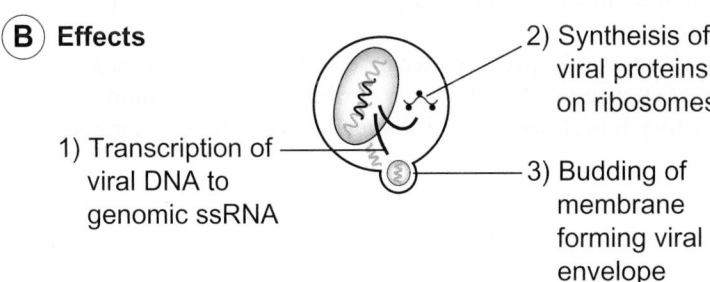

1) Transcription of viral DNA to genomic ssRNA

2) Syntheisis of viral proteins on ribosomes

3) Budding of membrane forming viral envelope

4) Virions that can infect other cells
Infected cells have a half-life of around 15 days

*Note*: Individuals with certain mutations in the CCR5 (C chemokine receptor 5) receptor are resistant to HIV. These mutations are more prevalent in Caucasian populations compared with African populations.

# AUTO-IMMUNE DISEASES

Auto-immune diseases result from, or are associated with, an immune response against the individual's own cells, or in some cases cell products. Although both humoral and cellular immunity are involved, it is thought that changes in the latter are of primary importance.

In auto-immunity, something occurs to destroy integrity of self-tolerance (see p. 140). The aetiology of auto-immunity is not fully established. Potential causes include:

1. **Genetic susceptibility**
   - Genetic predisposition to auto-immune disease in family members.
   - Susceptibility to auto-immune disease may be linked to specific MHC alleles, e.g. ankylosing spondylitis HLA B27.

2. **Environmental susceptibility**
   - Sequestered antigen – an antigen is exposed to the immune system following injury or infection, e.g. myocarditis after myocardial infarction.
   - Molecular mimicry – microbial antigens cross-react with self-antigens.
   - Polyclonal activation – infectious agents can act as superantigens triggering many B and T cell clones.

3. **Other triggers of auto-immunity**
   - Hormones, e.g. SLE (systemic lupus erythematosus) is more common in females and may be triggered by oestrogen.
   - Drugs – certain drugs may act as a **hapten** rendering a self-antigen immunogenic.
   - T suppressor cells – loss of suppressor T cells can contribute to auto-immunity, e.g. individuals with inflammatory bowel disease and diabetes have reduced numbers of T suppressor cells.

# AUTO-IMMUNE DISEASES

Auto-immune diseases were traditionally classified as organ specific and non-organ specific. However, since there is some crossover between these two groups, they can be classified by the predominant effector mechanism leading to organ damage.

## PREDOMINANTLY ANTIBODY-MEDIATED AUTO-IMMUNE DISEASE

| AUTOANTIGEN | TARGET ORGAN | DISEASE |
|---|---|---|
| Red blood cells | Red blood cells | Haemolytic anaemia |
| Acetylcholine receptor | Voluntary muscle | Myasthenia gravis |
| Thyroid stimulating hormone receptor | Thyroid | Graves disease |
| Nuclear constituents, e.g. DNA | Many – kidney, skin, blood vessels, joint, heart | Systemic lupus erythematosus |

## PREDOMINANTLY T CELL-MEDIATED AUTO-IMMUNE DISEASE

| AUTOANTIGEN | TARGET ORGAN | DISEASE |
|---|---|---|
| Myelin basic protein | Central nervous system | Multiple sclerosis |
| β-Islet cells | Pancreas | Type 1 insulin-dependent diabetes mellitus |
| Thyroglobulin Microsomal antigens Thyroid peroxidase | Thyroid | Hashimoto thyroiditis |
| IgG | Synovium/joints | Rheumatoid arthritis |

# AUTO-IMMUNE DISEASES

Primary thyrotoxicosis (Graves disease) and myasthenia gravis are of particular interest. In these diseases, specific auto-immune antibodies combine with antigen on the cell surface and either stimulate or block the action of the physiological agent which would normally turn on the activity of the cell.

## Stimulatory effect

In Graves disease, excessive amounts of thyroid hormone are produced. LATS (long acting thyroid stimulator), an IgG auto-antibody, combines with antigen on the thyroid cell surface and produces changes mimicking those produced by TSH (thyroid stimulating hormone) physiologically manufactured by the pituitary.

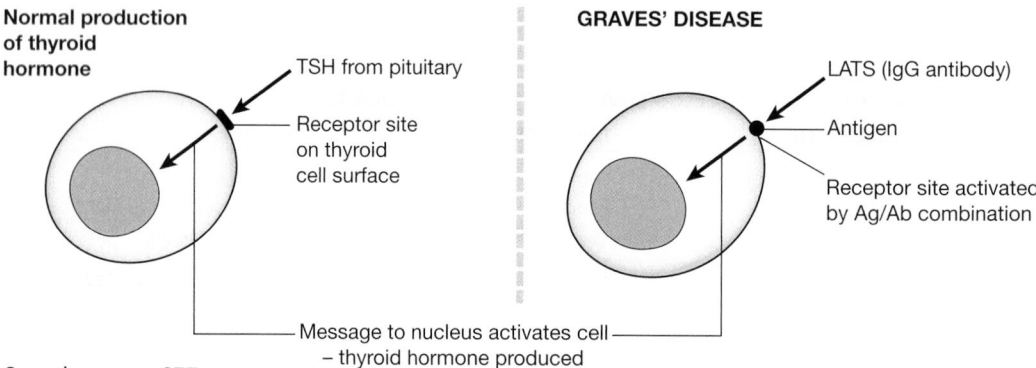

*See also page 677.*

See also page 677.

## Blocking effect

In myasthenia gravis the acetylcholine formed at the motor nerve endings is prevented from stimulating the muscle motor end plate due to the antibody blocking the specific acetylcholine receptors. The end plate is also damaged (Ag/Ab + complement).

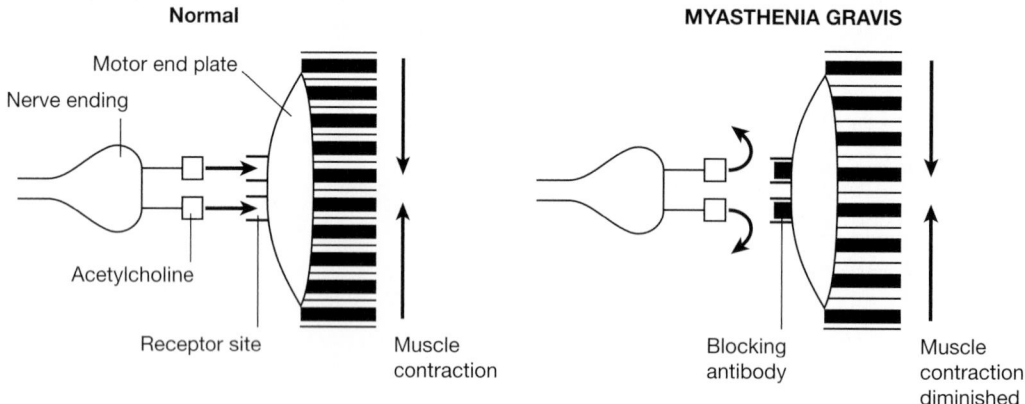

# APPLIED IMMUNOLOGY

## Immunohistochemical identification

Immunohistochemistry is now well established and allows identification of specific substances in histological sections.

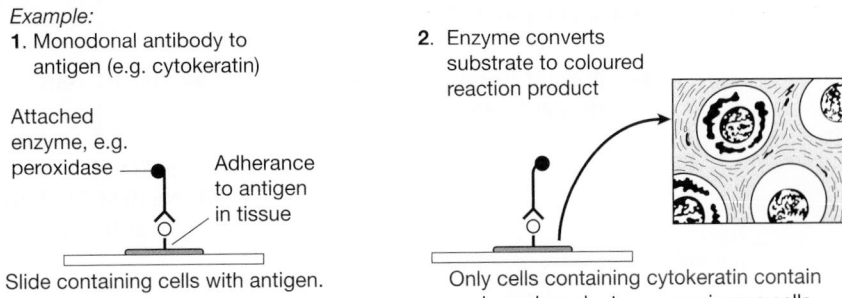

*Example:*

**1.** Monodonal antibody to antigen (e.g. cytokeratin)

Attached enzyme, e.g. peroxidase —

Adherance to antigen in tissue

Slide containing cells with antigen.

**2.** Enzyme converts substrate to coloured reaction product

Only cells containing cytokeratin contain coloured product, e.g. carcinoma cells.

This or similar techniques are used to identify a wide range of substances. Immunohistochemistry is now a major ancillary technique used in the pathology laboratory to subtype cancers.

## Flow cytometry

In this technique, cells in suspension are labelled by fluorescent markers, excited by a laser and counted electronically by passing them through a flow cytometer. This is the technique employed, among others, for monitoring CD4+ counts in HIV.

## Prophylaxis and treatment of infections

1. **Passive immunisation** is the term used when antibody formed in one individual is given to another individual who is at risk of infection – the protection is temporary. Examples include:

   Pooled human γ-globulin → general protection → particularly useful in cases of immune deficiency in agammaglobulinaemia.

2. **Active immunisation** is the term used when the infective agent is modified in some way to eliminate its harmful effects without loss of antigenicity. The subject's own immune response is activated. Examples include:

   TOXOID – e.g. tetanus toxin modified chemically.

   KILLED ORGANISMS – e.g. TAB (typhoid, paratyphoid A and B) vaccine.

   ATTENUATED ORGANISMS – e.g. viruses; cowpox, polio, measles.

   GENETICALLY ENGINEERED – e.g. hepatitis B (HBV) where recombinant DNA technology is used to manufacture specific HBV proteins.

## Monoclonal antibodies

These are formed by immortalising a single clone of plasma cells, by fusion with myeloma cells, so that a large amount of identical antibody is produced.

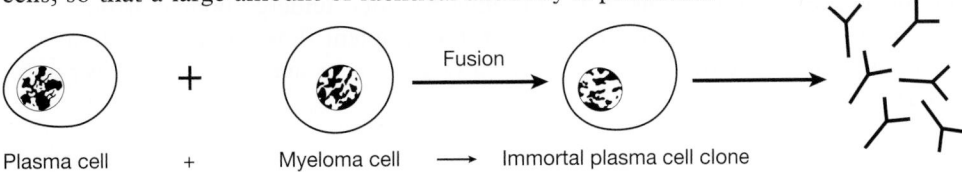

Plasma cell    +    Myeloma cell  ⟶  Immortal plasma cell clone

Fusion

*Note*: Monoclonal antibodies can now be constructed from Ig gene libraries.

# APPLIED IMMUNOLOGY – TISSUE TRANSPLANTATION

In the past, allografting (transplanting of tissues or organs from one individual to another of the same species) inevitably led to rejection of the graft by the host. Understanding of the mechanisms has allowed intervention so that nowadays successful survival of grafts is usual (e.g. 90% survival of renal transplants after 1 year).

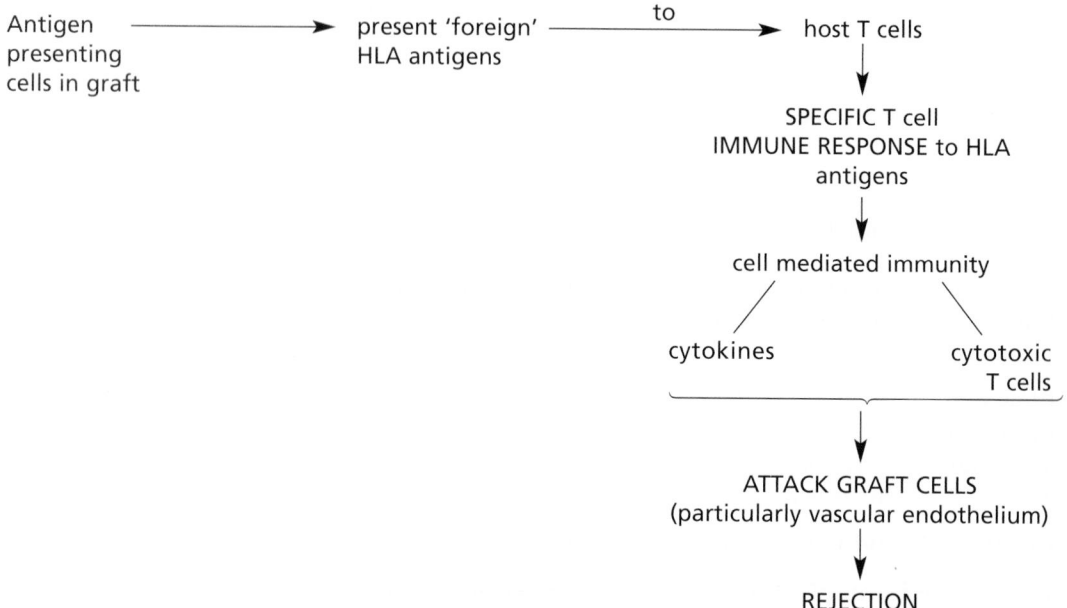

Rejection may also occur, very rapidly, if pre-existing antibodies are present (e.g. due to previous incompatible blood transfusion or pregnancy) – leading to activation of complement with haemolysis.

Usually rejection takes weeks while the cell mediated immune response is building up.

The remarkable improvement in transplant prognosis is due to:

(a) Careful matching of HLA compatibility between donor and recipient.
(b) Use of immunosuppressive agents (particularly cyclosporin A).
(c) Screening for the presence of pre-existing HLA and cytotoxic antibodies.

Paradoxically the pre-transplant transfusion of compatible blood improves the chances of graft survival.

## GRAFT VERSUS HOST DISEASE

When immunosuppressed individuals (e.g. leukaemia patients) undergo bone marrow transplantation, T cells from the graft proliferate in the recipient (host) and establish an immune response against the host tissues: the main target organs are the skin, the liver and the alimentary tract.

# NEOPLASIA

## OBJECTIVES

1. To know the main pathological features and behaviour of benign and malignant tumours.
2. To classify malignant tumours according to tissue of origin.
3. To understand how tumours spread.
4. To have knowledge of the utility of tumour markers.
5. To know about oncogenes and tumour suppressor genes and their role in carcinogenesis.
6. To understand the stepwise process of carcinogenesis.

# NEOPLASIA

Cancer is the second commonest cause of death (25%) in the Western world after heart disease. Knowledge of non-neoplastic proliferation is helpful in understanding neoplasia.

Physiological proliferation occurs:

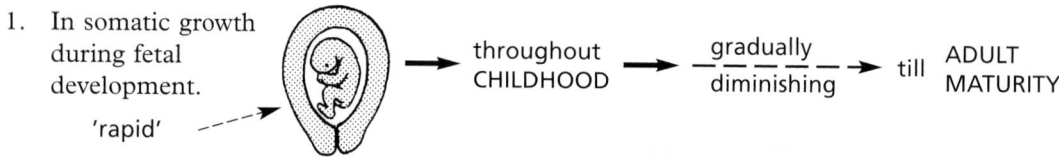

1. In somatic growth during fetal development.
   'rapid'
   throughout CHILDHOOD → gradually diminishing → till ADULT MATURITY

2. In tissues where constant proliferation is needed in RAPID CELL TURNOVER from stem cells (p. 59), e.g. in:

   (a) bone marrow          (b) gut epithelium          (c) skin

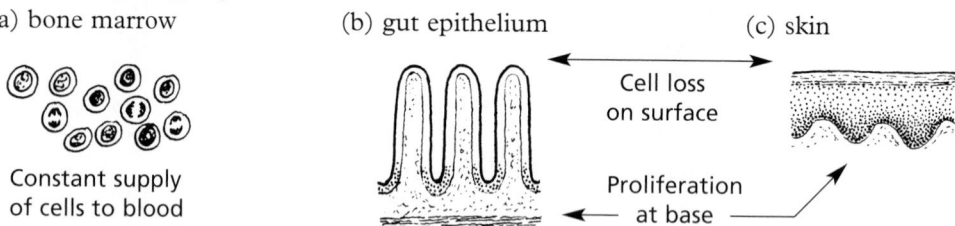

   Constant supply of cells to blood

   Cell loss on surface

   Proliferation at base

3. Proliferation at a much slower rate occurs in tissues where cell turnover is low, e.g. LIVER, but will increase rapidly following injury.

ENLARGEMENT of an organ due to increase in the parenchymal cell mass may be due to:
   (1) an increase in the size of the individual cells – **hypertrophy**
   or (2) an increase in the number of cells – **hyperplasia**
   or (3) commonly a combination of (1) and (2).

The stimuli responsible are:   (a)   increase in functional demand
                                (b)   increased trophic hormonal activity
*Physiological enlargement* of organs is common. An example of this is the increase in muscle bulk which occurs during training and the enlargement of uterus and breasts in pregnancy.
*Pathological* enlargement is the result of disease processes.

## HYPERTROPHY

Enlargement of the heart as a result of hypertension is a good example of hypertrophy. There is an increase in the size of the myocardial cells as a result of the increased functional demand required to maintain the high blood pressure.

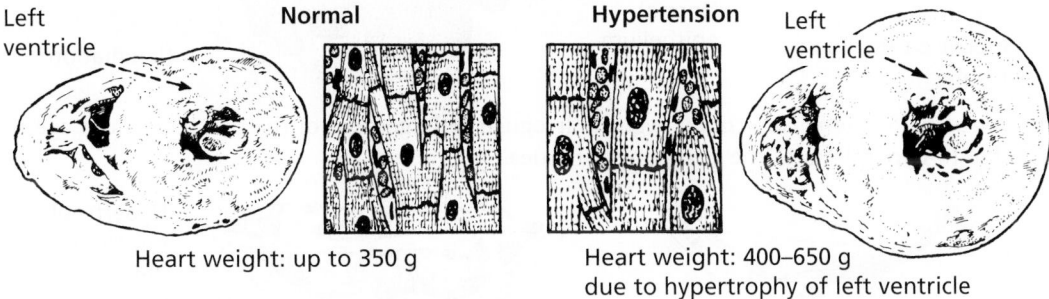

Left ventricle
**Normal**
**Hypertension**
Left ventricle

Heart weight: up to 350 g

Heart weight: 400–650 g due to hypertrophy of left ventricle

# NON-NEOPLASTIC PROLIFERATION

### HYPERPLASIA

The two main causes are:

(a) *Chronic irritation* (and inflammation), e.g. in the skin, increased thickness results.

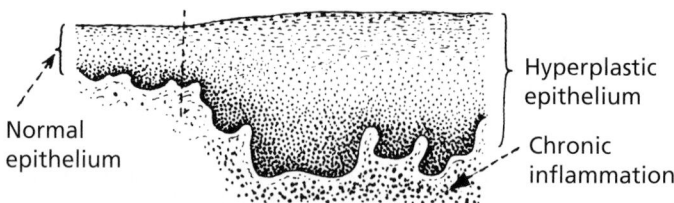

Normal epithelium

Hyperplastic epithelium

Chronic inflammation

(b) *Imbalance of hormonal activity*, e.g. the irregular enlargement of the prostate in old age is due to hyperplasia of the component tissues.

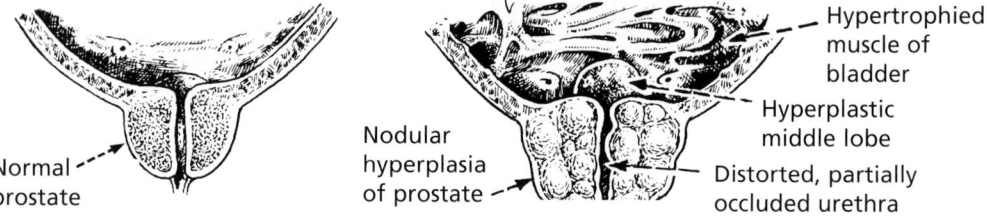

Normal prostate

Nodular hyperplasia of prostate

Hypertrophied muscle of bladder

Hyperplastic middle lobe

Distorted, partially occluded urethra

*Note*: If the abnormal stimulus is removed, the affected organ can return to normal.

### METAPLASIA

This is a change from one type of differentiated tissue to another, usually of the same broad class but often less well specialised. The change is commonly seen in lining epithelia but occurs also in connective tissues. There is frequently an associated hyperplasia.

Reflux of acid results in metaplasia of the squamous epithelium of the lower oesophagus to glandular mucosa (Barrett oesophagus p. 324)

Change from mucus-secreted epithelium to stratified squamous epithelium as in the bronchial irritation associated with smoking

Chronic inflammation

**Bronchus**

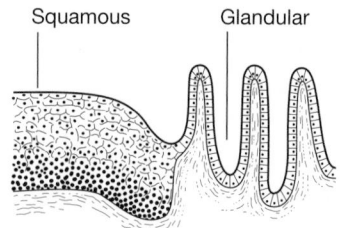

Squamous   Glandular

**Oesophagus**

### DYSPLASIA

This term refers to disordered growth which is frequently the precursor of malignancy. It is described on page 190.

# NEOPLASTIC PROLIFERATION

A tumour is a proliferation of cells which persists after the stimulus which initiated it has been withdrawn, i.e. it is autonomous. It is:

1. **Progressive**

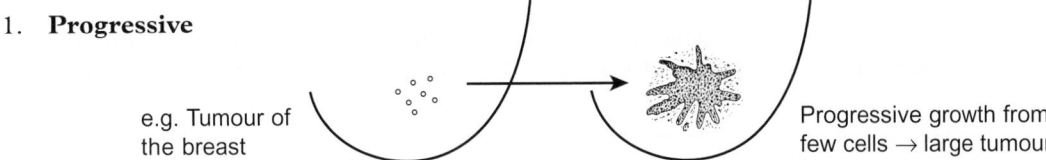

e.g. Tumour of the breast

Progressive growth from few cells → large tumour

2. **Purposeless**

e.g. Tumour of fibrous tissue

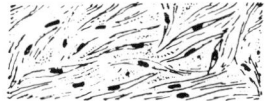   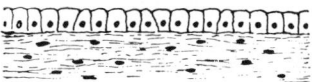

The fibres of a tumour of fibrous tissue have no regular arrangement and serve no useful purpose.

In normal fibrous tissue, the strands have a definite arrangement, supporting some structure such as an epithelial surface.

3. **Regardless of surrounding tissue**

e.g. Smooth muscle tumour of uterus compresses normal tissues and distorts uterine cavity.

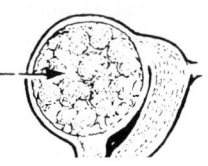

4. **Not related to needs of the body**

e.g. In leukaemia: these tumours of bone marrow produce needlessly, enormous numbers of leucocytes which fill the marrow, and then enter the blood stream.

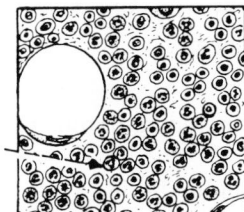   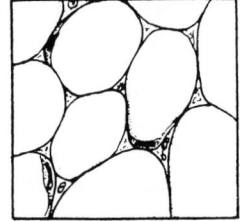

**Normal marrow**

5. **Parasitic**

The tumour draws its nourishment from the body while contributing nothing to its function. It induces the body to provide a blood supply and, in the case of epithelial tumours, a supporting stroma.

# NEOPLASMS – CLASSIFICATION

Tumours may be classified in two ways: (1) clinical behaviour and (2) histological origin.

## 1. CLINICAL BEHAVIOUR

The tumour is classified according to its morbid anatomy and behaviour. Two main groups are recognised – *benign* (simple) and *malignant*. The contrast between these two groups is as follows:

| | BENIGN | MALIGNANT |
|---|---|---|
| **Spread (the most important feature)** | Remains localised | Cells transferred via lymphatics, blood vessels, tissue planes and serous cavities to set up satellite tumours (metastases) |
| **Rate of growth** | Usually slow | Usually rapid |
| **Boundaries** | Circumscribed, often encapsulated | Irregular, ill-defined and non-encapsulated |
| **Relationship to surrounding tissues** | Compresses normal tissue | Invades and destroys normal tissues |
| **Effects** | Produced by pressure on vessels, tubes, nerves, organs, and by excess production of substances, e.g. hormones. Removal will alleviate these | Destroys structures, causes bleeding, forms strictures |

In practice, there is a spectrum of malignancy. Some tumours may grow locally and invade normal tissues but never produce metastases. Others will produce metastases only after a very considerable time, while at the other end of the spectrum, there are tumours which metastasise very early in their development.

## 2. HISTOLOGICAL ORIGIN

Tumours may arise from any tissue in the body and they can be conveniently accommodated in five groups:

1. Epithelia
2. Mesenchymal tissues including fibrous tissue, bone, cartilage and vessels
3. Neuroectoderm
4. Haemopoietic and lymphoid cells
5. Germ cells.

The commonest tumours arise from tissues which have a rapid turnover of cells and which are exposed to environmental mutagens, e.g. epithelium of mucous membranes, skin, breast and reproductive organs, as well as lymphoid and haemopoietic tissues.

# BENIGN TUMOURS – HISTOLOGY

In general, the cells of benign tumours are well differentiated. They:

1. **Mimic the structure of their parent tissue.**

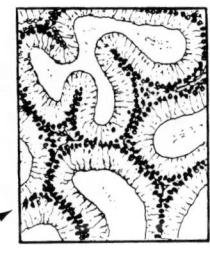

e.g. In an adenoma (simple gland-forming tumour) of colon the cells arrange themselves in acini.

In a skin papilloma (wart) the squamous epithelium still forms a covering for underlying connective tissue

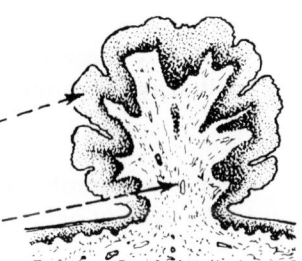

2. **Resemble the cells of their tissue of origin.**

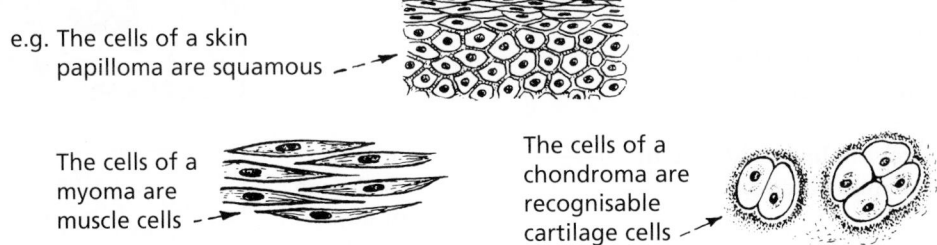

e.g. The cells of a skin papilloma are squamous

The cells of a myoma are muscle cells

The cells of a chondroma are recognisable cartilage cells

3. As in normal tissue, **show a remarkable uniformity in size, shape and nuclear configuration.**

4. **Show evidence of normal function.**

This may be useless, e.g.

or

pathological, e.g. excess secretion of parathyroid hormone by a parathyroid adenoma.

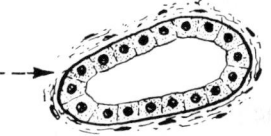

Mucous secretion in acinus of an adenoma

5. **Have relatively infrequent mitotic figures:** these are of normal type.

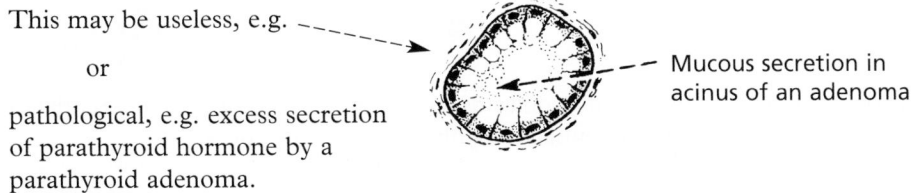

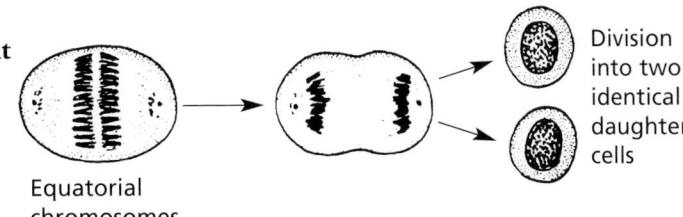

Division into two identical daughter cells

Equatorial chromosomes

# MALIGNANT TUMOURS – HISTOLOGY

The cells of malignant tumours tend to be less well differentiated than those of benign tumours.

They:

1. **Generally show a haphazard arrangement.** —————→ e.g. Carcinoma of breast

2. **Bear less resemblance to the cells of origin.**

3. **Tend to vary widely in size, shape and nuclear configuration, reflecting an increase in chromosomal number and DNA content (aneuploidy).** —————→ e.g. Pleomorphic sarcoma

4. **Provide less evidence of normal function.** —————→ e.g. Adeno carcinoma of bowel (secretory activity limited)

5. **Show frequent mitoses often of abnormal type.**

Three daughter cells

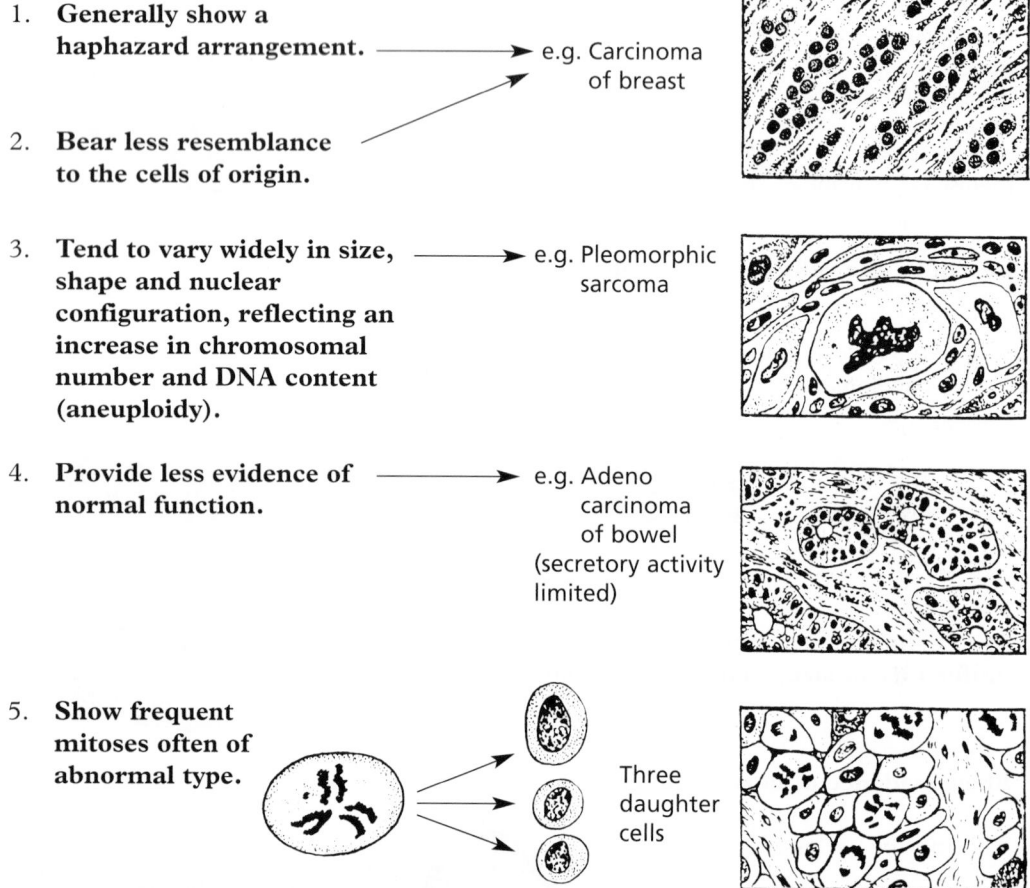

There is a spectrum within malignant neoplasms from slowly growing well-differentiated examples to rapidly growing undifferentiated highly malignant tumours.

# BENIGN EPITHELIAL TUMOURS

Benign epithelial tumours are essentially of two types: (1) papillomas and (2) adenomas.

## PAPILLOMA

Papillomas take origin from an epithelial surface. As the epithelium proliferates it is thrown into folds which become increasingly complex.

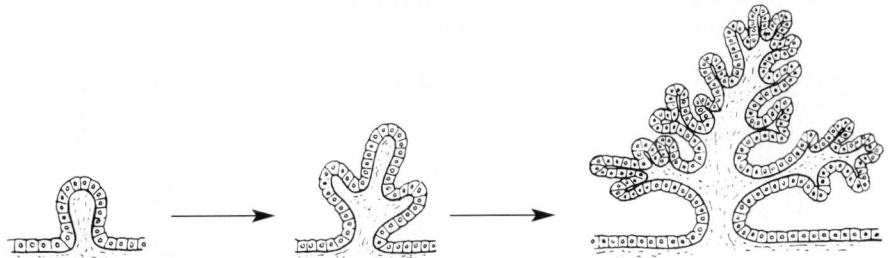

The epithelial proliferation is accompanied by a corresponding growth of supporting connective tissue and blood vessels.

Typical examples are found in the skin, e.g. the common wart.

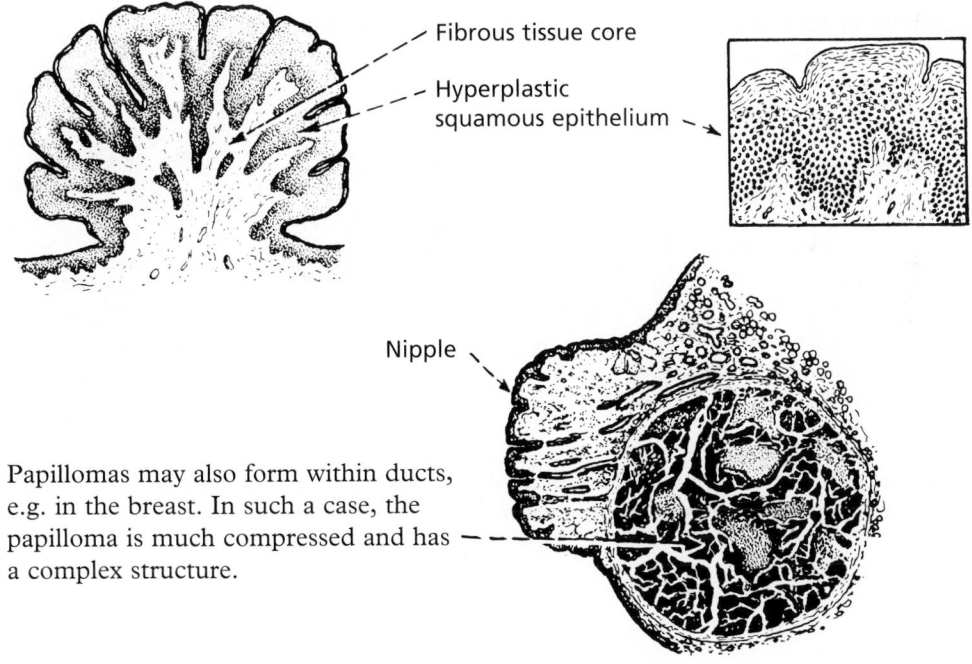

Fibrous tissue core

Hyperplastic squamous epithelium

Nipple

Papillomas may also form within ducts, e.g. in the breast. In such a case, the papilloma is much compressed and has a complex structure.

In these benign tumours:

(a) The normal arrangement of epithelial cells is maintained, e.g. in skin papillomas the surface cells are squamous and proliferation is confined to the deepest layers.
(b) The relationship of epithelium to connective tissue is normal.
(c) Blood vessels are well formed.

# BENIGN EPITHELIAL TUMOURS

### ADENOMA

Adenomas are derived from the ducts and acini of glands, although the name is also used to cover simple tumours arising in solid epithelial organs.

Again the proliferation of epithelium of a gland causes the formation of tubules which ramify and become compound. The original communication with the parent gland duct or acinus tends to become lost.

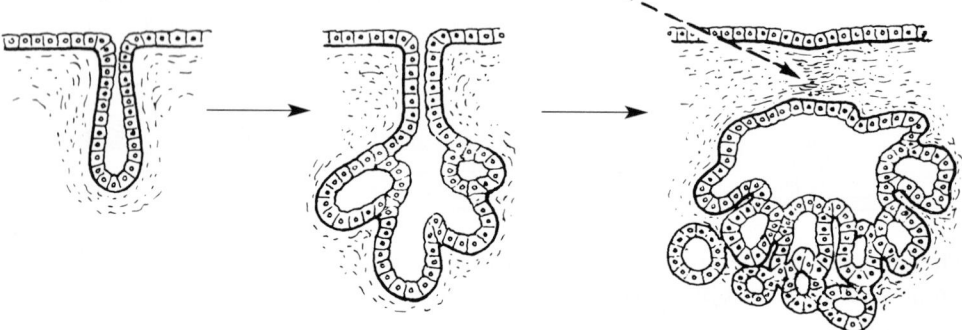

In the case of a hollow viscus, such as the intestine, the adenomatous proliferation, instead of growing down into the underlying connective tissue, is usually pushed upwards into the lumen of the viscus.

The growth therefore combines the features of a papilloma and an adenoma. The term adenomatous polyp is often applied in such a case.

# BENIGN EPITHELIAL TUMOURS

In the type which grows into the subjacent connective tissue, the progressive budding of the epithelium results in new acini which become nipped off from the parent acini.

In cases in which retention of secretion is marked, a cyst forms and the tumour is then called a **CYSTADENOMA** which may reach an enormous size, e.g. some cystadenomas of the ovary may be 30–40 cm in diameter, particularly those which secrete mucus.

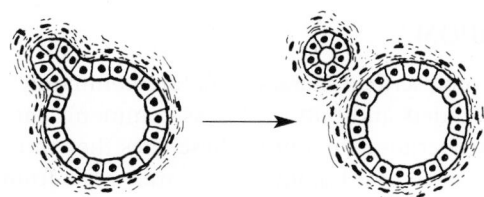

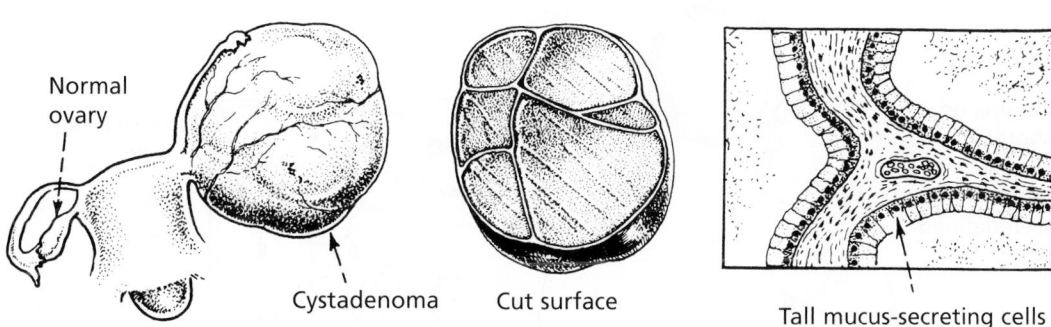

Normal ovary

Cystadenoma    Cut surface

Tall mucus-secreting cells

As in a hollow viscus, the proliferating epithelium may be heaped to form papillomas and the tumour then becomes a **PAPILLARY CYSTADENOMA**. These are also common in the ovary (see p. 549).

## FIBROADENOMA

In the breast, the term is clinically useful for a small nodule consisting of a mixture of acinar elements and prominent supporting fibrous tissue. The histological appearances are variable depending on the distribution of the fibrous tissue (see also p. 560).

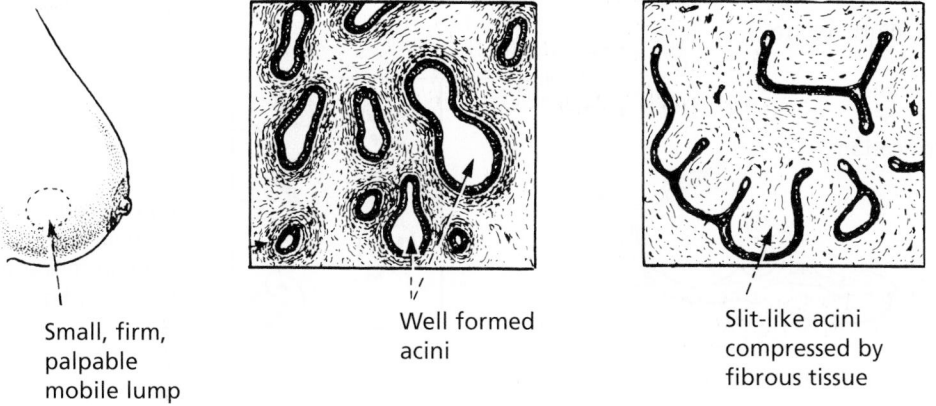

Small, firm, palpable mobile lump

Well formed acini

Slit-like acini compressed by fibrous tissue

# BENIGN CONNECTIVE TISSUE TUMOURS

Benign connective tissue tumours are composed of mature connective tissues – fat, cartilage, bone and blood vessels. They tend to form encapsulated rounded or lobulated masses which compress the surrounding tissues.

## LIPOMA

Circumscribed masses of fat are commonly found in the subcutaneous tissue of the arms, shoulders and buttocks. Less commonly they occur in the deep soft tissues of the limbs or retroperitoneum, but at these sites they must be carefully distinguished from low-grade liposarcomas. Lipomas very rarely arise from the viscera.

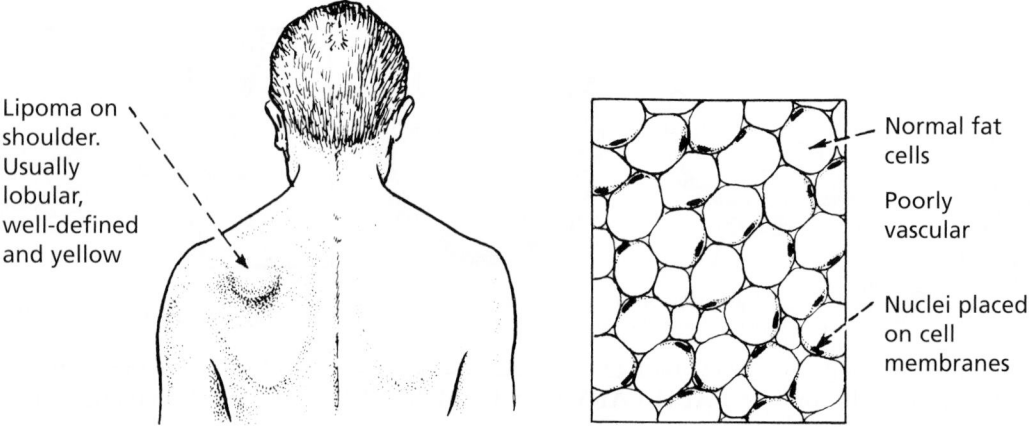

Lipoma on shoulder. Usually lobular, well-defined and yellow

Normal fat cells

Poorly vascular

Nuclei placed on cell membranes

## CHONDROMA

A chondroma usually arises within the medullary cavity of the tubular bones of the hands and feet. It grows slowly, causing gradual expansion of the bone. Less commonly it occurs in long bones. Rarely multiple enchondromas appear in children and are associated with deformity. They occasionally become malignant.

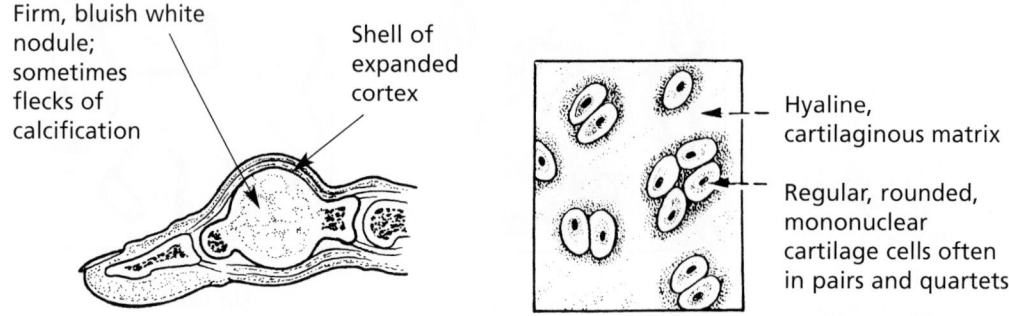

Firm, bluish white nodule; sometimes flecks of calcification

Shell of expanded cortex

Hyaline, cartilaginous matrix

Regular, rounded, mononuclear cartilage cells often in pairs and quartets

# BENIGN CONNECTIVE TISSUE TUMOURS

## OSTEOMA

This tumour is mainly found in the bones of the skull, although it may occur in long bones. Osteomas are relatively small but may produce severe symptoms because of their situation.

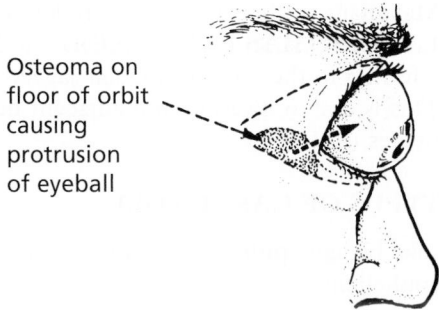

Osteoma on floor of orbit causing protrusion of eyeball

## LEIOMYOMA (FIBROID)

The majority of benign smooth muscle tumours occur in the wall of the uterus where they are extremely common, but may lie within the uterine cavity or attached to the serosa. They are firm, rounded masses which usually begin in the myometrium.

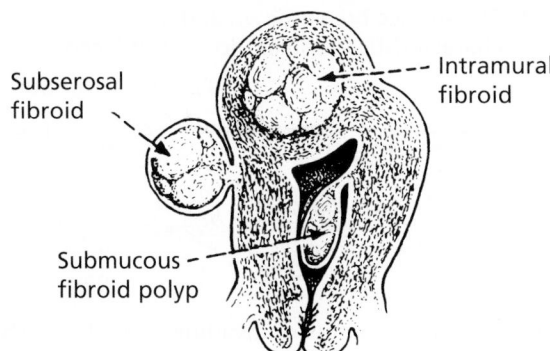

Subserosal fibroid

Intramural fibroid

Submucous fibroid polyp

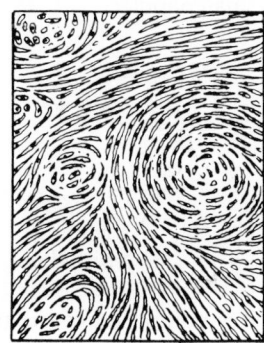

Cells and fibres in parallel bundles which in turn are whorled

## TUMOURS OF FIBROUS TISSUE

So-called 'fibromas' are rare, but tumour-like growths are fairly common. An example is a FIBROMATOSIS.

***Palmar fibromatosis***, at first nodular, causes flexion deformities of fingers (Dupuytren's contracture) due to contraction of fibrous tissue within the palmar fascia. A similar condition may affect the plantar fascia. Deeply located fibromatoses behave in a locally aggressive manner.

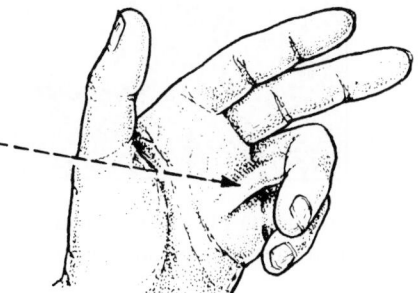

Benign tumours of PERIPHERAL NERVE and of VESSELS are described on pages 267 and 624.

# MALIGNANT EPITHELIAL TUMOURS

Malignant epithelial tumours are known as **CARCINOMAS** (Greek '*karkinos*': a crab), referring to the typical irregular jagged shape. This is due to invasion into adjacent normal tissues (p. 180).

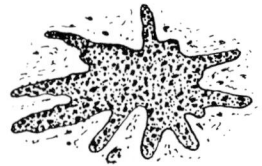

## TYPES OF CARCINOMA

Like benign epithelial tumours, carcinomas can arise from squamous or glandular epithelium.

## SQUAMOUS CELL CARCINOMA

This is commonly found on the skin, especially exposed surfaces, but also develops in other sites covered by stratified squamous epithelium, e.g. lips, tongue, pharynx, oesophagus and vagina. In addition, it may occur on surfaces covered by glandular-type epithelium through metaplastic transformation as in the bronchus, gall bladder and uterine cervix. It frequently arises from areas of carcinoma-in-situ (p. 189).

1. It starts as a small papular mass

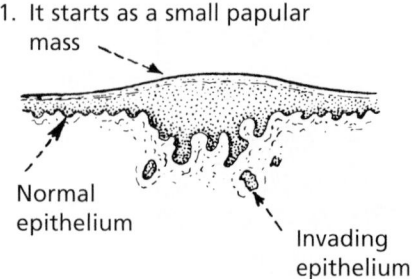

2. The surface breaks down and a characteristic irregular ulcer is produced.

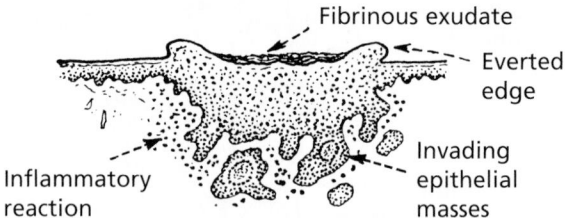

Histologically, it is composed of irregular strands and columns of invading epithelium which infiltrate the underlying connective tissue. If well differentiated, the central cells of the invading masses show conversion into eosinophilic keratin, while the outer layer consists of young basophilic cells. In cross section, the appearance is typical.

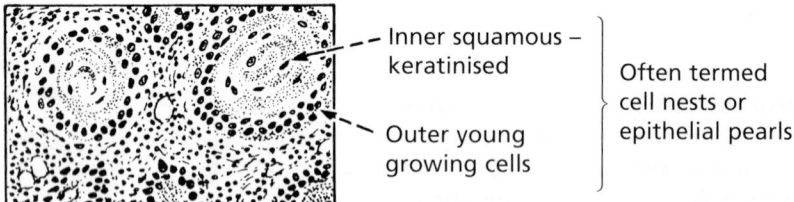

Squamous carcinoma of skin is typically well differentiated and slow growing. In contrast, uterine cervical carcinomas can be poorly differentiated and spread early to draining lymph nodes.

# TYPES OF CARCINOMA

## BASAL CELL CARCINOMA (RODENT ULCER)

This tumour may arise in any part of the skin but is most common in the face, near the eyes and nose.

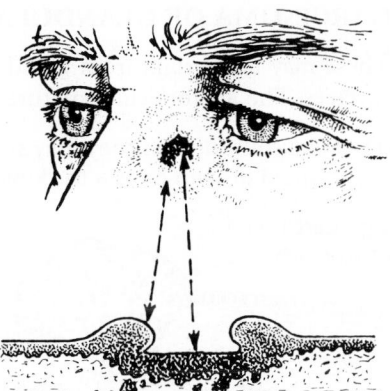

### First stage

It starts as a flattened papilloma which slowly enlarges over months or years.

### Second stage

The surface breaks down and a shallow, ragged ulcer with pearly edges is formed.

Usually the malignant tissue spreads slowly but progressively. It is composed of cells resembling those of the basal layer of the skin. It has a characteristic histological appearance.

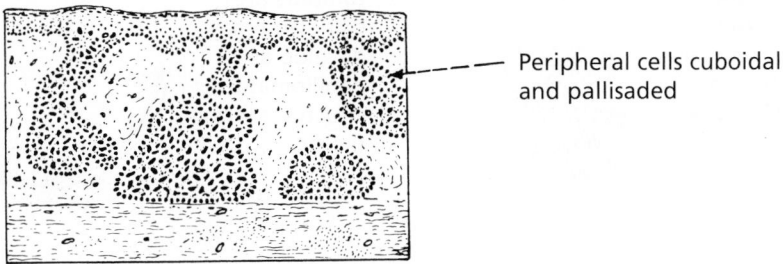

Peripheral cells cuboidal and pallisaded

There are many histological variants.

Basal cell carcinoma is a locally invasive growth which can be extremely destructive (hence its name: Rodent ulcer). It almost never metastasises. Thus the two processes of local invasion and distant metastases are not necessarily linked.

# TYPES OF CARCINOMA

### CARCINOMA OF GLANDULAR ORGANS

These may take origin from gland acini, ducts or the glandular epithelium of mucous surfaces. The anatomical structure varies.

(a) On mucous surfaces they may start as a polypoid growth or as a thick plaque.

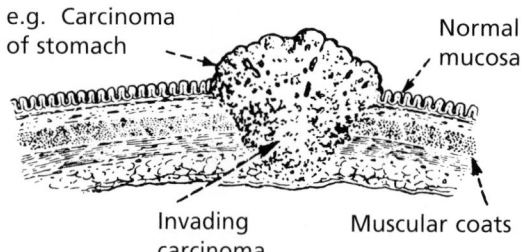

e.g. Carcinoma of stomach

Normal mucosa

Invading carcinoma

Muscular coats

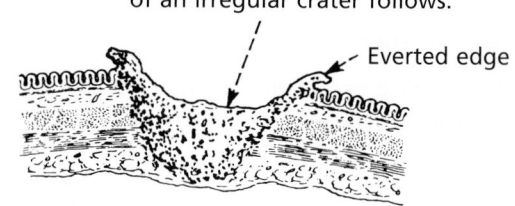

Ulceration with the formation of an irregular crater follows.

Everted edge

(b) In compound glands, e.g. the breast, the cancer forms an irregular penetrating mass – the typical crablike appearance.

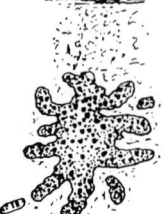

(c) Some malignant tumours are cystic and may develop as papillomatous structures within the cyst.

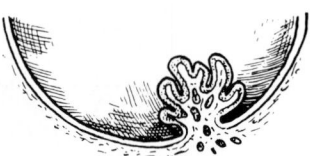

# TYPES OF CARCINOMA

Histologically, carcinomas of glandular tissue have three basic forms.

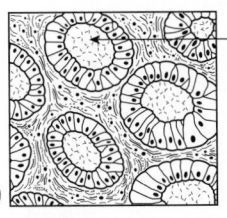

Adenocarcinoma: the tumour cells usually form gland-like structures.

Typically seen in linitis plastica. These tumours consist of **signet ring cells.**

Extracellular mucin may also be present.

Globules of mucin push the nucleus to one side.

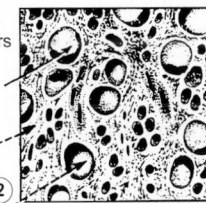

The individual cells may form intracellular gland-like structures. The resulting cell is known as a signet ring cell carcinoma.
– this is commonly seen in the stomach.

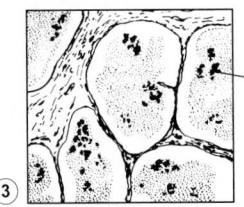

Occasionally a carcinoma will produce large quantities of mucus and merit the term mucoid carcinoma.
The tumours consist of only a few carcinoma cells in large lakes of mucus. They are commonest in organs normally containing large numbers of mucus-secreting cells, e.g. large intestine and stomach, but may also occur in the breast.

# MALIGNANT CONNECTIVE TISSUE TUMOURS

Malignant connective tissue tumours are referred to as Sarcomas (Greek '*sarkoma*': flesh). They arise in soft tissue, in bone and rarely in viscera.

Sarcomas are far less common than carcinomas, but are second in frequency to leukaemias and lymphomas in childhood and early adult life.

Unlike the ill-defined infiltrative carcinomas, sarcomas are large well-defined fleshy tumours. Naked eye assessment suggests that they are encapsulated, but histology shows that this is a false impression. Malignant cells do infiltrate between normal tissues at the margin, so that surgical 'shelling out' is almost inevitably followed by local recurrence from aggregates of cells remaining in the tumour bed.

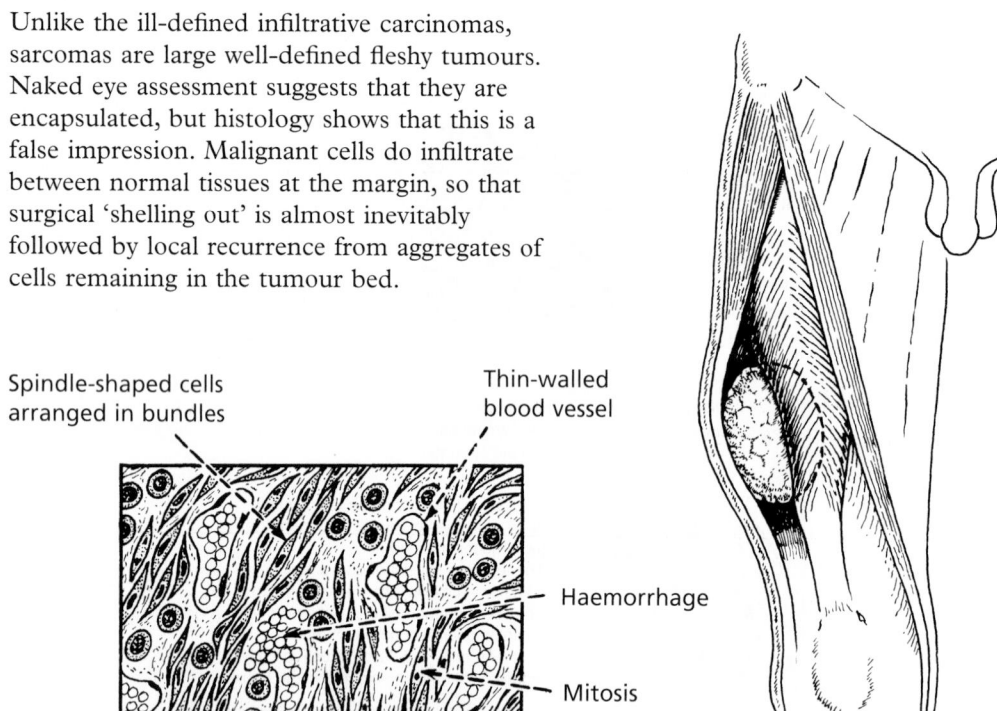

Spindle-shaped cells arranged in bundles

Thin-walled blood vessel

Haemorrhage

Mitosis

Most sarcomas consist of spindle-shaped cells, although some are of round cell type. They may be associated with the formation of many large thin-walled blood vessels which are easily invaded by sarcoma cells. Blood borne metastases to lung are common. In contrast, lymph node involvement is rare in most types of sarcoma.

# SARCOMAS

Many different histological types of sarcoma have been described. The nomenclature is based on adding the suffix 'sarcoma' to the type of differentiation shown, e.g. chondrosarcoma, liposarcoma, leiomyosarcoma (cartilage, adipose tissue, smooth muscle).

In general, the grade of the tumour is of more prognostic importance than the precise histological type. Some of the commoner forms of sarcoma are described here.

### Liposarcoma

This tumour arises in soft tissues of the limbs and retroperitoneum. A number of subtypes are described. Primitive fat containing cells (lipoblasts) are a feature.

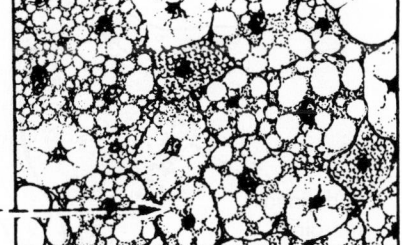

Pleomorphic cells with numerous droplets of lipid.

Well-differentiated liposarcoma has a good prognosis and rarely metastasises. Pleomorphic and round cell liposarcomas are highly aggressive tumours which metastasise early.

### Synovial sarcoma

This is a misnomer as the tumour does not arise from synovium. It has a typical microscopic appearance. Many tumours are biphasic – with both epithelioid and spindled forms. The majority are associated with a specific translocation t(X:18), which can be detected by molecular techniques.

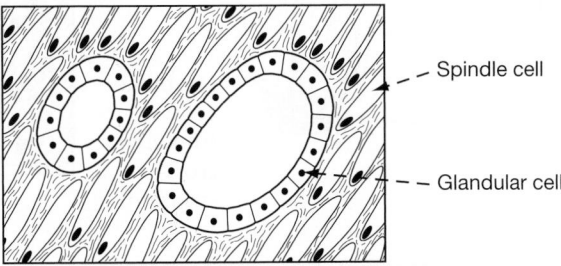

Spindle cell

Glandular cell

# SARCOMAS

### MYOSARCOMA (SARCOMA OF MUSCLE)

There are two varieties:

1. **Leiomyosarcoma**
   This is a malignant tumour of smooth muscle.
   These rare tumours arise in the skin, deep soft
   tissues and particularly in the uterus.

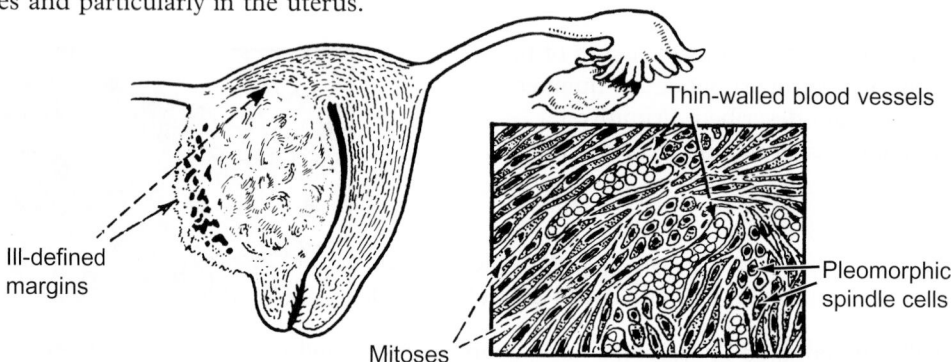

Thin-walled blood vessels

Ill-defined margins

Pleomorphic spindle cells

Mitoses

2. **Rhabdomyosarcoma**
   This is a malignant
   tumour of skeletal muscle.
   It is a rare tumour
   occurring mainly in
   children. It occurs very
   rarely in skeletal muscles.
   They may occur as
   polypoid tumours in the
   bladder, uterus and vagina,
   sometimes called sarcoma
   botryoides (grape-like).

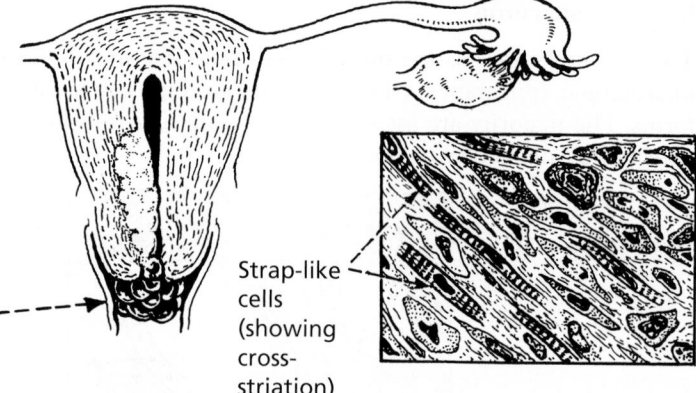

Strap-like cells (showing cross-striation)

### Pleomorphic or anaplastic sarcoma

Many highly malignant
sarcomas are so poorly
differentiated that their
specific type cannot be
determined.

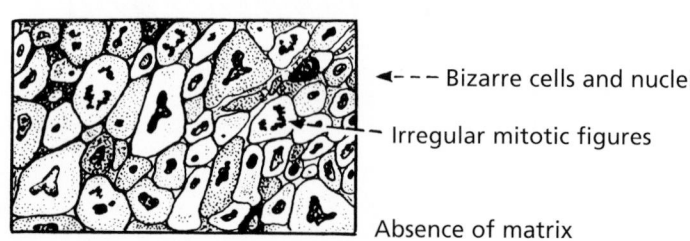

- - - Bizarre cells and nuclei

Irregular mitotic figures

Absence of matrix

Immunocytochemistry, electron microscopy and cytogenetic analysis (demonstrating typical chromosome translocations) all help in reaching more specific diagnoses than can be reached by conventional histology alone.

Sarcomas of bone are described on page 646.

# OTHER TUMOUR TYPES

### TERATOMA

This is a tumour derived from totipotent germ cells. Most arise in the **ovary (usually benign)** and **testis (almost always malignant)**. They may also occur at any site in the mid-line where germ cells have stopped in their migration to the gonads.

For example, **mature teratoma (**dermoid cyst**)** is typically seen in the ovary.

It consists mainly of ectodermal structures such as skin and its appendages and neural tissue. Frequently respiratory epithelium, intestinal epithelium, bone and cartilage are present.

**Sites**

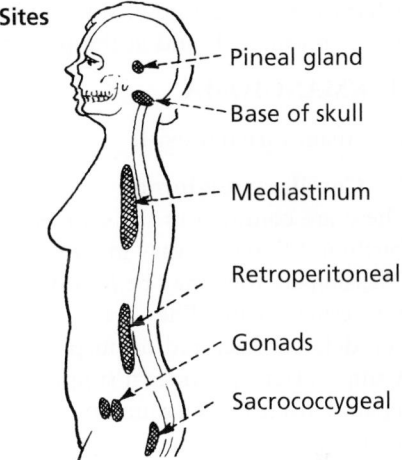

- Pineal gland
- Base of skull
- Mediastinum
- Retroperitoneal
- Gonads
- Sacrococcygeal

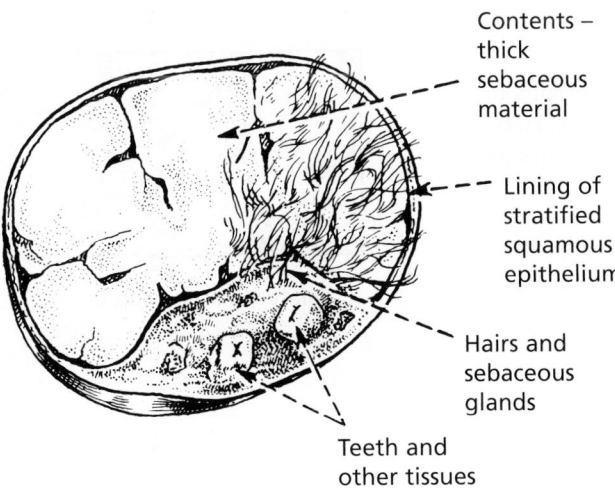

Contents – thick sebaceous material

Lining of stratified squamous epithelium

Hairs and sebaceous glands

Teeth and other tissues

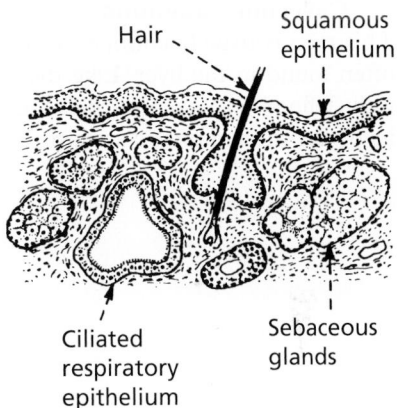

Hair

Squamous epithelium

Ciliated respiratory epithelium

Sebaceous glands

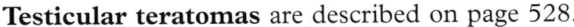

**Testicular teratomas** are described on page 528.

# OTHER TUMOUR TYPES

### HAMARTOMA

A hamartoma is a tumour-like but non-neoplastic malformation consisting of a mixture of tissues normally found at the particular site.

### HAEMANGIOMA

Two main varieties exist:

#### 1.   Capillary angioma
These are common in the skin as 'birthmarks', which vary in size. Occasionally they may be found in internal organs. They are well-defined, deep red or purple. A single artery provides a supply separate from the surrounding tissue.

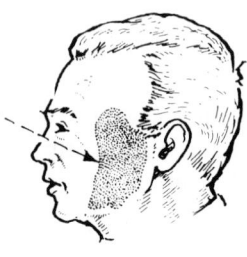

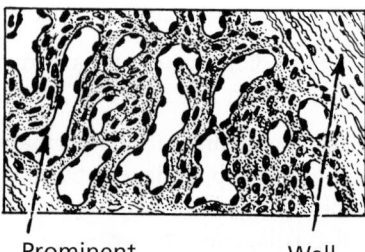

Prominent endothelial cells

Well-formed collagen

#### 2.   Cavernous angioma
This type is usually confined to internal organs and quite often found in the liver. Like the capillary variety they are well-defined and deep purple. Similar tumours are found involving the lymphatic system (lymphangioma).

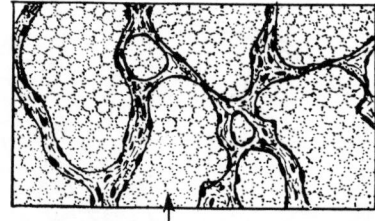

Dilated vascular spaces

# OTHER TUMOUR TYPES

## BENIGN PIGMENTED NAEVUS (MELANOCYTIC NAEVUS OR MOLE)

Benign pigmented naevus is extremely common. The term 'naevus' means a birthmark, but most naevi are acquired in childhood and adolescence.

During fetal life melanin-pigment-forming neuroectodermal cells migrate to the skin and are found in small numbers in the basal layer of the skin.

Melanocyte ‒ ‒ ‒

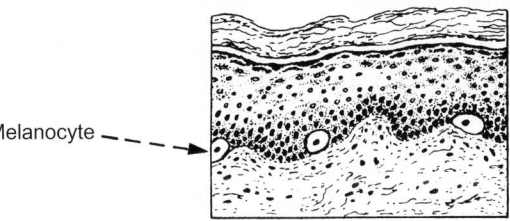

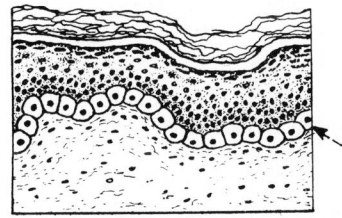

The common congenital pigmented mole is the result of an abnormality in migration, proliferation and maturation of these neuroectodermal cells. A continuous layer of pigmented cells is found adjacent to the basal epidermal cells.

The resulting naevi vary in size and appearance, from small flat macular brown areas or smooth papular lesions to warty hairy excrescences. Pigmentation is variable.

**Junctional naevus**
In this case proliferation is local and confined to the dermoepidermal junction.

**Compound naevus**
Proliferation is found in the dermis as well as the junctional area.

**Intradermal naevus**
Proliferation is wholly in the dermis.

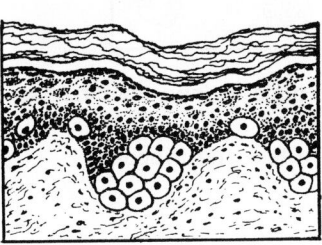

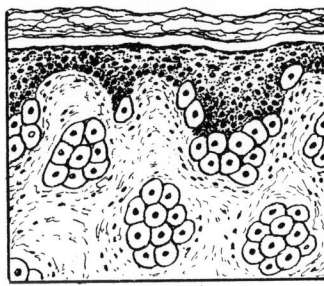

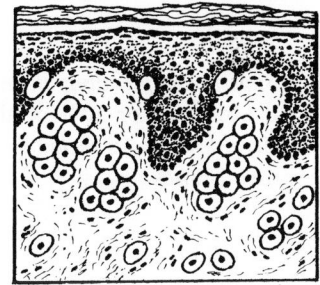

Blue naevus is another variation in which melanocytes are arrested in migration in the dermis.

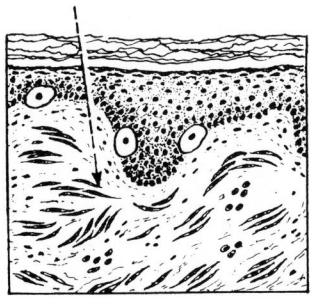

Active proliferative activity may extend into adult life, but the great majority of these lesions undergo a degree of involution. One feature which differentiates them from malignant change is that the deeper the cells penetrate the dermis, the smaller they become and the less active.

# OTHER TUMOUR TYPES

### MALIGNANT MELANOMA

Malignant proliferation of melanocytes usually arises de novo but some melanomas arise from pre-existing naevi. Exposure to SUNLIGHT (the UV component) is the most important aetiological factor.

1. *Chronic* – over many years – especially relevant in the elderly.
2. *Acute* – causing burning. This is particularly important.

### Sites

1. Skin of (a) face, soles of feet, palms of hands, nail beds, (b) legs (women) and (c) trunk (in men).
2. Mucous membranes of mouth, arms and genitalia – rare.
3. Eye and meninges – rare.

Some tumours are amelanotic (non-pigmented). The rate of growth is variable.

Four types of growth may occur:

1. *Lentigo maligna* – an 'in situ' lesion occurring on the face of the elderly. It may spread at one edge and regress at another.

Aberrant melanocytes spread along basal epidermal layer and round skin appendages.

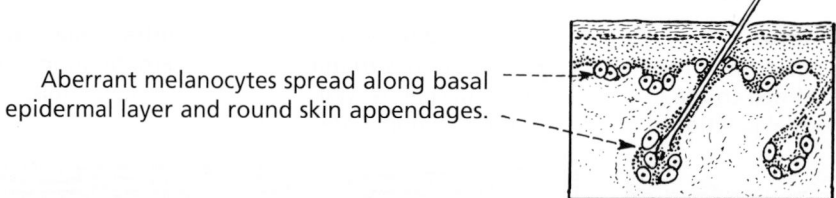

2. *Superficial spreading melanoma* – occurs most commonly on female leg and male trunk. It accounts for 50% of all skin melanomas in northern countries.
3. *Acral lentiginous melanoma* – found on palms of hands, soles of feet and mucous membranes.

# OTHER TUMOUR TYPES

4. *Nodular malignant melanoma* – usually on trunk. It invades early and ulceration is common.

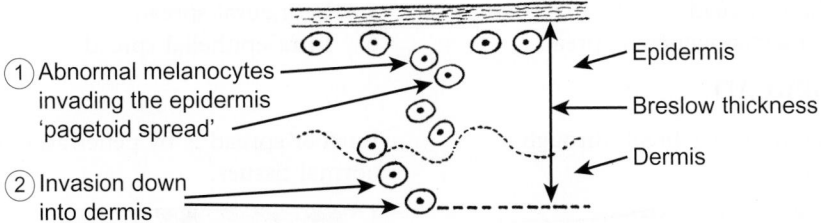

(1) Abnormal melanocytes invading the epidermis 'pagetoid spread'

(2) Invasion down into dermis

Epidermis

Breslow thickness

Dermis

The prognosis depends on depth of invasion. This measurement is known as the Breslow thickness.

| Thickness | 5 year survival |
|-----------|-----------------|
| <1 mm     | → 95–100%       |
| 1–2 mm    | → 80–95%        |
| 2–4 mm    | → 60–75%        |
| >4 mm     | → 50%           |

Activating mutations in the oncogene BRAF are present in around half of melanomas. Drugs which selectively inhibit mutant BRAF have been developed and induce dramatic responses in patients with metastatic disease. This is an example of molecularly targeted therapy.

# SPREAD OF TUMOURS

Tumours spread by several routes.

1. Local invasion.
2. Lymphatic spread.
3. Blood (haematogenous) spread.

4. Transcoelomic spread.
5. Perineural spread.
6. Intra-epithelial spread.

## LOCAL SPREAD

The proliferating cells break through normal barriers.

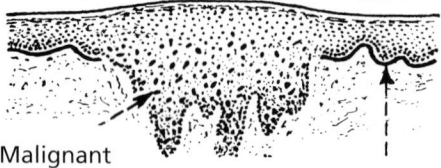

Malignant
cells break through basement membrane
into connective tissue

Further spread is by penetration between normal tissues.

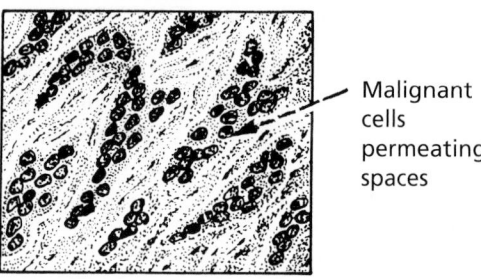

Malignant
cells
permeating
spaces

An important principle is that these permeating tumour cells take the line of least physical resistance.

Tumours may stimulate
the production of new collagen fibres
which are sometimes converted into
dense fibrous tissue → contracts and
fixes the tumour to surrounding structures.

e.g. Carcinoma of breast ⟶

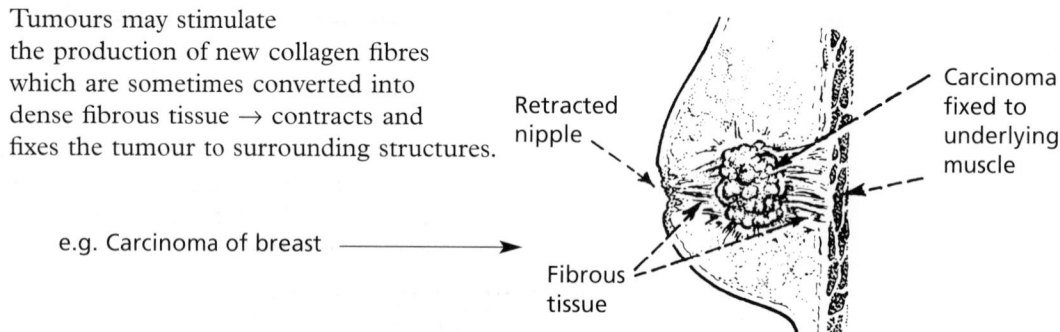

Retracted
nipple

Carcinoma
fixed to
underlying
muscle

Fibrous
tissue

The following diagram illustrates the basic mechanisms of cancer cell invasion.

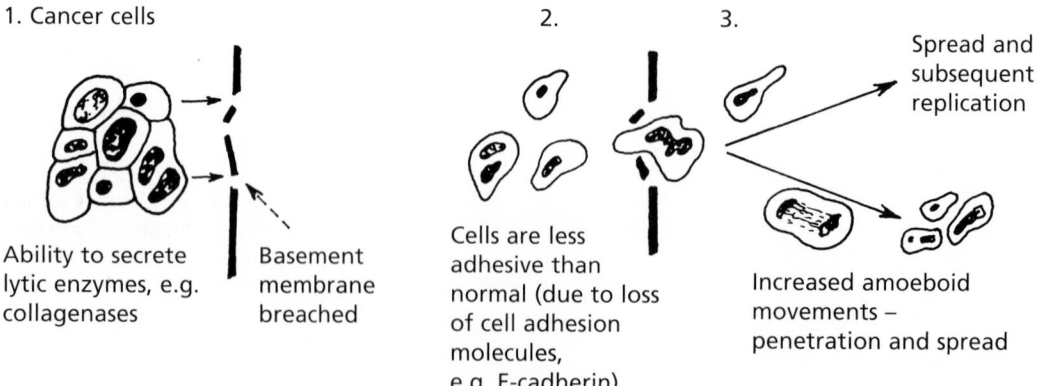

1. Cancer cells

Ability to secrete
lytic enzymes, e.g.
collagenases

Basement
membrane
breached

2.

Cells are less
adhesive than
normal (due to loss
of cell adhesion
molecules,
e.g. E-cadherin)

3.

Spread and
subsequent
replication

Increased amoeboid
movements –
penetration and spread

# LYMPHATIC SPREAD

## LYMPHATIC SPREAD

This is the commonest mode of spread of carcinomas and melanomas, but rarely of sarcomas. Malignant cells easily invade lymphatic channels from the tissue spaces.

Groups of cells form emboli in the lymph stream and are carried to the nearest node (the *sentinel node*).

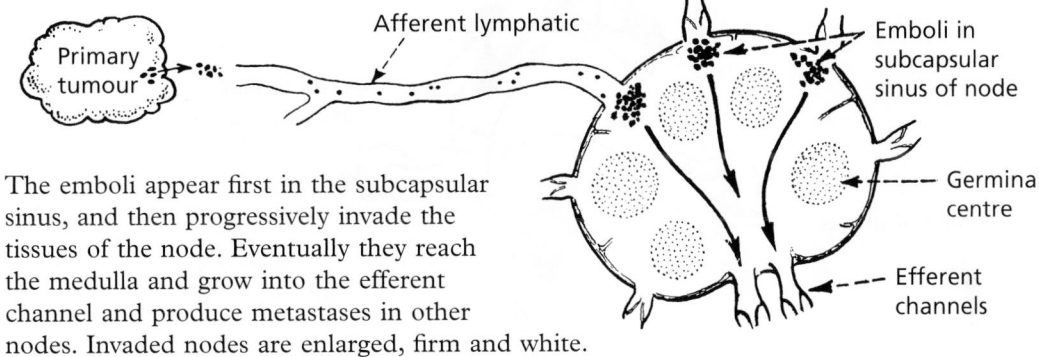

The emboli appear first in the subcapsular sinus, and then progressively invade the tissues of the node. Eventually they reach the medulla and grow into the efferent channel and produce metastases in other nodes. Invaded nodes are enlarged, firm and white.

Histological examination of the sentinel node is increasingly carried out to select the patients who require extensive lymph node dissection particularly in breast carcinoma and melanoma.

# LYMPHATIC SPREAD

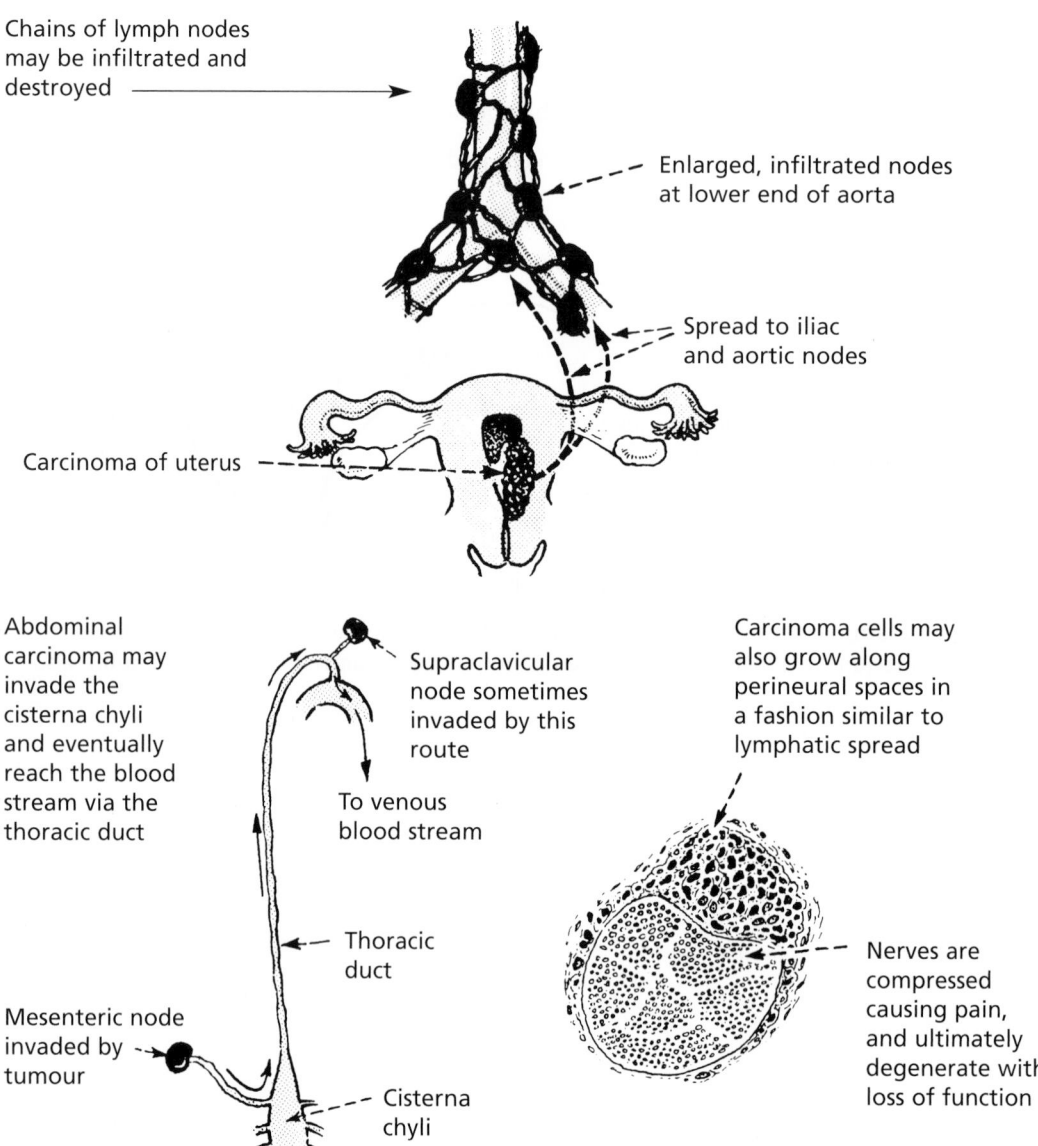

Chains of lymph nodes may be infiltrated and destroyed

Enlarged, infiltrated nodes at lower end of aorta

Spread to iliac and aortic nodes

Carcinoma of uterus

Abdominal carcinoma may invade the cisterna chyli and eventually reach the blood stream via the thoracic duct

Supraclavicular node sometimes invaded by this route

To venous blood stream

Carcinoma cells may also grow along perineural spaces in a fashion similar to lymphatic spread

Thoracic duct

Mesenteric node invaded by tumour

Cisterna chyli

Nerves are compressed causing pain, and ultimately degenerate with loss of function

# BLOOD SPREAD

Both carcinomas and sarcomas spread by the blood stream. The entry of malignant cells into the blood is via invasion of VENULES and by lymphatic embolism through the thoracic duct into the subclavian vein.

Carcinoma cells invading the thin wall of the vessel and entering the lumen.

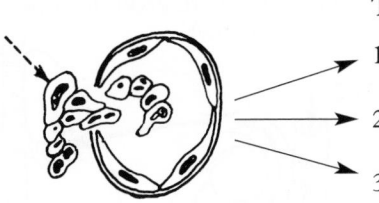

The following are possible sequels:

1. Tumour embolism to lungs (systemic circulation).
2. Embolism to liver (portal circulation).
3. Embolism via pulmonary veins to systemic ARTERIAL circulation. (Primary and secondary lung tumours.)

## VIA LARGER VEINS

Occasionally tumour thrombus is propagated from venules into larger veins. This is classically seen in RENAL CARCINOMA.

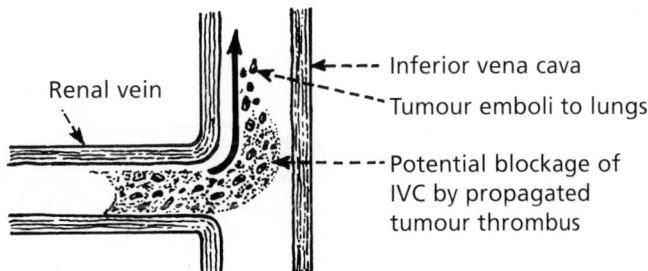

Renal vein

Inferior vena cava

Tumour emboli to lungs

Potential blockage of IVC by propagated tumour thrombus

Rarely, a malignant process may be complicated by thrombosis of distant veins (thrombophlebitis migrans). This is not due to malignant invasion of the veins but is caused by the action of circulating thromboplastins formed by the tumour.

## ARTERIAL SYSTEM

Direct invasion of arteries and arteriolar lumens is very rare because of the physical barrier provided by the thick muscular and elastic walls.

# BLOOD SPREAD

### DESTINATION OF EMBOLI

This depends on the anatomical drainage of the vessel invaded.

1. **Portal venous system** – emboli pass to liver

2. **Systemic venous system** – emboli pass to lungs. There are exceptions (see 'Retrograde Spread' below).

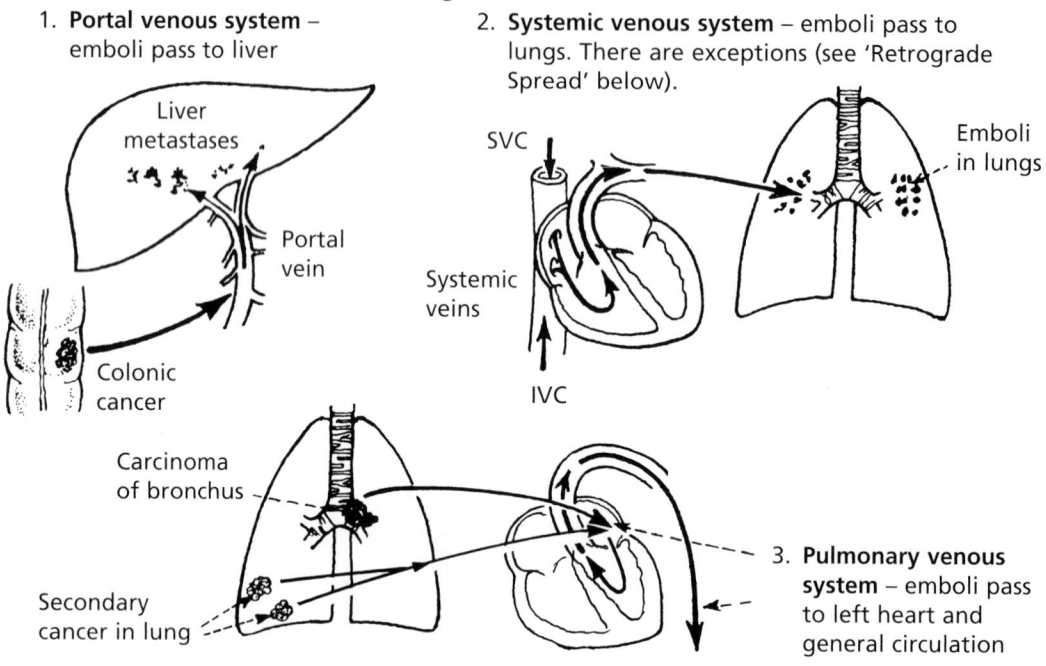

3. **Pulmonary venous system** – emboli pass to left heart and general circulation

### RETROGRADE VENOUS SPREAD

As in lymphatics, growth of tumour within a vein may cause reversal of blood flow. Reversal of flow is more likely to happen in certain areas of the body where veins form a rich plexus and are deficient in valves, e.g. in the pelvis and around vertebrae. Changes in intra-abdominal and intrathoracic pressures easily induce changes in blood flow in these channels. It is for this reason that secondary tumours are relatively common in vertebral bodies.

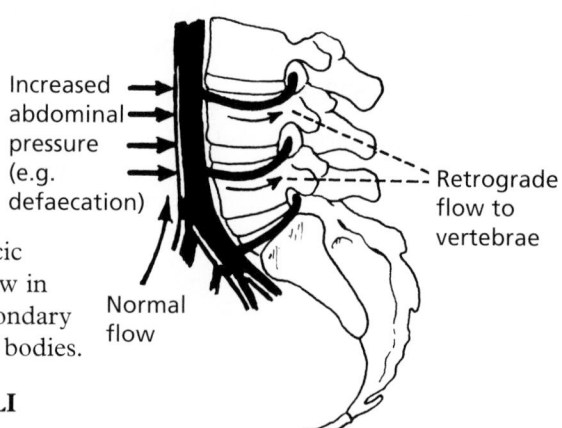

### FATE OF CARCINOMATOUS EMBOLI

#### Seed and soil analogy

The distribution of carcinomatous emboli is determined in part by anatomy, but many complex factors both in the 'seed' (the cancer cell) and the 'soil' (the potential metastatic site) are at play in the establishment of metastases at particular sites. They include surface properties of the cancer cells, e.g. increased expression of **integrins** and their **receptors** present in the endothelial cells at the metastatic site. Variation in the host IMMUNE RESPONSE is also important.

# OTHER MODES OF SPREAD OF TUMOURS

## TRANSCOELOMIC SPREAD (VIA SEROUS SACS)

This is an important and frequent route of spread in the peritoneal and pleural cavities. It also takes place in the pericardial sac.

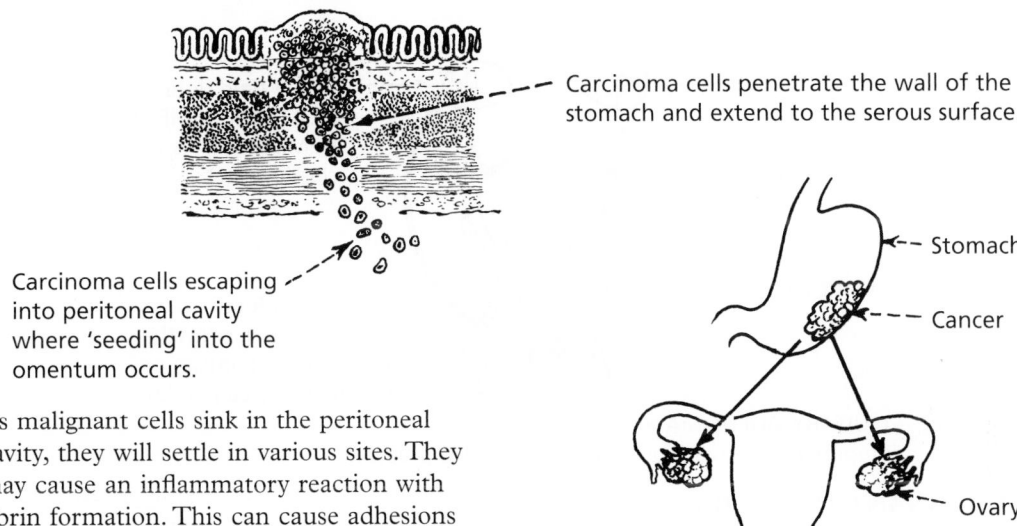

Carcinoma cells penetrate the wall of the stomach and extend to the serous surface.

Carcinoma cells escaping into peritoneal cavity where 'seeding' into the omentum occurs.

— Stomach

— — Cancer

— — Ovary

As malignant cells sink in the peritoneal cavity, they will settle in various sites. They may cause an inflammatory reaction with fibrin formation. This can cause adhesions between organs, e.g. loops of bowel.

Tumourous adhesions

Gastric cancer can spread to both ovaries (so-called 'KRUKENBERG TUMOUR'). An unusual but classic manifestation.

## INTRA-EPITHELIAL SPREAD

This form of spread may occur where carcinoma develops in a gland or its duct, e.g. in the breast. Carcinoma cells spread in the areolar skin (Paget's disease of the nipple).

Skin epithelium

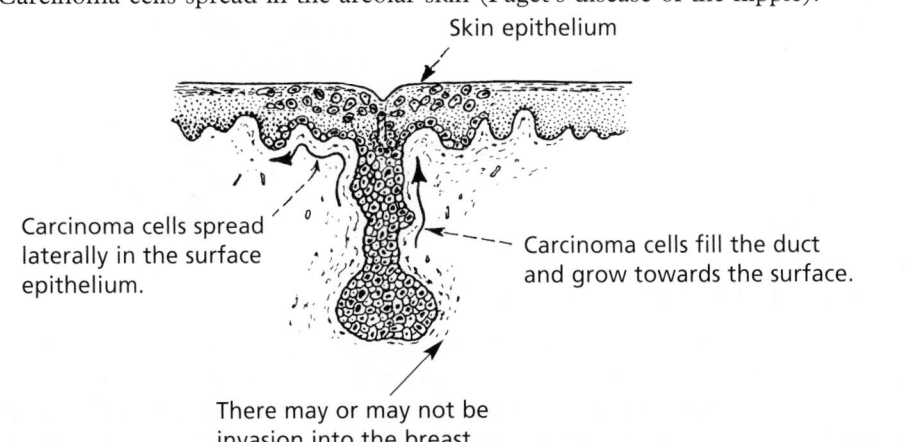

Carcinoma cells spread laterally in the surface epithelium.

Carcinoma cells fill the duct and grow towards the surface.

There may or may not be invasion into the breast.

# EFFECTS OF TUMOURS

### BENIGN TUMOURS

(a) The localised tumour mass may compress neighbouring structures causing loss of function and (b) benign endocrine tumours may produce excess hormones.

A pituitary adenoma is illustrative:

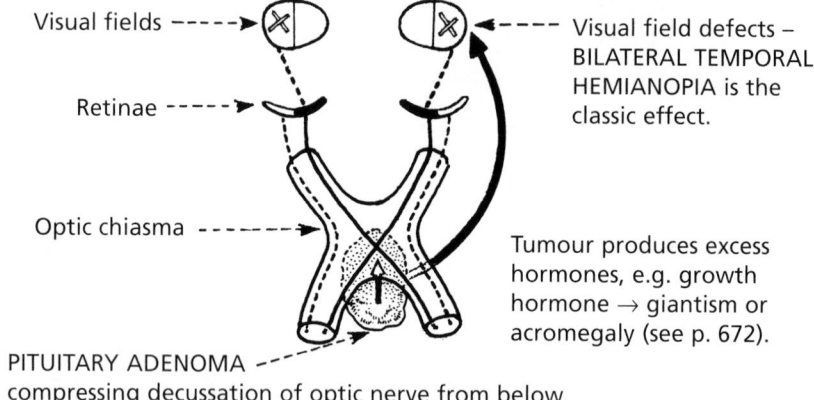

Visual fields

Retinae

Optic chiasma

Visual field defects –
BILATERAL TEMPORAL
HEMIANOPIA is the
classic effect.

Tumour produces excess
hormones, e.g. growth
hormone → giantism or
acromegaly (see p. 672).

PITUITARY ADENOMA
compressing decussation of optic nerve from below.

### MALIGNANT TUMOURS

(a) Local effects
    A tumour may narrow a hollow viscus, e.g. causing intestinal
    obstruction, ulceration and bleeding leading to anaemia.
                    E.g. stenosing cancer of colon
(b) Involvement of neighbouring structures
    Direct spread compresses adjacent viscera, blood vessels and
    nerves – LUNG CARCINOMA is illustrative (see p. 307–308).
(c) Effects of distant metastases

These are very numerous and variable. Two illustrative examples are given.

bleeding

(i) Metastases to bone cause pain and
    pathological fracture.

(ii) Metastases to the brain causing
    epilepsy, stroke, raised intracranial
    pressure, etc. (see p. 620).

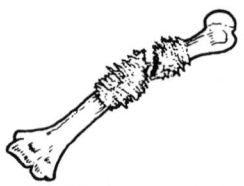

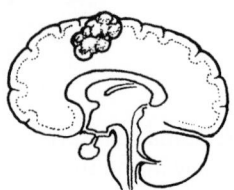

### NON-METASTATIC COMPLICATIONS

Patients with cancer often have severe weight loss (cachexia), loss of appetite and fever. These are probably due to release of cytokines (e.g. TUMOUR NECROSIS FACTOR) from tumour cells. Other complications include myopathy and neuropathy. Relapsing thrombosis of distant veins (thrombophlebitis migrans) is due to release of thromboplastins.

# TUMOUR MARKERS

Tumour cells produce substances, many of which are proteins. These can be helpful in diagnosis and monitoring of treatment.

(a) Product enters blood stream (and/or urine) where it can be measured.

Vein

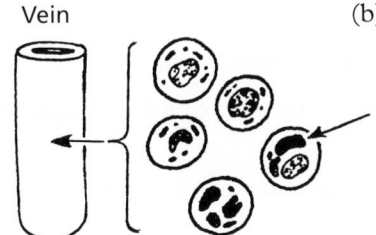

(b) Histological diagnosis is improved by identifying the specific product using immunostaining in the cytoplasm of the tumour cells.

Some examples are:

| TUMOUR MARKER | TUMOUR |
|---|---|
| Human chorionic gonadotrophin (HCG) | Choriocarcinoma, teratoma of testis |
| α-Fetoprotein (αFP) | Hepatocellular carcinoma, teratoma of testis |
| Prostate specific antigen, prostatic acid phosphatase | Prostatic carcinoma |
| Carcino-embryonic antigen (CEA) | Gastrointestinal and other cancers |
| Calcitonin | Medullary thyroid carcinoma |
| 5-hydroxyindole-acetic acid (5HIAA) in URINE (metabolite of 5-hydroxytryptamine [5HT-SEROTONIN]) | Intestinal carcinoid |

## Monitoring treatment

Blood levels of tumour markers reflect the effects of treatment. Example: **testicular teratoma**

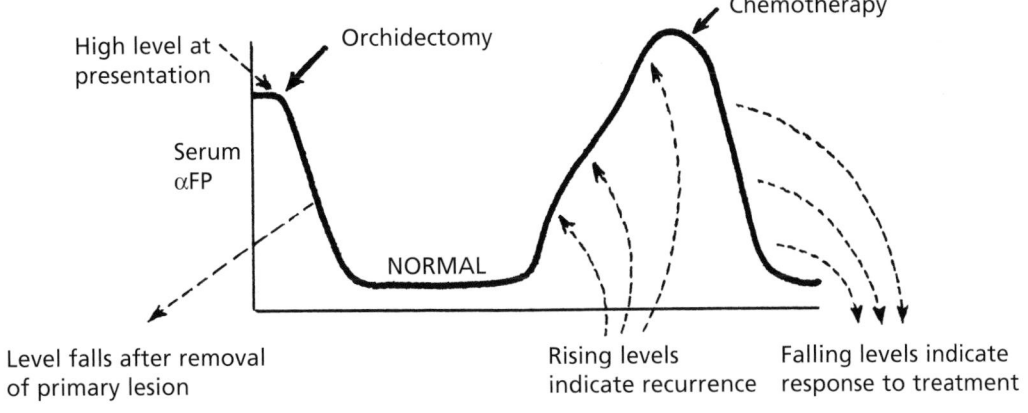

# DIAGNOSIS OF TUMOURS IMMUNOCYTOCHEMISTRY

Diagnosis of tumours is made by combining clinical information with pathological information of several types:

1.  *Gross examination.*
2.  *Conventional histological assessment.*
3.  *Immunocytochemical staining and molecular testing.*

Different immunocytochemical panels are used to help address specific histological dilemmas.

Thus for a metastatic adenocarcinoma of unknown origin, the pathologist may request:

| | |
|---|---|
| Cytokeratin profiling | CK 7, 20 |
| Transcription factors | Wilms tumour 1 (WT1), thyroid transcription factor 1 (TTF-1), CDX2 |
| Hormone receptors | Oestogen (ER), progesterone (PR) receptors |
| 'Tumour markers' | Prostate specific antigen (PSA), Ca125, Carcinoembryonic antigen |
| An adenocarcinoma with this profile is likely to be of pulmonary origin | CK7 +, CK20 − |
| | TTF1 +ve, WT1 −ve, CDX2 −ve |
| | ER −ve, PR −ve |
| | Ca125 −ve |
| | PSA −ve |

# PRE-MALIGNANCY

The pathological conditions which are associated with the development of malignancy fall into three groups: (1) benign tumours, (2) chronic inflammatory conditions and (3) intra-epithelial neoplasia.

## 1. MALIGNANT TRANSFORMATION OF BENIGN TUMOURS

(a) **Colonic cancer** is a good example in that most arise from a benign adenoma.

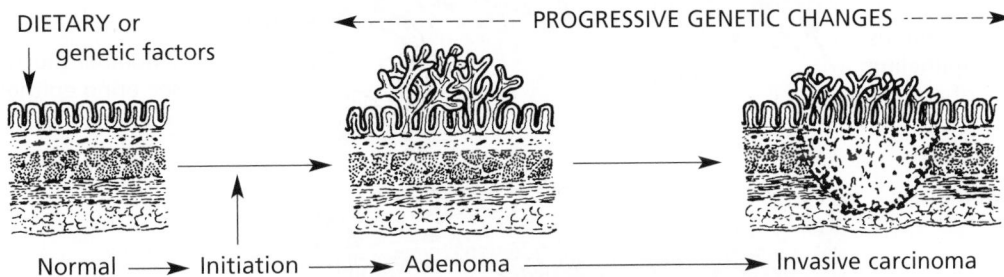

DIETARY or genetic factors ←‑‑‑‑‑‑‑‑‑‑ PROGRESSIVE GENETIC CHANGES ‑‑‑‑‑‑→

Normal ⟶ Initiation ⟶ Adenoma ⟶ Invasive carcinoma

(b) In familial adenomatous polyposis (polyposis coli), transformation to cancer in one or more of the very numerous adenomas is inevitable (p. 330).

## 2. CHRONIC INFLAMMATORY CONDITIONS

The inflammation has to be very long standing and transformation to cancer is RARE. Examples are:

(a) In **ulcerative colitis**, repeated epithelial damage and repair increase the risk of cancer.

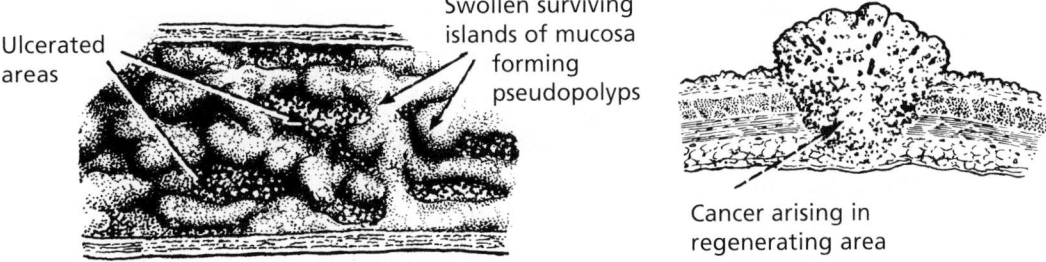

Ulcerated areas

Swollen surviving islands of mucosa forming pseudopolyps

Cancer arising in regenerating area

(b) In **Hashimoto disease** – an auto-immune thyroiditis – the uniformly enlarged thyroid contains many proliferating lymphoid follicles and lymphocytes.

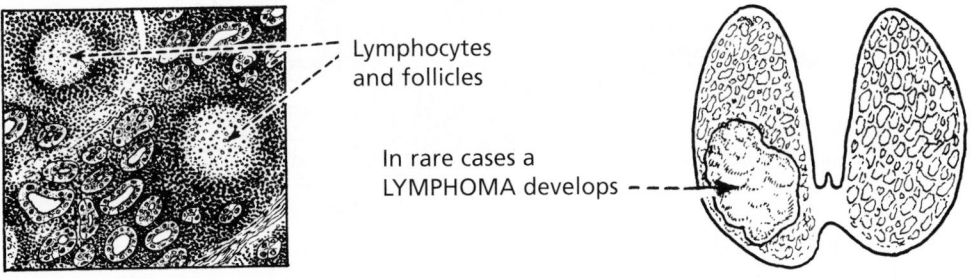

Lymphocytes and follicles

In rare cases a LYMPHOMA develops ‑‑‑

## 3. INTRA-EPITHELIAL NEOPLASIA (carcinoma in situ) is common and a very important pre-cancerous condition at several sites.

# CARCINOMA IN SITU (INTRA-EPITHELIAL NEOPLASIA)

This represents an intermediate stage in the production of a cancer. All the cytological features of malignancy are present, but the cells have not invaded the surrounding tissues. It is frequently found in the cervix uteri at the junction of ecto and endocervix.

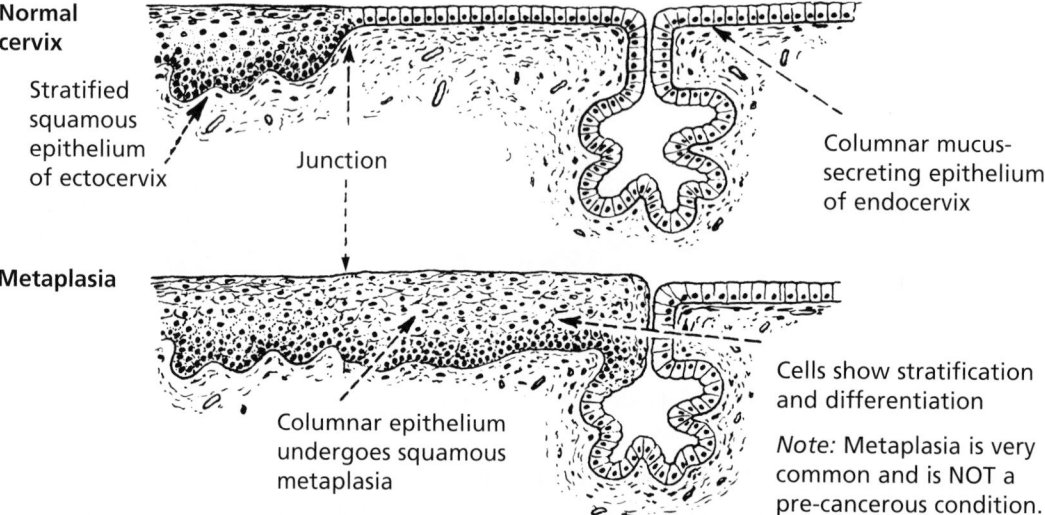

**Normal cervix**

Stratified squamous epithelium of ectocervix

Junction

Columnar mucus-secreting epithelium of endocervix

**Metaplasia**

Columnar epithelium undergoes squamous metaplasia

Cells show stratification and differentiation

*Note:* Metaplasia is very common and is NOT a pre-cancerous condition.

In the cervix, the abbreviation CIN (cervical intra-epithelial neoplasia) is used. There are three grades of severity.

1. CIN 1 (mild dysplasia).

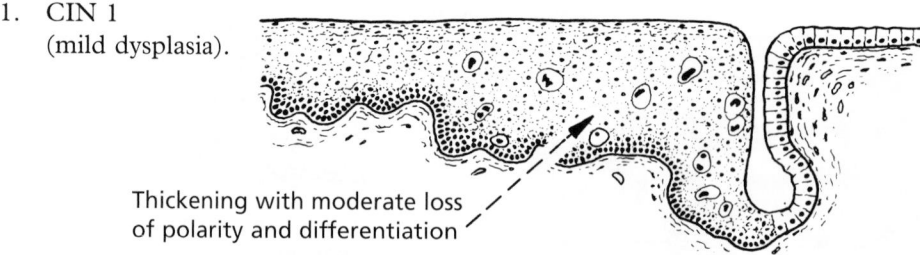

Thickening with moderate loss of polarity and differentiation

2. CIN 2 – appearances intermediate between Grades 1 and 3.
3. CIN 3 (carcinoma in situ).

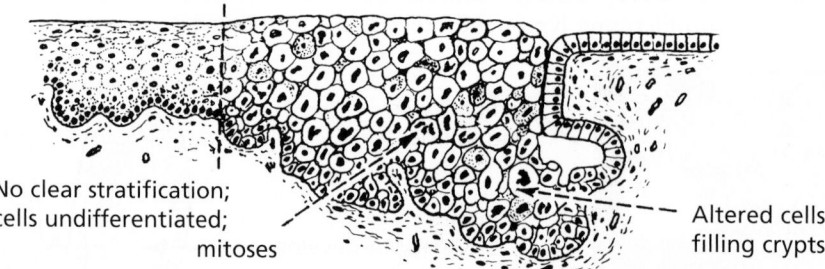

No clear stratification; cells undifferentiated; mitoses

Altered cells filling crypts

These premalignant conditions may revert to normal, but most commonly they become truly malignant and invade the surrounding tissues.

The concept of progressive pre-malignant proliferation applies equally in other organs (e.g. breast, stomach, oesophagus, bronchus, prostate, mouth, vulva).

# CARCINOGENESIS

Malignant tumours are due to UNCONTROLLED PROLIFERATION of cells. Most tumours are MONOCLONAL, i.e. are derived from a single transformed cell.

This concept is well illustrated in MULTIPLE MYELOMA – a malignant tumour of plasma cells.

All of the tumour cells produce the same immunoglobulin – including the same light chain.

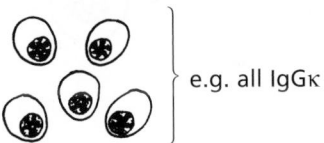

e.g. all IgGκ

See also page 136.

In contrast, an inflammatory infiltrate of plasma cells is POLYCLONAL...

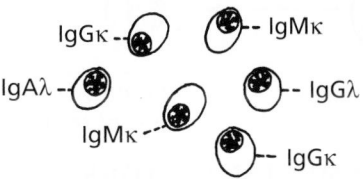

… producing various immunoglobulins and light chains.

## CLONAL EVOLUTION

In time, some cells undergo further mutations which are passed on to their progeny. This is called clonal evolution or progression and explains the morphological variations seen in tumours. Some of the subclones grow more rapidly and metastasise more readily while others are so abnormal that proliferation is not possible and the clone dies out.

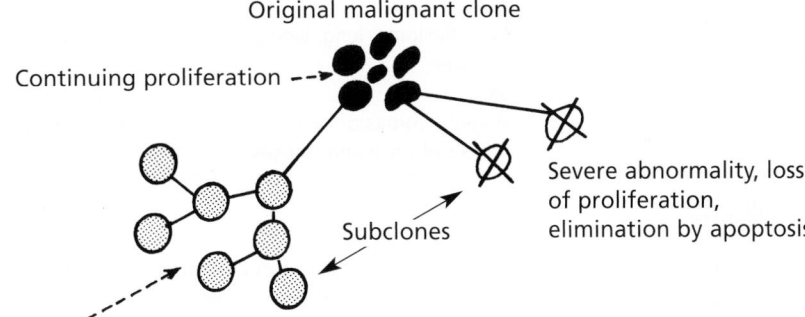

Original malignant clone

Continuing proliferation

Severe abnormality, loss of proliferation, elimination by apoptosis

Subclones

Increased proliferation and malignant characteristics increased

### Nuclear morphology and DNA content

In histological sections these abnormalities are indicated by variations in nuclear density (usually increased), size and shape (i.e. PLEOMORPHISM).

The term 'POLYPLOIDY' is used when the nuclear DNA is increased by exact multiples of the normal.

'ANEUPLOIDY' indicates irregular increases in DNA content. →

# CARCINOGENESIS

A number of factors, both environmental and genetic, contribute to a cell undergoing malignant change. This should be regarded as a multistep sequence (see p. 199).

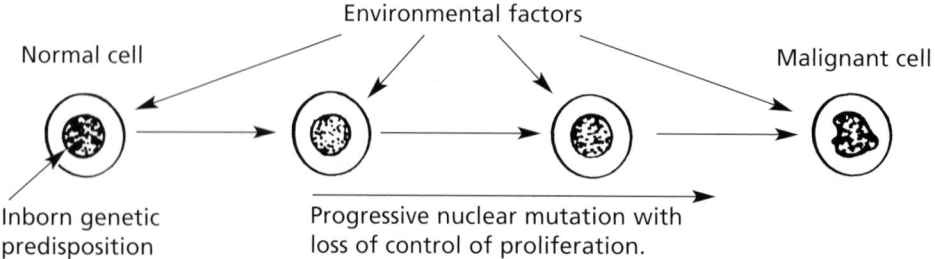

## ENVIRONMENTAL FACTORS

The three major environmental factors which induce tumours are (1) chemical carcinogens, (2) radiation and (3) viruses.

## CHEMICAL CARCINOGENESIS

Historically, chemical agents were the first to be associated with cancer. Now, many are recognised in (a) industrial processes, (b) social habits and (c) diet.

| INDUSTRY | TUMOUR | CHEMICAL RESPONSIBLE |
|---|---|---|
| Aniline dyes | Bladder cancer | Naphthylamine |
| Insulation, e.g. shipbuilding, building | Mesothelioma, lung, laryngeal cancer | Asbestos |
| Mineral oil and tar | Skin cancers | Benzpyrene and other hydrocarbons |
| Plastics | Angiosarcomas of liver | Vinyl chloride monomer |
| Wood dust | Cancer of nose and sinuses | ? |

### Social habits

Cigarette smoking is strongly associated with the development of many cancers, including lung, mouth, larynx and bladder. Chewing tobacco greatly increases the risk of oral cancer. It is likely that air pollution, e.g. combustion products of petrol and diesel, also contributes to carcinogenesis. Obesity is associated with an increased risk of cancer, e.g. of the uterus and colon.

### Diet

Chemicals in food may be carcinogenic. Nitrosamines may be formed by the action of bacteria on ingested nitrites. AFLATOXINS produced by fungi (*Aspergillus flavus*) and contaminating foodstuffs, may cause liver cancer.

*Note:* Chemical carcinogens may act in two ways:

1. Directly at the site of application or portal of entry, e.g. skin and lung cancers.
2. After modification, either at the sites of metabolism or excretion, e.g. liver and urinary tract tumours.

# CARCINOGENESIS

This is a multistep process of long duration.

The stages of **initiation** and **promotion** are important and were identified in classic experiments of skin carcinogenesis.

1. **Normal skin**

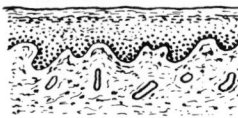

Application of carcinogen, e.g. Benzpyrene (a mutagen).

2. **INITIATION** – Skin appears normal but important changes have occurred in the cell's DNA.

3. **PROMOTION** – initiated by co-carcinogens, e.g. croton oil, turpentine. (These agents are not mutagenic but act by stimulating cell proliferation.) Visible surface and histological changes are seen.

(a) Keratosis and papilloma formation

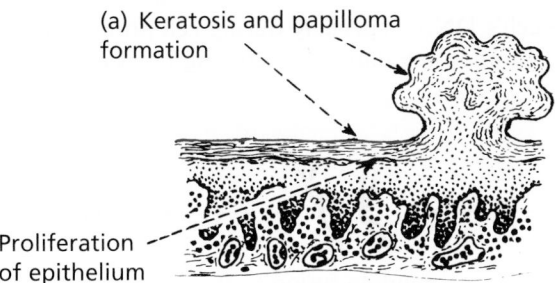

Proliferation of epithelium

(b) Dysplasia, i.e. cytological features of malignancy, but no invasion (see p. 144).

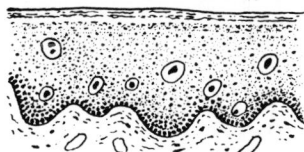

These stages are reversible.

4. **Appearance of MALIGNANT TUMOUR** (An irreversible change)

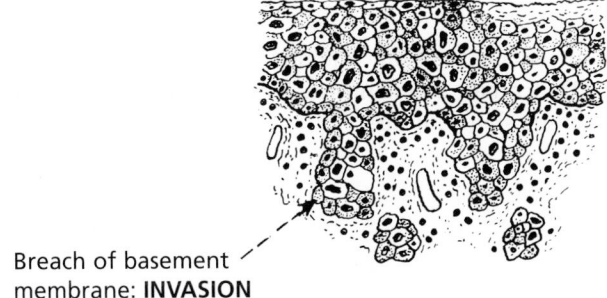

Breach of basement membrane: **INVASION**

The order of application of these agents is important. No tumour follows application of promotor alone, or promotor followed by initiator.

In rodents, these changes take months. In humans the time scale is years and is exemplified in the skin, cervix uteri, bronchus, urinary bladder, colon and breast.

# CARCINOGENESIS

## RADIANT ENERGY

The potential dangers from irradiation give much cause for concern.

| SOURCE OF RADIATION | TUMOURS | TYPE OF RADIATION |
|---|---|---|
| Sunlight | Melanoma, carcinoma of skin | UV (non-ionising) |
| Nuclear explosions (e.g. atom bombs, Chernobyl) | Leukaemia, carcinomas of lung, breast, thyroid | Ionising |
| Therapeutic irradiation | Various carcinomas, sarcomas, leukaemia | Ionising |
| Mining radioactive substances (e.g. uranium) | Lung carcinomas | Ionising |
| X-ray workers (historical) | Skin cancer, leukaemia | X-rays: ionising |

## Effects of irradiation on cells

The ionising effect of radiation damages the cell's DNA, especially during cell proliferation, ranging from single gene mutation to major chromosome damage, including breaks, deletions and translocations.

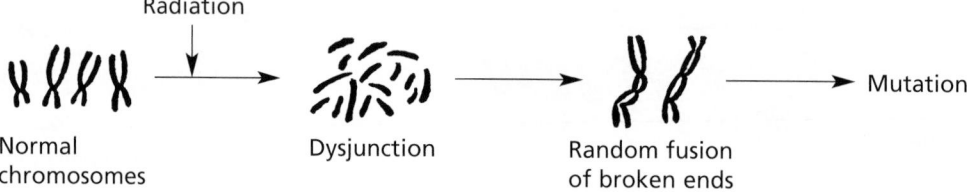

Normal chromosomes — Dysjunction — Random fusion of broken ends — Mutation

Proliferating cells are particularly vulnerable. Bone marrow and gastrointestinal mucosa are highly sensitive.

UV light is of low energy and mainly affects the skin. The 'PYRIMIDINE DIMERS' formed by UV light are normally excised by DNA repair mechanisms. In **xeroderma pigmentosum**, these are deficient, leading to numerous skin tumours.

# CARCINOGENESIS – VIRUSES

Viruses have long been known to cause cancer in animals (e.g. Rous sarcoma virus and the mouse mammary tumour virus – the Bittner milk factor).

In recent years viruses have been shown to contribute to the development of some human cancers.

| VIRUS | TYPE | TUMOUR TYPE |
| --- | --- | --- |
| Epstein–Barr (EBV) | DNA | Burkitt lymphoma, nasopharyngeal cancer, Hodgkin disease, post-transplantation lymphoma |
| Human herpes virus 8 (HHV-8) | DNA | Kaposi sarcoma |
| Hepatitis 'B' | DNA | Hepatocellular carcinomas |
| Human papilloma virus (HPV) | DNA | Cervical, penile, anal carcinoma |
| Human 'T' cell leukaemia virus (HTLV-1) | RNA (retrovirus) | T lymphoblastic leukaemia |

## Mode of action of oncogenic viruses

The essential feature is addition of new DNA to the nucleus of host cells resulting in mutants, but the way in which this is achieved differs in the two types of virus.

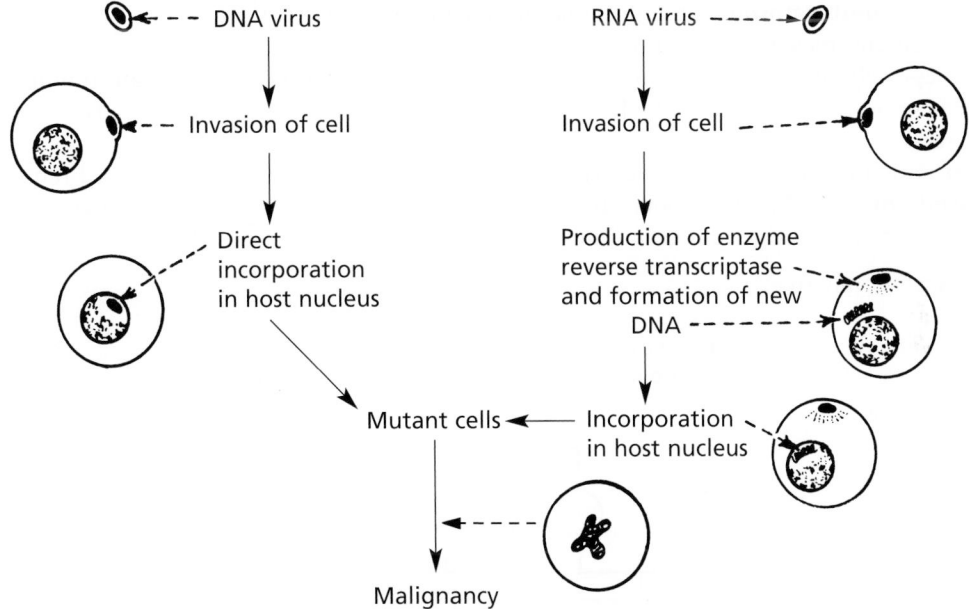

# CARCINOGENESIS – HEREDITY

The inherited genetic influences in cancer are now well recognised.

1.  There is a high risk of cancer in some uncommon syndromes inherited as Mendelian traits. Illustrative examples are:
    (a) **Familial adenomatous polyposis coli** (APC). 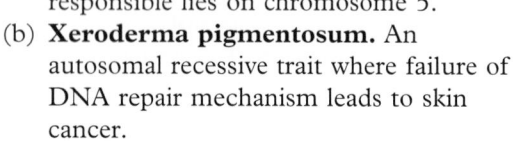 **(APC)**. An autosomal dominant condition. Numerous polyps occur in the colon in late childhood (10–14 years) and inevitably lead to adenocarcinoma in early middle age (30–45 years). The APC gene responsible lies on chromosome 5.
    (b) **Xeroderma pigmentosum.** An autosomal recessive trait where failure of DNA repair mechanism leads to skin cancer.
    (c) **Neurofibromatosis** – multiple neurofibromas (NF) – with a 1% risk of sarcoma, is due to a defect of NF-1 gene on chromosome 17.
    (d) **Retinoblastoma** – an autosomal dominant condition (Rb gene on chromosome 13), (p. 198).
2.  A less well-defined, but strong familial tendency is seen with some common tumours. For some the gene is identified, e.g. BRCA-1 gene, chromosome 17, – 60% risk of breast or ovarian cancer by 50 years.
3.  In some families, there is a high risk of several types of cancer. In the rare Li-Fraumeni syndrome, childhood sarcomas, breast cancer in young women and many other cancers are seen. This is due to a germ-line mutation of the p53 gene (p. 198).

Illustrative family tree:

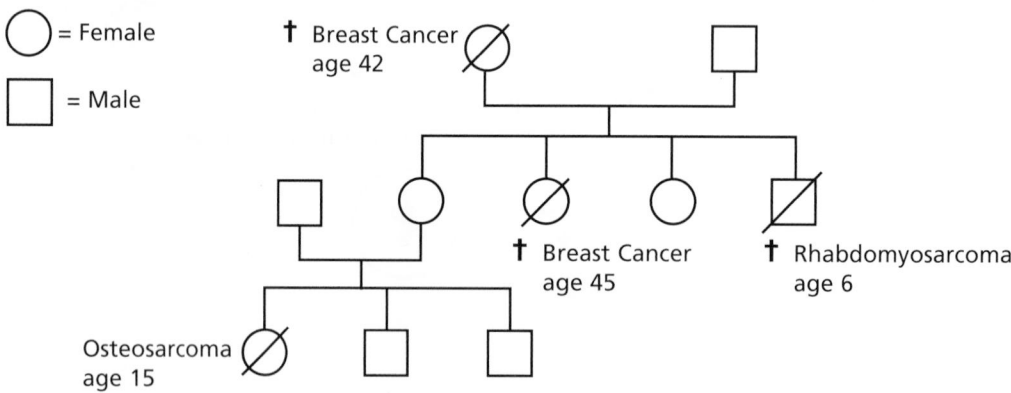

◯ = Female

▢ = Male

† Breast Cancer age 42

† Breast Cancer age 45

† Rhabdomyosarcoma age 6

Osteosarcoma age 15

/ = denotes affected.

# ONCOGENES AND TUMOUR SUPPRESSOR GENES

Cellular proto-oncogenes are NORMAL genes which STIMULATE cell division. Tumour suppressor genes are NORMAL genes which INHIBIT cell division. Their normal activity during somatic growth and in regeneration and repair takes place during the $G_0$–$G_1$ phase of the cell cycle and is strictly controlled.

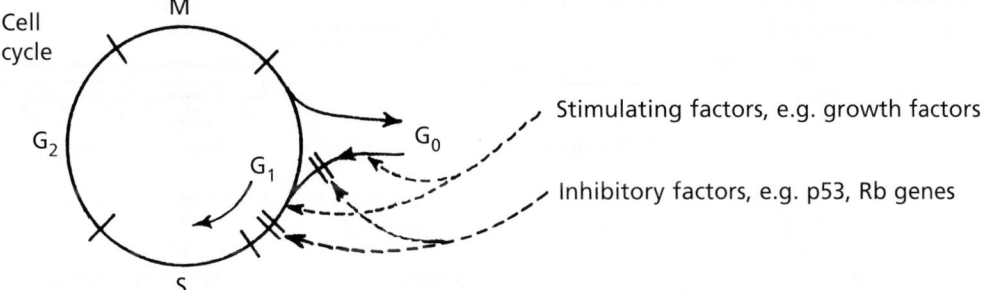

In cancer cells the normal controls are defective so that the balance between factors stimulating and inhibiting cell growth is permanently lost, resulting in increased proliferation.

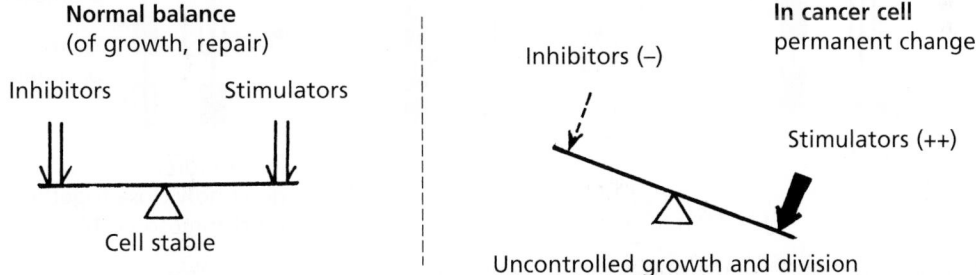

Cellular proto-oncogenes code for a number of proteins involved in cell proliferation:

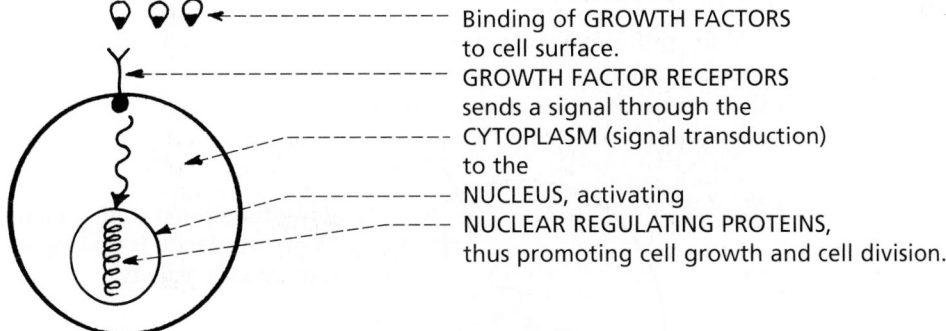

Binding of GROWTH FACTORS to cell surface.
GROWTH FACTOR RECEPTORS sends a signal through the CYTOPLASM (signal transduction) to the NUCLEUS, activating NUCLEAR REGULATING PROTEINS, thus promoting cell growth and cell division.

In the cancer cell, these normal genes are permanently changed to ONCOGENES and proliferation is uncontrolled.

Mutation or overexpression of genes which normally control APOPTOSIS (p. 5) are increasingly recognised in many tumours, e.g. overexpression of *bcl-2* inhibits apoptosis in follicular lymphoma (p. 469).

# ONCOGENES

The production and activity of ONCOGENES is complex and there are many ways in which they are activated.

The following are examples.

1.  **Production of excess NORMAL protein**

    (a) Gene amplification, e.g. neuroblastoma (*myc* type gene)

    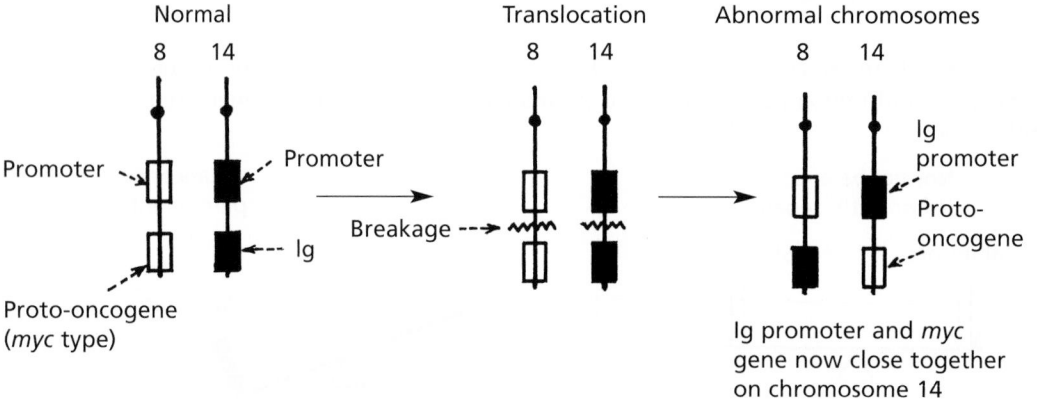

    (b) Increased mRNA transcription due to chromosomal translocation, e.g. in Burkitt LYMPHOMA chromosomes 8 and 14 are involved.

    The *myc* oncogene is now under the influence of the Ig gene control and is permanently switched on.

2.  **Production of FUNCTIONALLY ABNORMAL PROTEIN**

    A point mutation of the proto-oncogene produces a protein with an altered function so that over-stimulation occurs.
    Altered **growth factor receptor function** is an example.

    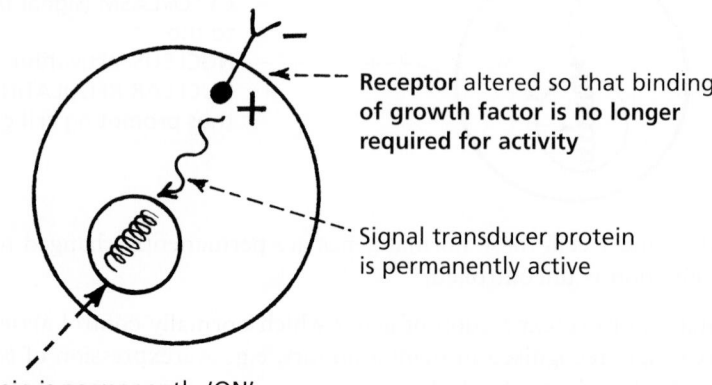

# TUMOUR SUPPRESSOR GENES

Tumour suppressor genes are normal genes which switch off cell proliferation by acting on the cell cycle in $G_1$. Their biological role is much broader than simply suppressing tumour function, but the name reflects how they have been discovered.

Loss of *both* copies of a tumour suppressor gene is required for cancer to develop. In contrast, only one copy of a given oncogene needs to be activated to cause excess proliferation.

Examples are:

| TUMOUR SUPPRESSOR GENE | CHROMOSOME | TUMOURS |
| --- | --- | --- |
| p53 | 17 | Carcinoma of lung and breast: sarcoma |
| Retinoblastoma (Rb) | 13 | Retinoblastoma, sarcoma: some carcinomas |
| NF1 | 17 | Neurofibromas, malignant peripheral nerve tumours |
| APC | 5 | Colonic carcinoma |
| WT1 | 11 | Wilms tumour, bladder cancer |

**p53 gene:** this gene codes for a nuclear phosphoprotein, which is expressed in increased amounts following cellular damage, e.g. **irradiation**.

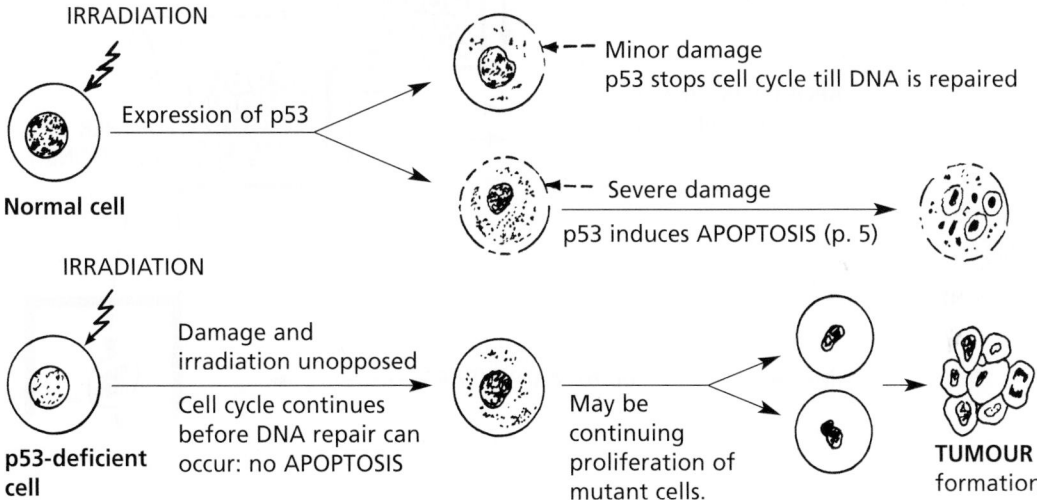

IRRADIATION

Expression of p53

Normal cell

Minor damage
p53 stops cell cycle till DNA is repaired

Severe damage
p53 induces APOPTOSIS (p. 5)

IRRADIATION

Damage and irradiation unopposed

Cell cycle continues before DNA repair can occur: no APOPTOSIS

p53-deficient cell

May be continuing proliferation of mutant cells.

TUMOUR formation

p53 has been called the 'guardian of the genome'. Abnormalities of p53 are found in at least 30% of all cancers.

Germ line p53 mutation is a feature of the Li-Fraumeni syndrome.

# CARCINOGENESIS – SUMMARY

## THE MULTISTEP STAIRWAY TO MALIGNANCY

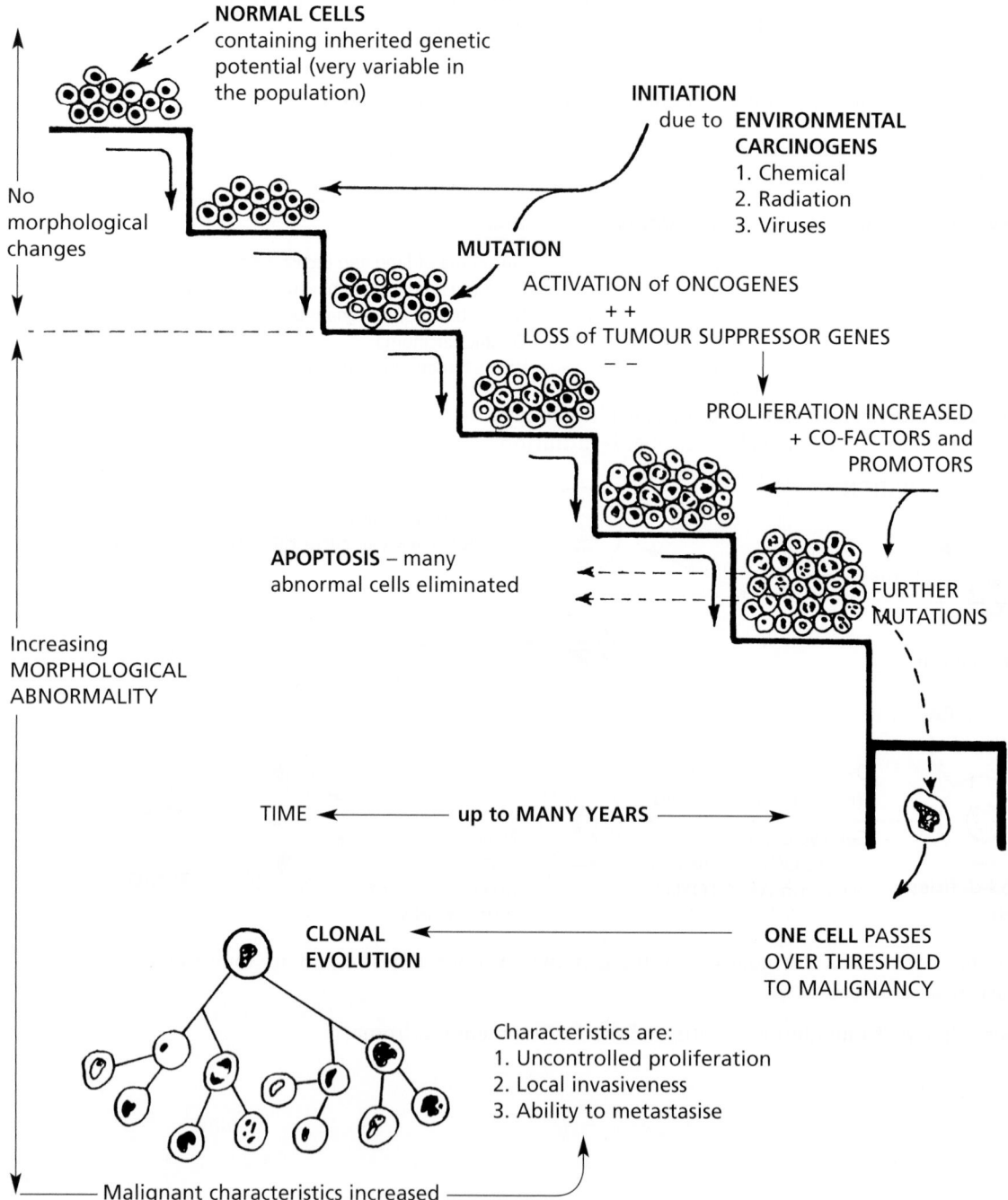

**NORMAL CELLS**
containing inherited genetic
potential (very variable in
the population)

**INITIATION**
due to **ENVIRONMENTAL
CARCINOGENS**
1. Chemical
2. Radiation
3. Viruses

No
morphological
changes

**MUTATION**

ACTIVATION of ONCOGENES
+ +
LOSS of TUMOUR SUPPRESSOR GENES

PROLIFERATION INCREASED
+ CO-FACTORS and
PROMOTORS

**APOPTOSIS** – many
abnormal cells eliminated

Increasing
MORPHOLOGICAL
ABNORMALITY

FURTHER
MUTATIONS

TIME ◄──────── **up to MANY YEARS** ────────►

**ONE CELL** PASSES
OVER THRESHOLD
TO MALIGNANCY

**CLONAL
EVOLUTION**

Characteristics are:
1. Uncontrolled proliferation
2. Local invasiveness
3. Ability to metastasise

──── Malignant characteristics increased ────

# CARDIOVASCULAR DISEASES

## OBJECTIVES

1. Describe the normal function of the heart and the effects of heart failure.
2. Describe the key processes in atherosclerosis and hypertension.
3. Describe the spectrum of ischaemic heart disease and its complications.
4. Briefly describe the key causes and effects of valvular heart disease and endocarditis.
5. Briefly describe the key causes and effects of vasculitis.

# CARDIAC FUNCTION

The main function of the heart is to provide the pumping action in a closed circulation.

Comparison with a simple mechanical system is useful and valid, provided that it is appreciated that the human heart is infinitely more sophisticated, with delicate built-in controls and balances which influence the inotropic (intrinsic contractility) activity of the heart.

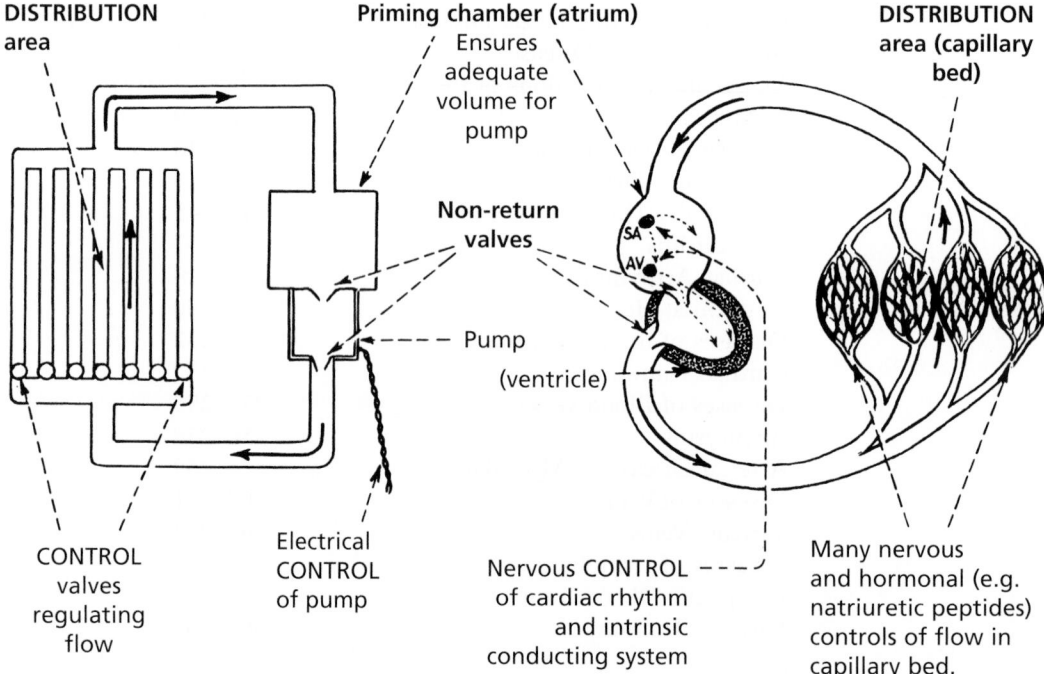

**DISTRIBUTION area**

**Priming chamber (atrium)** Ensures adequate volume for pump

**DISTRIBUTION area (capillary bed)**

**Non-return valves**

Pump (ventricle)

CONTROL valves regulating flow

Electrical CONTROL of pump

Nervous CONTROL of cardiac rhythm and intrinsic conducting system

Many nervous and hormonal (e.g. natriuretic peptides) controls of flow in capillary bed.

The pump is the essential part of the system: it has to be flexible to accommodate any changes required in the distribution side of the system.

In the human circulation, reserves of ventricular muscle power are available to meet the wide range of metabolic activity required in the distribution area.

# HEART FAILURE

**Heart failure** is very common and occurs when the **_ventricular muscle_** is incapable of maintaining a circulation adequate for the needs of the body, producing symptoms on exercise and at rest.

Causes of heart failure can be separated into two main groups:

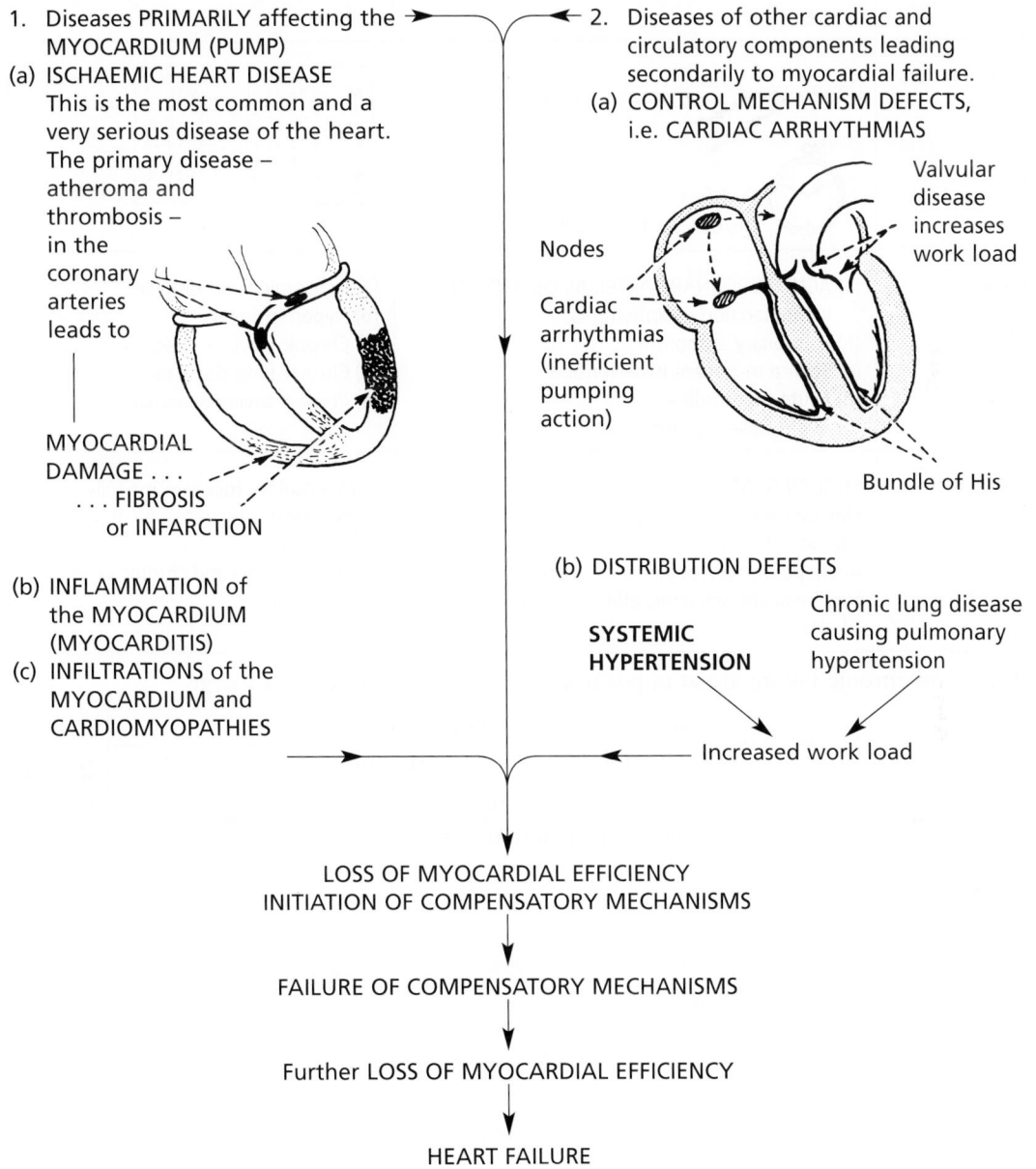

1. Diseases PRIMARILY affecting the MYOCARDIUM (PUMP)
(a) ISCHAEMIC HEART DISEASE
This is the most common and a very serious disease of the heart. The primary disease – atheroma and thrombosis – in the coronary arteries leads to

MYOCARDIAL DAMAGE . . .
. . . FIBROSIS or INFARCTION

(b) INFLAMMATION of the MYOCARDIUM (MYOCARDITIS)
(c) INFILTRATIONS of the MYOCARDIUM and CARDIOMYOPATHIES

2. Diseases of other cardiac and circulatory components leading secondarily to myocardial failure.
(a) CONTROL MECHANISM DEFECTS, i.e. CARDIAC ARRHYTHMIAS

Valvular disease increases work load

Nodes

Cardiac arrhythmias (inefficient pumping action)

Bundle of His

(b) DISTRIBUTION DEFECTS

SYSTEMIC HYPERTENSION

Chronic lung disease causing pulmonary hypertension

Increased work load

LOSS OF MYOCARDIAL EFFICIENCY
INITIATION OF COMPENSATORY MECHANISMS

FAILURE OF COMPENSATORY MECHANISMS

Further LOSS OF MYOCARDIAL EFFICIENCY

HEART FAILURE

# HEART FAILURE

### ACUTE AND CHRONIC

This depends on the **suddenness of onset** and **rate of development**.

The causes and effects are different.

| | ACUTE | CHRONIC |
|---|---|---|
| Time factors | Instantaneous Sudden (hours – a few days) | Weeks Months |
| Causes | (a) ACUTE CORONARY ARTERIAL OCCLUSION with infarction or arrhythmia <br> (b) Pulmonary embolism <br> (c) Severe malignant hypertension <br> (d) Acute myocarditis <br> (e) Acute valve rupture | (a) Ischaemic heart disease <br> (b) Hypertension <br> (c) Chronic valvular diseases <br> (d) Chronic lung diseases <br> (e) Chronic severe anaemia |
| Effects | SUDDEN DEATH <br> May be no time for compensatory mechanisms to be initiated <br> Acute pulmonary oedema is common <br> May be acute ischaemic effects in brain and kidneys | Compensatory mechanisms fully developed – hypertrophy and dilatation <br> Chronic oedema and chronic venous congestion |

Acute and chronic failure are at opposite ends of a spectrum but may merge.

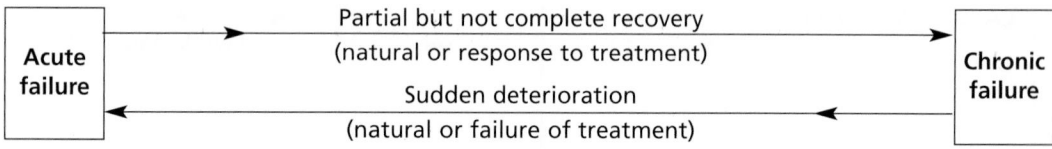

Acute failure → Partial but not complete recovery (natural or response to treatment) → Chronic failure

Chronic failure → Sudden deterioration (natural or failure of treatment) → Acute failure

# HEART FAILURE

## LEFT, RIGHT AND COMBINED VENTRICULAR FAILURE

From a clinical point of view it is convenient to consider heart failure as affecting one or the other side of the heart.

**The pulmonary circulation**
A low pressure system
Systolic arterial pressure = 24 mmHg
Pressure gradient, artery/vein = 8 mmHg

**The systemic circulation**
A high pressure system
Systolic arterial pressure = 120 mmHg
Pressure gradient, artery/vein = 90 mmHg

Right ventricular mass and    Left ventricular mass and
coronary blood supply   <   coronary blood supply
1:4 (approx.)

**MAIN CAUSES OF:**

**Right ventricular (RV) failure**

Usually secondary to disease elsewhere, causing obstruction to pulmonary blood flow.

(a) LUNG DISEASE –
   e.g. emphysema, fibrosis

(b) Some forms of cardiac valve disease, esp. MITRAL STENOSIS

(c) Congenital heart disease

(d) As a CONSEQUENCE of LV FAILURE

**Left ventricular (LV) failure**

1. Muscle weakness –
   ISCHAEMIC HEART DISEASE (due to coronary artery disease)

2. Excessive work load –
   SYSTEMIC HYPERTENSION
   Since these causes are so prevalent, LV failure is much more common than RV failure.

Less common causes are:
   Aortic valve disease
   Mitral incompetence
   Congenital heart disease.

Although left-sided and right-sided failure can occur independently, because their actions are closely integrated, failure of one cannot exist for long without eventually leading to failure of the other (combined ventricular failure).

# HEART FAILURE

### COMPENSATORY MECHANISMS

The onset of heart failure is preceded by compensatory changes:

1. **Increased rate of pumping**
2. **Dilatation**
3. **Hypertrophy**

### DILATATION

In physiological conditions, the volume of the ventricular chamber at the end of diastole (pre-load) directly influences the pumping force of the ventricular muscle, therefore:

This physiological dilatation also occurs in cardiac disease.

The larger the chamber size
(i.e. the longer the initial fibre length
and the greater the fibre stretch)
} the greater the contracting force.

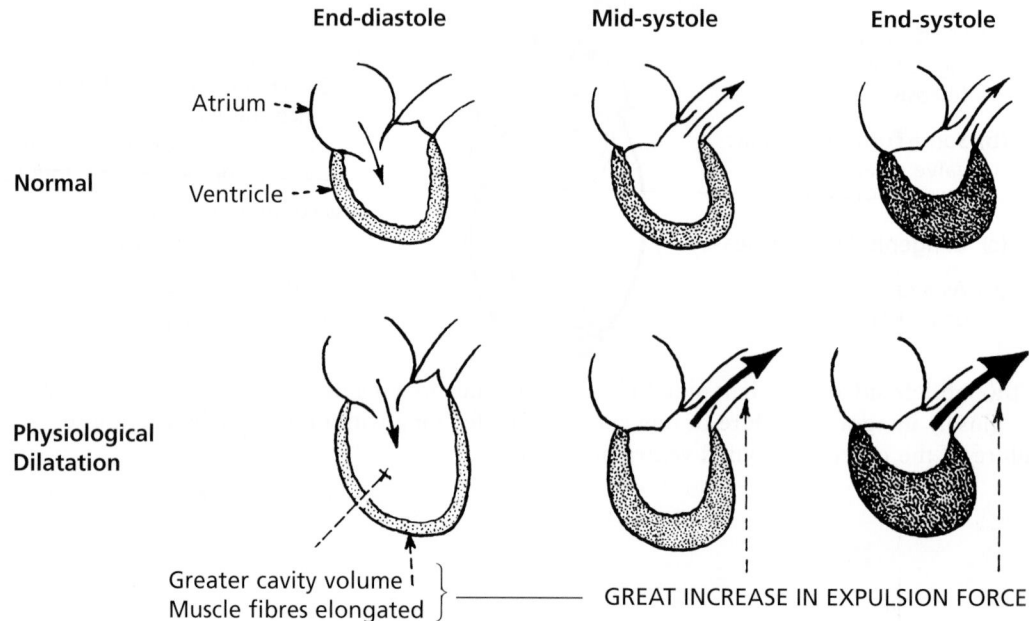

Greater cavity volume
Muscle fibres elongated
} ——————— GREAT INCREASE IN EXPULSION FORCE

# HEART FAILURE

In cardiac disease, particularly in cases of valvular incompetence, dilatation which occurs passively to accommodate the regurgitated blood is an important factor.

Aortic valve incompetence is a good example:

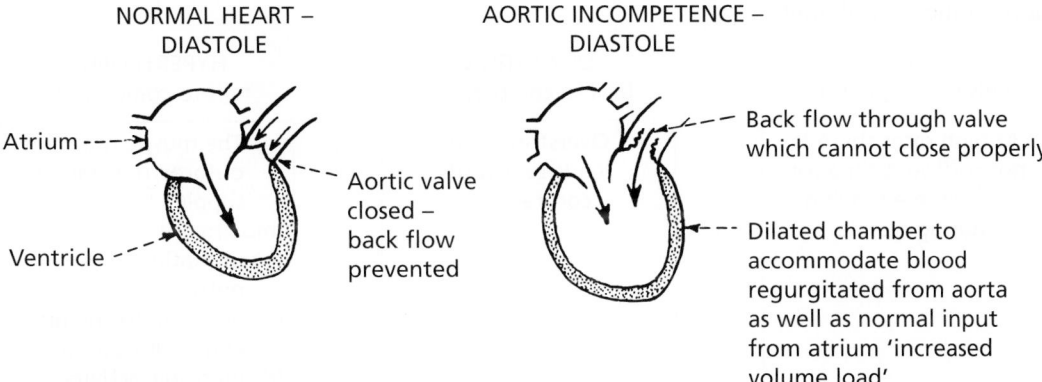

HYPERTROPHY involves an increase in muscle fibre bulk; the increased muscle mass is able to deal with a greater work load. In its pure form, hypertrophy is seen best in cases of increased pressure load.

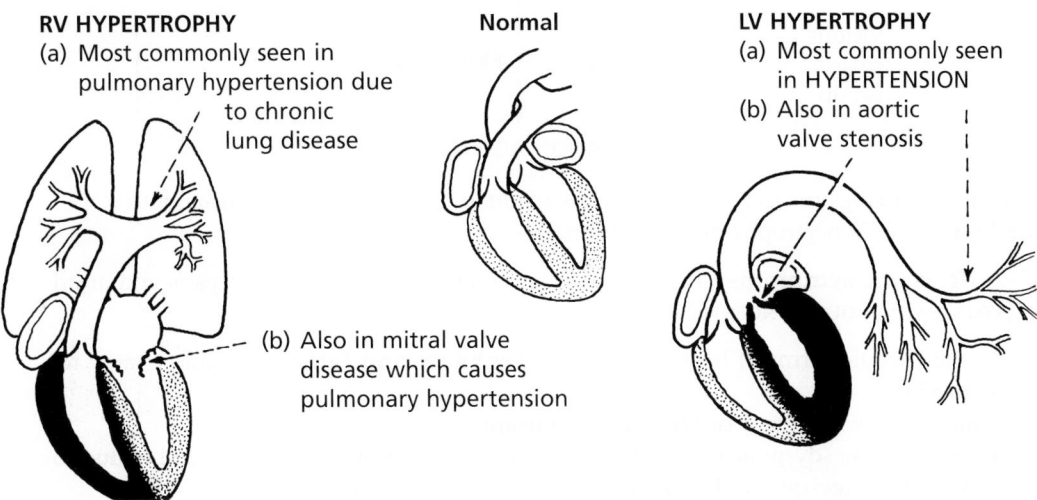

At first the blood supply to the hypertrophied muscle increases to meet the increased metabolic requirements. Later, however, the increased muscle bulk is detrimental as it places greater demands on the cardiac blood supply.

# HEART FAILURE

### FAILURE OF COMPENSATORY MECHANISMS

The increased efficiency derived from all three mechanisms is limited, and beyond this limit heart failure develops.

Beyond the critical limit:

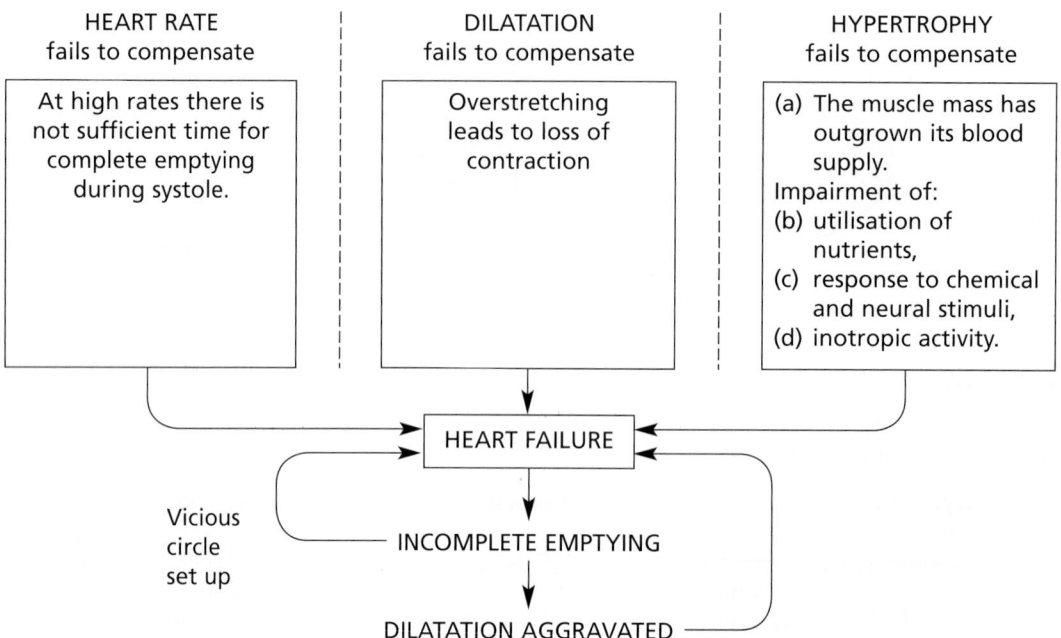

| HEART RATE fails to compensate | DILATATION fails to compensate | HYPERTROPHY fails to compensate |
|---|---|---|
| At high rates there is not sufficient time for complete emptying during systole. | Overstretching leads to loss of contraction | (a) The muscle mass has outgrown its blood supply. Impairment of: (b) utilisation of nutrients, (c) response to chemical and neural stimuli, (d) inotropic activity. |

HEART FAILURE

Vicious circle set up

INCOMPLETE EMPTYING

DILATATION AGGRAVATED

Thus in most cases of heart failure there is CARDIAC ENLARGEMENT due usually to a combination of hypertrophy and dilatation.

The **effects** and **symptoms** of heart failure are seen in the peripheral organs and are due to HYPOXIA and VENOUS CONGESTION.

(a) In the chronic forms of heart failure, the **weakness and fatigue** are due mainly to **hypoxia**.
(b) Venous congestion and oedema are important.
Breathlessness (dyspnoea) is almost a constant feature of heart failure and is due to venous congestion and fluid retention within the lungs.
In severe failure, particularly when bed rest is obligatory, *hypostatic pneumonia* and *pulmonary embolism* (from leg vein thrombosis) may be serious and terminal complications.

# EFFECTS OF HEART FAILURE

**LV** is the initiating event in most cases of combined failure.

The main effects are the results of:
(a) Low output
(b) 'Backward' pressure.*

**Cyanosis** is the result of excess reduced haemoglobin in capillaries and venules.

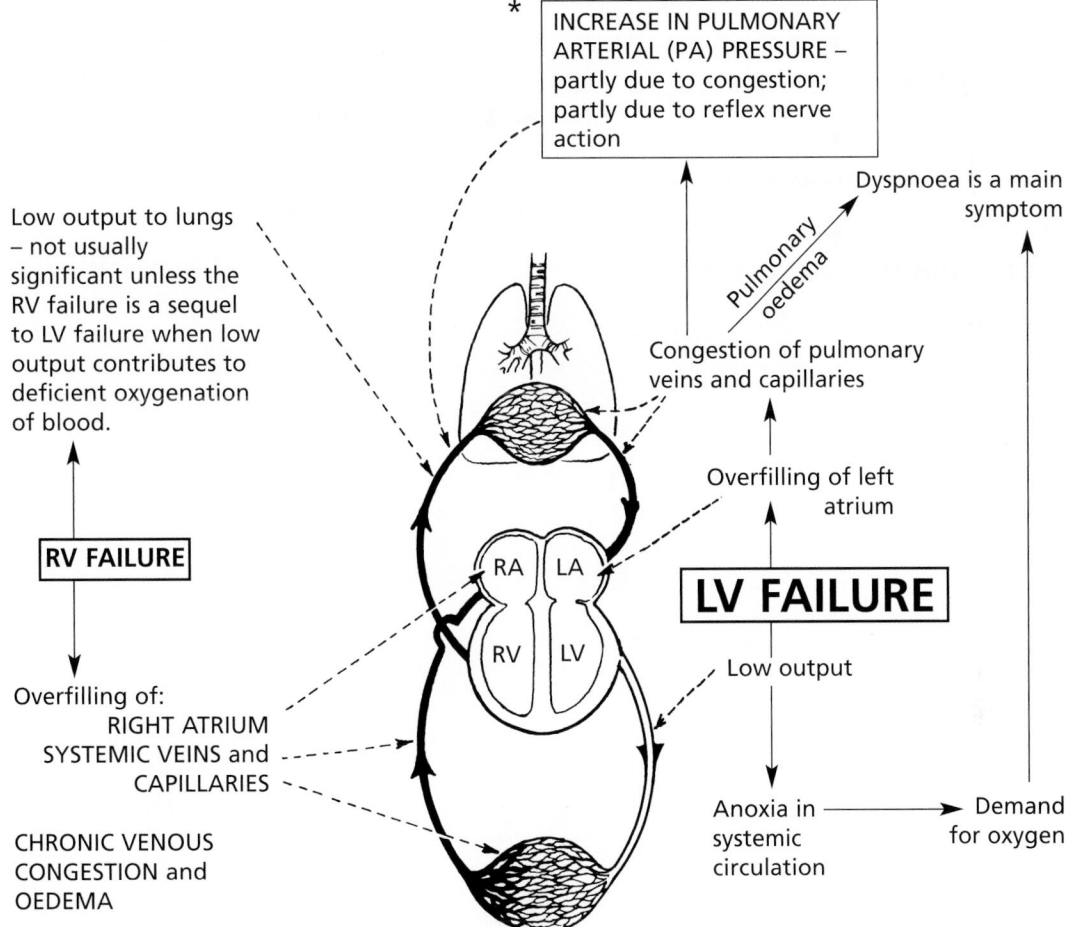

\* INCREASE IN PULMONARY ARTERIAL (PA) PRESSURE – partly due to congestion; partly due to reflex nerve action

Dyspnoea is a main symptom

Low output to lungs – not usually significant unless the RV failure is a sequel to LV failure when low output contributes to deficient oxygenation of blood.

Pulmonary oedema

Congestion of pulmonary veins and capillaries

Overfilling of left atrium

RV FAILURE

LV FAILURE

Overfilling of:
RIGHT ATRIUM
SYSTEMIC VEINS and
CAPILLARIES

Low output

CHRONIC VENOUS CONGESTION and OEDEMA

Anoxia in systemic circulation ⟶ Demand for oxygen

**Cyanosis** is the result of excess reduced haemoglobin in capillaries and venules.

\* The increase in pulmonary arterial pressure is important because in most cases of chronic LV failure it eventually leads to RV failure (combined failure).
RV – Right Ventricular; LV – Left Ventricular

## ACUTE PULMONARY OEDEMA

In **acute left ventricular failure**, accumulation of fluid results in dyspnoea and hypoxaemia.

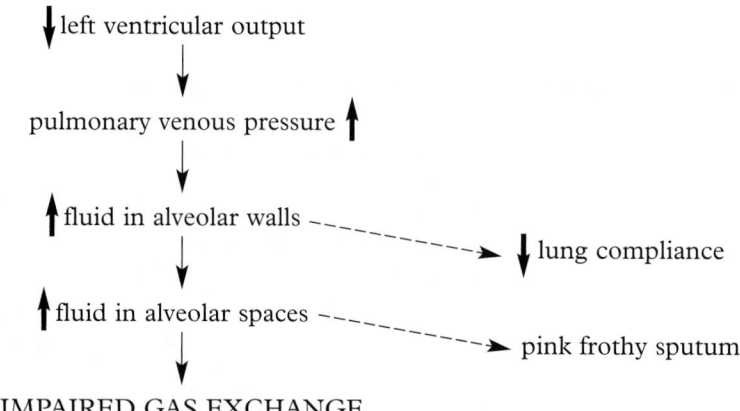

# CHRONIC PULMONARY OEDEMA

## CHRONIC VENOUS CONGESTION OF THE LUNGS

The results of chronic combined (congestive) failure and/or chronic left ventricular failure:

The lungs are bulky, congested and brownish in colour.

Cardiac failure

Hypoxia

Pulmonary venous engorgement

Hyperventilation

Pulmonary oedema

Alveolar haemorrhage

Breakdown of haemoglobin to haemosiderin and bilirubin

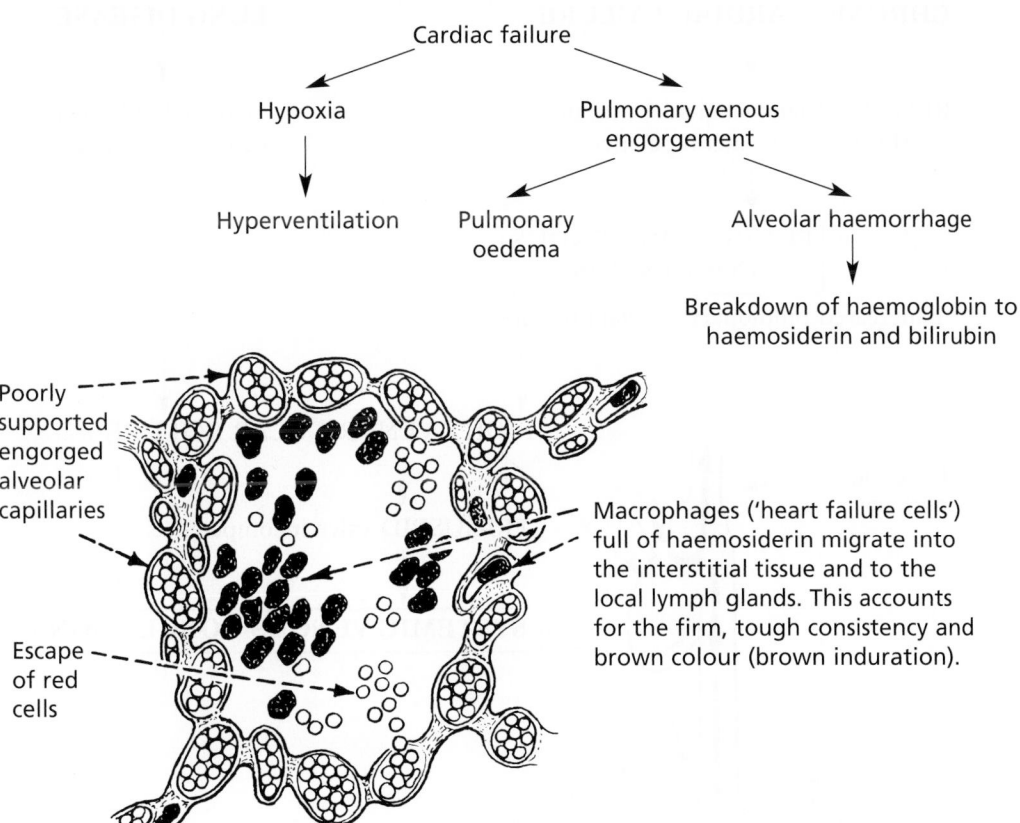

Poorly supported engorged alveolar capillaries

Escape of red cells

Macrophages ('heart failure cells') full of haemosiderin migrate into the interstitial tissue and to the local lymph glands. This accounts for the firm, tough consistency and brown colour (brown induration).

# CONGESTIVE CARDIAC FAILURE

Congestion of the systemic venous circulation is a result of right heart failure whether secondary to left heart failure or lung disease (cor pulmonale).

The basic mechanism is:

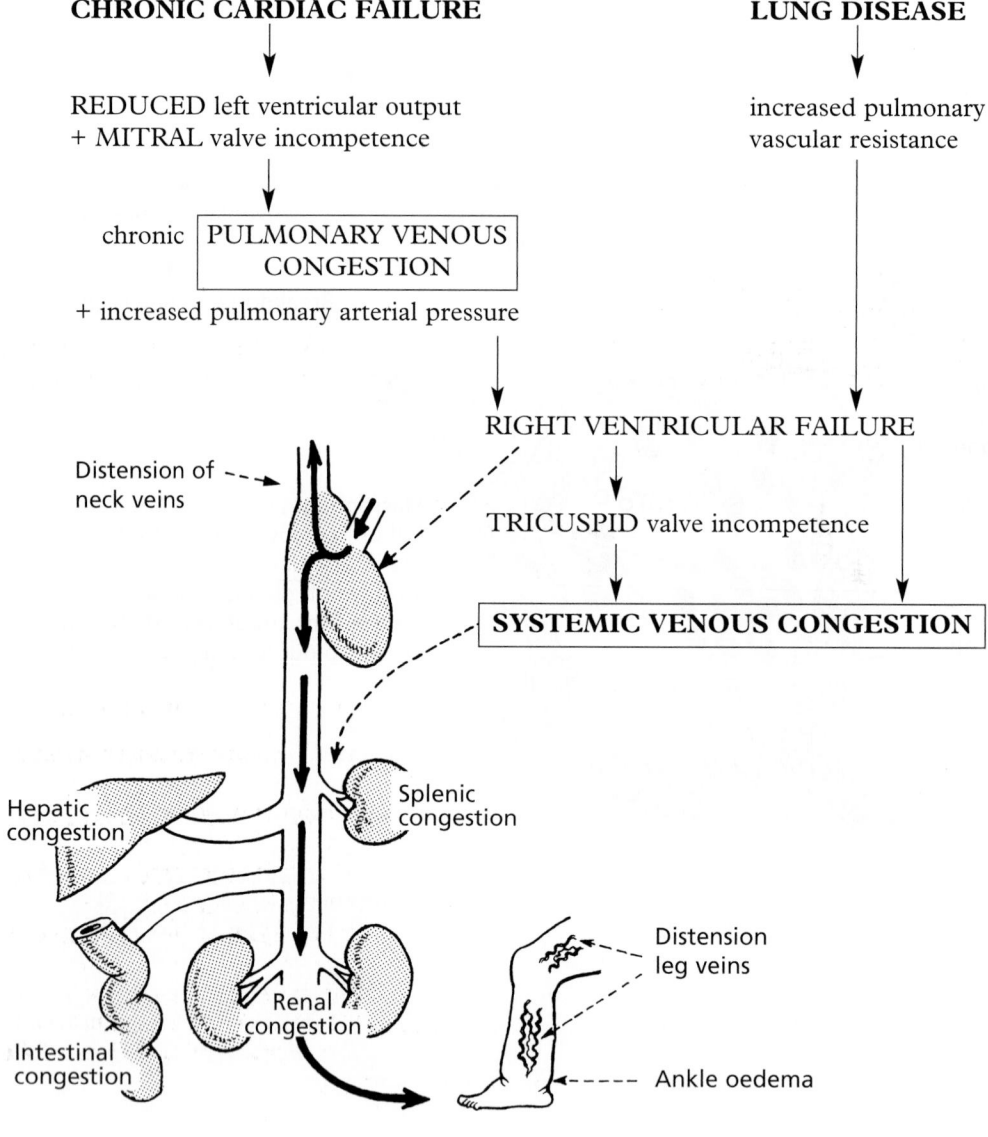

**CHRONIC CARDIAC FAILURE**

REDUCED left ventricular output
+ MITRAL valve incompetence

chronic | PULMONARY VENOUS CONGESTION

+ increased pulmonary arterial pressure

**LUNG DISEASE**

increased pulmonary vascular resistance

RIGHT VENTRICULAR FAILURE

TRICUSPID valve incompetence

SYSTEMIC VENOUS CONGESTION

Distension of neck veins

Hepatic congestion

Splenic congestion

Intestinal congestion

Renal congestion

Distension leg veins

Ankle oedema

# CONGESTIVE CARDIAC FAILURE

The **liver** shows striking changes: distension of the veins causes enlargement of the liver so that it can be felt below the costal margin.

The parenchymal cells furthest from the arterial blood supply, i.e. around the hepatic venules, undergo degeneration with atrophy and ultimately disappear. Cells nearer the arteries show an accumulation of fat.

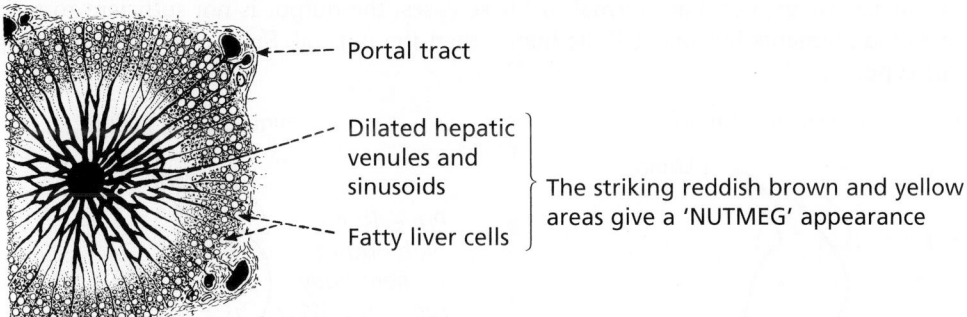

Portal tract

Dilated hepatic venules and sinusoids

Fatty liver cells

The striking reddish brown and yellow areas give a 'NUTMEG' appearance

## FLUID RETENTION

This is related to the REDUCED OUTPUT from the LV: the mechanism involves retention of sodium and water. Pleural effusion (p. 313) and ascites (p. 87) are also common effects of fluid retention in congestive cardiac failure.

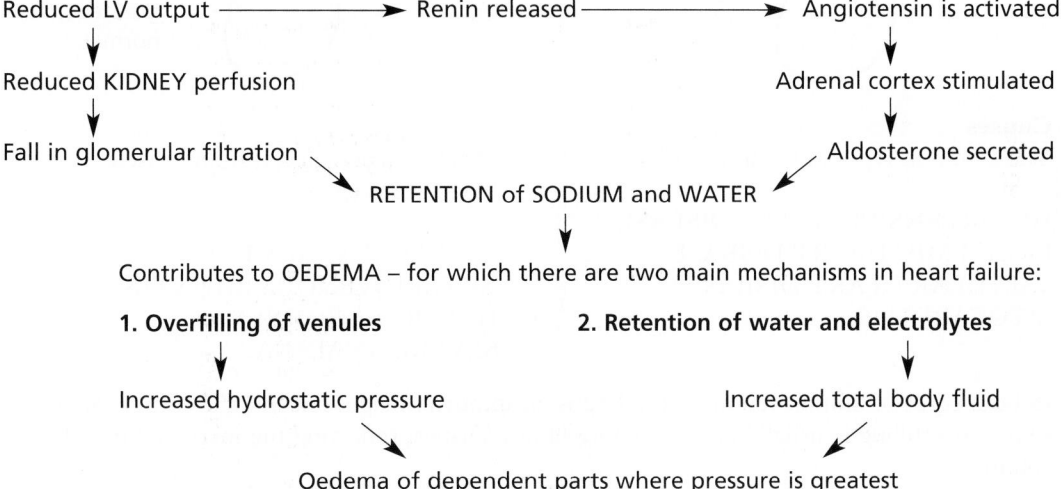

Reduced LV output ⟶ Renin released ⟶ Angiotensin is activated

Reduced KIDNEY perfusion → Adrenal cortex stimulated

Fall in glomerular filtration → Aldosterone secreted

RETENTION of SODIUM and WATER

Contributes to OEDEMA – for which there are two main mechanisms in heart failure:

**1. Overfilling of venules**

Increased hydrostatic pressure

**2. Retention of water and electrolytes**

Increased total body fluid

Oedema of dependent parts where pressure is greatest

# HIGH OUTPUT CARDIAC FAILURE

### LOW AND HIGH OUTPUT FAILURE

By definition, in cardiac failure output is low with respect to body requirements, and in most cases this output is lower than the normal output. Such cases are called **low output type.**

In a few conditions, the cardiac failure complicates a pre-existing state in which the output before failure was greater than normal. In these cases, the output is not sufficient to meet the body requirements but may still be higher than the normal. Such cases are called **high output type**.

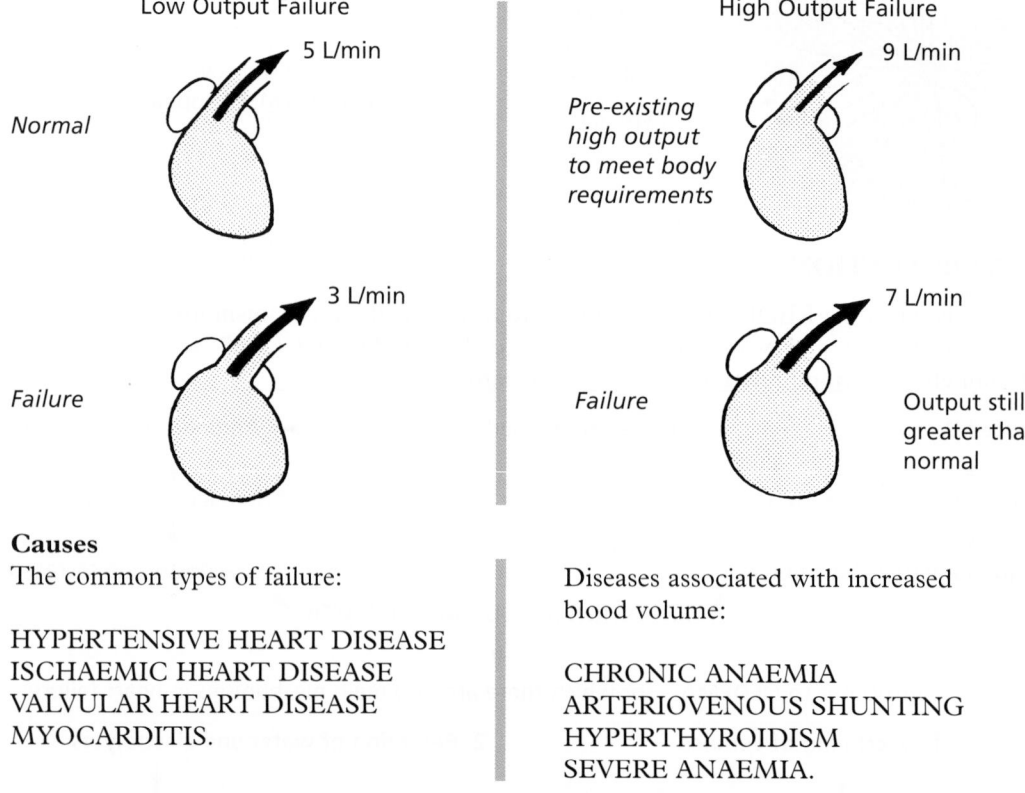

**Causes**

The common types of failure:

HYPERTENSIVE HEART DISEASE
ISCHAEMIC HEART DISEASE
VALVULAR HEART DISEASE
MYOCARDITIS.

Diseases associated with increased blood volume:

CHRONIC ANAEMIA
ARTERIOVENOUS SHUNTING
HYPERTHYROIDISM
SEVERE ANAEMIA.

In both types of failure, venous overfilling is an important sign, but in high output failure venous overfilling is usually present before failure ensues, reflecting the increased blood volume.

# DISEASES OF ARTERIES – ARTERIOSCLEROSIS

Arterial diseases are very common and are important because of their serious effects, especially on the heart and brain.

Normal age-related vascular changes:

**ARTERIOSCLEROSIS** (hardening of the arteries)

This is a generalised degeneration of the specialised muscle and elastic tissue of the media of the vessel wall, and replacement by fibrous tissue, proteoglycan and calcium salts. There is also proliferation of the inner layer of the vessel (intima).

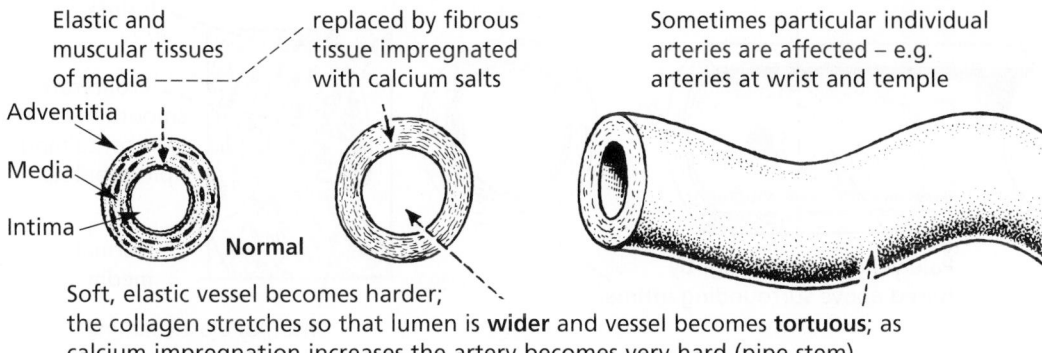

Elastic and muscular tissues of media ----- replaced by fibrous tissue impregnated with calcium salts

Sometimes particular individual arteries are affected – e.g. arteries at wrist and temple

Adventitia

Media

Intima

**Normal**

Soft, elastic vessel becomes harder; the collagen stretches so that lumen is **wider** and vessel becomes **tortuous**; as calcium impregnation increases the artery becomes very hard (pipe stem).

**HYALINE ARTERIOLOSCLEROSIS** affects the small branches of the arterial system (arterioles) – especially in the kidney.

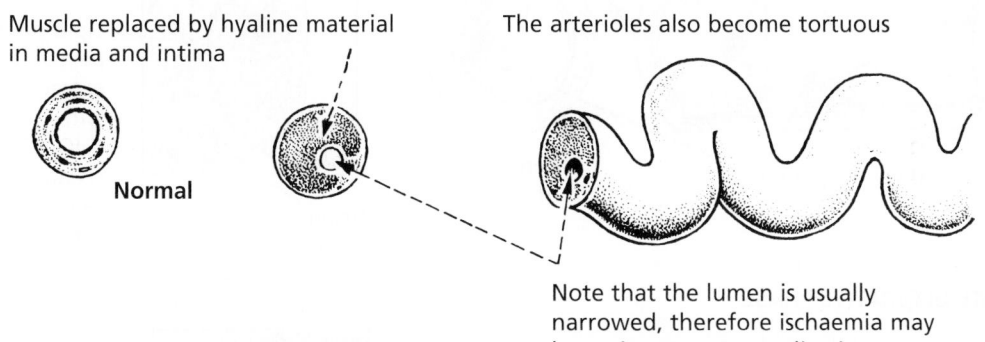

Muscle replaced by hyaline material in media and intima

The arterioles also become tortuous

**Normal**

Note that the lumen is usually narrowed, therefore ischaemia may be an important complication.

This is due to entry of blood plasma under the endothelium with protein deposition; gradual replacement by collagen occurs. The process is called **plasmatic vasculosis**.

*Note:* Arteriosclerosis is aggravated by HYPERTENSION and DIABETES MELLITUS.

In a variant of arteriosclerosis (Monckeberg), seen in the very elderly, calcium salts are very heavily deposited in the media particularly of the leg arteries. The X-ray appearances are striking but there is no significant loss of lumen unless atheroma co-exists.

# ATHEROMA (ATHEROSCLEROSIS)

Atheroma is a common disease in Westernised countries; it is of gradual onset but is progressive. It is commonly seen in the middle-aged and elderly people, but the earliest changes are present in adolescents. It is often asymptomatic but it may cause serious disease or death from complicating thrombosis. The lesions represent patchy deposition of lipid within plaques deep in the intima.

(Vessel opened longitudinally)

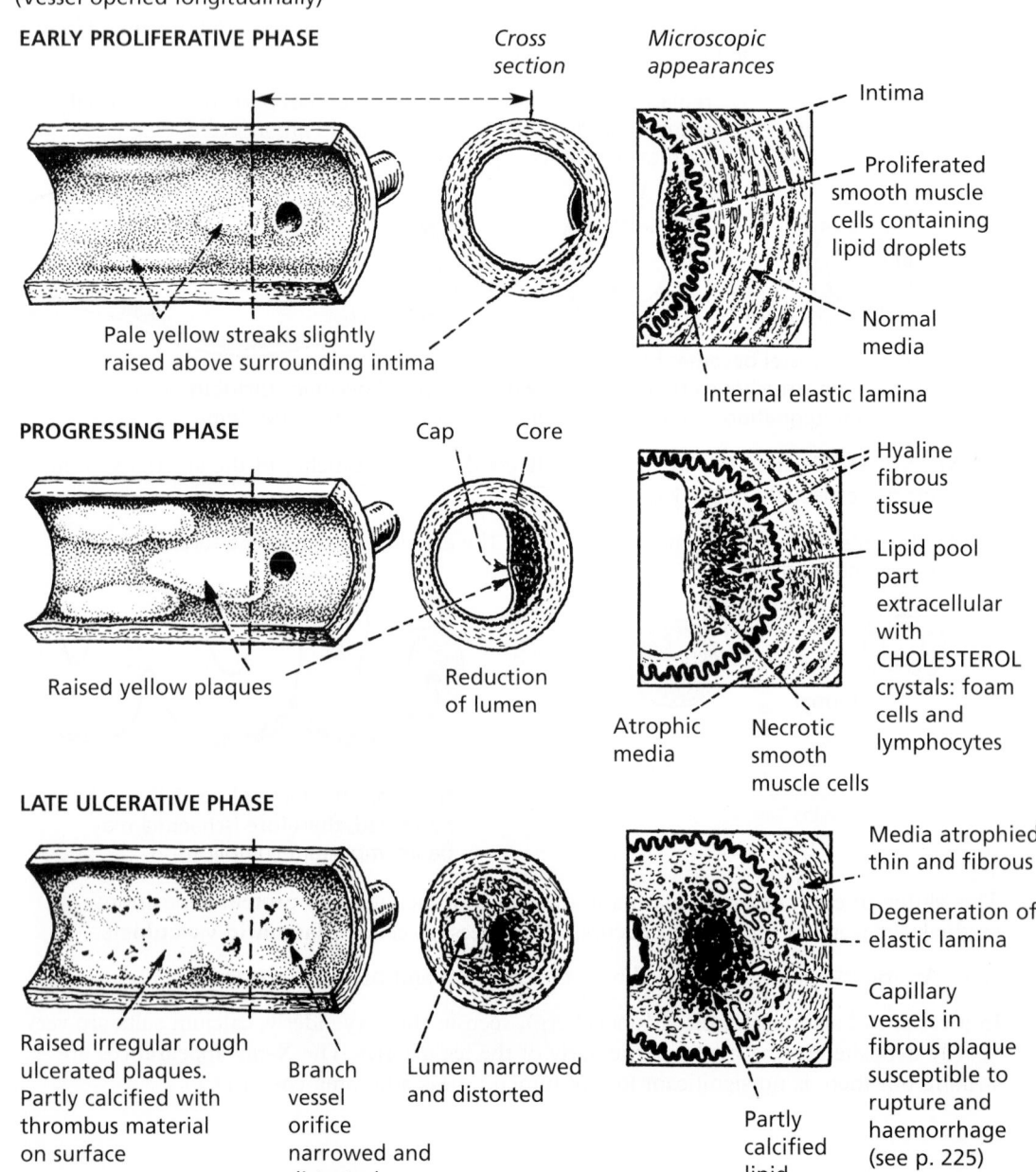

**EARLY PROLIFERATIVE PHASE**

Cross section

Microscopic appearances

Intima

Proliferated smooth muscle cells containing lipid droplets

Normal media

Pale yellow streaks slightly raised above surrounding intima

Internal elastic lamina

**PROGRESSING PHASE**

Cap          Core

Hyaline fibrous tissue

Lipid pool part extracellular with CHOLESTEROL crystals: foam cells and lymphocytes

Raised yellow plaques

Reduction of lumen

Atrophic media     Necrotic smooth muscle cells

**LATE ULCERATIVE PHASE**

Media atrophied, thin and fibrous

Degeneration of elastic lamina

Capillary vessels in fibrous plaque susceptible to rupture and haemorrhage (see p. 225)

Raised irregular rough ulcerated plaques. Partly calcified with thrombus material on surface

Branch vessel orifice narrowed and distorted

Lumen narrowed and distorted

Partly calcified lipid

# ATHEROMA – COMPLICATIONS

Fibrosis in the intima and media weaken the wall and may lead to aneurysm formation (see p. 256), but the most important complication of atheroma is THROMBOSIS.

Local factors at the site of the atheromatous plaque are important:

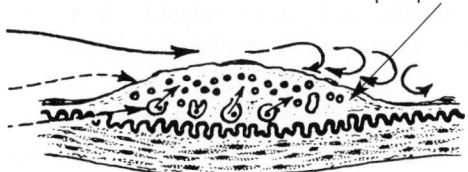

Atheromatous plaque

1.  Intimal roughening or distortion with eddying of flow.
2.  Thin, easily damaged intimal surface.
3.  Rupture of new capillaries in plaque with haemorrhage into the plaque

In addition, general factors influencing blood coagulability are important, e.g. smoking affecting vessel contractility and platelet function.

*Results*

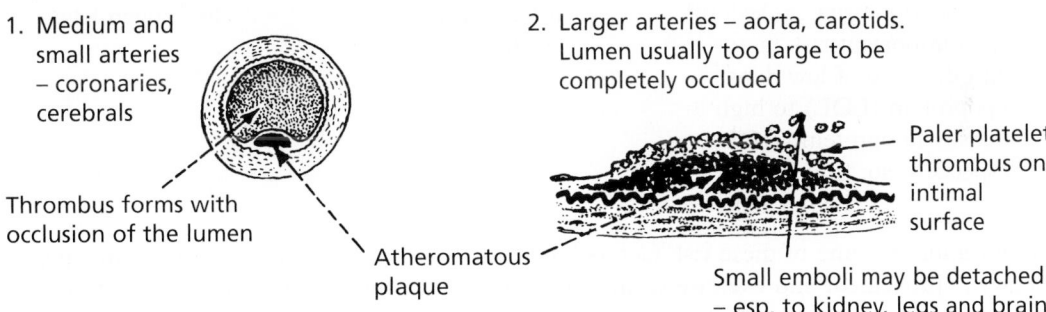

1. Medium and small arteries – coronaries, cerebrals

Thrombus forms with occlusion of the lumen

Atheromatous plaque

2. Larger arteries – aorta, carotids. Lumen usually too large to be completely occluded

Paler platelet thrombus on intimal surface

Small emboli may be detached – esp. to kidney, legs and brain

The important sites of atheroma and the effects due to complications are:

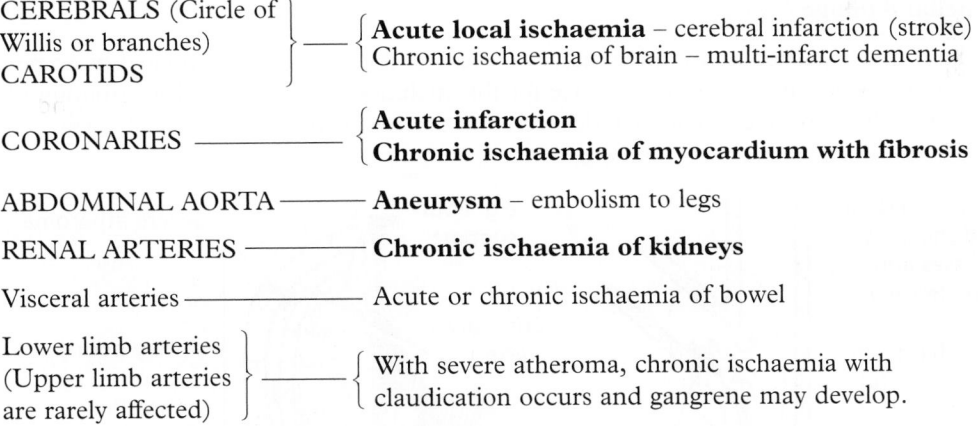

CEREBRALS (Circle of Willis or branches) CAROTIDS — { **Acute local ischaemia** – cerebral infarction (stroke) <br> Chronic ischaemia of brain – multi-infarct dementia

CORONARIES — { **Acute infarction** <br> **Chronic ischaemia of myocardium with fibrosis**

ABDOMINAL AORTA — **Aneurysm** – embolism to legs

RENAL ARTERIES — **Chronic ischaemia of kidneys**

Visceral arteries — Acute or chronic ischaemia of bowel

Lower limb arteries (Upper limb arteries are rarely affected) — { With severe atheroma, chronic ischaemia with <br> claudication occurs and gangrene may develop.

In severe cases of atheroma, most of these sites may be affected.

# ATHEROMA – AETIOLOGY

The cause of atheroma is complex and multifactorial.

The risk factors can be defined as fixed or modifiable. Modifiable risk factors can be further considered as environmental and disease related. The various risk factors exponentially increase with AGE.

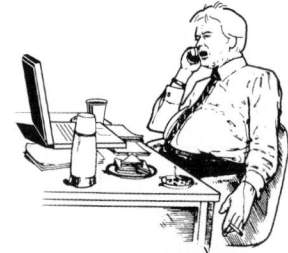

1. **FIXED**
   (a) SEX – male > female
   (b) HEREDITY
      (i) Family history of premature heart disease
      (ii) Familial hyperlipidaemias
   Increased plasma cholesterol is an important risk factor and the ratio of low density lipoprotein (LDL) to high density lipoprotein (HDL) especially, so: LDL↑ risk↑↑
              HDL↑ risk↓

2. **MODIFIABLE**
   *ENVIRONMENTAL*
   (a) SMOKING
   (b) DIET – rich in saturated fats and cholesterol and low in fruit and vegetables
   (c) Lack of exercise

3. **DISEASES**
   (a) HYPERTENSION
   (b) Hyperlipidaemia
   (c) Diabetes mellitus
   (d) Obesity
   (e) Increased fibrinogen levels

Modification of some of these risk factors has led to a fall in incidence. Avoiding smoking, dietary improvement and exercise seem most important, while treating raised cholesterol with statins is now widely used.

## PATHOGENESIS OF ATHEROSCLEROSIS

### Endothelial damage

Atheroma is now regarded as an inflammatory disease of the arterial wall initiated by some form of injury to the endothelium. Evidence for this includes the preferential distribution of lesions, e.g. arch of aorta, coronary arteries, cerebral arteries, carotids, abdominal aorta where local mechanical stress is common.

e.g. **Areas of lateral and shearing stresses and turbulence** at acute bends or branching – in aorta, carotids, abdominal aortic branches.

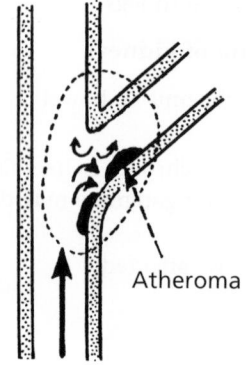

Atheroma

e.g. **Poor support**

Coronary artery

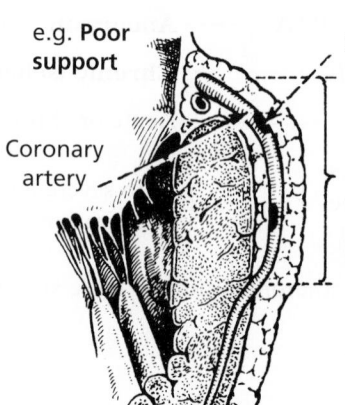

Severe atheroma

Artery poorly supported by pericardial tissues

Similarly in cerebral arteries, mesenterics, etc.

# ATHEROMA – AETIOLOGY AND PROGRESSION

## Pathogenesis

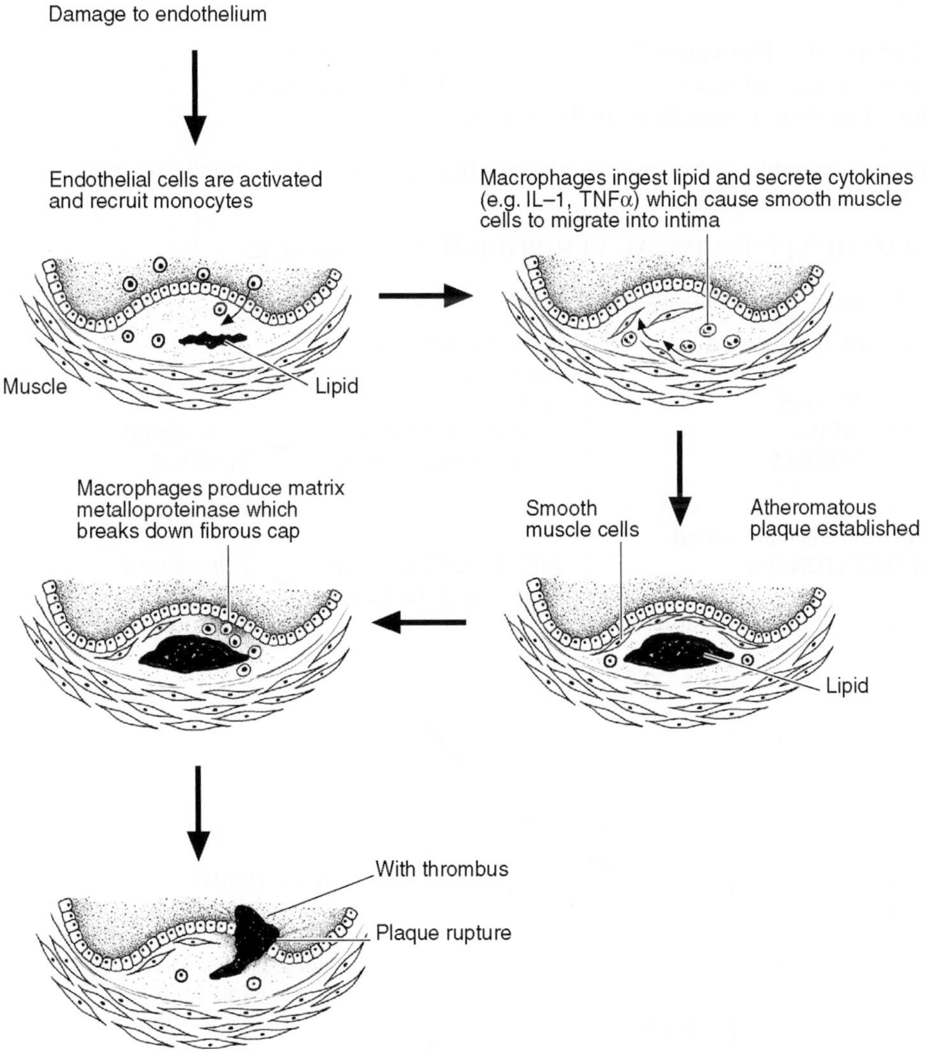

Damage to endothelium

Endothelial cells are activated
and recruit monocytes

Muscle — Lipid

Macrophages ingest lipid and secrete cytokines
(e.g. IL–1, TNFα) which cause smooth muscle
cells to migrate into intima

Macrophages produce matrix
metalloproteinase which
breaks down fibrous cap

Smooth
muscle cells

Atheromatous
plaque established

Lipid

With thrombus

Plaque rupture

# HYPERTENSION

High blood pressure (BP) is important because it increases the risk of cardiovascular disease, especially:

1. **Left Ventricular Hypertrophy** ⎫ ——————→ Cardiac failure.
2. **Ischaemic Heart Disease** ⎭ ——————→ Sudden death.
3. **Stroke** – Cerebral haemorrhage or Infarction.

BP is a continuous variable within the population. It is determined essentially by two variables:

BP = CARDIAC OUTPUT × TOTAL PERIPHERAL RESISTANCE.

**Mechanisms of normal maintenance of BP and the effect of age**

| | |
|---|---|
| The systolic pressure is governed by<br>(a) cardiac action<br>(b) the ELASTICITY and DISTENSIBILITY of the CONDUCTING ARTERIES | Increasing AGE is normally associated with<br>ARTERIOSCLEROSIS – loss of distensibility ↗ ∴ Increased SYSTOLIC pressure |
| The diastolic pressure is maintained by the **RESISTANCE (TONE)** of arterioles<br>(a subsidiary factor is blood viscosity) | ARTERIOLOSCLEROSIS – increased resistance ↗ ∴ Increased DIASTOLIC pressure |

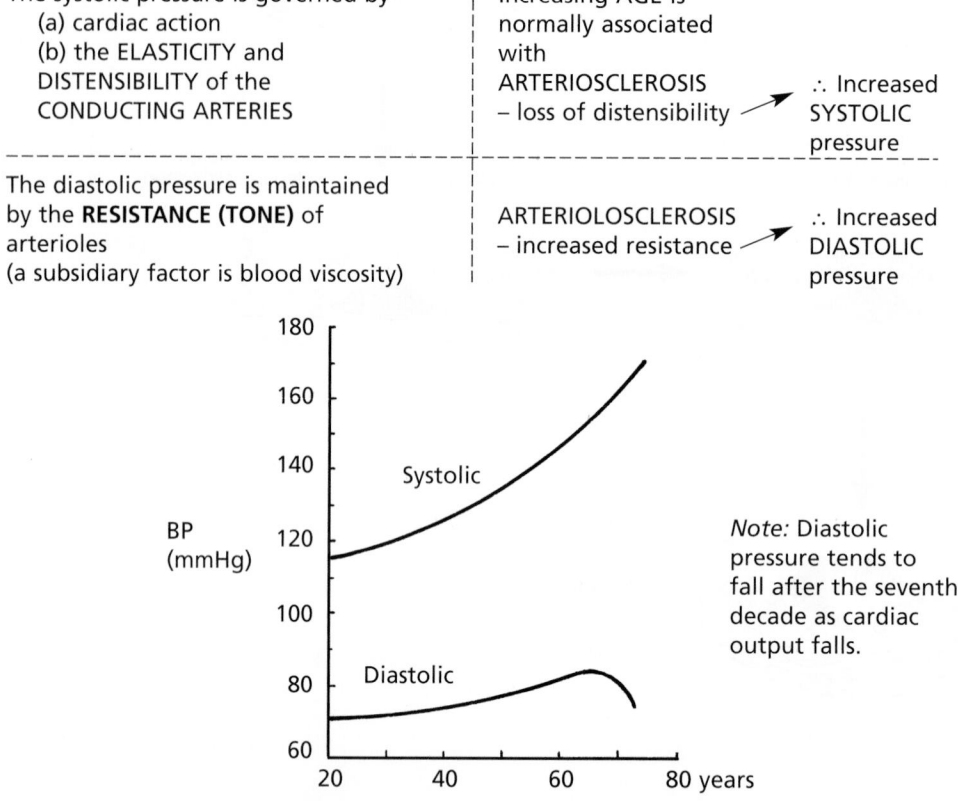

*Note:* Diastolic pressure tends to fall after the seventh decade as cardiac output falls.

Because of the wide range in the normal population, the definition of high BP is arbitrary. The risk of complications progressively increases with BP, including within the normal range. The levels of **systolic** and **diastolic** pressure are both risk factors.

Systolic BP>160 mmHg and diastolic BP>95 mmHg are generally accepted as **hypertension**.

Modern therapy is effective in lowering BP. The decision whether or not to treat depends on the level of BP and the presence of other risk factors for cardiovascular disease.

# HYPERTENSION – MECHANISMS

## Aetiology

The following diagram illustrates the physiological mechanisms controlling BP. They are presented in two groups but are complex and interconnected with feedback controls.

1. **Autonomic nervous system**
   (a) External environment
   (b) Internal environment, e.g. baroreceptors

2. **Hormones**
   (a) Pituitary/adrenal
   (b) Renal

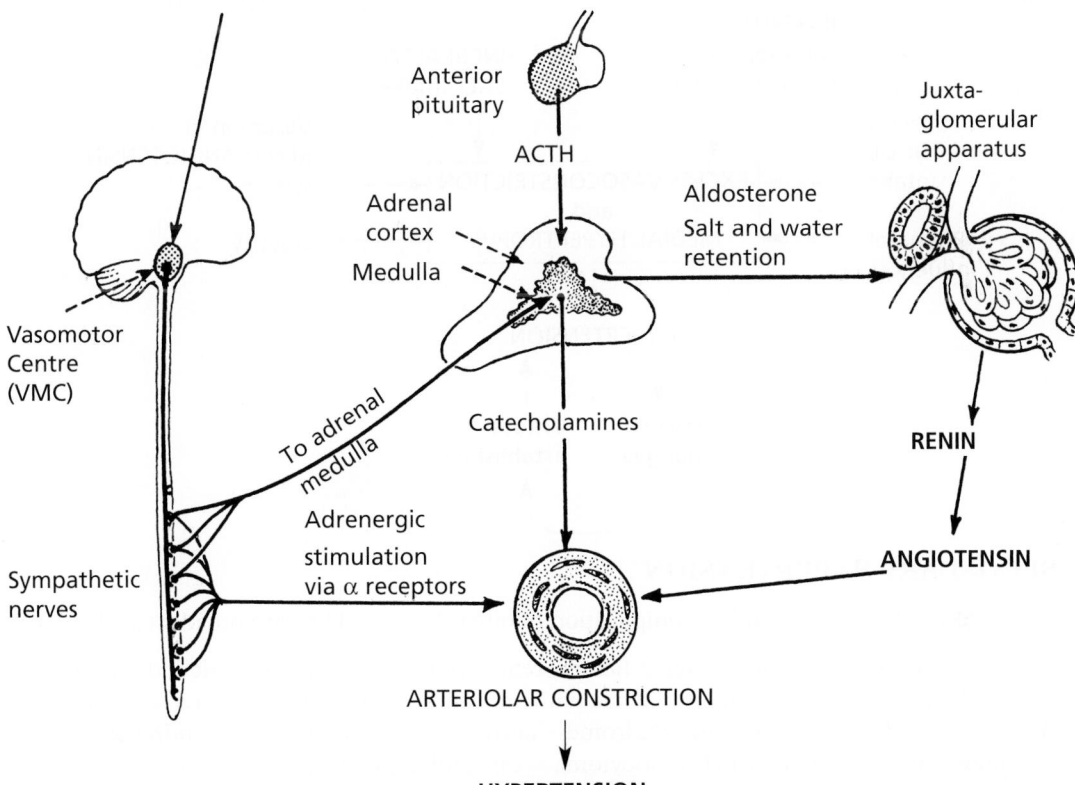

Anterior pituitary

ACTH

Juxta-glomerular apparatus

Adrenal cortex

Medulla

Aldosterone Salt and water retention

Vasomotor Centre (VMC)

To adrenal medulla

Catecholamines

RENIN

Sympathetic nerves

Adrenergic stimulation via α receptors

ANGIOTENSIN

ARTERIOLAR CONSTRICTION

**HYPERTENSION**

*Note:* **Nitric oxide** (NO) and **endothelin** are both produced physiologically by endothelial cells. They have powerful and opposite effects.

Nitric oxide _____ vasodilatation (short acting).
Endothelin _____ vasoconstriction (long acting).

Their role in hypertension is not yet clear.

# HYPERTENSION – ESSENTIAL AND SECONDARY

### ESSENTIAL HYPERTENSION

In 95% of cases of hypertension no obvious cause is found – this is ESSENTIAL hypertension – (a diagnosis of exclusion).

A number of aetiological factors may be implicated:
1. Genetic predisposition – polygenic inheritance.
2. Racial, e.g. black > white.
3. Sodium homeostasis: increased **salt intake.**
4. Lack of exercise.

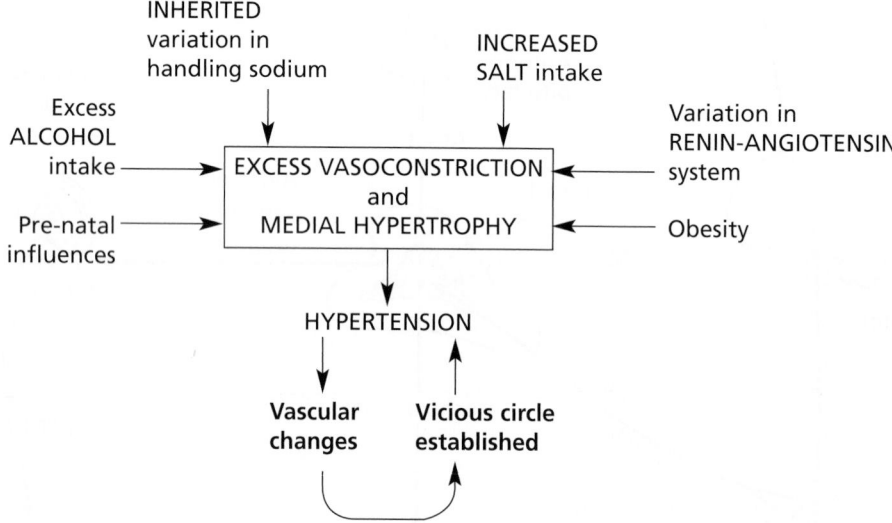

### SECONDARY HYPERTENSION

Five percent of hypertension is a complication of other diseases. They are broadly classified as:

(a) *Kidney diseases,* e.g. chronic renal failure, renal artery stenosis, polycystic kidneys. The mechanism is usually renal ischaemia with activation of the renin-angiotensin system.
(b) *Endocrine disorders* – Cushing syndrome – corticosteroid excess; Conn syndrome – aldosterone excess; Phaeochromocytoma – catecholamine excess.
(c) *Coarctation of aorta* – aortic narrowing → renal perfusion impaired → renin-angiotensin activation.
(d) *Eclampsia* and pre-eclampsia in pregnancy.
(e) *Drugs,* e.g. steroids, oral contraceptives.

# HYPERTENSION – ESSENTIAL AND SECONDARY

## CLASSIFICATION – BENIGN AND MALIGNANT

In the classification of hypertension, in addition to the aetiology, two other main factors are considered.

| 1. Rate of Progress | | 2. Height and rapidity of rise of the BP | |
|---|---|---|---|
| Chronic – over many years | + | Usually only mild or moderate very slow rise. (*Note:* The very old may have considerably higher BP without ill-effects) | **Benign –** during long course but eventually may have serious effects |
| Rapid (acute) – months or 1–2 years | + | Usually very high and rapidly rising BP, e.g. 120 + diastolic | **Malignant –** serious damaging effects |

**Summary**

Essential (95%)

Benign   or   Malignant

Secondary (5%)

Benign   or   Malignant

## COMPARISON OF BENIGN AND MALIGNANT HYPERTENSION

| | BENIGN | MALIGNANT |
|---|---|---|
| **Aetiology** | Usually ESSENTIAL If secondary, commonly of endocrine type | A few cases arise from benign essential Majority are SECONDARY TO RENAL DISEASE |
| **Age** | Begins younger than 45 years but is prolonged into sixth and seventh decades of life | Young adults 25–35 years |
| **Sex** | Female > Male | Female = Male |
| **Prevalence** | VERY COMMON – at least 15% of population in Western societies | Rare |
| **Course** | VERY SLOW – many years | RAPID – months to 1–2 years |
| **BP** | Diastolic 90–120 mmHg Very slow rise | Diastolic >120 mmHg Rapid rise |

# HYPERTENSION – ESSENTIAL AND SECONDARY

## VASCULAR CHANGES

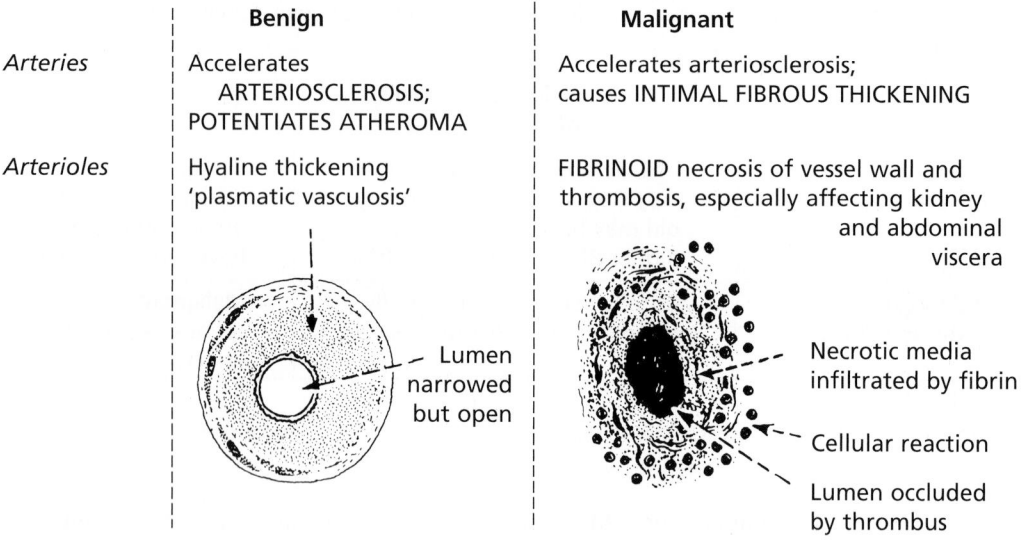

|  | **Benign** | **Malignant** |
|---|---|---|
| *Arteries* | Accelerates ARTERIOSCLEROSIS; POTENTIATES ATHEROMA | Accelerates arteriosclerosis; causes INTIMAL FIBROUS THICKENING |
| *Arterioles* | Hyaline thickening 'plasmatic vasculosis' | FIBRINOID necrosis of vessel wall and thrombosis, especially affecting kidney and abdominal viscera |

Lumen narrowed but open

Necrotic media infiltrated by fibrin

Cellular reaction

Lumen occluded by thrombus

## EFFECTS AND MAIN COMPLICATIONS IN VARIOUS ORGANS

| | | |
|---|---|---|
| *Heart* | Hypertrophy of left ventricle | Hypertrophy of left ventricle ± focal myocardial necrosis |
| *Heart failure* | Common | Acute heart failure |
| *Cerebral haemorrhage* | Due to rupture of damaged artery | Encephalopathy (fits and loss of consciousness) due to cerebral oedema and haemorrhage |
| *Kidney* | Varying degrees of NEPHROSCLEROSIS but usually not serious | Severe renal damage – death in uraemia |
| *Eyes* | Arterial narrowing – retinal exudation | Papilloedema; arterial narrowing; haemorrhage and exudates |

The effects and complications are proportional to the height of the BP. Therefore drug treatment which lowers the BP lowers the incidence of complications, but the diseased vessels do not return to normal and organ perfusion may be inadequate at levels of BP which would usually be considered physiological.

*Note:* Modern drug therapy has greatly reduced the morbidity and mortality from malignant hypertension.

# ISCHAEMIC HEART DISEASE

Cardiac ischaemia is a major cause of death in affluent Western societies. It is almost always due to **atheroma** of the **coronary arteries** causing narrowing or occlusion. The effects may be sudden or of gradual onset.

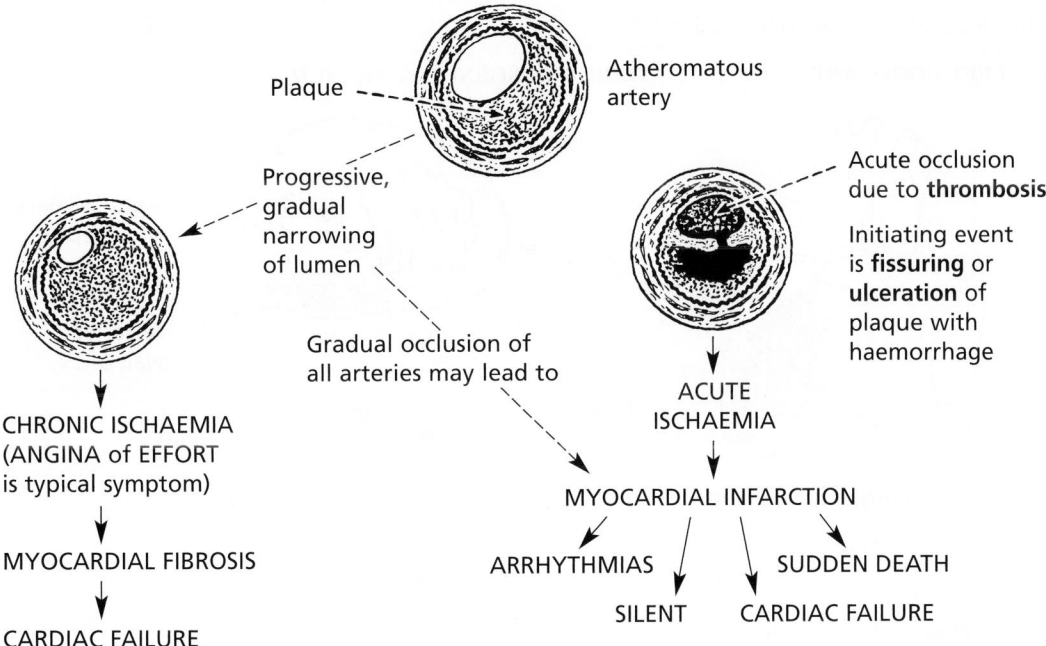

Plaque

Atheromatous artery

Progressive, gradual narrowing of lumen

Acute occlusion due to **thrombosis**

Initiating event is **fissuring** or **ulceration** of plaque with haemorrhage

Gradual occlusion of all arteries may lead to

ACUTE ISCHAEMIA

CHRONIC ISCHAEMIA (ANGINA of EFFORT is typical symptom)

MYOCARDIAL INFARCTION

MYOCARDIAL FIBROSIS

ARRHYTHMIAS

SUDDEN DEATH

CARDIAC FAILURE

SILENT

CARDIAC FAILURE

## Distribution of atheromatous plaques

1. There may be only a few plaques, but because the sites of predilection are in the proximal parts of the arteries (usually within 3 cm of the origin from the aorta), the effects of occlusion are serious.

or 2. Very numerous plaques.
*Note*: The small terminal arteries penetrating the myocardium are usually not affected.

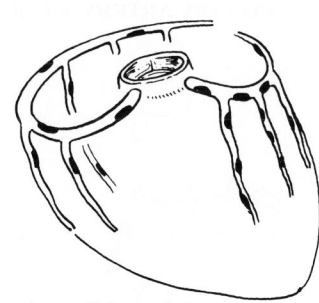

L. circumflex artery

R. cor. artery

L. ant. desc. artery

Aortic valve

3. Any combination of 1. and 2.

The site of ischaemic damage usually represents the distribution area of the diseased arterial branch.

# MYOCARDIAL INFARCTION

Ninety percent of cardiac infarcts are regional in distribution. The remaining 10% are subendocardial.

### REGIONAL INFARCTION

The three commonest regions are:

1. **LEFT CORONARY ARTERY – ANTERIOR DESCENDING BRANCH**

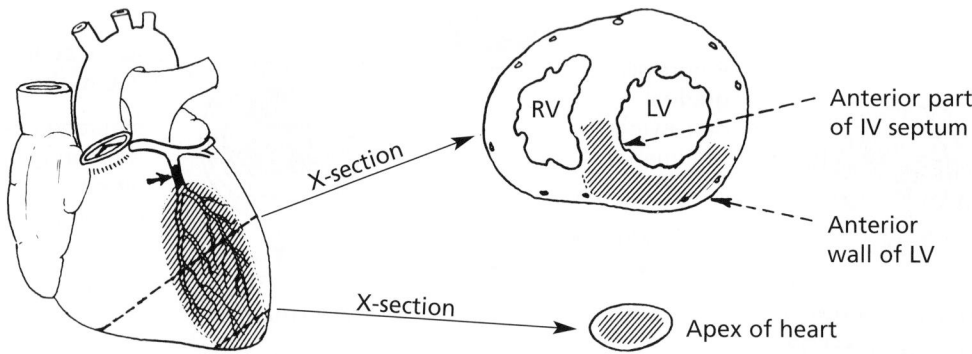

2. **RIGHT CORONARY ARTERY**

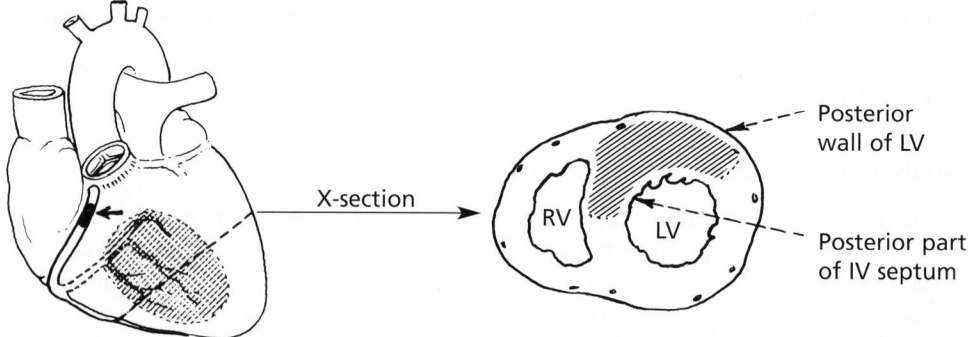

3. **LEFT CORONARY ARTERY – CIRCUMFLEX BRANCH**

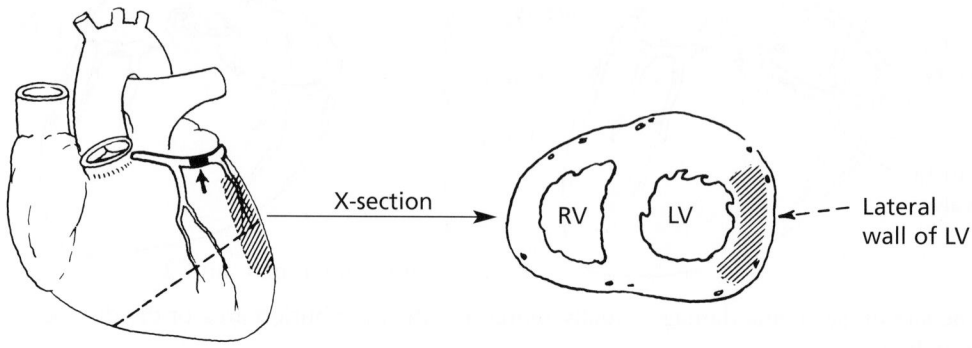

# MYOCARDIAL INFARCTION

## EXTENT OF DAMAGE

This depends on:

1. The inherited individual anatomical variation in distribution area, e.g. the calibres of the right coronary artery and the circumflex branch of the left coronary artery show considerable variation and are usually inversely related.

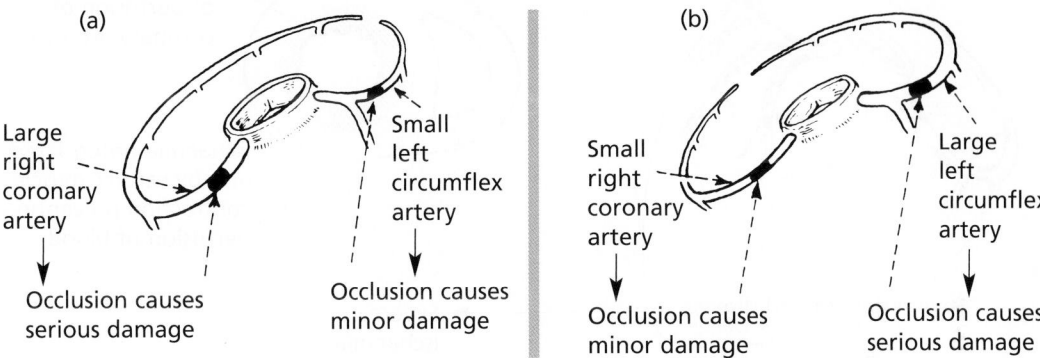

(a)

Large right coronary artery

Small left circumflex artery

Occlusion causes serious damage

Occlusion causes minor damage

(b)

Small right coronary artery

Large left circumflex artery

Occlusion causes minor damage

Occlusion causes serious damage

2. The efficiency of any anastomosis in the deprived distribution area. Gradual narrowing of an artery allows time for increased anastomosis to the deprived distribution area to develop, and so old age tends to be associated with improved anastomoses.

(a)
ACUTE OCCLUSION supervening on MINIMAL STENOSIS OF LUMEN

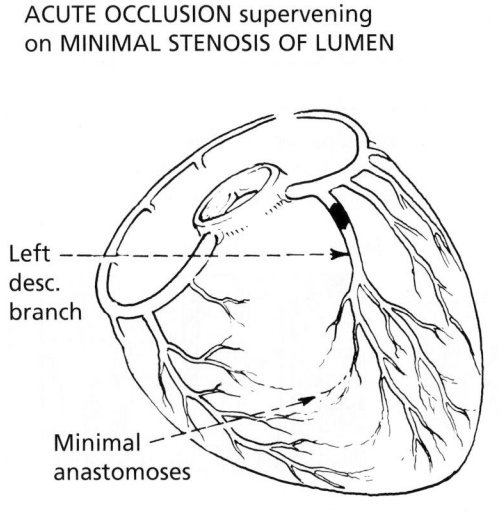

Left desc. branch

Minimal anastomoses

COMPLETE OCCLUSION is usually accompanied by myocardial infarction.

(b)
ACUTE OCCLUSION following GRADUAL STENOSIS of left desc. branch

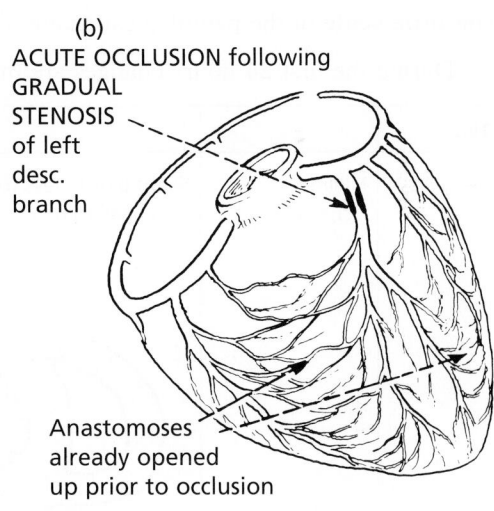

Anastomoses already opened up prior to occlusion

COMPLETE OCCLUSION may be accompanied by only minor damage.

# MYOCARDIAL INFARCTION

### SUBENDOCARDIAL INFARCTION

This type occurs round the circumference of the left ventricle under the endocardium in cases of severe stenosis of all the coronary arteries and is often due to hypotension. The coronaries are usually not thrombosed.

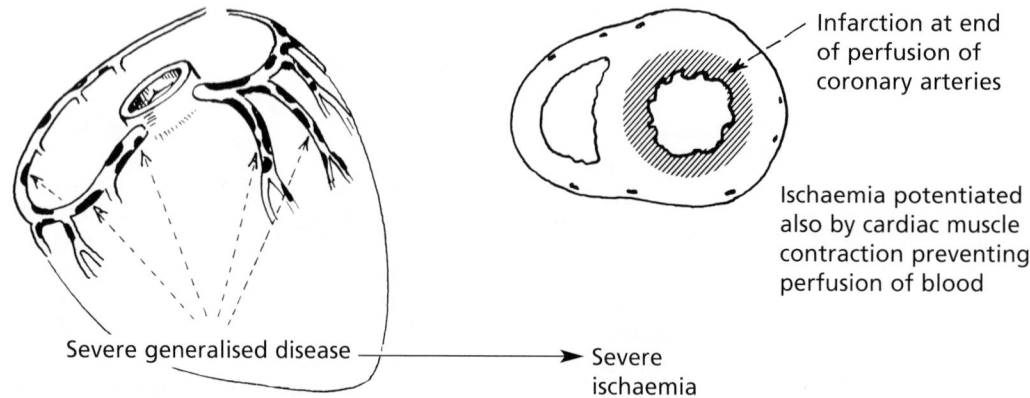

Infarction at end of perfusion of coronary arteries

Ischaemia potentiated also by cardiac muscle contraction preventing perfusion of blood

Severe generalised disease ⟶ Severe ischaemia

**Microscopic focal infarction** is necrosis of single or small groups of muscle fibres at the margins of areas of myocardium previously damaged by ischaemia and is a component of progressive chronic ischaemia.

The **time scale** of the pathological changes following acute infarction is illustrated.

1. During the first 24 hours changes are minimal.

| Time | | | |
|---|---|---|---|
| *0–24 hrs* | Minimal change | Slight blotchiness (congestion and pallor) of infarcted area | Slight separation of fibres; slight increase of leucocytes between fibres; slight disturbance of cell cytoplasm<br><br>*Normal     Affected fibres* |

# MYOCARDIAL INFARCTION

| Time | | | |
|------|---|---|---|
| *24 hrs – 3 days* | Definite changes in dead muscle | Dead muscle, paler yellow<br>*Note:* Usually a thin layer of healthy muscle under the endocardium | Dead muscle fibres have lost striations and nuclei; cytoplasm glassy pink (H & E staining); capillary congestion at margin; neutrophils and macrophages increasing in number |
| *3–10 days* | Healing (organisation) commencing | Margin of congestion (redness) appearing around dead muscle and resorption of muscle becoming visible at the edges | Muscle fibres splitting up and being resorbed; granulation tissue at edges; neutrophils still present |
| *Weeks– months* | Scar tissue – healing complete | White fibrous tissue | Scar tissue – may be occasional surviving muscle fibres embedded |

These changes represent the uncomplicated continuous process of healing and can be altered by the administration of early thrombolytic therapy, e.g. streptokinase. Streptokinase therapy can lead to revascularisation of the heart muscle with haemorrhage in any necrotic muscle. Complications of myocardial infarction are frequent, producing serious, often fatal, effects.

# MYOCARDIAL INFARCTION

| TIME | COMPLICATIONS |
|------|---------------|
| *Minutes, hours* | 1. **ARRHYTHMIAS**<br>(a) *Ventricular fibrillation*, i.e. cardiac arrest (especially liable at onset of infarction and during first few days)<br>(b) *Heart block of impulse* conduction in Bundle of His and/or its branches – usually causes slowing of ventricular rhythm or upsets the balance of ventricular contraction<br><br>2. **CARDIAC FAILURE**<br><br>3. **CARDIOGENIC SHOCK**<br>Associated with large infarcts |
| *Days* | 4. **THROMBOTIC COMPLICATIONS**<br><br>(a) **MURAL THROMBOSIS**<br><br>Thrombus may form on endocardium over site of infarction: potential EMBOLISM to<br>Brain<br>Intestine<br>Kidney<br>Lower limbs<br><br>(b) **ATRIAL THROMBOSIS**<br><br>Thrombus may form in atrial appendages – especially if atrial rhythm is disturbed<br><br>(c) **LEG VEIN THROMBOSIS**<br><br>Due to bed rest and venous stasis    →    **Pulmonary embolism** may be FATAL |

# MYOCARDIAL INFARCTION

| TIME | COMPLICATIONS (continued) |
|------|---------------------------|
| 3–14 days | 5. **RUPTURE OF HEART** Potentiated by:<br>(a) infarction of whole wall thickness<br>(b) unusual increased neutrophil activity before organisation is established → softening of dead muscle (myomalacia cordis)<br><br>**Sites affected and results**<br>(i) *MURAL MYOCARDIUM*<br><br><br><br>Infarct      Blood passing through ventricular wall into pericardial sac      Pericardial sac is distended with blood (tamponade); heart action impeded – DEATH<br><br>(ii) *PAPILLARY MUSCLE*<br><br><br><br>Infarct      Rupture of muscle      Sudden incompetence of mitral valve. Serious aggravation of cardiac pumping load; acute failure → often DEATH<br><br>(iii) *INTERVENTRICULAR SEPTUM*<br><br><br><br>Infarct      Rupture with interventricular communication ⟶ Rapid combined ventricular failure ↓ DEATH |

# MYOCARDIAL INFARCTION

| TIME | COMPLICATIONS *(continued)* |
|---|---|
| *3–14 days* | 6. **ACUTE PERICARDITIS** |
| *Weeks* | 7. **CHRONIC HEART FAILURE**<br>At the stage of fibrosis, chronic heart failure may supervene (+ ANGINA PECTORIS)<br><br>8. **DRESSLER SYNDROME**<br>An auto-immune disorder with pericarditis and pleurisy, related to the release of antigens from damaged heart muscle |
| *Months* | 9. **CARDIAC ANEURYSM**<br><br><br><br>Gradual stretching of thin fibrous scar   Bulging aneurysm formed   Laminated mural thrombus may cause embolism<br><br>Chronic heart failure |
| *At any time* | 10. **RECURRENCE OF INFARCTION**<br>Due to further thrombotic occlusion of a coronary arterial branch |

# CHRONIC ISCHAEMIC HEART DISEASE

With chronic ischaemia there is replacement of the myocardial fibres by fibrous tissue which is laid down in two main ways depending on whether the coronary insufficiency is due to severe generalised stenosis or is the result of local infarction following thrombosis.

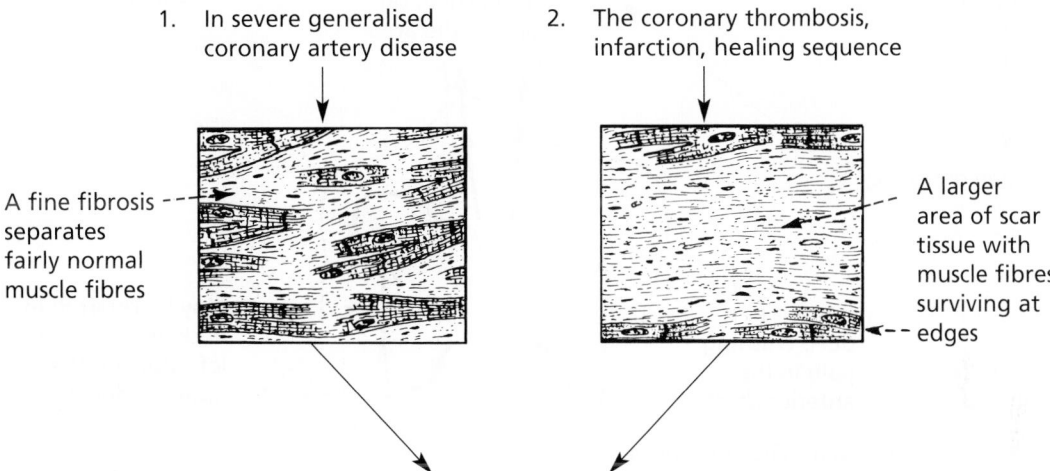

1. In severe generalised coronary artery disease

A fine fibrosis separates fairly normal muscle fibres

2. The coronary thrombosis, infarction, healing sequence

A larger area of scar tissue with muscle fibres surviving at edges

However, in many cases both mechanisms are present and lesions merge.

Myocardial fibrosis tends to be progressive, reflecting the progression of the atheromatous narrowing of the arteries.

Myocardial hypertrophy from any cause is an important contributory factor in many cases.

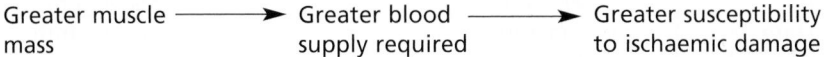

Greater muscle mass ⟶ Greater blood supply required ⟶ Greater susceptibility to ischaemic damage

Thus hypertension, which causes left ventricular hypertrophy, is an important background factor.

233

# ISCHAEMIC HEART DISEASE

### CLINICAL, LABORATORY AND ELECTROCARDIOGRAPH (ECG) EFFECTS

Cardiac pain is caused by muscle ischaemia as follows:

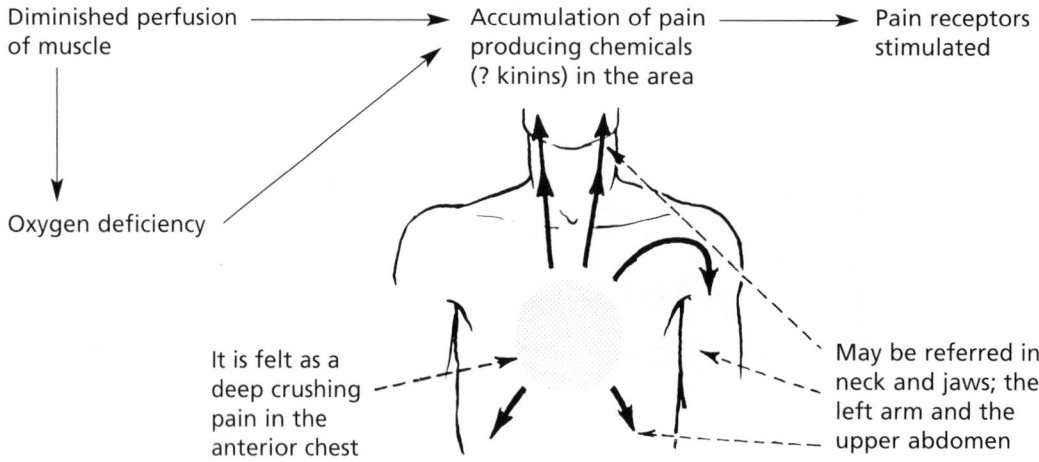

It occurs in three main circumstances:

1. **In acute infarction** – especially in the early phases before necrosis is complete. It is usually a continuous pain – not relieved by rest.
2. **In chronic myocardial ischaemia without infarction,** e.g. ANGINA PECTORIS – episodes of cardiac pain brought on by temporary ischaemia.

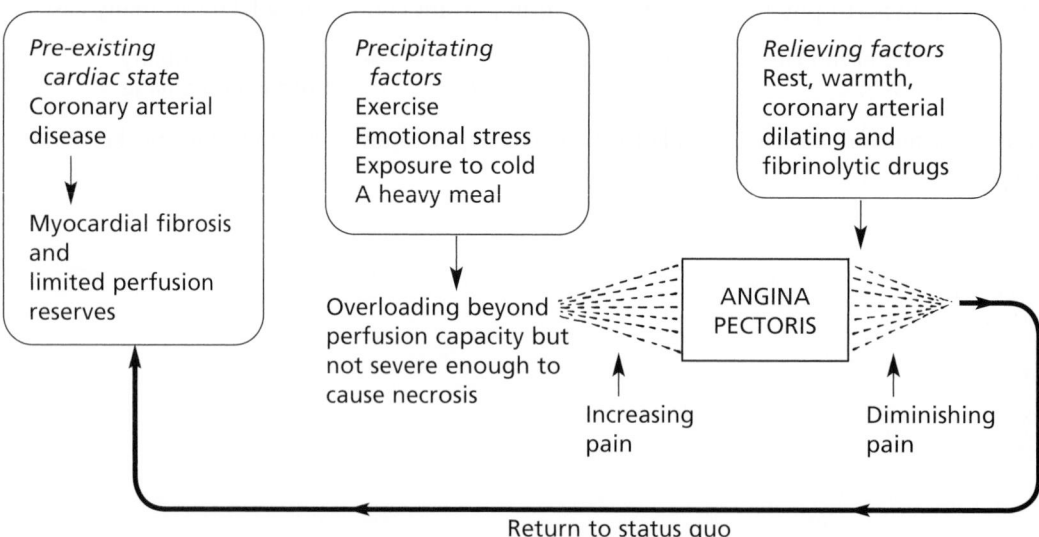

3. *Note:* The term 'crescendo' or 'unstable angina' refers to rapidly increasing anginal pain over a period of a few days without treatment, usually leading to myocardial infarction. It is due to developing thrombus or plaque rupture.

# ISCHAEMIC HEART DISEASE

## The blood in myocardial infarction

*Leucocytosis*

12 000–15 000/mm$^3$
lasting not more
than one week

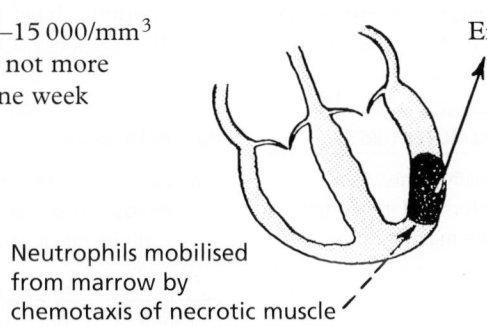

Neutrophils mobilised
from marrow by
chemotaxis of necrotic muscle

*Enzyme changes*

Enzymes liberated from necrotic muscle.
Two commonly used in diagnosis:

1. Troponin, within 12 hours of onset.
2. Myocardial creatine kinase (CKMB)
   is specific for cardiac muscle. Peak
   in 24 hours; falls in 72 hours.

These changes do not occur in angina pectoris since by definition necrosis has not occurred.

## The electrocardiogram (ECG)

The ventricular changes in ischaemia are reflected in the portion of ECG representing
ventricular activity, i.e. the QRST complex. During excitation, contraction and restitution,
the electrical potentials across the membranes of necrotic muscle fibres are strikingly
different from healthy muscle. The ECG changes may be subtle but three common patterns
are illustrated.

**Normal**

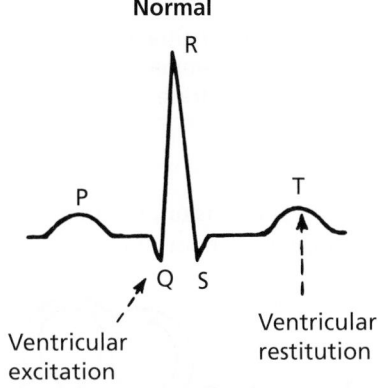

Ventricular
excitation

Ventricular
restitution

**Infarction**

1.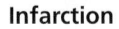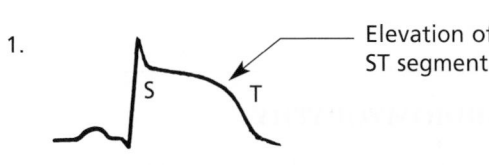

Elevation of
ST segment

2.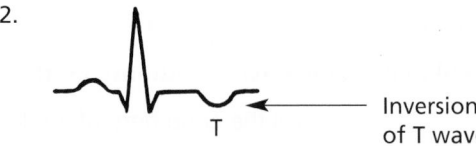

Inversion
of T wave

3.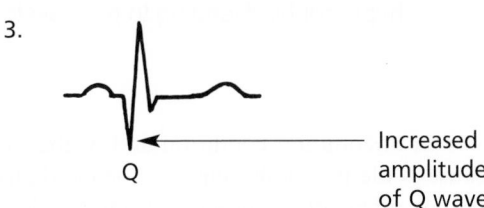

Increased
amplitude
of Q wave

# MISCELLANEOUS AFFECTIONS OF THE MYOCARDIUM

## MYOCARDITIS

Inflammation of the myocardium is rare. It may be caused by a variety of agents. The process is usually acute and may be generalised, regional or focal; most patients have chest pain but recover: less commonly heart failure develops. Some patients die suddenly. Others go on to develop cardiomyopathy years later.

| AGENTS | SPECIAL FEATURES | BASIC PATHOLOGY |
|---|---|---|
| **Viruses**<br>e.g. Coxsackie B group and influenza virus | Usually generalised: interstitial inflammation the main feature | Muscle fibre damage – necrosis and lysis of individual or small groups |
| **Bacteria,**<br>e.g. Lyme disease –*Borrelia burgdorferi* | | |
| **Toxins (incl. chemicals)**<br>Classic example – diphtheria toxin circulating in blood. Also in other severe infections, e.g. typhoid, pneumonia | Usually generalised: muscle damage the main feature | |
| **Immunological,**<br>e.g. rheumatic fever – myocarditis is an important component of the disease (see p. 214 for details of special features). | | Interstitial oedema and inflammatory cellular infiltrate |

## CARDIOMYOPATHY

This term refers to diseases of cardiac muscle when ischaemia, hypertension, valvular disease and inflammation have been excluded. Genetic influences are important.

Three main forms are recognised:

1. **Dilated (congestive) cardiomyopathy**

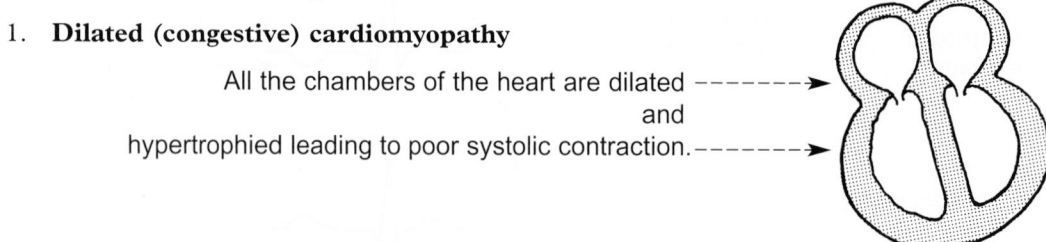

All the chambers of the heart are dilated ------> and hypertrophied leading to poor systolic contraction. ------>

This is an uncommon condition and in the majority of cases no cause is identified although end-stage damage from myocarditis, alcohol or pregnancy is often suspected. It is familial in a minority of cases often due to mutations affecting cytoskeletal proteins. Patients present clinically with unexplained heart failure usually between the ages of 30 and 60 years.

# MISCELLANEOUS AFFECTIONS OF THE MYOCARDIUM

### 2a. Hypertrophic cardiomyopathy

This can occur at any age, but young adults are often affected. There is often a family history presenting usually as an autosomal dominant pattern. Several genes encoding contractile protein may be involved, e.g. β-myosin heavy chain.

The effects include: sudden death, often following exercise, arrhythmias and cardiac failure.

*Muscle hypertrophy* without dilatation occurs. There is disproportionate thickening of the interventricular septum. Histologically the enlarged muscle fibres are arranged irregularly.

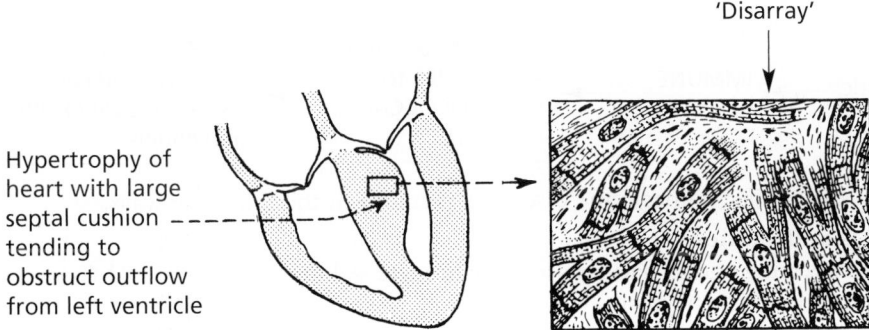

'Disarray'

Hypertrophy of heart with large septal cushion tending to obstruct outflow from left ventricle

### 2b. Restrictive cardiomyopathy

In this form the myocardium does not relax properly in diastole; this restricts ventricular filling and **cardiac output is reduced. It may be primary as in endomyocardial fibroelastosis** – a rare disease of childhood – or in Loeffler endocarditis where there is accompanying eosinophilia or secondary to infiltration of the myocardium as in amyloidosis, haemochromatosis or sarcoidosis.

# MISCELLANEOUS AFFECTIONS OF THE MYOCARDIUM

### RHEUMATIC FEVER

In rheumatic fever (acute rheumatism), a disease of children and young adults, inflammation affects the connective tissues at many sites, of which the **heart** is the most important. The incidence in Western countries has fallen dramatically, but it is common in parts of Africa and Asia.

### Aetiology

There is a strong association with streptococcal sore throat. *Streptococcus* is important because it shares antigens with human tissues, particularly heart muscle.

### Mechanism

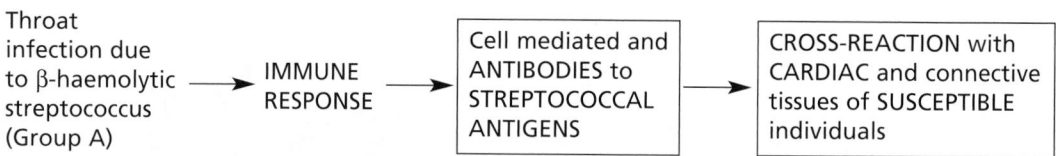

Throat infection due to β-haemolytic streptococcus (Group A) → IMMUNE RESPONSE → Cell mediated and ANTIBODIES to STREPTOCOCCAL ANTIGENS → CROSS-REACTION with CARDIAC and connective tissues of SUSCEPTIBLE individuals

In addition to the cardiac damage, the disease is manifest in the following ways:

1. **General manifestations** include:
   Fever with sweating and malaise: raised Erythrocyte sedimentation rate and C-reactive protein: neutrophil leucocytosis.
2. **Localised inflammation**
   (a) *Joints and adjacent musculofascial tissues* – causing POLYARTHRITIS with effusion, muscle pains and weakness.
   (b) *Serous membranes* – pericardial and sometimes pleural effusion.
   (c) *Skin*  (i)  a rash (erythema marginatum).
             (ii) small subcutaneous palpable nodules over bony prominences subject to pressure.
   (d) *Central nervous system* – chorea (involuntary spasmodic muscular movements).

### CARDIAC MANIFESTATIONS

The inflammation is widespread throughout the heart (PANCARDITIS) – affecting the pericardium, myocardium and endocardium.

1. **Pericarditis** occurs during the acute phase of the illness and is an important cause of pericardial effusion.
2. **Myocarditis** is common during the acute phase and is usually mild: it is rarely severe enough to cause cardiac failure. The histological picture is striking and the presence of the Aschoff body is characteristic.

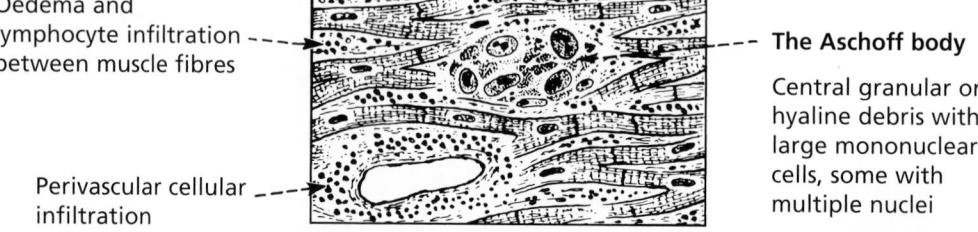

Oedema and lymphocyte infiltration between muscle fibres ---

Perivascular cellular --- infiltration

--- **The Aschoff body**

Central granular or hyaline debris with large mononuclear cells, some with multiple nuclei

# MISCELLANEOUS AFFECTIONS OF THE MYOCARDIUM

3. **Endocarditis.** Although there is a widespread histological inflammation, gross changes are seen usually on the endocardial sites subject to the greatest pressures and traumas, i.e. in the left side of the heart at the points of valve closure and at any sites of jet effect in the blood flow. The inflammation is complicated by ulceration of the valve surface followed by platelet and fibrin thrombosis in the form of small 'vegetations'.

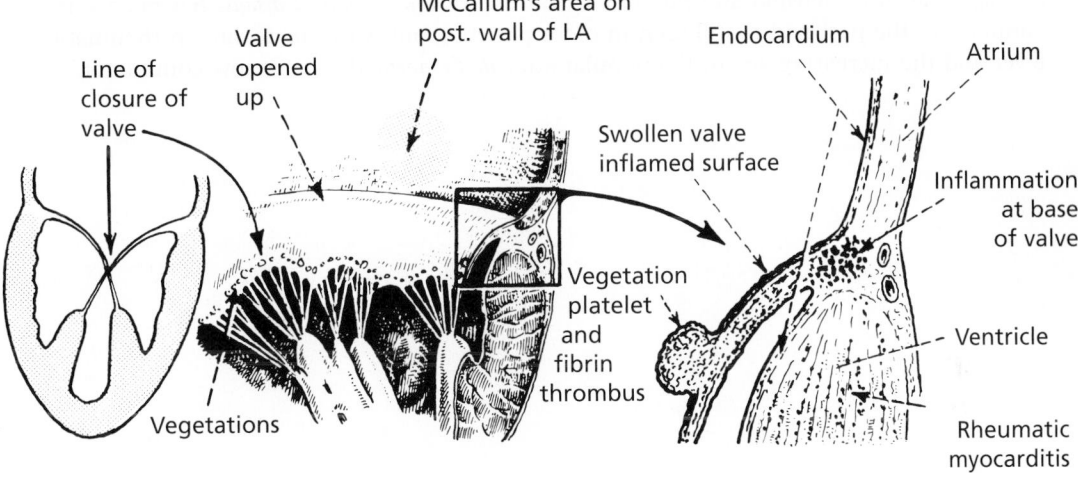

## Progression of the disease

In most cases the acute phase passes off and is followed by healing with various degrees of scarring. In a significant number of cases, no florid acute phase is noticed, and in a small number, a low-grade chronic inflammation is present for long periods. Repeated episodes lead to chronic valvular heart disease in about 50% of patients.

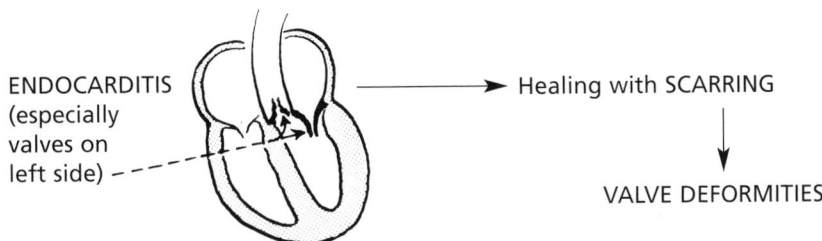

# VALVULAR HEART DISEASE

The main causes are RHEUMATIC FEVER, degenerative changes including DYSTROPHIC CALCIFICATION and congenital heart disease. Inherited deficiencies of the ground substance of the valve are rare causes. Nowadays, with the advent of powerful antibiotics, the late effects of healed infective endocarditis are assuming greater importance.

The MITRAL and AORTIC valves, subjected to much greater pressures, are more susceptible to damage than the tricuspid and pulmonary valves. *Rheumatic mitral disease* has been very common in the past and is still seen in older patients, but with the decline in rheumatic fever and the increasing age of the population, *calcific aortic disease* is now commoner.

# MITRAL VALVE DISEASE

**Mitral valve stenosis** is most commonly the result of post-inflammatory scarring as a consequence of rheumatic fever.

**Normal valve**
Note thin delicate curtains and chordae tendinae.

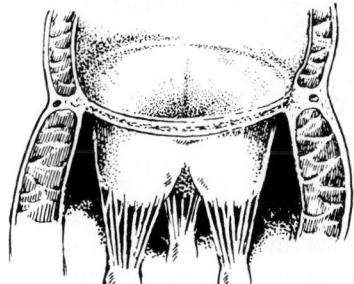

**Stenosis**
Simple adherence of curtains: a diaphragm formed (balloon valvuloplasty or valvotomy may be possible).

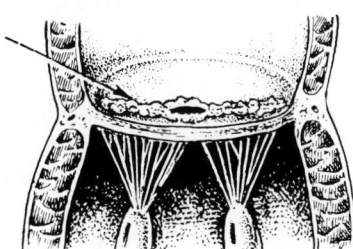

OR

Adherence and distortion, thickening, shortening, calcification of valve curtains and chordae resulting in 'funnel' stenosis.

(Whole valve replacement required.)

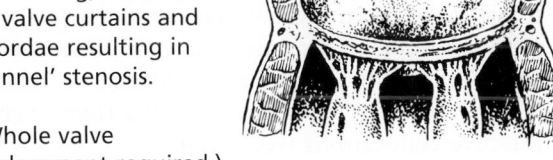

**Normal valve**

Note thin delicate curtains and chordae tendinae.

**Stenosis**

Simple adherence of curtains: a diaphragm formed (balloon valvuloplasty or valvotomy may be possible).

OR

Adherence and distortion, thickening, shortening, calcification of valve curtains and chordae resulting in 'funnel' stenosis.

(Whole valve replacement required.)

# MITRAL VALVE DISEASE

Mitral value incompetence has many causes:

1. Post-inflammatory scarring, i.e. rheumatic fever.
2. In cases of left ventricular failure when severe dilatation occurs.

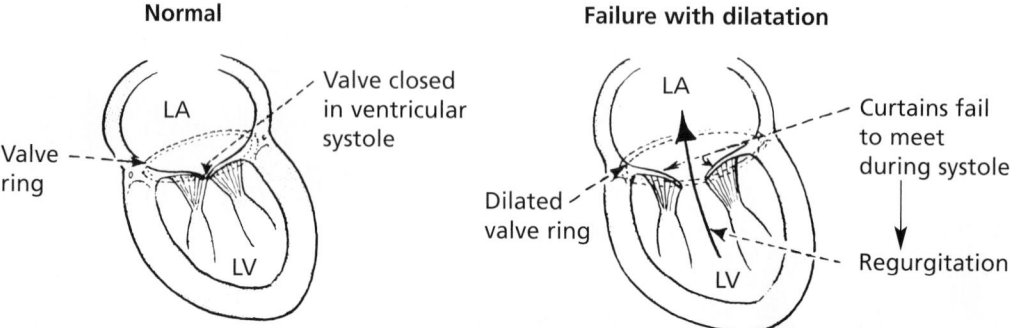

**Normal**        **Failure with dilatation**

3. Necrosis with rupture of papillary muscle in acute myocardial infarction.
4. It may result from myxoid degeneration of the valve. This may be primary – the 'floppy valve syndrome'. This most commonly affects young women. It may also occur secondary to conditions such as Marfan or Ehlers–Danlos syndrome. The enlarged 'floppy' valve prolapses into the left atrium during systole.
5. Infective endocarditis (see p. 246).

**The mechanical effects of mitral disease**

*Chronic stenosis – pure*        *Chronic incompetence – pure*

Dilatation and hypertrophy of left atrium

Left ventricle *not* affected

Back flow through damaged valve causes DILATATION and hypertrophy of *left ventricle*

**Diastolic** murmur        **Systolic** murmur

In rheumatic heart disease, combined stenosis and incompetence are often seen.

# MITRAL VALVE DISEASE

In mitral disease, the back pressure in the left atrium is transmitted to the pulmonary veins, and by raising pulmonary arterial pressure it causes effects on the right side of the heart.

## (a) Compensated phase

1. Left atrial dilatation

2. Pulmonary congestion

3. Right ventricular hypertrophy

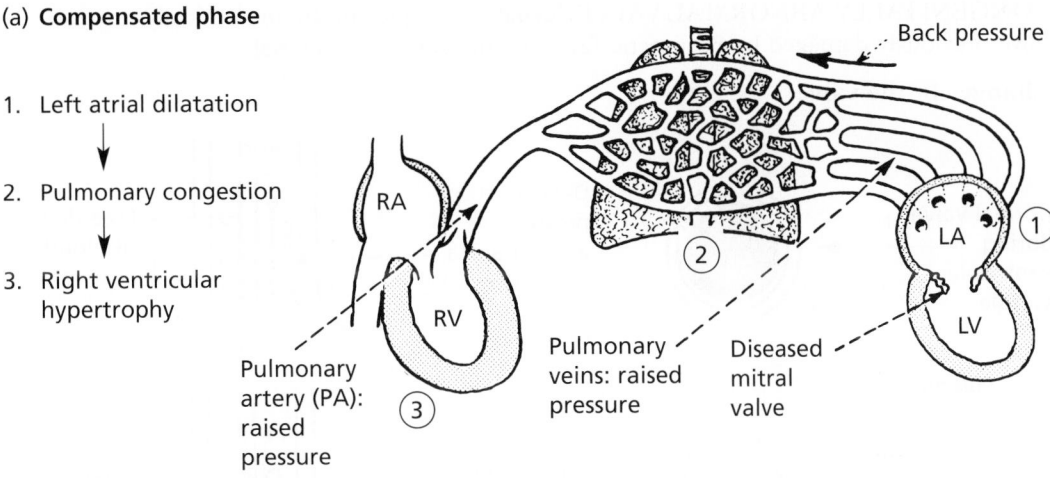

## (b) Congestive cardiac failure

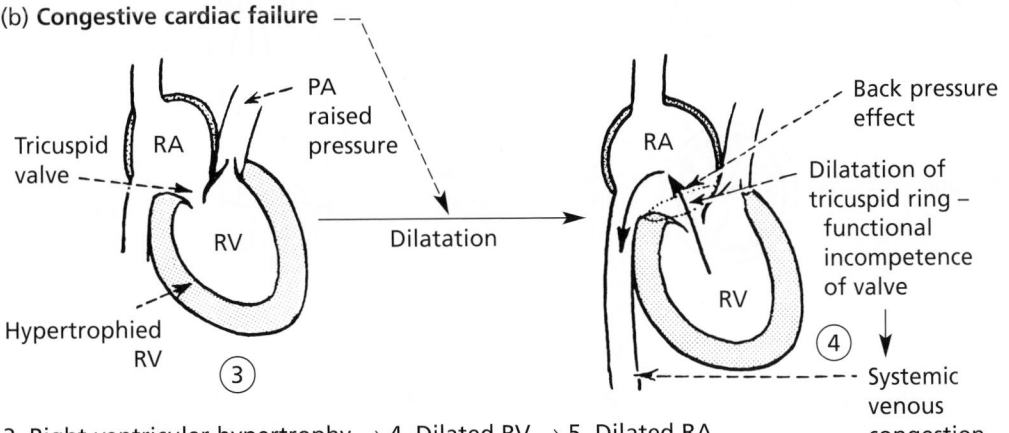

3. Right ventricular hypertrophy → 4. Dilated RV → 5. Dilated RA

In the acute types of mitral incompetence, the sudden change in the intracardiac haemodynamics very seriously aggravates the heart failure already present due to the primary disease.

## Complications of chronic mitral disease

1. Atrial fibrillation is common.
   Fibrillation → thrombosis in atrial appendage → systemic embolism
2. Infective endocarditis.

# AORTIC VALVE DISEASE

### STENOSIS

The main causes are SCARRING and CALCIFICATION occurring in a CONGENITALLY ABNORMAL VALVE (usually bicuspid) or an anatomically normal valve previously damaged by rheumatic fever or endocarditis (bacterial).

### Changes in the valve

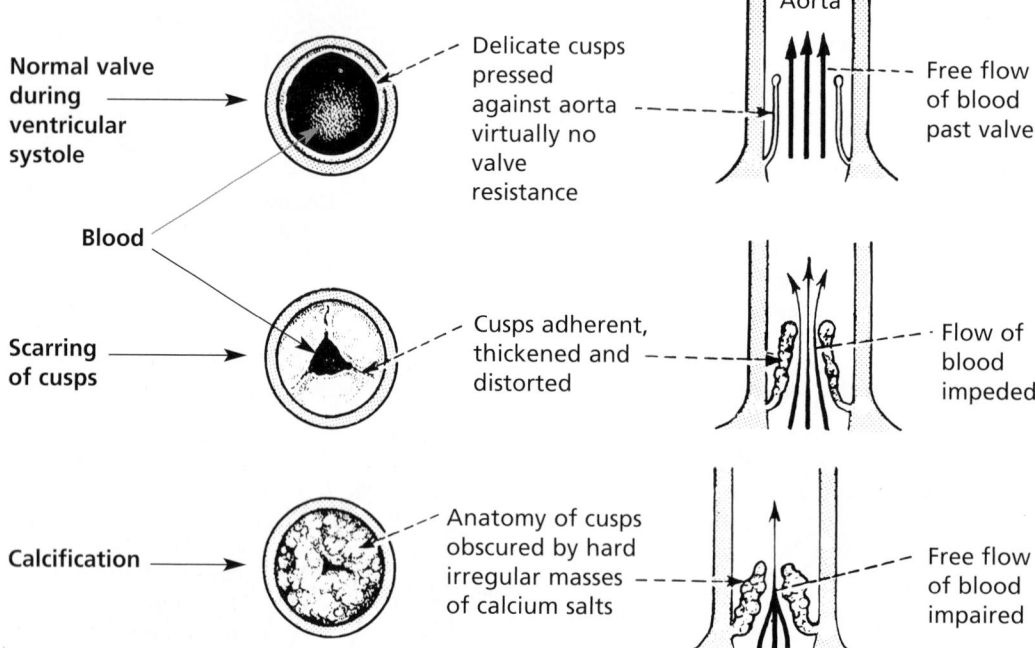

Normal valve during ventricular systole

Blood

Delicate cusps pressed against aorta virtually no valve resistance

Aorta

Free flow of blood past valve

Scarring of cusps

Cusps adherent, thickened and distorted

Flow of blood impeded

Calcification

Anatomy of cusps obscured by hard irregular masses of calcium salts

Free flow of blood impaired

### Effects
The main effect is HYPERTROPHY of the left ventricle to overcome the valve resistance, e.g. 600 g (normal – 300 g)

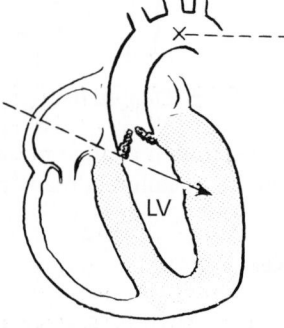

Ejection systolic murmur

Low pulse pressure may reduce flow in the coronary arteries. The hypertrophied muscle is therefore susceptible to ischaemic damage.

The heart often remains in this 'compensated' state for years, but eventually failure develops with dilatation.

SUDDEN DEATH (without pre-existing signs of failure) is a definite risk at any time, but particularly during exercise.

In adults, severe aortic stenosis usually requires valve replacement.

# AORTIC VALVE DISEASE

## INCOMPETENCE

The main causes are scarring of the cusps due to rheumatic fever or infective endocarditis, or less commonly dilatation of the valve ring due to disease (e.g. in ankylosing spondylitis: Marfan syndrome) or degeneration in old age.

### Changes in the valve

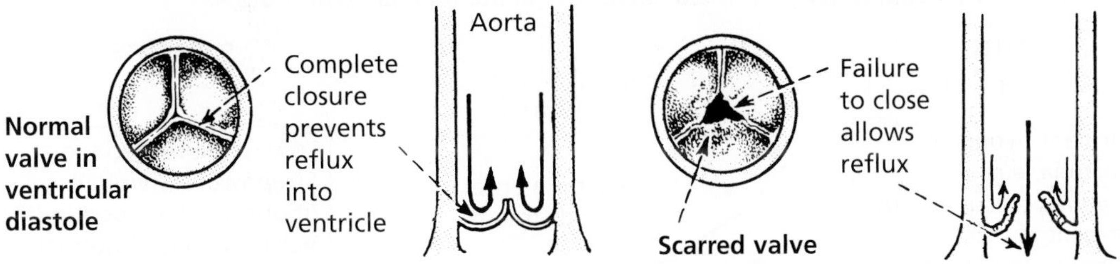

**Normal valve in ventricular diastole**

Aorta

Complete closure prevents reflux into ventricle

Failure to close allows reflux

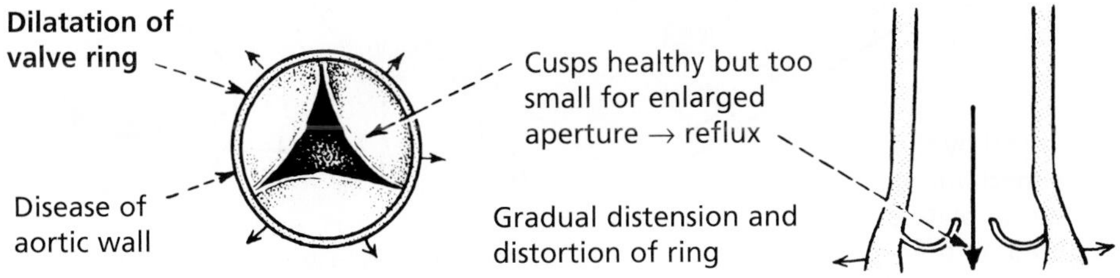

**Scarred valve**

**Dilatation of valve ring**

Disease of aortic wall

Cusps healthy but too small for enlarged aperture → reflux

Gradual distension and distortion of ring

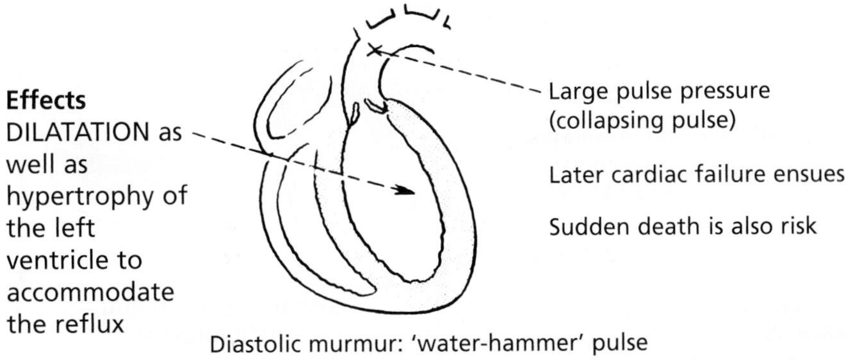

**Effects**
DILATATION as well as hypertrophy of the left ventricle to accommodate the reflux

Large pulse pressure (collapsing pulse)

Later cardiac failure ensues

Sudden death is also risk

Diastolic murmur: 'water-hammer' pulse

Aortic stenosis and incompetence often exist together and the effects are compounded.

## TRICUSPID AND PULMONARY VALVES

Diseases of these valves are not common. However, functional tricuspid incompetence due to severe cardiac dilatation is an important end stage in progressive cardiac failure.

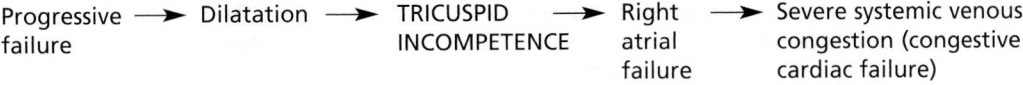

Progressive failure ⟶ Dilatation ⟶ TRICUSPID INCOMPETENCE ⟶ Right atrial failure ⟶ Severe systemic venous congestion (congestive cardiac failure)

# ENDOCARDITIS

### INFECTIVE ENDOCARDITIS

In this disease, there is colonisation or invasion of the heart valves by micro-organisms leading to the formation of friable vegetations. In many cases the values have been previously damaged, e.g. by rheumatic fever. In other cases, normal values may be affected by particularly virulent organisms, e.g. intravenous drug users.

Endocarditis has traditionally been classified into acute and subacute forms.

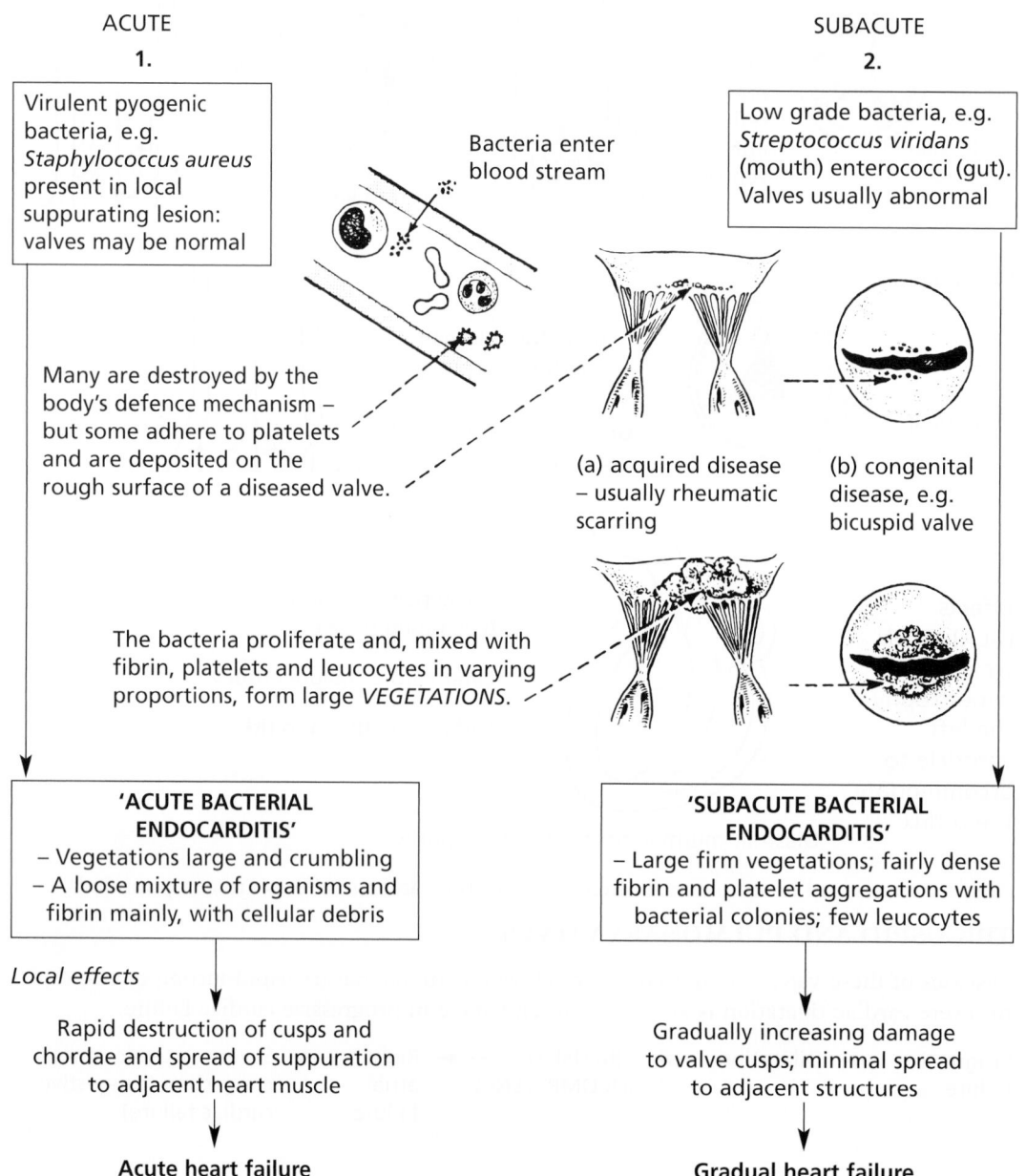

ACUTE

**1.**

Virulent pyogenic bacteria, e.g. *Staphylococcus aureus* present in local suppurating lesion: valves may be normal

Bacteria enter blood stream

SUBACUTE

**2.**

Low grade bacteria, e.g. *Streptoccocus viridans* (mouth) enterococci (gut). Valves usually abnormal

Many are destroyed by the body's defence mechanism – but some adhere to platelets and are deposited on the rough surface of a diseased valve.

(a) acquired disease – usually rheumatic scarring

(b) congenital disease, e.g. bicuspid valve

The bacteria proliferate and, mixed with fibrin, platelets and leucocytes in varying proportions, form large *VEGETATIONS*.

**'ACUTE BACTERIAL ENDOCARDITIS'**
– Vegetations large and crumbling
– A loose mixture of organisms and fibrin mainly, with cellular debris

**'SUBACUTE BACTERIAL ENDOCARDITIS'**
– Large firm vegetations; fairly dense fibrin and platelet aggregations with bacterial colonies; few leucocytes

*Local effects*

Rapid destruction of cusps and chordae and spread of suppuration to adjacent heart muscle

Gradually increasing damage to valve cusps; minimal spread to adjacent structures

**Acute heart failure**

**Gradual heart failure**

# ENDOCARDITIS

In addition to the local effects, there may be systemic complications:

1) Embolism
   – Embolic infarction and pyaemic abscesses may occur in the brain or kidneys.
   – Glomerulonephritis, retinal haemorrhages and fingernail splinter haemorrhages due to antigen–antibody complexes becoming trapped in small vessels.

2) Pyrexia
3) Leucocytosis

Valves in immunocompromised patients may be colonised by opportunistic organisms, e.g. fungi.
Cardiac prostheses and catheter lines act as a focus for bacterial growth and infective endocarditis is a serious complication.

## OTHER

MARANTIC ENDOCARDITIS – in debilitated patients (often with disseminated malignancy), thrombus may form on the closure line of the valve cusps.
LIBMAN-SACKS DISEASE – thrombotic vegetations can occur in systemic lupus erythematosus (SLE) and cause embolic complications
CARCINOID SYNDROME – excess 5-hydroxytrptamine secretion for metastatic carcinoid tumours can result in right heart endocardial fibrosis leading to stenosis or incompetence of the tricuspid valve.

# CARDIAC ARRHYTHMIAS

### CARDIAC ARRHYTHMIAS AND DISEASES OF THE CONDUCTING SYSTEM

Of the wide variety of cardiac arrhythmias which have now been studied in detail using the electrocardiograph, the majority are due to (A) functional disturbances of the intrinsic excitability of the cardiac muscle at various sites or of the cardiac neurohumoral controls; only a minority are due to (B) organic disease of the conducting system itself.

(A) **Important disorders of cardiac muscle excitability**
1. **Atrial fibrillation**
   This is a common condition in which there is irregular, rapid and ineffective atrial contraction.
   There are two main effects:

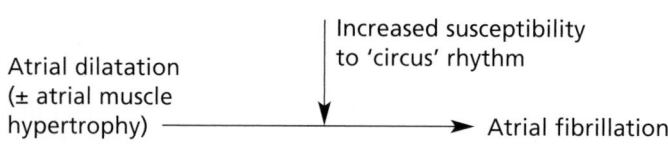

**Predisposing conditions**
Ischaemic heart disease ⎫
Rheumatic heart disease ⎪ Atrial dilatation          Increased susceptibility
Hypertension            ⎬ (± atrial muscle            to 'circus' rhythm
Thyrotoxicosis          ⎭ hypertrophy) ──────────────────────→ Atrial fibrillation

There are two main effects:

(a) *Contribution to cardiac failure*

(i) loss of atrial contraction to priming of ventricles

(ii) *Note:* Causes increased irregular ventricular rate

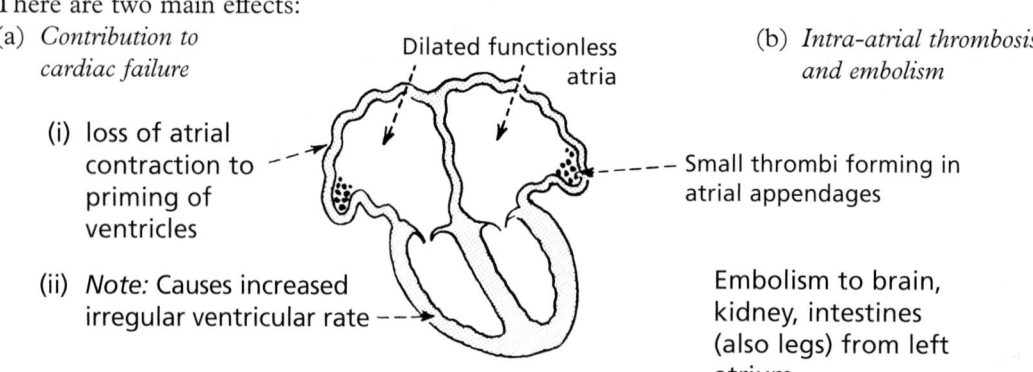

Dilated functionless atria

(b) *Intra-atrial thrombosis and embolism*

Small thrombi forming in atrial appendages

Embolism to brain, kidney, intestines (also legs) from left atrium.

2. **Ventricular paroxysmal tachycardia and fibrillation**
   These usually occur in association with ischaemic heart disease. In fibrillation, a form of cardiac 'arrest', cardiac function ceases.

# CARDIAC ARRHYTHMIAS

## (B) Diseases of the conducting system

This is usually due to disease in the adjacent heart tissue. The heart rate is slow.

*Associated conditions*

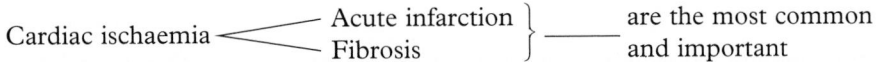

Cardiac ischaemia ——< Acute infarction ⎱ ——— are the most common
　　　　　　　　　　　　 Fibrosis ⎰ 　　　　　　　and important

Others are myocarditis, calcification around the valve rings and drugs, e.g. digitalis, propranolol.

**Sites of disorder**　　　　　　　　　　　　　　　　　　　　**Effects**

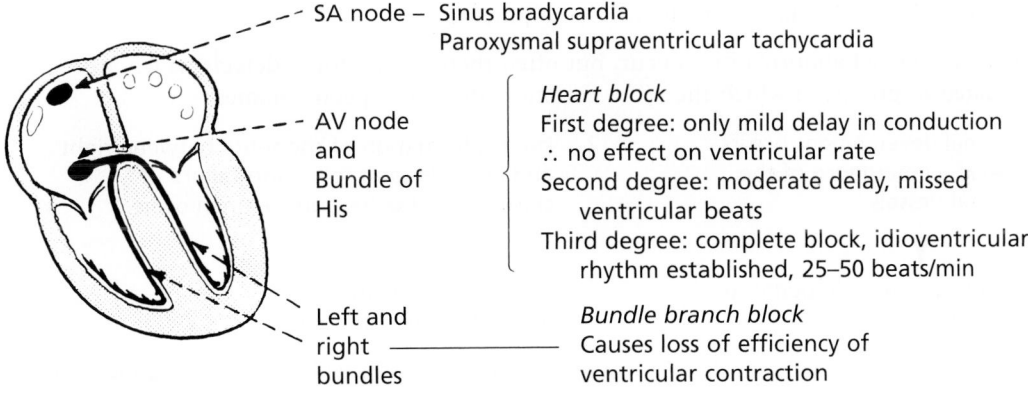

SA node – Sinus bradycardia
　　　　　　Paroxysmal supraventricular tachycardia

AV node
and
Bundle of
His

*Heart block*
First degree: only mild delay in conduction
∴ no effect on ventricular rate
Second degree: moderate delay, missed
　　　　ventricular beats
Third degree: complete block, idioventricular
　　　　rhythm established, 25–50 beats/min

Left and
right ————————
bundles

*Bundle branch block*
Causes loss of efficiency of
ventricular contraction

The three important components of arrhythmias are:

Tachycardia
Bradycardia
Irregularity

The effect of any arrhythmia on cardiac function depends essentially on its effect on ventricular output.

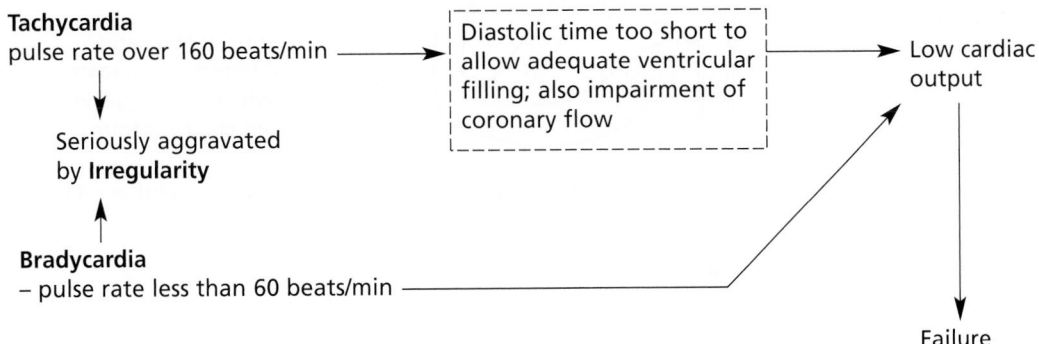

**Tachycardia**
pulse rate over 160 beats/min ——→ Diastolic time too short to
allow adequate ventricular
filling; also impairment of
coronary flow ——→ Low cardiac
output

↓

Seriously aggravated
by **Irregularity**

↑

**Bradycardia**
– pulse rate less than 60 beats/min ———————

Failure

# CONGENITAL HEART DISEASE

Developmental abnormalities of the heart are relatively common; clinically significant defects occur in 7–11 per 1000 live births and the rate is significantly higher in stillbirths. The severity varies from minor aberrations to complex distortions incompatible with life. Many patients now live normal lives after cardiac surgery.

**Aetiology**

This is often obscure. Hereditary factors are of limited importance, Down syndrome often causes septal defects. Possible environmental factors are complex and numerous.

Examples include: virus infection, e.g. rubella; teratogen, e.g. thalidomide (historically); altitude at birth (patent ductus arteriosus is commoner at high altitudes).

The initial damage, which is sustained during the first trimester of pregnancy, is modified by later fetal and postnatal growth and development.

Single anatomical abnormalities occur, but often there are multiple defects which are associated in groups of which the more common are given specific names.

Abnormal development occurs:

1. At the emergence of the great vessels

↓

Stenoses cause impedence to blood flow

2. During formation of the septa between right and left sides and following failure of closure, e.g. ductus and foramen ovale.

↓

Abnormal apertures allow shunting of blood

**Fallot tetralogy** is an example of congenital heart disease in which there is cyanosis. There are four components:

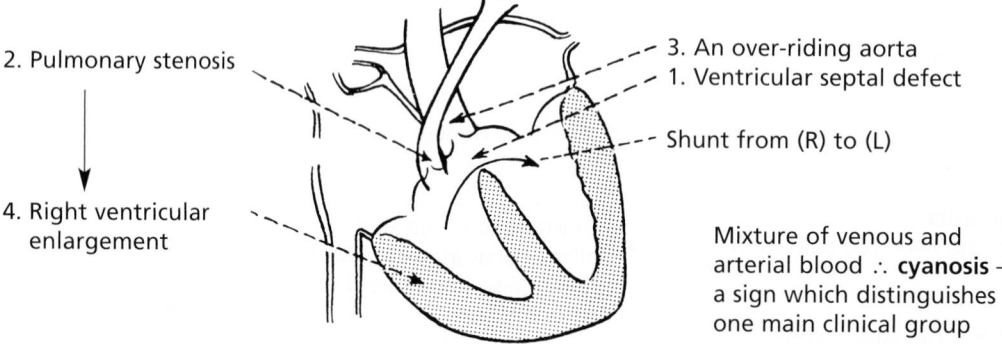

2. Pulmonary stenosis

↓

4. Right ventricular enlargement

3. An over-riding aorta
1. Ventricular septal defect

Shunt from (R) to (L)

Mixture of venous and arterial blood ∴ **cyanosis** – a sign which distinguishes one main clinical group

Often complications – pulmonary hypertension, increased blood volume, polycythaemia, and infective endocarditis – increase the disability.

Surgical repair is the ideal treatment.

# DISEASES OF THE PERICARDIUM

## PERICARDITIS

Pericarditis is a complication of diseases of the heart or adjacent structures or of generalised disorders. In some cases no cause can be found.

**Acute pericarditis** may be:
1. Fibrinous – this is the commonest form and is seen in acute myocardial infarction and anaemia.
2. Serous – e.g. in rheumatic fever, scleroderma, SLE.
3. Purulent – due to invasion of the pericardial space by infectious organisms.
4. Haemorrhagic – e.g. with trauma or tumour.

**Fibrinous pericarditis**                    **Pericarditis with effusion**

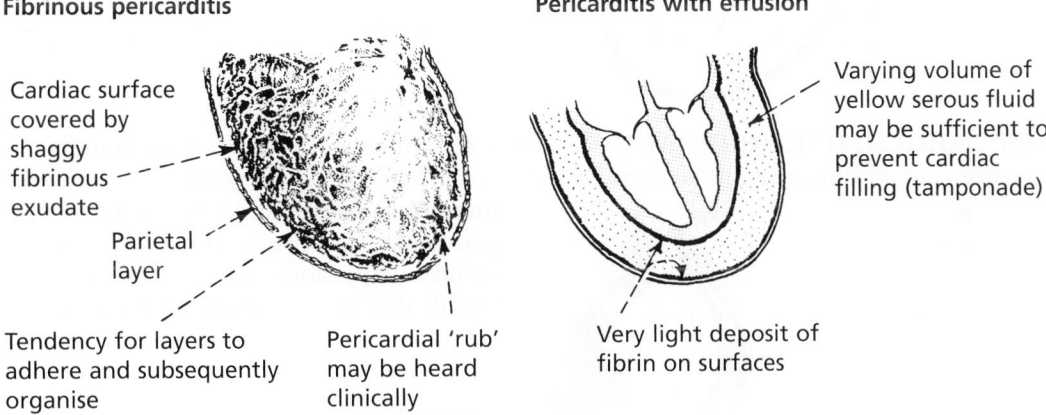

Cardiac surface covered by shaggy fibrinous exudate

Parietal layer

Tendency for layers to adhere and subsequently organise

Pericardial 'rub' may be heard clinically

Varying volume of yellow serous fluid may be sufficient to prevent cardiac filling (tamponade)

Very light deposit of fibrin on surfaces

**Diseases which may lead to pericarditis**

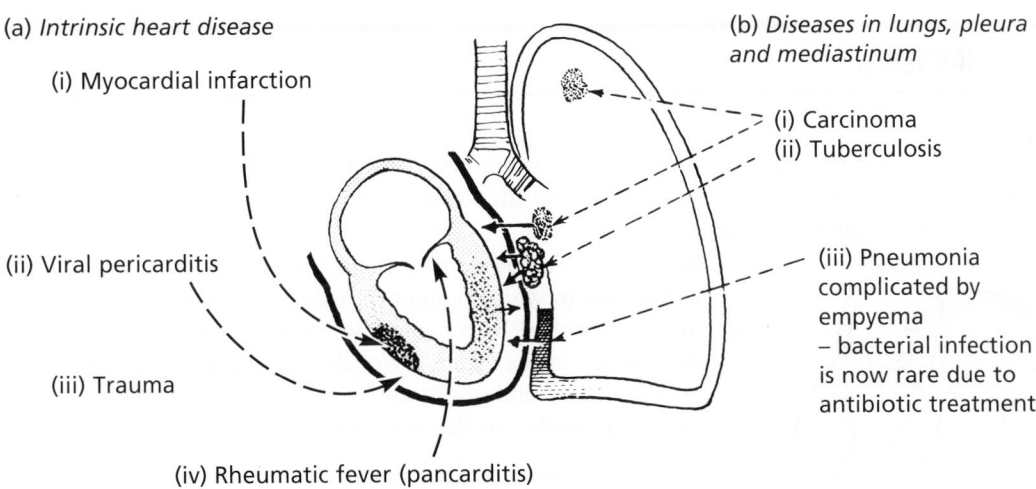

(a) *Intrinsic heart disease*

   (i) Myocardial infarction

   (ii) Viral pericarditis

   (iii) Trauma

       (iv) Rheumatic fever (pancarditis)

(b) *Diseases in lungs, pleura and mediastinum*

   (i) Carcinoma
   (ii) Tuberculosis

   (iii) Pneumonia complicated by empyema – bacterial infection is now rare due to antibiotic treatment

(c) *Generalised disorders*

  (i) Uraemia
  (ii) Connective tissue diseases, e.g. SLE, rheumatoid disease

# DISEASES OF THE PERICARDIUM

**CHRONIC PERICARDITIS** may be due to tuberculosis, viral infection or rheumatoid arthritis; sometimes the cause cannot be determined. The basic changes are organisation and calcification. In extreme cases, cardiac function is impaired.

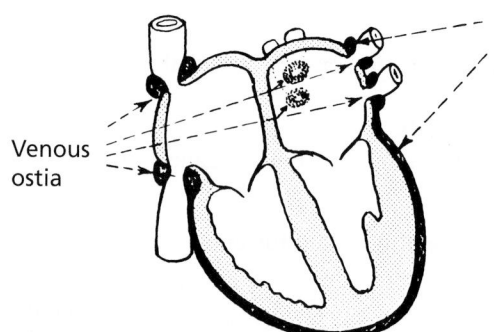

Venous ostia

Dense fibrous calcified tissues – causing close adherence of the pericardial layers; preventing proper cardiac filling; – this extreme condition is called **constrictive pericarditis.**

**PERICARDIAL HAEMORRHAGE** occurs most commonly as a result of **cardiac rupture** complicating acute infarction. The other main cause is rupture of dissecting **aortic aneurysm** back into the pericardium. The pericardial sac becomes distended with blood (tamponade) and death follows rapidly due to compression of the heart.

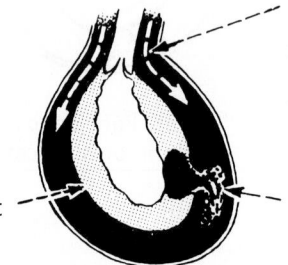

Compression of heart

Cardiac rupture into pericardium

# CARDIAC TUMOURS

Primary tumours in the heart are very rare. Secondary tumours, especially from the lungs, affecting the pericardium by direct spread and the heart by blood spread are fairly common in advanced malignant disease.

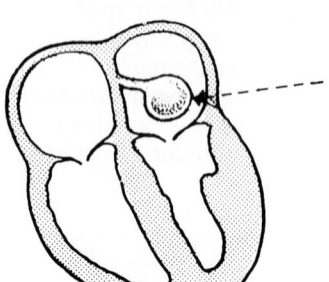

Atrial 'myxoma' is a rare benign tumour affecting usually the left atrium in which a smooth, pale, soft, rounded mass is attached by a pedicle to the endocardium. It can cause serious effects by occluding the mitral valve opening or by embolisation. Mesothelioma may present primarily in the pericardium.

Rhabdomyomas are occasionally seen in childhood, and are associated with tuberous sclerosis.

# DISEASES OF BLOOD VESSELS

## VASCULITIDES

The term vasculitis refers to a group of conditions with inflammation of the blood vessel wall, usually due to immune mechanisms. Vessels of any size may be affected.

## LARGE VESSEL VASCULITIS

### Temporal arteritis (Giant-cell arteritis/cranial arteritis)

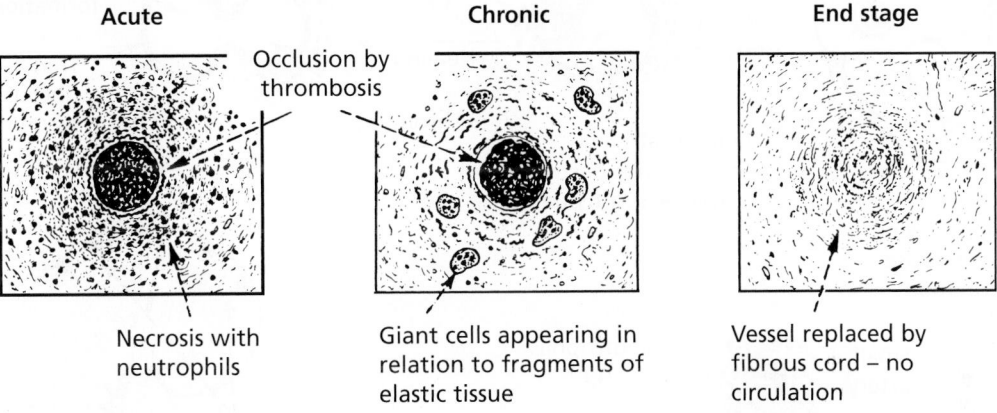

**Acute** — Occlusion by thrombosis — Necrosis with neutrophils

**Chronic** — Giant cells appearing in relation to fragments of elastic tissue

**End stage** — Vessel replaced by fibrous cord – no circulation

This disease of unknown aetiology affects elderly people (over 65 years). It may cause severe facial pain, jaw claudication and headache, and may be associated with ocular symptoms and cause blindness. In a significant number of old people, there are no symptoms.

Some cases occur along with polymyalgia rheumatica – a disease in which there are generalised muscle pains and systemic malaise. Commonly, branches of the external carotid arteries are affected, but sometimes other caudal arteries and even the aortic arch may also be involved.

There is inflammation of the vessel wall complicated by thrombosis.

### Takayasu disease

This rare disease, typically affects young females (20–30 years). The patchy arteritis is more severe and affects the aorta and its primary branches, leading to ischaemia of BRAIN (cerebral arteries), EYES (ophthalmic arteries), FACE (carotid arteries), ARMS ('pulseless' disease), HEART (coronary orifices), and KIDNEYS (causing HYPERTENSION) in varying combinations.

# DISEASES OF BLOOD VESSELS

## MEDIUM VESSEL VASCULITIS

### Polyarteritis nodosa (PAN)

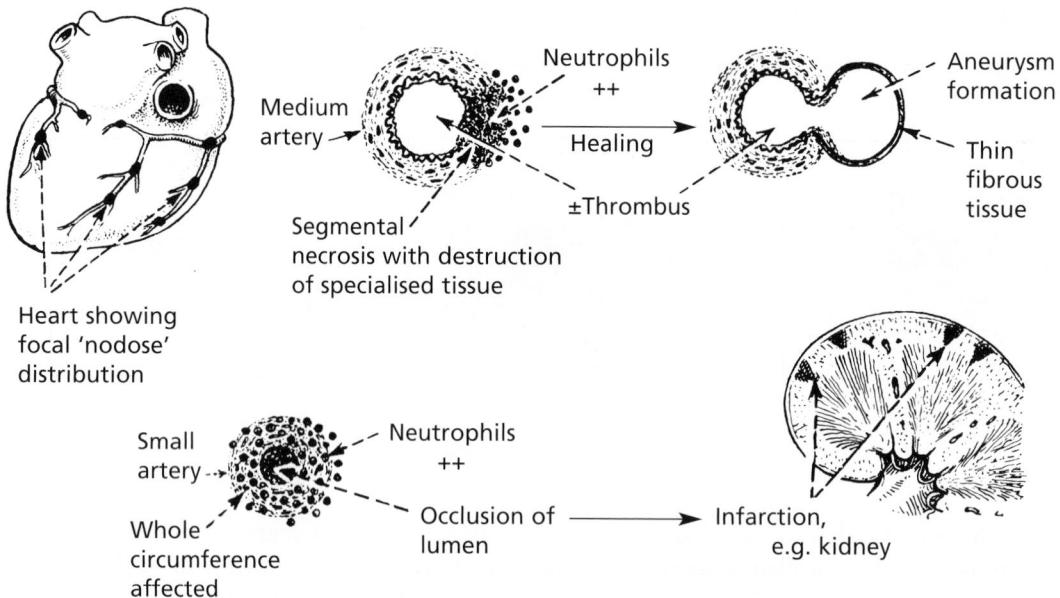

This is a disease affecting the medium and small arteries and arterioles. In the acute phase, there are signs of generalised illness with fever etc., but the disease often becomes chronic and relapsing.

Typically there is a focal necrosis of the arterial wall.

Any artery may be affected, but damage to the HEART, KIDNEYS, BRAIN and GUT is particularly important. When the arteries supplying peripheral nerves are affected symptoms of 'neuritis' may be striking.

### Kawasaki disease

This is a disease of infants which affects the main aortic branches particularly the coronary arteries.

# DISEASES OF BLOOD VESSELS

## SMALL VESSEL VASCULITIS

### Anti-neutrophil cytoplasmic antibodies (ANCA) associated

ANCA occur in various forms of vasculitis. A perinuclear pattern of staining (p-ANCA) is seen in microscopic polyarteritis and about 50% of cases of eosinophilic granulomatosis with polyangiitis (Churg-Strauss syndrome). Cytoplasmic staining (c-ANCA) is seen in granulomatosis with polyangiitis (Wegener granulomatosis).

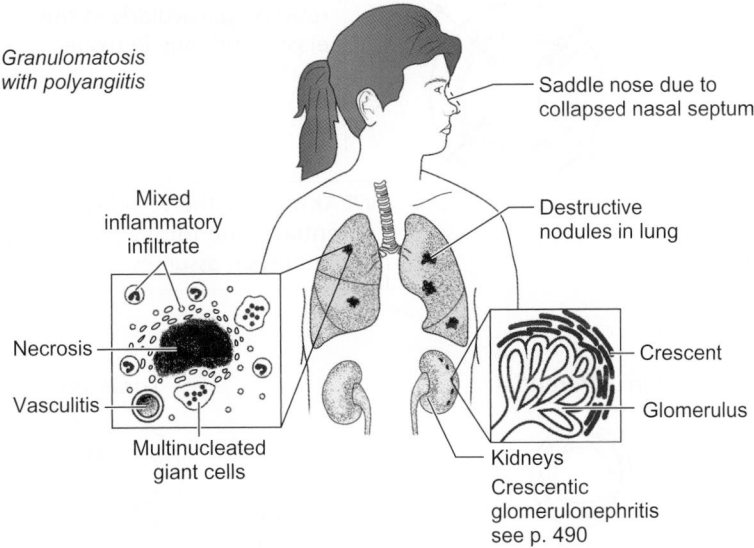

*Granulomatosis with polyangiitis*

Saddle nose due to collapsed nasal septum

Mixed inflammatory infiltrate

Destructive nodules in lung

Necrosis

Vasculitis

Crescent

Glomerulus

Multinucleated giant cells

Kidneys

Crescentic glomerulonephritis see p. 490

In **microscopic polyarteritis**, there is a form of glomerulonephritis due to involvement of afferent arterioles as well as pulmonary capillaritis. In **granulomatosis with polyangiitis** destructive lesions of the nasal mucosa, the lungs and the kidneys are seen. In **eosinophilic granulomatosis with polyangiitis** there is vasculitis with peripheral eosinophilia, asthma and sinusitis sometimes associated with peripheral neuropathy.

### Immune complex associated

The best known example of this is **IgA vasculitis** (Henoch-Schonlein purpura). This is characterized by deposition of immune complexes containing IgA which results in purpura, arthritis and abdominal pain due to intestinal involvement. Renal involvement may also occur.

# ANEURYSMS

A local enlargement of an artery is called an **aneurysm**. Although localised, it often reflects the presence of more widespread arterial disease.

## MECHANISM OF FORMATION

The two main forces that maintain the integrity of the shape of an artery are:

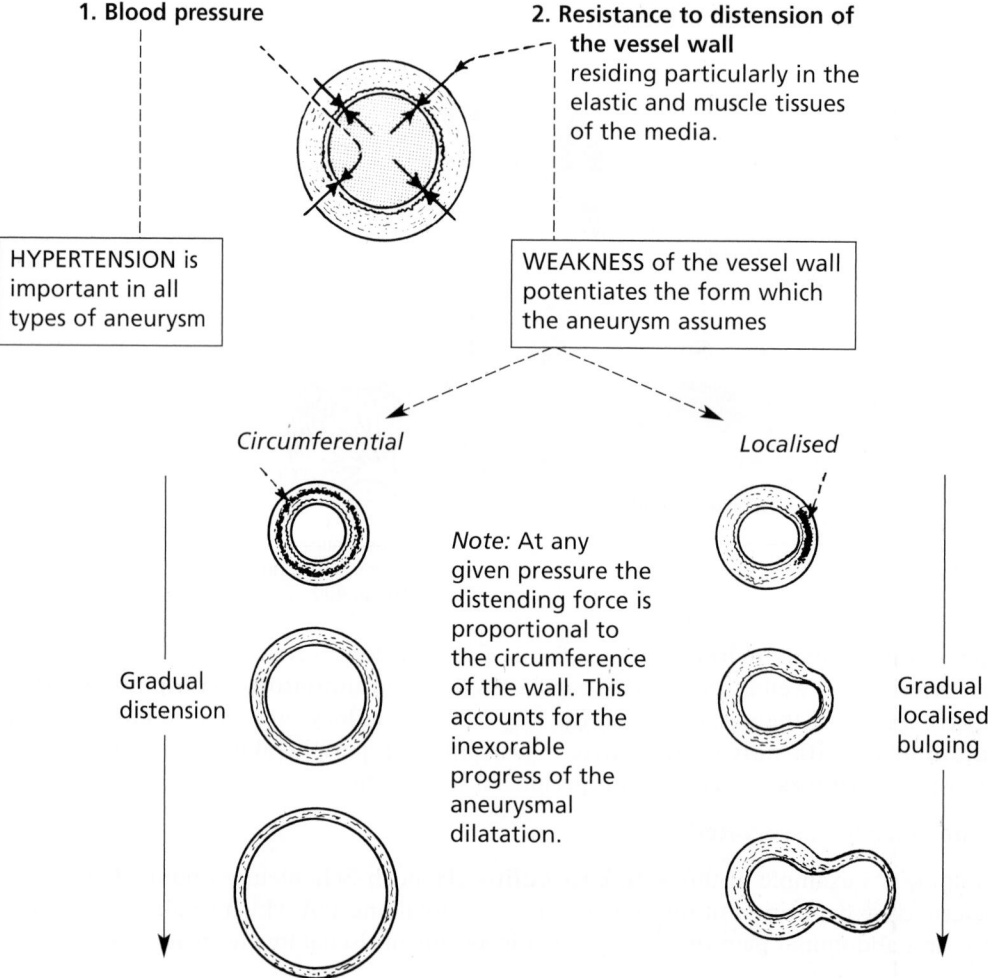

**1. Blood pressure**

**2. Resistance to distension of the vessel wall**
residing particularly in the elastic and muscle tissues of the media.

HYPERTENSION is important in all types of aneurysm

WEAKNESS of the vessel wall potentiates the form which the aneurysm assumes

*Circumferential*

*Localised*

Gradual distension

Gradual localised bulging

*Note:* At any given pressure the distending force is proportional to the circumference of the wall. This accounts for the inexorable progress of the aneurysmal dilatation.

## Causes

Aneurysms may be due to: acquired diseases of vessel wall (atheroma, arteritis, syphilis [now rare]); congenital weakness ('berry aneurysms', p. 582); hypertension; trauma.

# ANEURYSMS

## TYPES OF ANEURYSM

There are two main varieties:

### 1. FUSIFORM

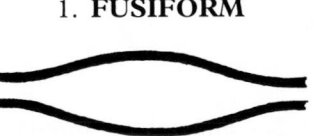

### 2. SACCULAR

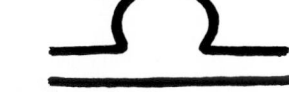

These are well illustrated in the aorta.

**Fusiform aneurysm** of abdominal aorta – usually due to atheroma; often below renal arteries and may also affect iliac arteries.

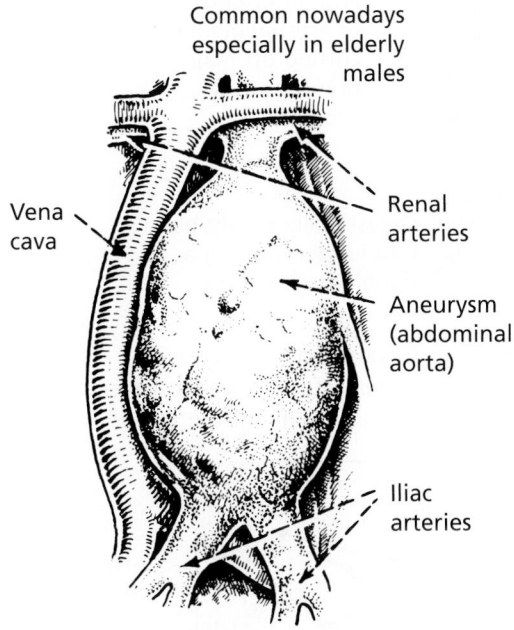

Common nowadays especially in elderly males

Vena cava

Renal arteries

Aneurysm (abdominal aorta)

Iliac arteries

**Saccular aneurysm** of aortic arch – now usually due to atheroma; in the past, syphilis.

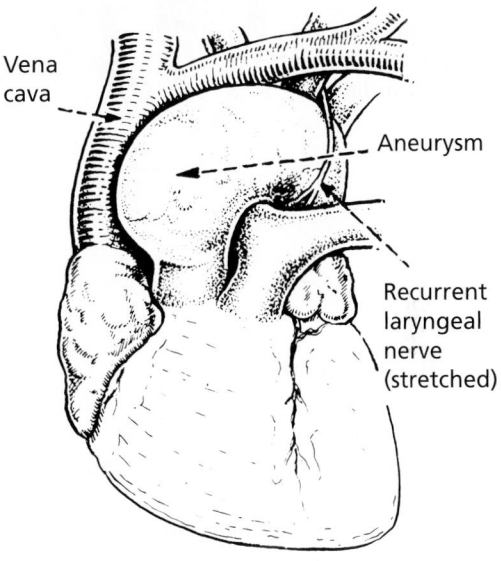

Vena cava

Aneurysm

Recurrent laryngeal nerve (stretched)

COMPLICATIONS
1. Local pressure effects – usually not serious.
2. Thrombosis with embolism to legs.
3. Rupture with fatal retroperitoneal or intraperitoneal haemorrhage.

COMPLICATIONS
1. Pressure effects:
   (a) On nerves, e.g. recurrent laryngeal nerve paralysis.
   (b) On bones, e.g. vertebral, sternal or rib erosion.
   (c) On neighbouring viscera, e.g. oesophagus, heart, lungs.
2. Fatal haemorrhage.

# ANEURYSMS

### OTHER VARIETIES OF ANEURYSM

1.  **Dissecting aneurysm**
    Classically begins in the arch of aorta.

    *Predisposing causes:* (a) HYPERTENSION (common)
    (b) Atheroma
    (c) Medial degeneration (rare) seen in Marfan syndrome due to mutation of the fibrillin gene.

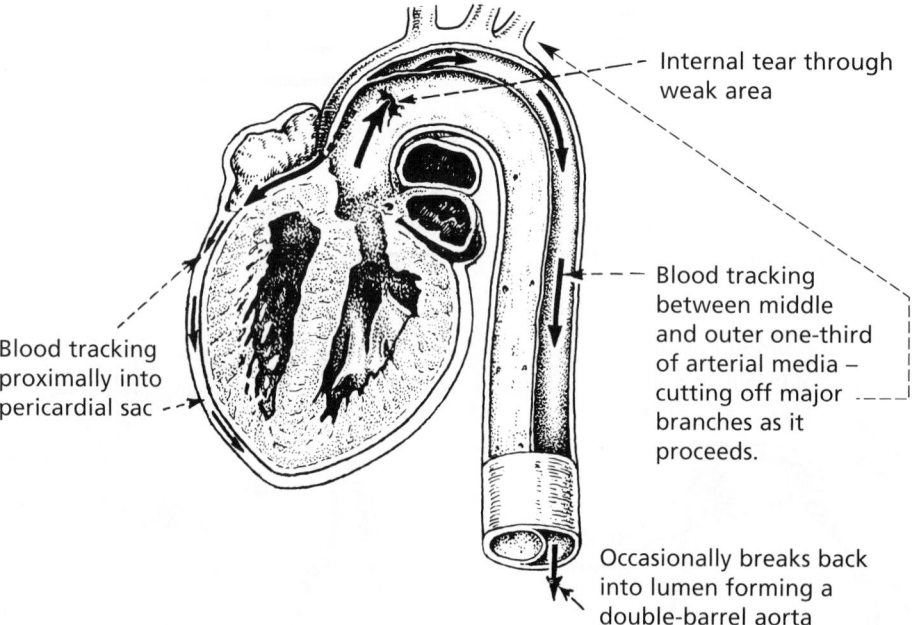

Internal tear through weak area

Blood tracking between middle and outer one-third of arterial media – cutting off major branches as it proceeds.

Blood tracking proximally into pericardial sac

Occasionally breaks back into lumen forming a double-barrel aorta

2.  **'Berry' aneurysm** occurs in medium-sized vessels at the base of the brain, e.g. on Circle of Willis. Associated with congenital deficiency of arterial media. Rupture causes subarachnoid haemorrhage.

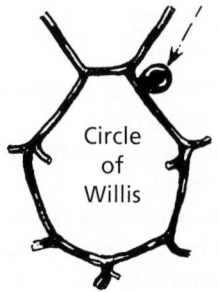

Circle of Willis

3.  **Microaneurysm** – associated with hypertension and affects smaller arteries and arterioles, especially in the brain.

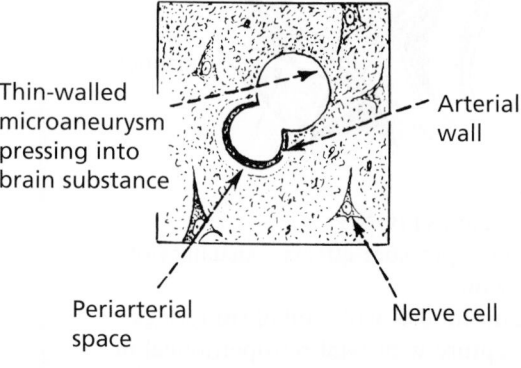

Thin-walled microaneurysm pressing into brain substance

Arterial wall

Periarterial space

Nerve cell

Rupture causes intra-cerebral haemorrhage.

# ARTERIAL DISEASES – MISCELLANEOUS

## RAYNAUD PHENOMENON

There are spasmodic attacks of pallor of the fingers (the toes, ears and nose may also be affected) due to intense constriction of the small arteries and arterioles in response to cold. The cause is not known.

The condition affects 5–10% of young women in temperate climates.

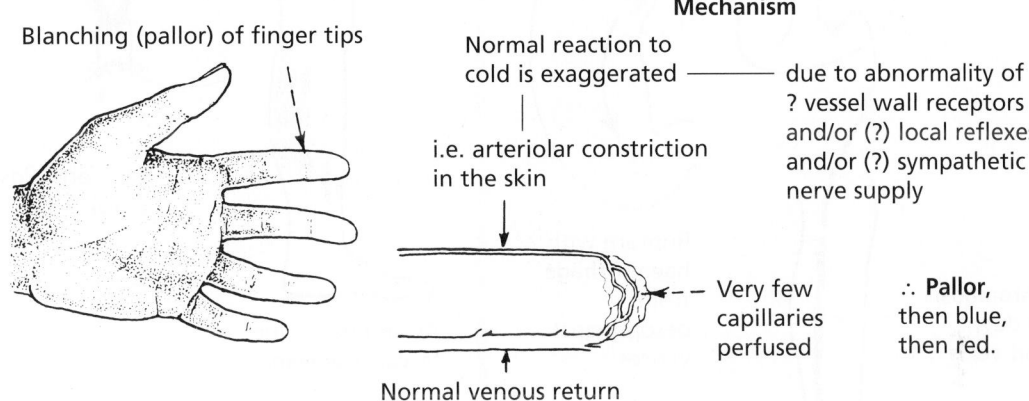

**Mechanism**

Blanching (pallor) of finger tips

Normal reaction to cold is exaggerated —— due to abnormality of ? vessel wall receptors and/or (?) local reflexes and/or (?) sympathetic nerve supply

i.e. arteriolar constriction in the skin

Very few capillaries perfused

∴ **Pallor**, then blue, then red.

Normal venous return

This condition may continue for many years and NO PERMANENT DAMAGE RESULTS.

A **secondary form** of Raynaud phenomenon may occur as a symptom in other conditions. Examples include the 'collagen diseases', systemic sclerosis (see p. 659) and SLE; cold agglutinins causing vascular blockage due to agglutination of red cells; the use of heavy pneumatic drills disturbing neurovascular controls in the hands.

In these circumstances the disease is serious and disabling, the trophic changes adding significantly to the damage caused by the primary diseases elsewhere in the body.

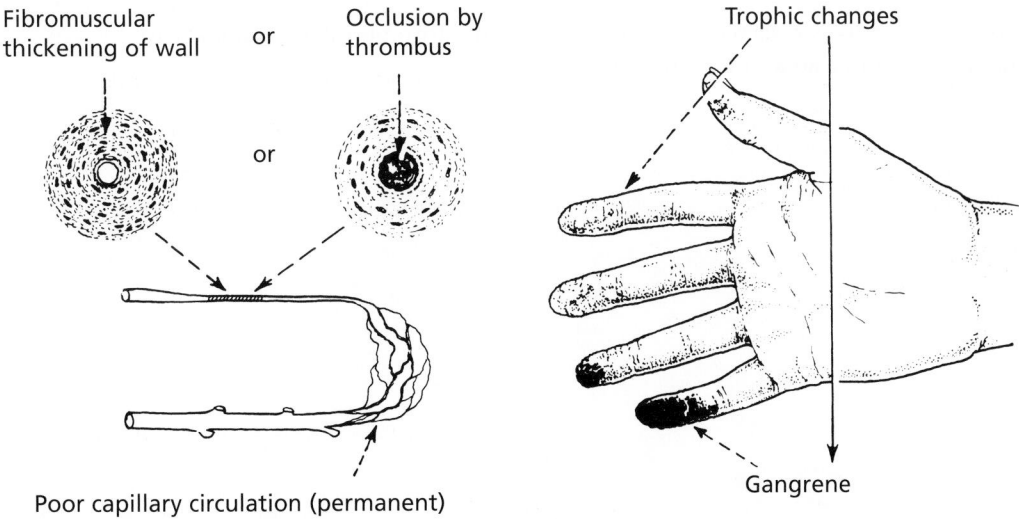

Fibromuscular thickening of wall    or    Occlusion by thrombus

or

Trophic changes

Poor capillary circulation (permanent)

Gangrene

# DISEASES OF VEINS

Diseases of the veins are important because they can be associated with:

1. *Acute* severe, sometimes fatal, complications

2. *Chronic* disability

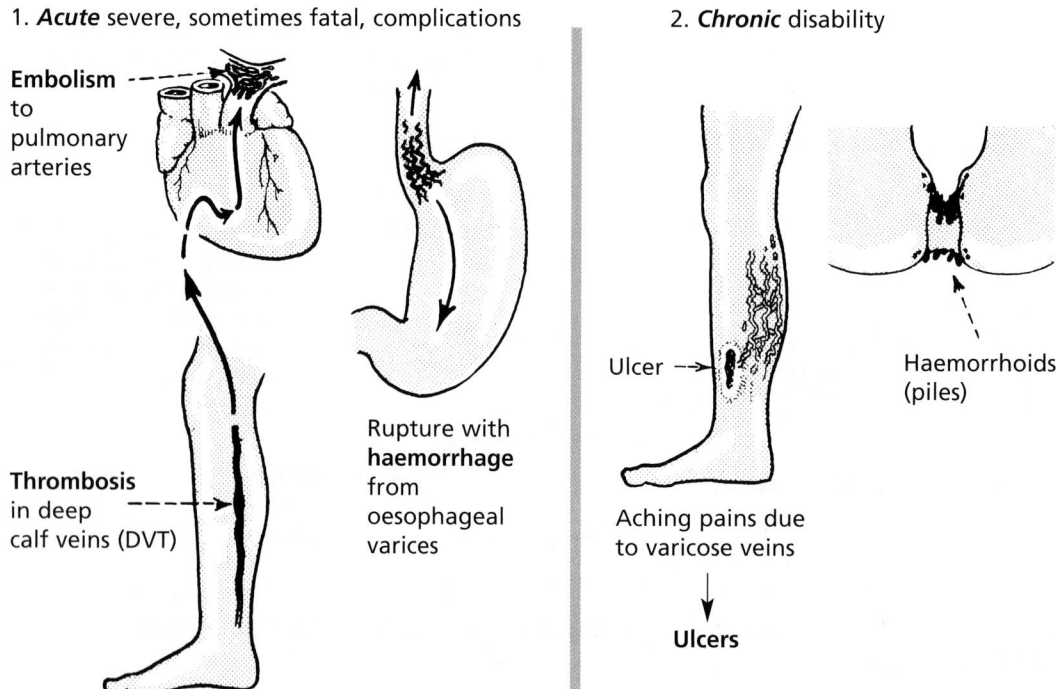

**Embolism** to pulmonary arteries

**Thrombosis** in deep calf veins (DVT)

Rupture with **haemorrhage** from oesophageal varices

Ulcer →

Aching pains due to varicose veins

↓

**Ulcers**

Haemorrhoids (piles)

## DEEP VEIN THROMBOSIS AND THROMBOPHLEBITIS

The veins of the lower limbs are very common sites of acute thrombosis, especially after surgical operations and during illnesses with enforced bed rest.

In the majority of cases the thrombosis is the primary event and mild inflammation follows as a reaction.

Thrombophlebitis is reserved for cases in which the thrombosis is secondary to inflammation in or adjacent to the vein.

# DISEASES OF VEINS

## ACUTE PHLEBITIS

### Suppurative (pyogenic)

Secondary to bacterial infection,
e.g. a very rare complication of appendicitis

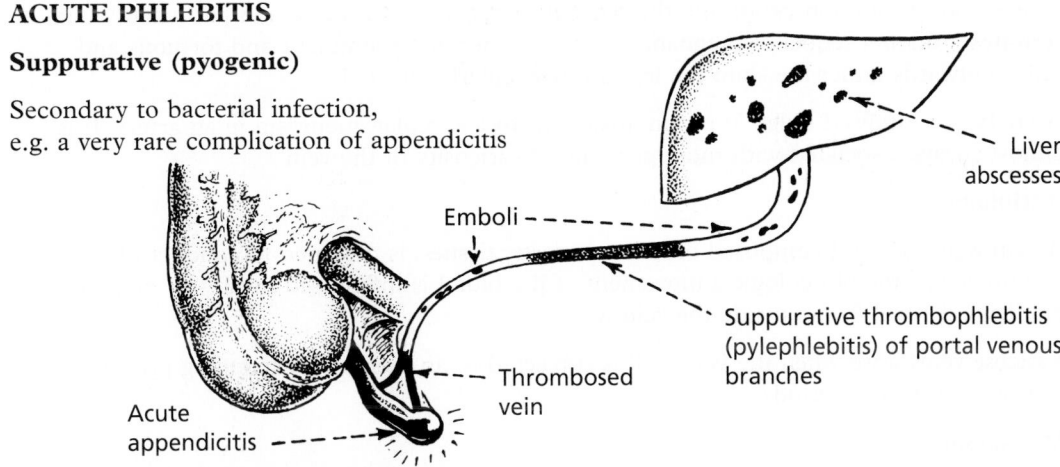

## VEINS IN MALIGNANT DISEASE

(a) Venules are easily invaded and infiltrated by carcinoma and are an important route in the metastatic spread of the tumour.
(b) Large veins, particularly in the mediastinum and pelvis, may be compressed from outside by the tumour – the resulting obstruction causing serious effects.

## SUPERIOR VENA CAVA OBSTRUCTION

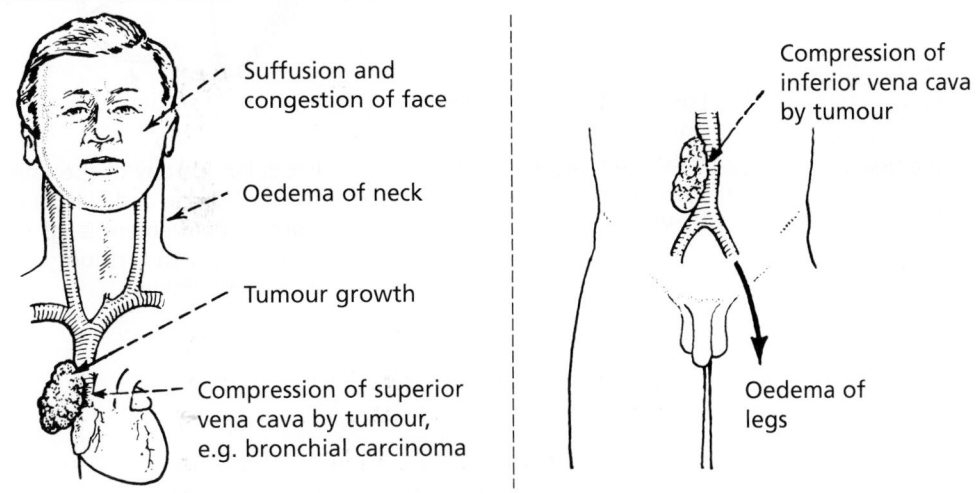

### Migratory thrombophlebitis (thrombophlebitis migrans)

In this rare condition the thrombosis is not confined to the lower limb veins and can affect veins anywhere in the body. A striking feature is the appearance and disappearance of thrombosis, apparently at random sites.

The mechanism is not fully understood but usually a **malignant tumour** is in the background – sometimes the phlebitis is the first clinical sign of an occult tumour but more often it complicates the terminal stages of tumour growth.

# VARICOSE VEINS

This is a very common condition, the incidence increasing with **age** and particularly high in **females** – often a sequel of pregnancy. The veins become prominent and tortuous and bulge outwards under the skin; the legs are particularly affected.

A **varix** is a localised bulge in a vein analogous to a saccular aneurysm in an artery. It is almost always associated with more generalised varicosity of the vein.

### Aetiology

A vein wall, thin and composed of musculoelastic tissues, is designed to conduct blood at low pressures: the physiological movement of the blood is influenced mostly by pressure gradients derived from outside the vein wall.

Varicose veins arise when the vein wall is subjected to an increased expanding pressure (tension) over long periods.

### Mechanism

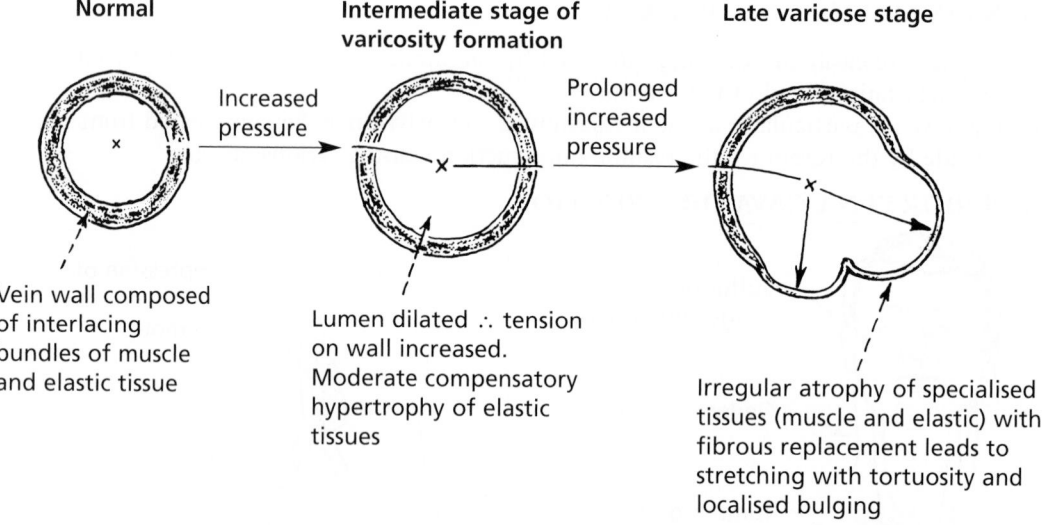

**Normal**

**Intermediate stage of varicosity formation**

**Late varicose stage**

Increased pressure

Prolonged increased pressure

Vein wall composed of interlacing bundles of muscle and elastic tissue

Lumen dilated ∴ tension on wall increased. Moderate compensatory hypertrophy of elastic tissues

Irregular atrophy of specialised tissues (muscle and elastic) with fibrous replacement leads to stretching with tortuosity and localised bulging

# VARICOSE VEINS

## FACTORS WHICH INFLUENCE THE BASIC MECHANISM

1. **Acting on the vein wall.**

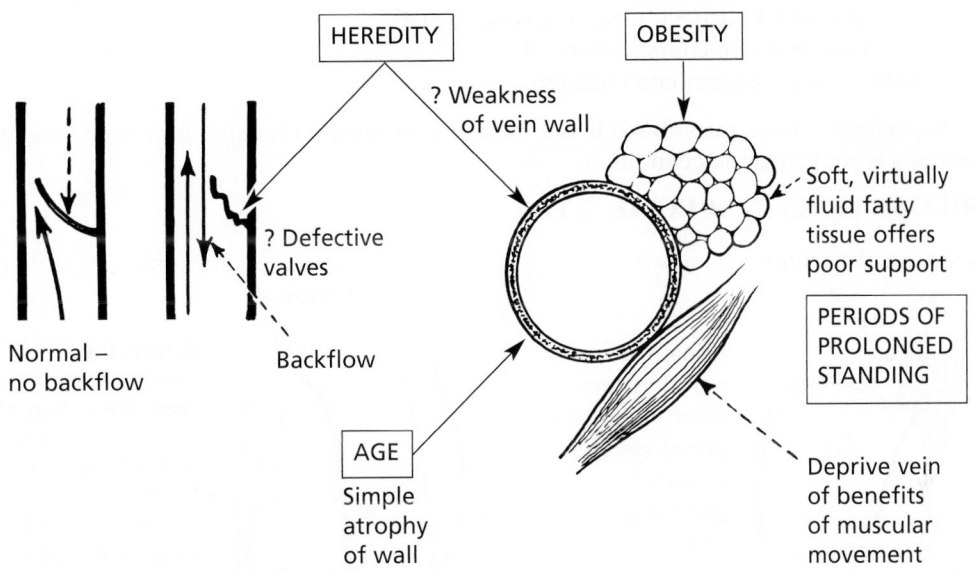

HEREDITY

OBESITY

? Weakness of vein wall

? Defective valves

Normal – no backflow

Backflow

Soft, virtually fluid fatty tissue offers poor support

PERIODS OF PROLONGED STANDING

AGE
Simple atrophy of wall

Deprive vein of benefits of muscular movement

2. **Increasing the intraluminal pressure**

(a) Obstruction to venous flow
– usually in the pelvis – by:
   Pregnancy
   Tumour
   Constipation with
      loaded colon
   Thrombosis in veins
      (also may destroy valves)
   Constrictions on limbs

(b) Special anatomical considerations.

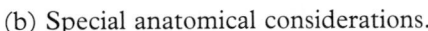

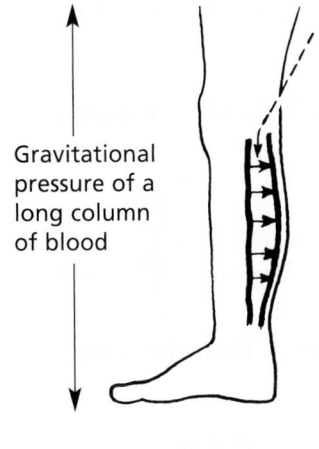

Gravitational pressure of a long column of blood

Special communicating veins between deep and superficial systems, if valves not competent, cause backflow into superficial veins greatly increasing the pressure within them.

# VARICOSE VEINS

### Effects

1. Fatigue and aching in legs.
2. Trophic changes – varicose eczema with pigmentation due to haemosiderin deposition may proceed to ULCERATION: very slow to heal.
3. Haemorrhage is a rare complication.
4. Thrombosis is a frequent complication.

*Note:* Superficial venous thrombosis is not usually associated with embolism; deep venous thrombosis is the dangerous condition.

## VARICOSE VEINS IN SPECIAL SITES

### Oesophageal varices

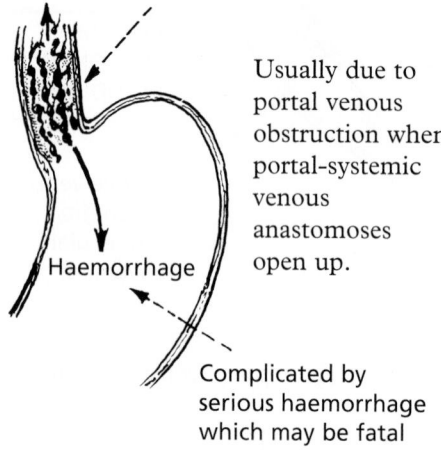

Haemorrhage

Usually due to portal venous obstruction when portal-systemic venous anastomoses open up.

Complicated by serious haemorrhage which may be fatal

**Varicocele**

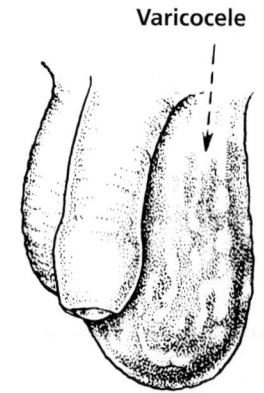

Affects the pampiniform plexus: feels like a 'bag of worms'. It may cause dull aching and, because the increased vascularity raises the scrotal temperature, the condition has been associated with infertility.

### Haemorrhoids

Varices of the anorectal veins; usually associated with constipation.

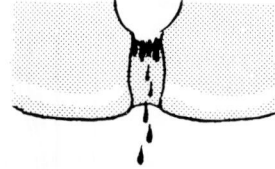

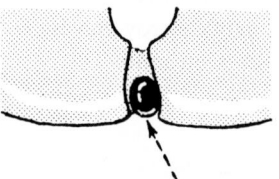

Complications are: 1. Rectal bleeding

3. Prolapse

2. Acute pain due to local haematoma (not a true haemorrhoid)

# DISEASES OF LYMPHATICS

The lymphatic vessels participate in disease processes in two main ways:

1. They afford a natural route by which diseases can spread.
2. They may become obstructed, with serious results.

### 1. LYMPHATICS as a mechanism by which DISEASE SPREADS

Small lymphatics are thin-walled vessels which have a simple endothelial layer and readily allow entry of tumour cells, bacteria and foreign material often within phagocytes.

The mechanism is important in the spread of (a) infection and (b) tumours.

Malignant cells

### Acute lymphangitis

The lymphatics draining an area infected by pyogenic bacteria (especially *streptococci*) may themselves become acutely inflamed.

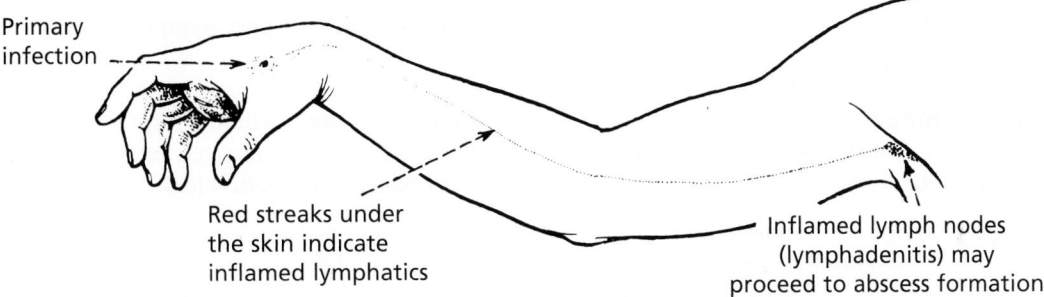

Primary infection

Red streaks under the skin indicate inflamed lymphatics

Inflamed lymph nodes (lymphadenitis) may proceed to abscess formation

**Chronic infections** such as tuberculosis also spread by lymphatics.

### Spread of tumours

This is an important route of spread of malignant tumours, especially carcinoma.

### Disposal of particulate matter

This was formerly seen in the lungs where inhaled soot could be seen clearly indicating the lymphatic system under the pleura.

Soot (carbon) is relatively inert, but other dusts may cause serious disease.

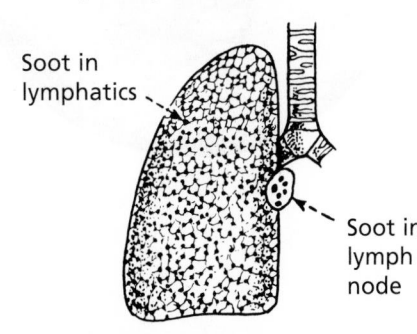

Soot in lymphatics

Soot in lymph node

# LYMPHATIC OBSTRUCTION

## LYMPHATIC OBSTRUCTION

This is usually due to acquired disease but rarely there is a congenital deficiency of lymphatics (Milroy syndrome).

The main causes of acquired obstruction are:

### (a) Tumour growth

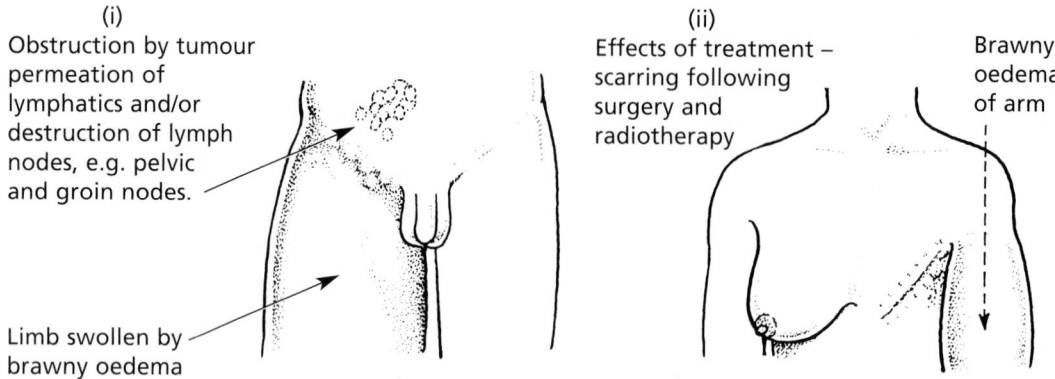

(i)
Obstruction by tumour permeation of lymphatics and/or destruction of lymph nodes, e.g. pelvic and groin nodes.

Limb swollen by brawny oedema

(ii)
Effects of treatment – scarring following surgery and radiotherapy

Brawny oedema of arm

### (b) Blocking by parasites – e.g. adult worms of filariasis in the tropics.

### Effects of chronic lymphatic obstruction:
– accumulation of fluid in the tissues causes swelling of the affected part (lymphoedema).

### Special varieties of lymphoedema

***Peau d'orange*** – where the lymphatics of the skin are blocked by tumour.

Peau d'orange surrounding ulcerated cancer of breast

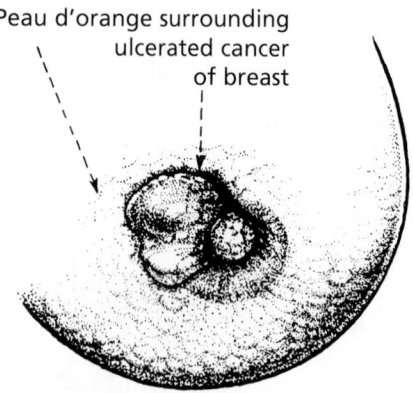

***Elephantiasis*** – where a limb and/or the scrotum is massively enlarged due to filarial lymphatic blockage.

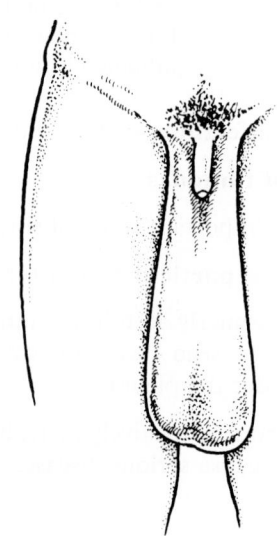

# VASCULAR TUMOURS

Benign tumours of endothelial cells – ANGIOMAS – illustrate the difficulty in defining the borderline between the tumours (neoplasms) and hamartomas (developmental abnormalities). These are discussed on p. 176.

Other varieties include:

## 1. PYOGENIC GRANULOMA

This lesion appears on the skin at a site subject to trauma and infection, e.g. around the finger nails, the nostrils or the tongue.

It commonly occurs during pregnancy.

It grows over several days to form a small red nodule up to about 1 cm in diameter and is usually ulcerated.

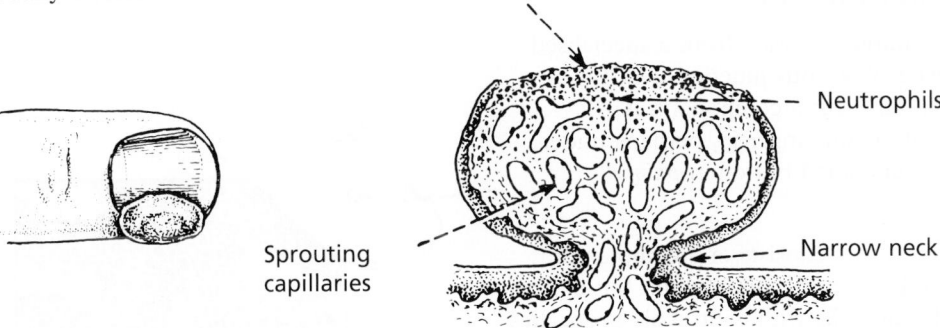

The lesion is benign despite its rapid evolution, and is cured by simple removal.

## 2. TELANGIECTASIS

Small localised dilatations of small blood vessels. There are two main types: congenital and acquired.

(a) *Congenital.* In the rare hereditary haemorrhagic telangiectasia, the small lesions occur in the skin and mucous membranes and may be associated with bleeding (especially from the nose).

(b) *Acquired.* The small lesions, affecting the face and neck, are known as **spider naevi**.

The mechanism of their development is probably related to oestrogen excess, since they occur in pregnancy and in serious liver disease (oestrogen catabolism diminished) where they are a diagnostic sign.

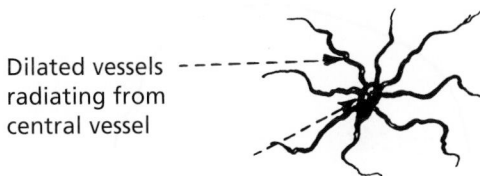

Telangiectasia may be seen in skin damaged by radiotherapy.

# VASCULAR TUMOURS

### 3. LYMPHANGIOMA

Lymphangiomas are much rarer
than haemangiomas and are usually
without serious pathological significance.

Occasionally the abnormal lymphatic vessels become
distended and form fluctuant swellings with local
pressure effects, e.g. 'cystic hygroma' of neck of
babies and children.

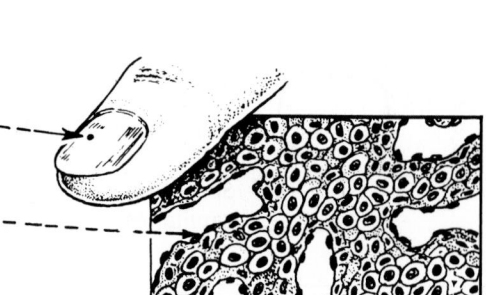

Gradually
expanding
'cyst'

### 4. GLOMANGIOMA

(Glomus tumour) – arises from a specialised
type of arteriolovenous junction which
includes a rich neural component. A
common site is the fingertip, perhaps under
the nail; a very small but often *painful*
*tumour.*

Microscopically it consists of a complex of
blood vessels lined by endothelium but cuffed
by round clear cells with contractile properties
(myoid cells). It is rich in nerve fibres.

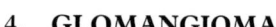

### ANGIOSARCOMAS

These are uncommon malignant tumours of endothelial cells. They may affect the skin.

Lesions of the scalp occur in the
elderly. They appear as spreading
'bruise-like' areas often with a
central nodule. Chronic sun
exposure is thought to be important.

Lesions often arise in the limbs in areas
of lymphoedema, e.g. in the past
following irradiation and lymph node
clearance for carcinoma of breast.

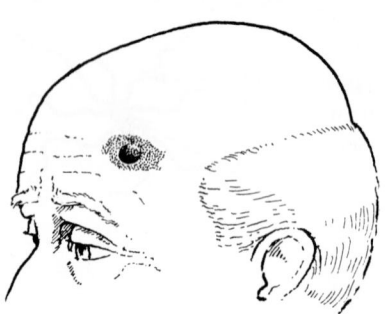

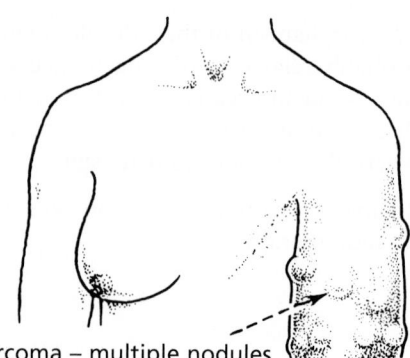

Angiosarcoma – multiple nodules

Angiosarcoma of the liver is associated with exposure to vinyl chloride monomer.

# VASCULAR TUMOURS

## KAPOSI SARCOMA

This tumour has increased in incidence with the spread of AIDS and HIV infection.

It is a tumour of endothelial cells due to infection by Herpes virus type 8, often occurring in immunocompromised patients.

It occurs in four groups of patients.

(a) **AIDS associated.**
(b) **Sporadic** (classic) – affecting elderly males (especially Ashkenazi Jews) living in the Mediterranean littoral.
(c) **Endemic** – mainly in central Africa, typically affecting young adults.
(d) **Iatrogenic** – in immunosuppression, e.g. transplant patients.

The disease presents as dark coloured (due to high blood content) **subcutaneous nodules** or plaques resembling bruises.

(a) The nodules may be **multiple** and fairly randomly distributed – this is seen particularly in AIDS cases.

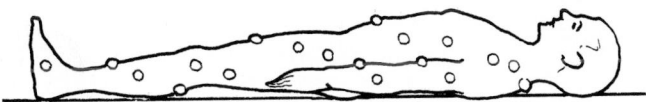

(b) In 'classic' Kaposi, the tumour begins as a **solitary** nodule particularly on the limbs.

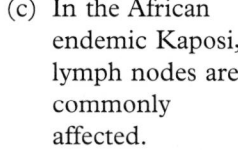

(c) In the African endemic Kaposi, lymph nodes are commonly affected.

The histological appearances are of malignant spindle cells lining a network of sieve-like spaces containing extravasated red cells.

Spindle cells

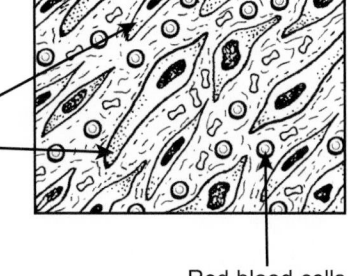

Red blood cells

# RESPIRATORY SYSTEM

## OBJECTIVES

To understand:
1. Common conditions of the upper respiratory tract.
2. The normal structure of the respiratory tract and how this relates to disease.
3. The pathology and aetiology of chronic obstructive pulmonary disease.
4. The aetiology, classification, pathology and complications of pneumonia.
5. The main types of lung cancer, including presentation and spread.

# UPPER RESPIRATORY TRACT

### INFLAMMATION

Infections of the nose, nasal sinuses, pharynx and larynx are common. They are usually mild and self-limiting. Most cases are due to viral infection, but this is often followed by bacterial superinfection.

**1. VIRAL INFECTION**

This phase is characterised by features of acute inflammation but without the exudation of neutrophils.

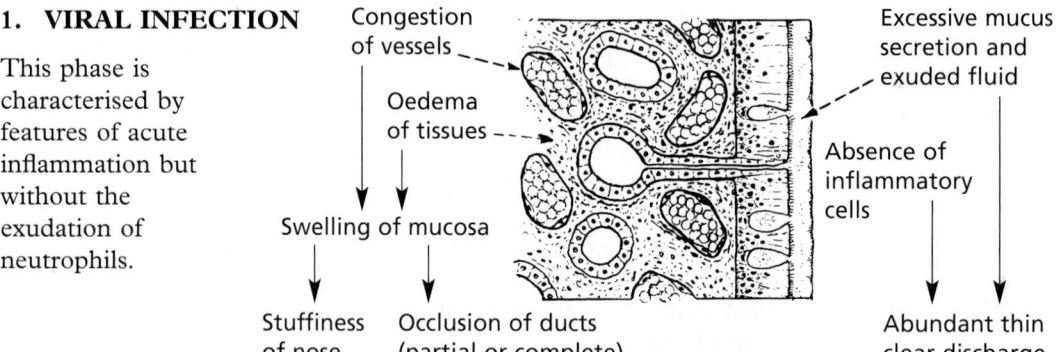

Congestion of vessels

Oedema of tissues

Swelling of mucosa

Stuffiness of nose

Occlusion of ducts (partial or complete)

Excessive mucus secretion and exuded fluid

Absence of inflammatory cells

Abundant thin clear discharge

# UPPER RESPIRATORY TRACT

**Viruses involved**

A wide variety, of which the major types are:

(i) **Rhinoviruses** ⎤
(ii) **Coronaviruses** ⎦ Responsible for more than half of cases of the common cold.

(iii) Adenovirus, influenza, parainfluenza and respiratory syncytial viruses can also invade the lower respiratory tract.

The viruses adhere to cell surface proteins, e.g. on cilia; ⟶ enter the cells and replicate ⟶ and kill them

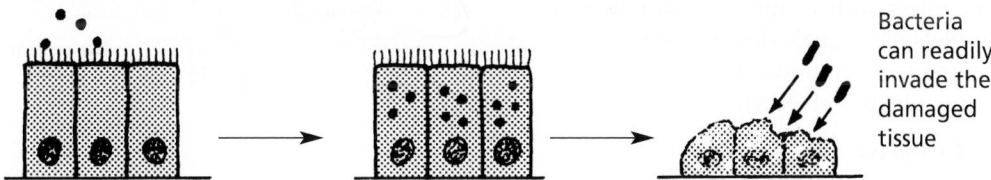

Bacteria can readily invade the damaged tissue

## 2. BACTERIAL PHASE

Many bacteria are commensal in the respiratory tract (e.g. *Streptococcus mutans, Haemophilus influenzae*) and can superinfect the damaged tissue, which then exhibits the typical features of acute inflammation including exudation of neutrophils.

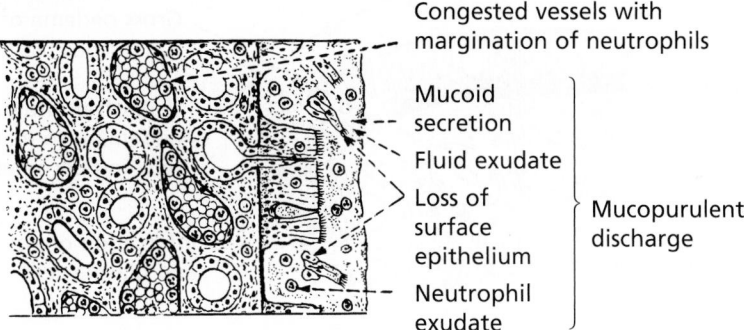

Congested vessels with margination of neutrophils

Mucoid secretion

Fluid exudate

Loss of surface epithelium

Neutrophil exudate

⎫
⎬ Mucopurulent
⎭ discharge

The wide variety of different viruses involved prevents protective immunity.

# RHINITIS

### INFECTIVE

Acute coryza (common cold) usually involves the nose and adjacent structures.

The two phases, *viral* and *bacterial*, are typically seen in this disease.

The drainage from the sinuses, especially the maxillary, is often blocked by swelling of the mucosa — giving rise to sinusitis.

The infection is acquired by airborne droplets (sneezing), direct contact with respiratory secretions or fomites (contaminated objects).

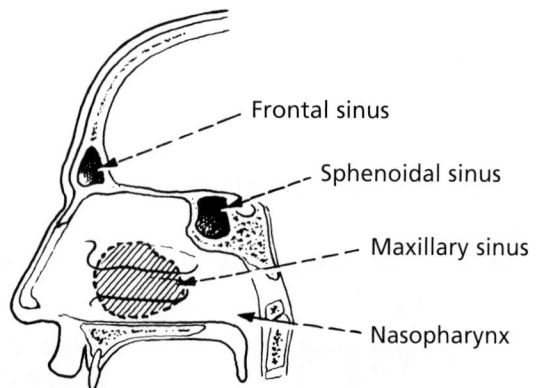

### ALLERGIC

Allergic rhinitis (hay fever) is a Type I hypersensitivity reaction (p. 141) to inhaled materials (e.g. seasonal – grass, pollen; non-seasonal – house dust mite, pets). Patients develop immediate symptoms of sneezing, itching and watery rhinorrhoea.

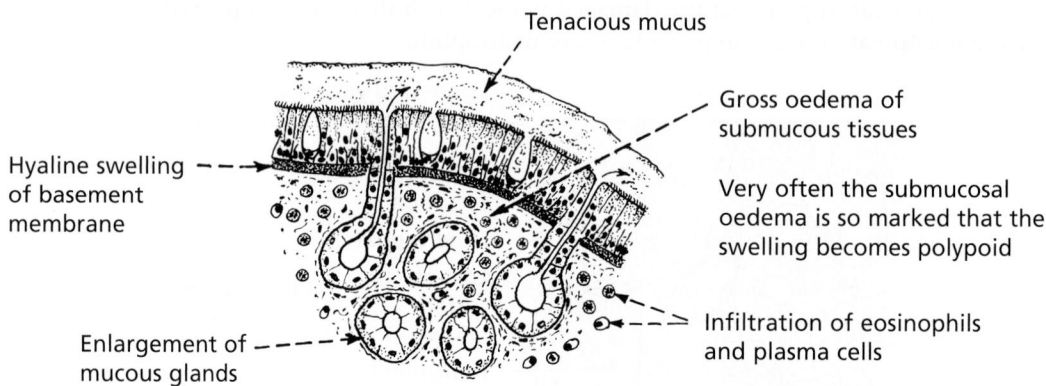

# RHINITIS

The repeated attacks frequently lead to chronic changes in the mucosa with polyp formation, particularly on the middle turbinate bones and within the maxillary sinuses.

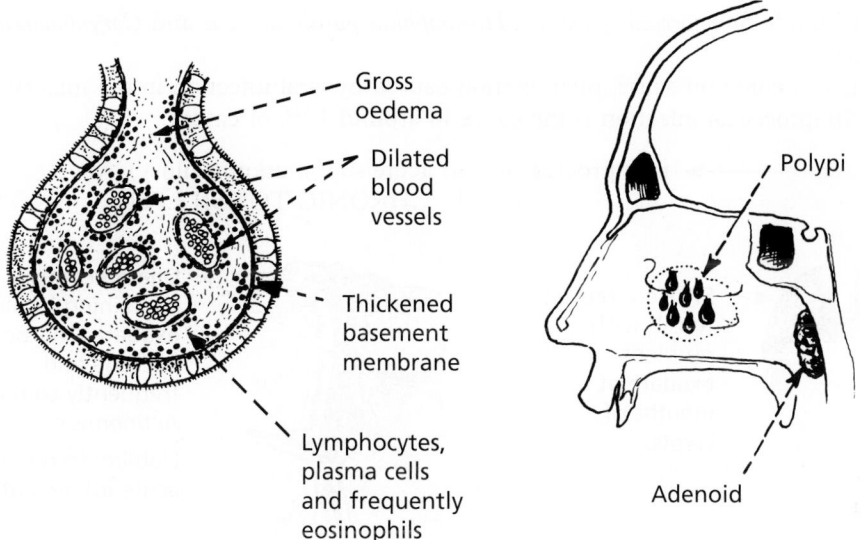

Gross oedema

Dilated blood vessels

Thickened basement membrane

Lymphocytes, plasma cells and frequently eosinophils

Polypi

Adenoid

## NON-ALLERGIC RHINITIS

This is an umbrella term for rhinitis of multiple causes including occupational exposure, smoking, hormonal and medication induced. In vasomotor rhinitis, non-allergic triggers (exercise, hormonal factors, spicy food, alcohol) are thought to cause dilatation of blood vessels in the nose.

# ACUTE PHARYNGITIS, TRACHEITIS AND LARYNGITIS

### ACUTE PHARYNGITIS AND TRACHEITIS

Most sore throats are caused by **viruses** – including adenovirus and Epstein–Barr virus.

**Bacteria** include *Streptococcus pyogenes*, *Haemophilus parainfluenzae* and *Corynbacterium diphtheriae*.

**Tonsillitis** is a common acute inflammation caused by viral infection in the majority of cases. Streptococcal infection is the cause in around 10% of cases.

Acute phase ──────▶ may progress to (a) acute suppuration (quinsy)
                             or (b) CHRONIC TONSILLITIS

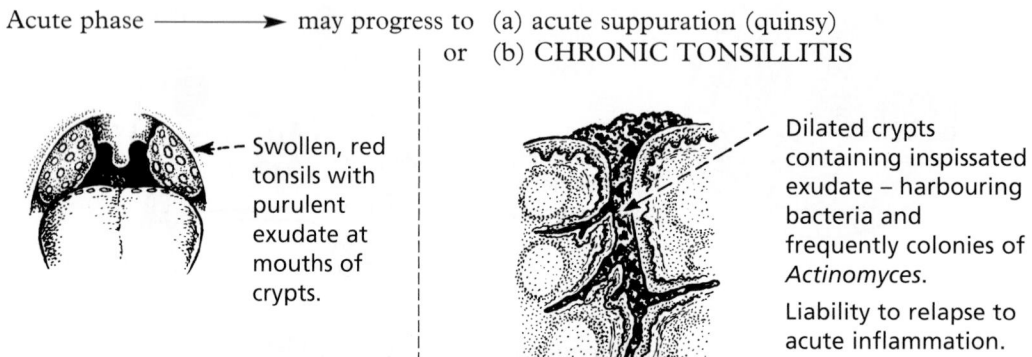

Swollen, red tonsils with purulent exudate at mouths of crypts.

Dilated crypts containing inspissated exudate – harbouring bacteria and frequently colonies of *Actinomyces*.

Liability to relapse to acute inflammation.

**Diphtheria**, now uncommon due to vaccination, is a serious infection. Symptoms begin with a sore throat and fever. In severe cases formation of a pseudomembrane is striking.

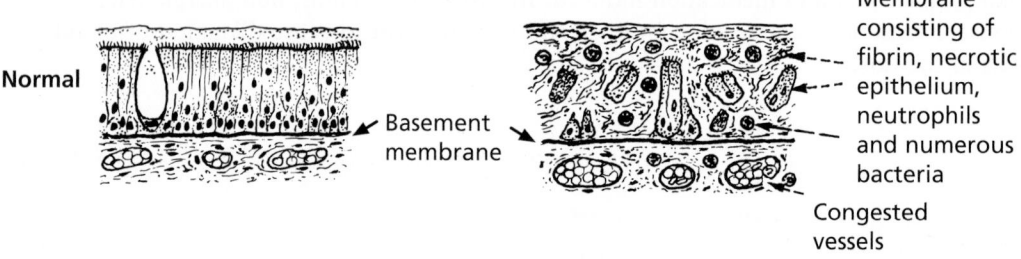

**Normal**

Basement membrane

Membrane consisting of fibrin, necrotic epithelium, neutrophils and numerous bacteria

Congested vessels

This pseudomembrane may spread to block the larynx, causing respiratory obstruction.

The EXOTOXIN of diphtheria is encoded by a bacteriophage (a virus which infects the bacterium). It can cause myocarditis (p. 236) and neuropathy (p. 613).

**Acute epiglottitis** was historically caused by *H. influenzae*. With vaccination it is now more often caused by other bacteria (e.g. *Staphylococcus aureus*). There is severe inflammation and oedema. In young children, the larynx becomes obstructed necessitating tracheostomy and administration of antibiotics.

**Acute laryngitis** is caused by viruses (e.g. rhinoviruses), bacteria (e.g. group A streptococcus) and irritants (e.g. cigarette smoke). Acute *oedema of the glottis* is seen in some cases of anaphylaxis (p. 141) and angioedema (which can be allergic, drug induced or hereditary).

# ACUTE PHARYNGITIS, TRACHEITIS AND LARYNGITIS

## CHRONIC LARYNGITIS

Cigarette smoking, repeated attacks of infection and atmospheric pollution may lead to chronic inflammation of the larynx.

Two main features are (a) changes in the lining epithelium and (b) increase in mucus secretion.

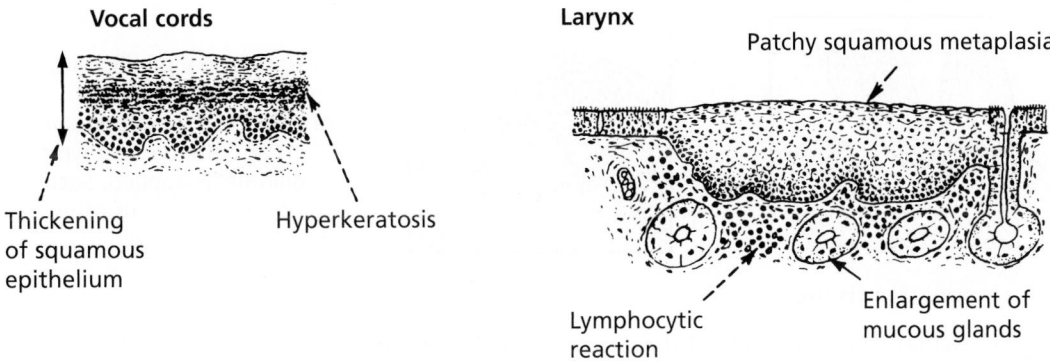

**Vocal cords**

Thickening of squamous epithelium

Hyperkeratosis

**Larynx**

Patchy squamous metaplasia

Lymphocytic reaction

Enlargement of mucous glands

The following sequence of events tends to take place:

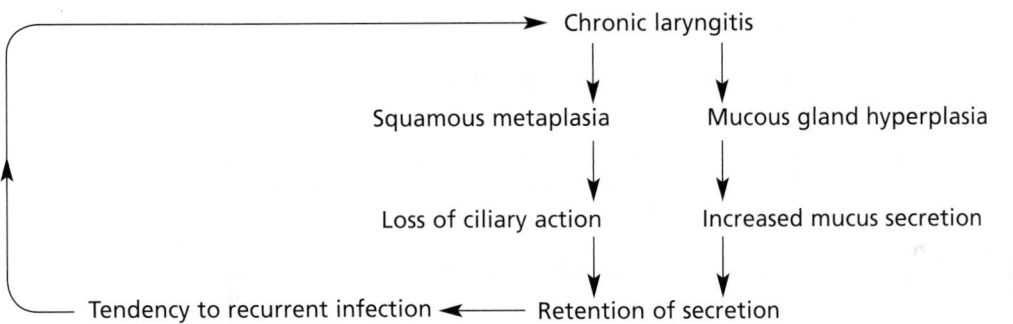

Chronic laryngitis

Squamous metaplasia → Mucous gland hyperplasia

Loss of ciliary action → Increased mucus secretion

Tendency to recurrent infection ← Retention of secretion

**Tuberculosis** – this can cause severe ulceration of the larynx and is usually secondary to pulmonary tuberculosis.

## Vocal cord polyps and singer's nodules

They consist of squamous epithelium overlying fibrin-rich and myxoid stroma. Vocal cord polyps more commonly affect men and are unilateral and associated with vocal abuse. Singer's nodules are more common in females and are bilateral.

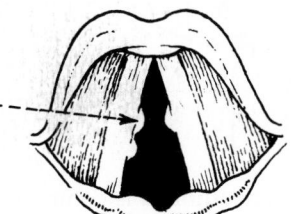

# TUMOURS OF THE UPPER RESPIRATORY TRACT

### BENIGN TUMOURS

(a) **Epithelial**

Papillomas may be single but are often multiple and due to infection by papilloma virus (HPV 11 and 16). The epithelium may be one of two types:

Squamous cell              Transitional cell

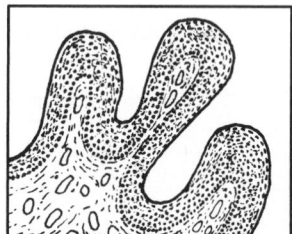 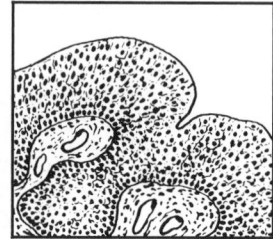

In transitional papillomas, the abnormal epithelium grows down the glandular ducts and the name 'inverted papilloma' is applied. Such tumours often recur after incomplete removal.

(b) **Connective tissue**

Haemangiomas, especially of the nasal septum, are a rare cause of persistent nose bleeds. A special form, angiofibroma, typically located in the nasal septum, affects male children. It is locally aggressive and grows throughout childhood but typically regresses.

### MALIGNANT TUMOURS

These are mainly squamous carcinomas and are commonly seen in the larynx. Intraepithelial neoplasia (carcinoma-in-situ) is a frequent precursor.

**Smoking** and alcohol consumption are aetiologically important. HPV (human papilloma virus) (particularly type 16) is a factor in cancers of the tonsils and hypopharynx but is rarely a factor in the larynx.

The rate of growth and spread is influenced by the site within the larynx.

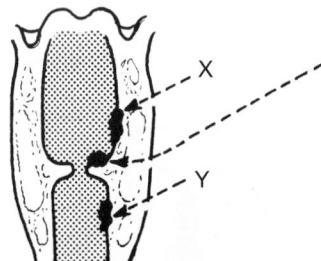

Tumours of the true cord tend to stay localised and have a better prognosis than supraglottic (X) and subglottic (Y) tumours – the looser surrounding tissues allow early local and cervical node spread.

**Nasopharyngeal carcinoma** is common in certain regions of East Asia and Africa and is associated with Epstein–Barr virus infection, which can usually be detected in tumour cells by PCR on in-situ hybridisation techniques.

Adenocarcinoma of the nose is a rare tumour, sometimes seen in woodworkers.

# LUNGS – ANATOMY

## ACINUS

This is the functional unit of the lung, where gas transfer takes place. It consists of the respiratory bronchiole and associated alveolar ducts and sacs supplied by one terminal bronchiole. There are approximately 25 000 acini in the normal adult male lung.

## LOBULE

This is served by one pre-terminal bronchiole and is the smallest anatomic compartment of lung that is grossly apparent. It contains 3 to 30 acini and is bound by connective tissue septa. These connective tissue septa may be accentuated in smokers.

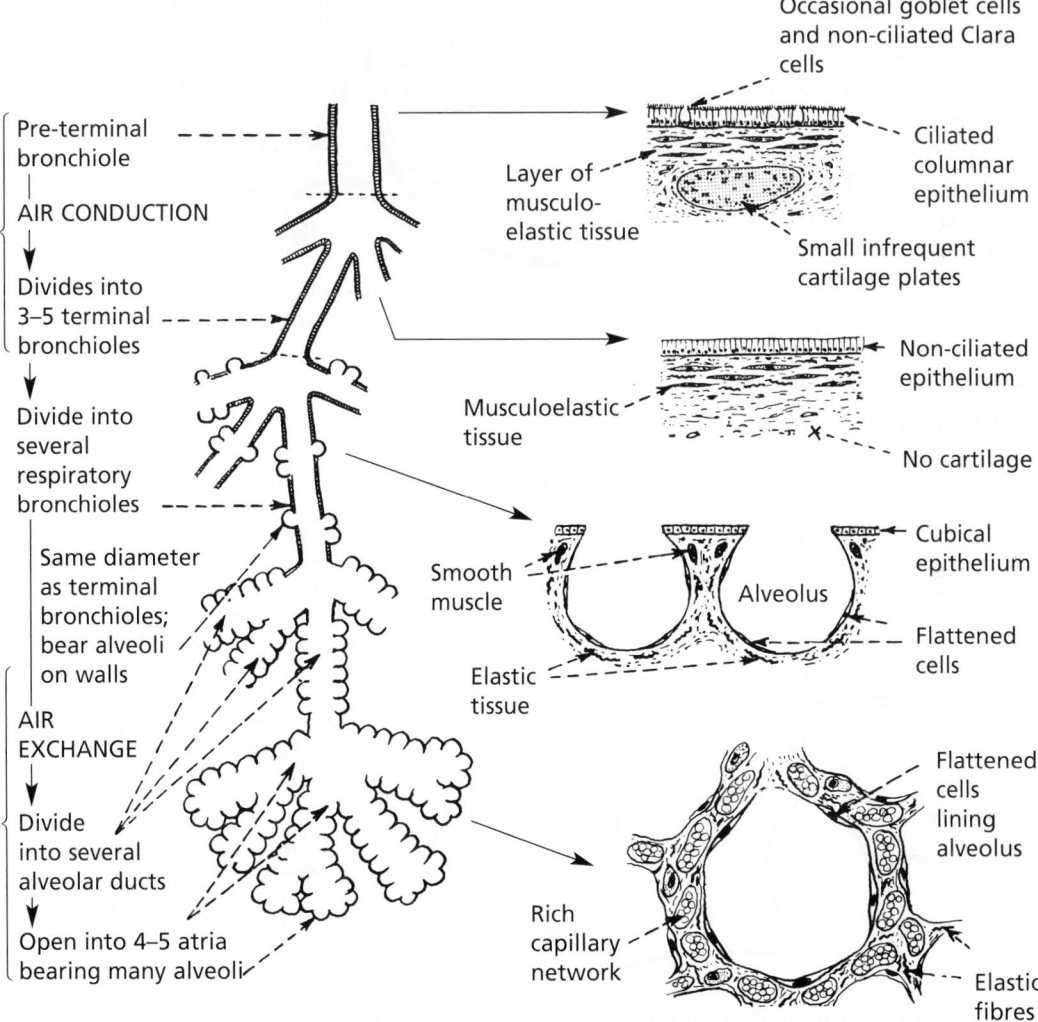

The total area for air exchange is very large (equivalent to a tennis court), allowing considerable reserve capacity.

# LUNGS – ANATOMY

### HISTOLOGY OF THE ALVEOLUS

Two types of cell (pneumocytes) line the alveoli:

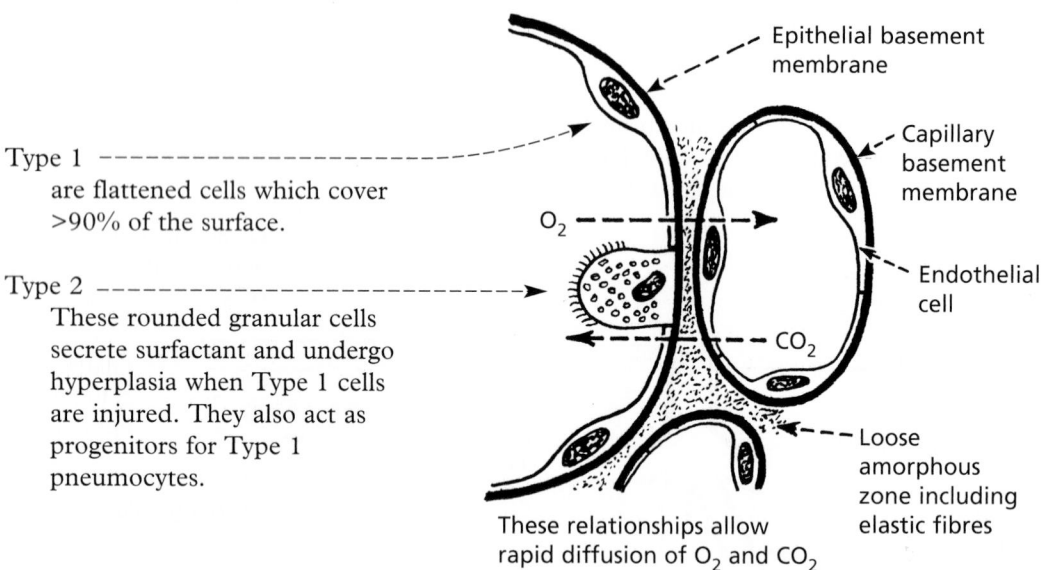

Type 1 ---------------------------
are flattened cells which cover
>90% of the surface.

Type 2 ----------------------------
These rounded granular cells
secrete surfactant and undergo
hyperplasia when Type 1 cells
are injured. They also act as
progenitors for Type 1
pneumocytes.

Epithelial basement membrane

Capillary basement membrane

Endothelial cell

Loose amorphous zone including elastic fibres

$O_2$

$CO_2$

These relationships allow rapid diffusion of $O_2$ and $CO_2$

Macrophages and mast cells are also present in the alveoli.

### PULMONARY VASCULATURE

Dual blood supply

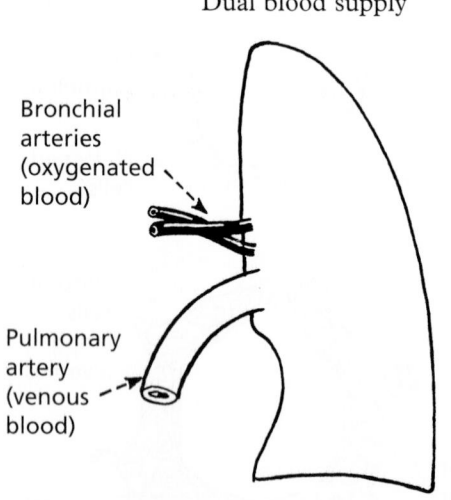

Bronchial arteries (oxygenated blood)

Pulmonary artery (venous blood)

This dual supply is of importance
when a pulmonary arterial branch
is blocked.

Lymph drainage

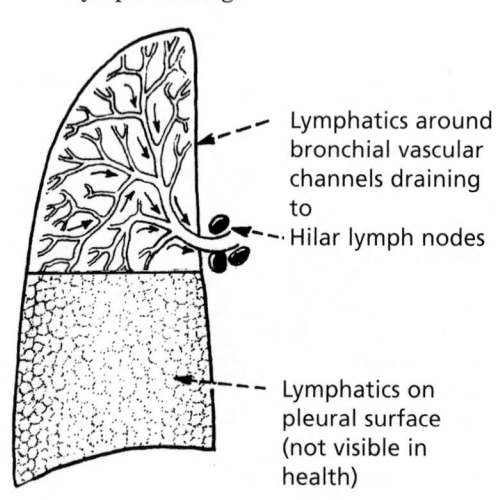

Lymphatics around bronchial vascular channels draining to Hilar lymph nodes

Lymphatics on pleural surface (not visible in health)

This fine network of lymphatics
becomes visible when pigmented dust
is inhaled over long periods.

# RESPIRATION

The normal intake of air is around 7 litres per minute; of this, after allowing for non-functioning dead space (trachea, bronchi, etc.), approximately 5 litres per minute is available for alveolar ventilation. A definite flow of air is maintained as far as the terminal bronchiole. Beyond this point the actual flow ceases and gas exchange is effected by diffusion.

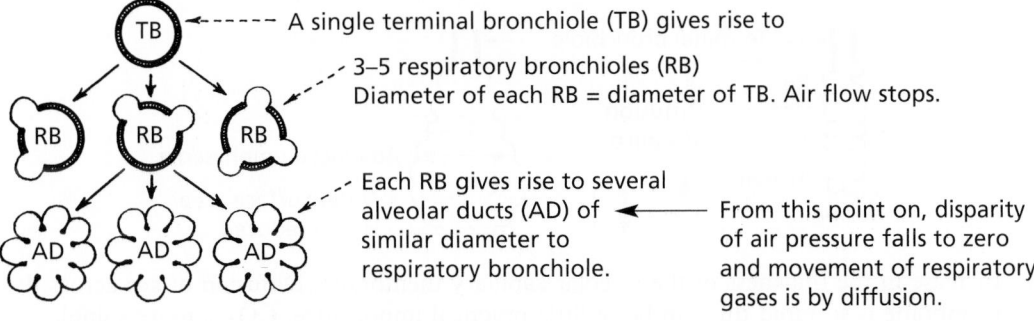

A single terminal bronchiole (TB) gives rise to

3–5 respiratory bronchioles (RB)
Diameter of each RB = diameter of TB. Air flow stops.

Each RB gives rise to several alveolar ducts (AD) of similar diameter to respiratory bronchiole.

From this point on, disparity of air pressure falls to zero and movement of respiratory gases is by diffusion.

Three factors are involved in the maintenance of adequate respiration:

1. Adequate intake of air ----------------------------------
2. Rapid diffusion along alveolar ducts
   and through alveolar walls ----------------------------
3. Adequate perfusion of pulmonary circulation

Interference with any of these factors will result in respiratory embarrassment (dyspnoea) and even respiratory failure.

## Inadequate air supply to alveoli (hypoventilation)

This may be due to lesions and diseases which interfere with the mechanics of respiration, such as central nervous lesions affecting the respiratory centre, paralysis of muscles of respiration as in poliomyelitis, injuries and deformities of the thoracic skeleton (e.g. fracture of ribs, kyphosis) and pleural disease preventing lung expansion as in pleural effusion or pneumothorax.

The most common cause of hypoventilation is bronchial obstruction. This may be reversible due to bronchial spasm, as in asthma, or irreversible in chronic obstructive pulmonary disease (COPD) (p. 286).

# RESPIRATION

### Impaired diffusion of gases

Three mechanisms may interfere with diffusion:

1.  Reduction in the total alveolar surface available for diffusion, e.g. consolidated airless lobe in pneumonia, fibrosis of lung or tumour growth.
2.  Increase in distance over which diffusion takes place as in emphysema.

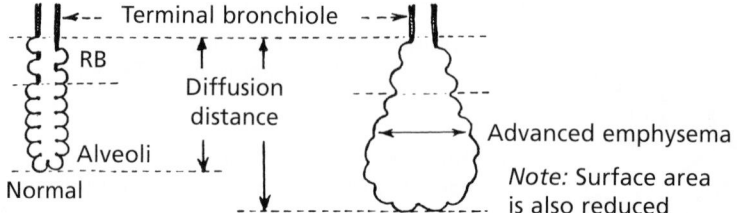

3.  Increase in the thickness of the alveolar capillary membrane. Diffusion of gas across the membrane is so rapid this can be of little practical importance. $CO_2$ is more soluble than $O_2$ and its diffusion through the alveolar wall is 20 times as rapid as $O_2$, therefore while blood $O_2$ progressively falls there is usually no retention of $CO_2$.

### Altered pulmonary perfusion

Interference with the pulmonary circulation may occur in four main ways:

1.  Occlusion of larger vessels by multiple emboli.
2.  Slowing of the pulmonary circulation as in venous congestion due to left heart lesions or congenital left-right shunts.
3.  Reduction in the pulmonary capillary bed by diffuse lung disease such as fibrosis or emphysema.
4.  Pulmonary vascular spasm due to hypoxia. Permanent changes can occur in the vessels if the hypoxia is unrelieved.

*Note*: In addition to hypoxaemia, inadequate perfusion tends to cause retention of carbon dioxide.

In chronic lung disease, ventilation, diffusion and perfusion disorders are present in varying degrees.

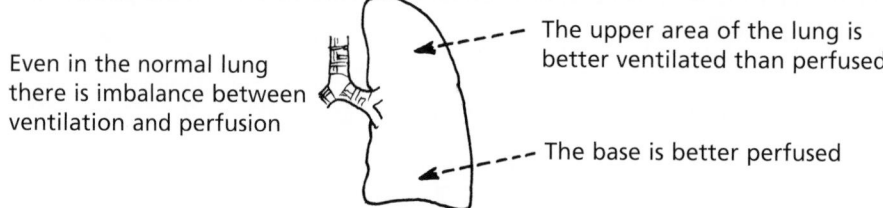

In many lung diseases this imbalance is increased. Admixture of well and poorly oxygenated blood results in hypoxaemia.

# ACUTE BRONCHITIS

This is an inflammation of the large and medium bronchi. The condition may be serious if associated with pre-existing respiratory disease. Mucous and serous glands in the walls of the bronchi provide abundant mucoid secretion during the inflammation. Ciliated epithelia lining the bronchi aid passage of the exudate upward and help prevent spread down to the bronchioles.

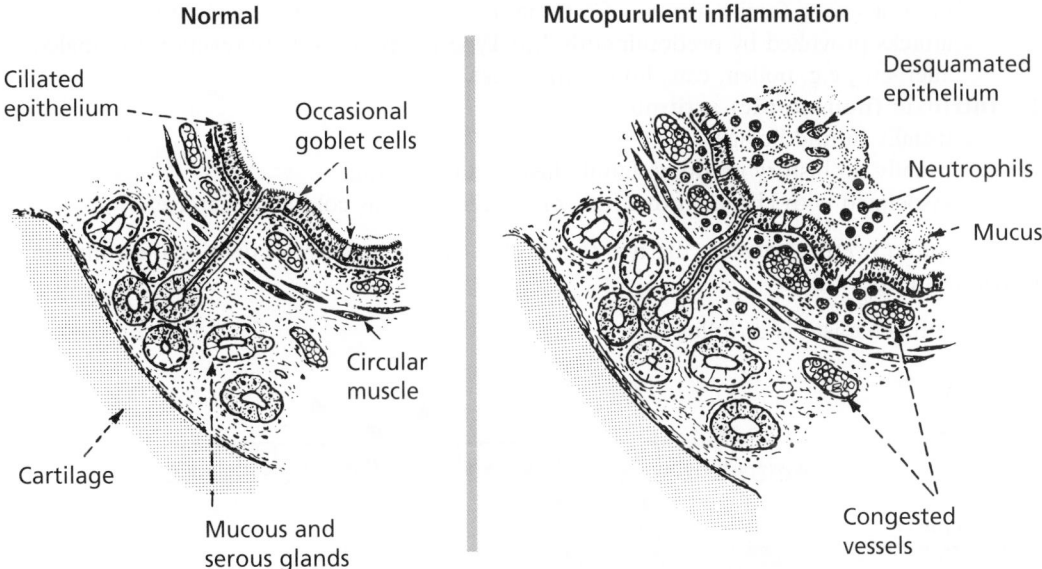

**Normal**

Ciliated epithelium

Occasional goblet cells

Circular muscle

Cartilage

Mucous and serous glands

**Mucopurulent inflammation**

Desquamated epithelium

Neutrophils

Mucus

Congested vessels

In most cases, the process is initiated by a viral or mycoplasmal infection. It is a common complication of influenza and measles. This initial phase is followed by bacterial invasion. *Streptococcus pneumoniae* and *H. influenzae* are commonest, but *S. aureus* and *S. pyogenes* may be found, especially in infants.

The condition is usually mild, and spread to the bronchioles is unusual in healthy adults due to the effective ciliary action of the bronchial epithelium. Spread may occur however in debilitated people. Bronchiolitis and bronchopneumonia result and can prove fatal. Equally important is the serious effect of repeated attacks of acute infection in patients with CHRONIC BRONCHITIS (p. 287).

In **children:**

1. Whooping cough (due to *Bordetella pertussis*) may cause permanent damage due to the severity of the infection and the stress on the airways during the coughing and whooping attacks.
2. **Bronchiolitis** in the very young (<2 years), in the majority of cases, is due to *respiratory syncytial virus* and the risk of progression to **bronchopneumonia** is high.

# BRONCHIAL ASTHMA

In asthma, there are spasmodic attacks of reversible bronchial obstruction with wheezing and dyspnoea and often a dry cough. The prevalence has markedly increased in recent years, although has now plateaued. There are two main patterns:

1. **Extrinsic (atopic) asthma** (p. 143)
   - typically starts in childhood.
   - often a strong family history of asthma or atopic conditions (e.g. eczema).
   - attacks provoked by predominantly IgE Type I hypersensitivity reaction to inhaled allergens, e.g. pollen, cats, house mite dust.
2. **Intrinsic (non-atopic) asthma**
   - usually in middle age.
   - usually no history of atopy: family history uncommon.
   - associated with chronic bronchitis or triggers such as cold and exercise.

There is often overlap between the two types. Other types include occupational asthma and aspirin-induced asthma.

The basic mechanism is as follows:

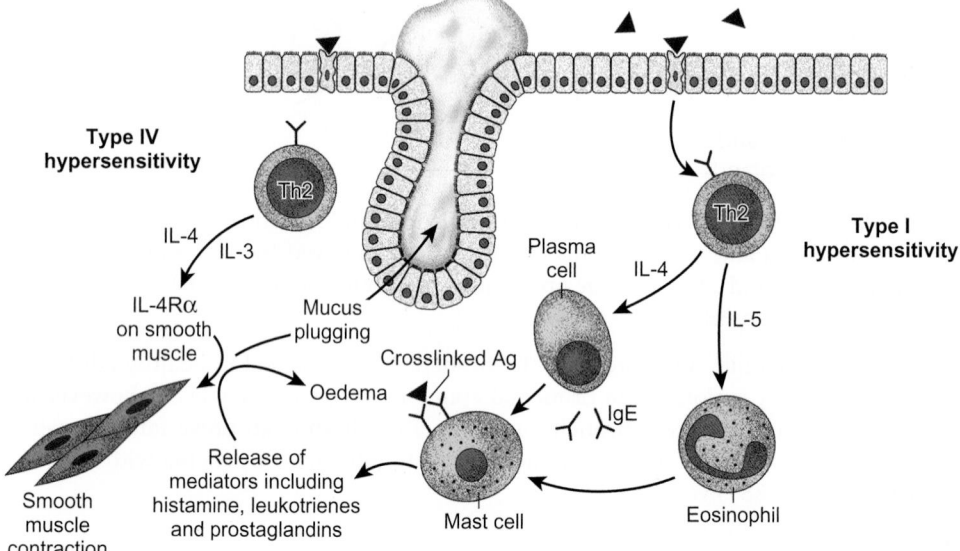

# BRONCHIAL ASTHMA

The **histological changes** are a combination of allergic reaction and muscular hypertrophy, the result of prolonged spasm.

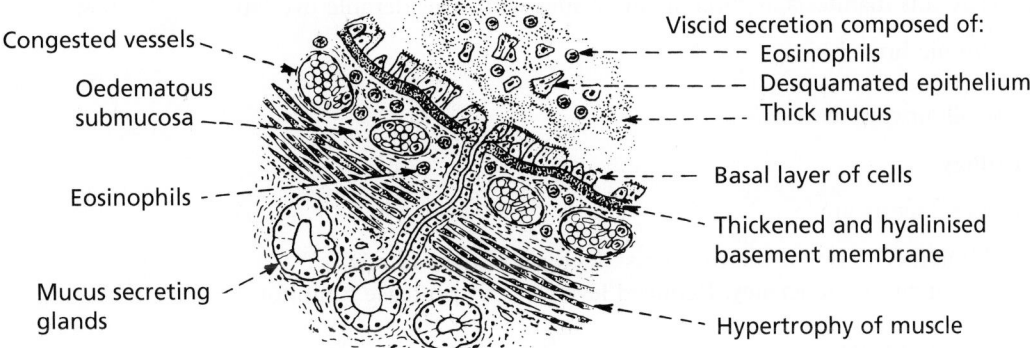

Congested vessels

Oedematous submucosa

Eosinophils

Mucus secreting glands

Viscid secretion composed of:
- Eosinophils
- Desquamated epithelium
- Thick mucus

Basal layer of cells

Thickened and hyalinised basement membrane

Hypertrophy of muscle

## Sputum

In some cases the following may be seen:

1. *Curschmann spirals* – appear as small white granules in sputum.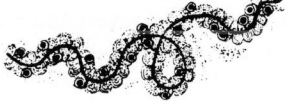

2. *Charcot–Leyden crystals* – in association with eosinophils.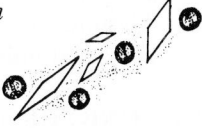

# CHRONIC OBSTRUCTIVE PULMONARY DISEASE (COPD)

COPD is a common slowly progressive disease characterised by poorly reversible airflow obstruction and an abnormal inflammatory response in the lungs.

Clinically this manifests as three main entities with considerable overlap:

1. Chronic bronchitis.
2. Emphysema.
3. Small airways disease.

**Aetiology**

The main factors are:

1. SMOKING – by far the major risk factor and dose related.
2. $\alpha_1$-Antitrypsin deficiency. Reduced levels of this protease inhibitor correlate with lung damage, especially in smokers.
3. OCCUPATION, especially exposure to dusts, e.g. coal mining.

**Pathogenesis**

1. Innate and adaptive immune response to long-term exposure to noxious particles and gases, particularly cigarettes.
2. This ongoing immune response leads to poorly reversible airflow obstruction and an abnormal inflammatory response in the lungs.

## CHRONIC BRONCHITIS

The clinical definition is based on the presence of a productive cough lasting at least 3 months and occurring annually for at least 2 years.

Pathologically the following changes are seen:

The increase in thickness of the mucous gland layer is striking: at post mortem the Reid index is measured, i.e. the ratio of the submucous layer (X) to the whole thickness (Y): a value greater than 1:2 is significant.

# CHRONIC OBSTRUCTIVE PULMONARY DISEASE (COPD)

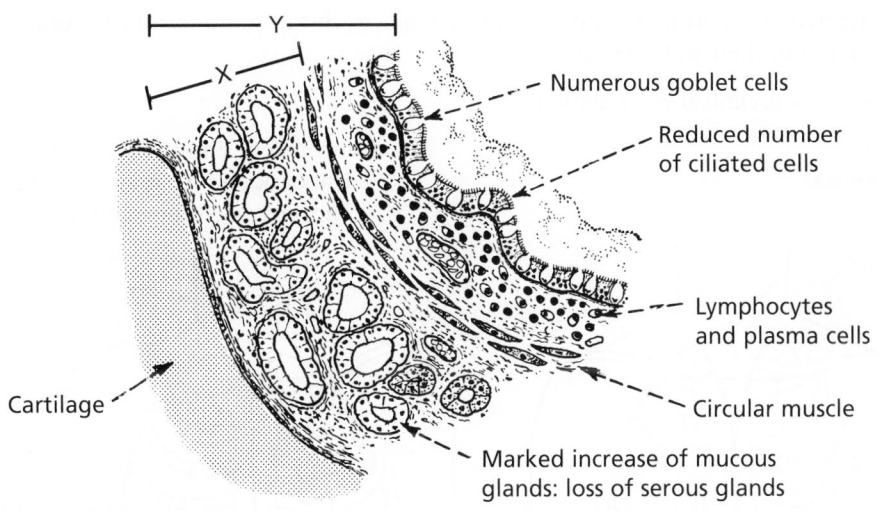

Numerous goblet cells

Reduced number of ciliated cells

Lymphocytes and plasma cells

Circular muscle

Cartilage

Marked increase of mucous glands: loss of serous glands

The effect of these changes is:

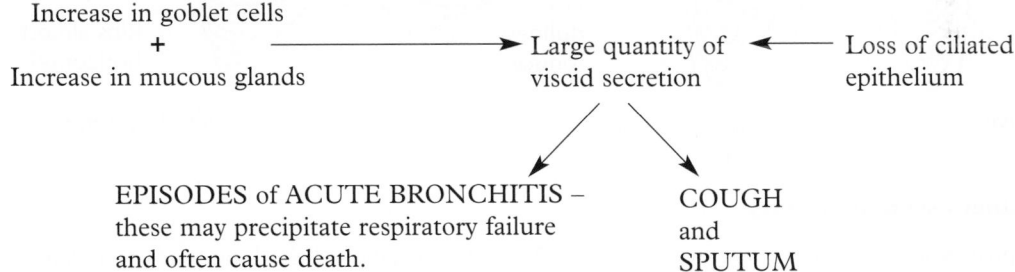

Increase in goblet cells
+
Increase in mucous glands — Large quantity of viscid secretion — Loss of ciliated epithelium

EPISODES of ACUTE BRONCHITIS – these may precipitate respiratory failure and often cause death.

COUGH and SPUTUM

# EMPHYSEMA

This is defined as a permanent dilatation of air spaces distal to the terminal bronchiole due to destruction of their walls without fibrosis.

Changes seen on clinical examination:

**Normal emphysema**

**Anatomical changes** due to increased use of accessory muscles of respiration and increased lung volume.

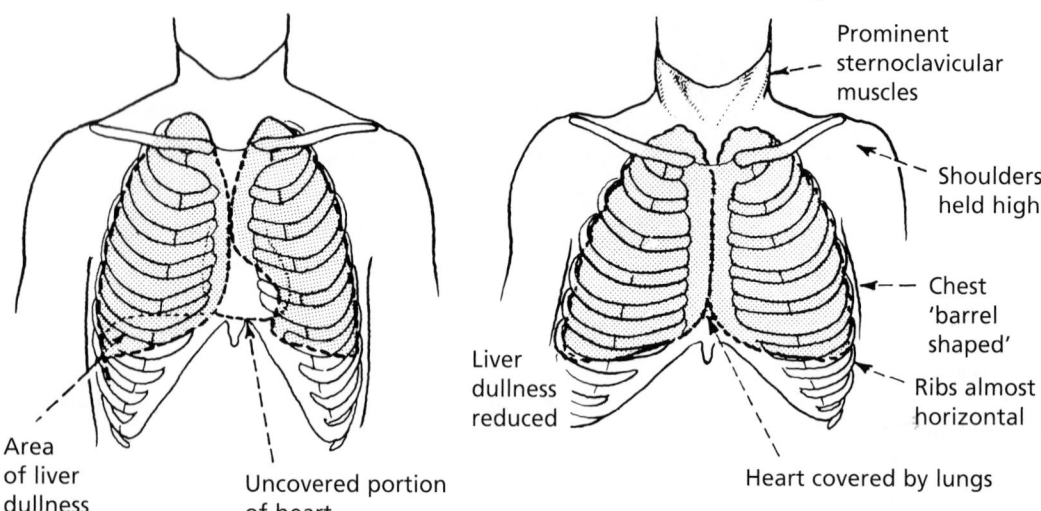

Prominent sternoclavicular muscles

Shoulders held high

Chest 'barrel shaped'

Ribs almost horizontal

Liver dullness reduced

Heart covered by lungs

Area of liver dullness

Uncovered portion of heart

**Changes seen at autopsy**

At post mortem the lungs are over-inflated. (*Note:* When removed the lung tends to collapse unless it is inflated with fixative and cut later.)

**External appearance**

**Cut surface**

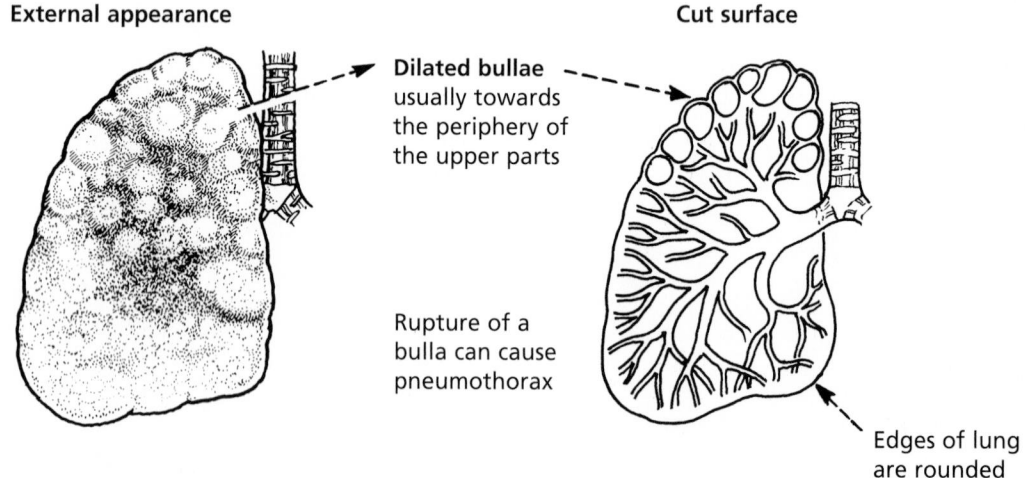

Dilated bullae usually towards the periphery of the upper parts

Rupture of a bulla can cause pneumothorax

Edges of lung are rounded

On the sectioned lung, two main patterns are seen.

1. **Centriacinar (centrilobular) emphysema**    2. **Panacinar emphysema**

# EMPHYSEMA

## CENTRIACINAR EMPHYSEMA

In this form the dilated air spaces immediately surround and involve the respiratory bronchioles.

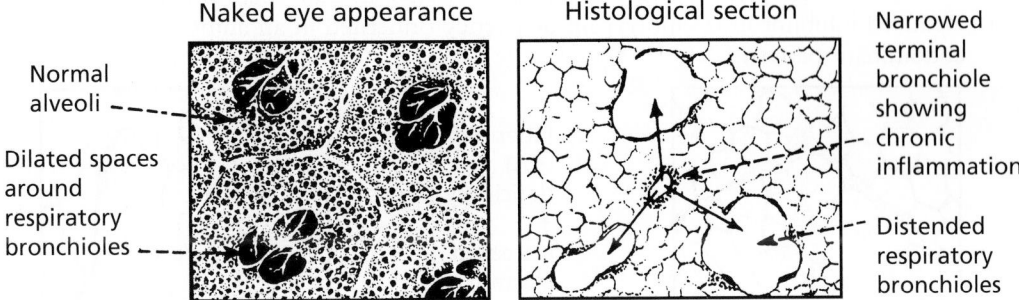

Naked eye appearance · Histological section

Normal alveoli

Dilated spaces around respiratory bronchioles

Narrowed terminal bronchiole showing chronic inflammation

Distended respiratory bronchioles

Chronic inflammation of the respiratory bronchioles is an important feature: eventually, in many cases, the distension extends to produce panacinar emphysema.

## PANACINAR EMPHYSEMA

The enlarged air spaces are distributed across the entire acinus.

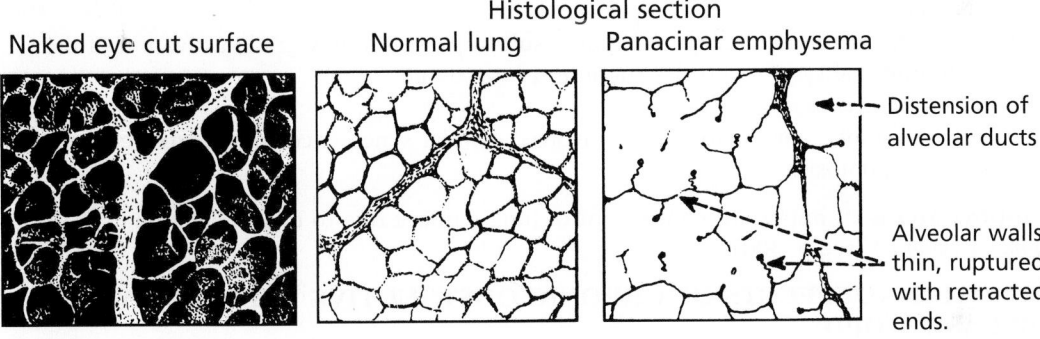

Histological section

Naked eye cut surface · Normal lung · Panacinar emphysema

Distension of alveolar ducts

Alveolar walls thin, ruptured with retracted ends.

Special stains show loss of elastic tissue. The capillaries are stretched and thinned. The reduction in blood supply is probably a factor leading to rupture of alveoli.

There is little evidence of bronchiolitis. The voluminous lungs produce characteristic radiological changes. The distension eventually spreads to involve the respiratory bronchiole, i.e. the whole acinus is affected – panacinar emphysema.

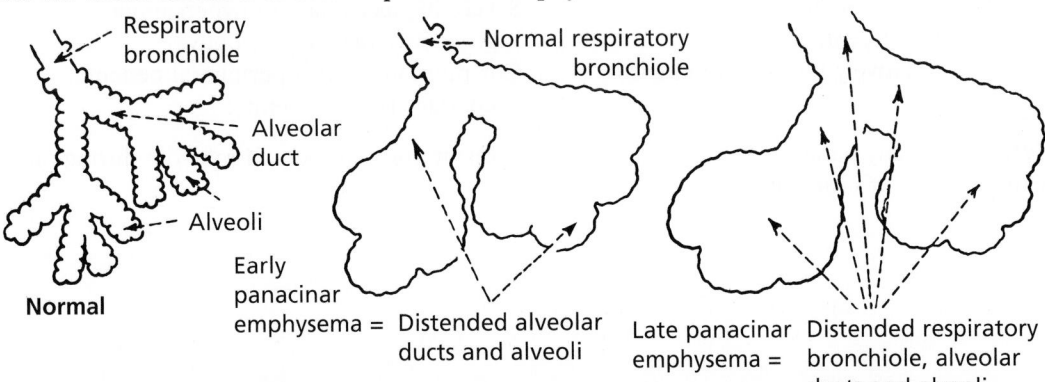

Respiratory bronchiole

Alveolar duct

Alveoli

**Normal**

Normal respiratory bronchiole

Early panacinar emphysema = Distended alveolar ducts and alveoli

Late panacinar emphysema = Distended respiratory bronchiole, alveolar ducts and alveoli

289

# EMPHYSEMA

### Pathogenesis

In emphysema alveolar destruction is the result of several processes:

(1) *An imbalance between protease and antiprotease activity.* This may occur due to:
    (a) Reduced inhibitor in $\alpha_1$-antitrypsin deficiency (inherited in an autosomal codominant pattern.

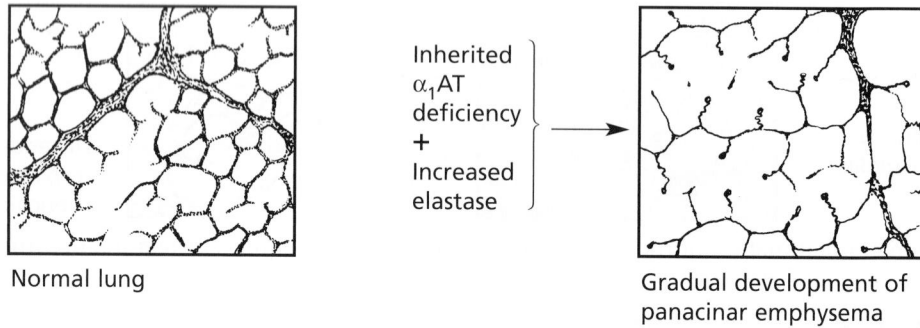

Normal lung

Inherited $\alpha_1 AT$ deficiency + Increased elastase

Gradual development of panacinar emphysema

    (b) Excess enzyme production, e.g. due to smoking $\rightarrow$ inflammation of bronchioles $\rightarrow$ $\uparrow$ proteases $\rightarrow$ centrilobular emphysema.

(2) *Innate immunity*
Alterations in Toll like receptor 4 may result in persistent low grade activation of the innate immune system and destruction of lung tissue.

(3) *Cellular senescence*
Cigarette smoke upregulates genes involved cellular senescence and affected cells may undergo apoptosis.

**Emphysema** is an important component of lung damage due to dust inhalation (*pneumoconiosis*) (see p. 300).

## FUNCTIONAL EFFECTS OF CHRONIC OBSTRUCTIVE PULMONARY DISEASE (COPD)

Patients with COPD tend to fall into two clinical groups depending on whether or not they tolerate hypoxia.

(a) PINK PUFFERS
    Do NOT tolerate hypoxia.
    Severe breathlessness.
    Hyperventilation.
    Relatively normal blood gases.

(b) BLUE BLOATERS
    Tolerate hypoxia.
    Severe hypoxaemia and hypercapnia.
    Right ventricular hypertrophy.
    Cor pulmonale with peripheral oedema.
    Secondary polycythaemia.

Eventually many patients develop severe chronic respiratory failure and may die during an acute episode of bronchitis.

# BRONCHIECTASIS

Bronchiectasis means a permanent dilatation of one or more bronchi. There are two main subdivisions:

1. ***Obstructive*** due to tumour, foreign body or enlarged lymph nodes.
2. ***Post-infective*** due to repeated respiratory infection, e.g. cystic fibrosis or immunodeficiency syndromes.

## Pathogenesis

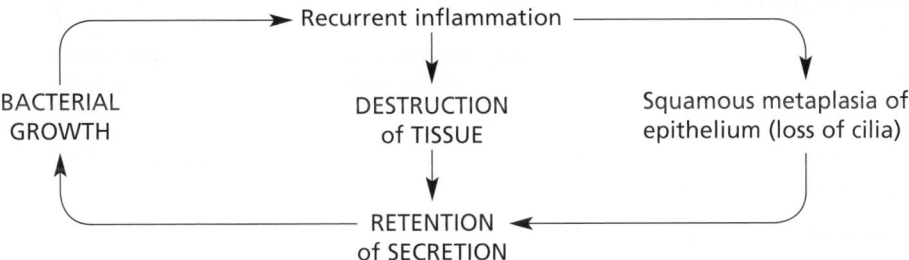

Recurrent inflammation → DESTRUCTION of TISSUE → RETENTION of SECRETION

Recurrent inflammation → Squamous metaplasia of epithelium (loss of cilia) → RETENTION of SECRETION

RETENTION of SECRETION → BACTERIAL GROWTH → Recurrent inflammation

## Effects

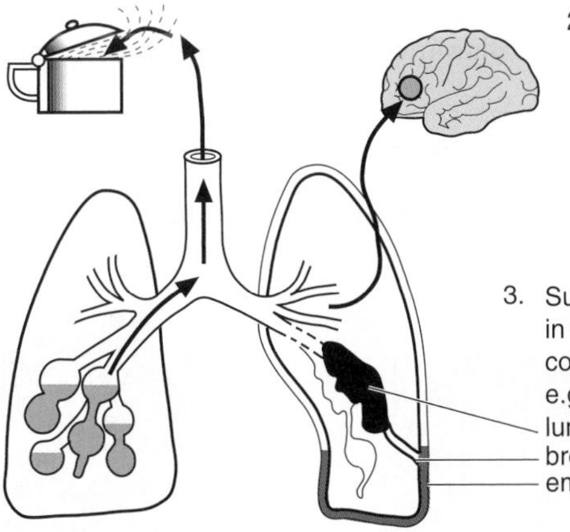

1. Large quantities of secretion are retained in the bronchi and putrefactive bacteria produce a foul smell
2. Pyaemia giving rise to brain abscess or meningitis may result from involvement of a pulmonary vein branch by the suppurative process
3. Suppuration is common in the cavities and local complications arise, e.g.
   - lung abscess
   - bronchopleural fistula
   - empyema
4. Clubbing of fingers (hypertrophic pulmonary osteoarthropathy – also occurs in COPD and lung cancer)

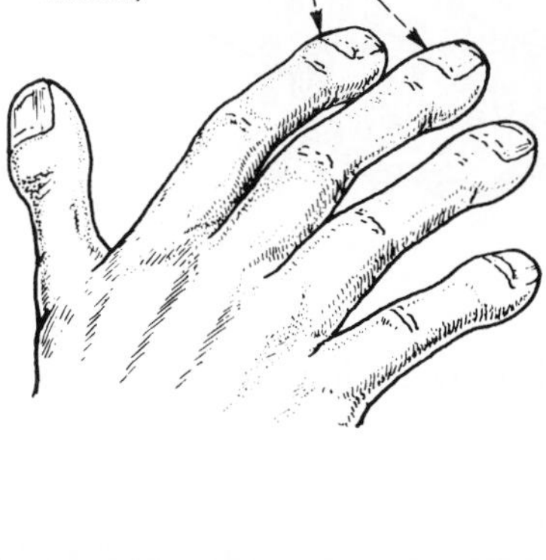

5. Pulmonary hypertension (p. 205) progressing to → Right heart failure
6. Development of amyloid disease, e.g. in kidney

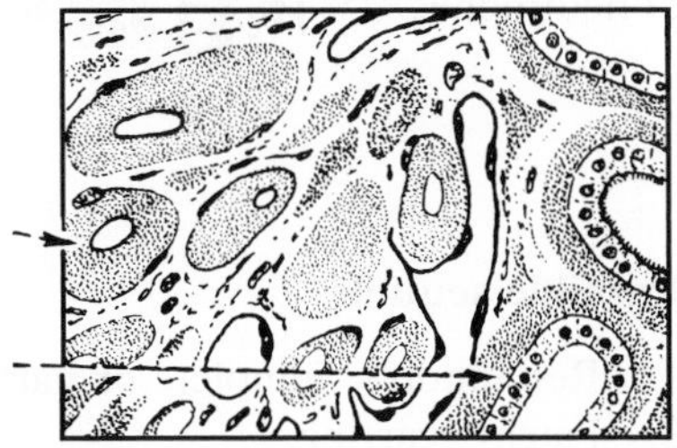

Amyloid around glomerular capillaries and tubule basement membranes

# PNEUMONIA – BRONCHOPNEUMONIA

Pneumonia is an inflammatory process involving the alveolar tissue of the lungs. There are many clinical classifications but in pathology it is discussed under three main headings:

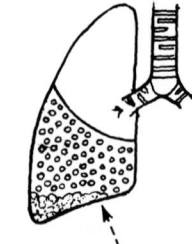

1. Bronchopneumonia
2. Lobar pneumonia
3. Miscellaneous pneumonias

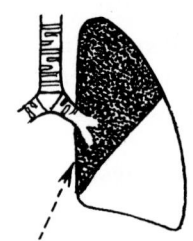

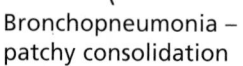

Bronchopneumonia – patchy consolidation

Lobar pneumonia – whole lobe affected

## 1. BRONCHOPNEUMONIA

Bronchopneumonia caused by a variety of bacteria is the commonest form. It may affect all ages, but it is particularly frequent in four circumstances:

    (a) As a terminal event in a chronic debilitating disease.
    (b) In infancy.
    (c) In old age.
    (d) As a manifestation of secondary infection in viral conditions, e.g. influenza, measles.

Bronchopneumonia is primarily an inflammation spreading from terminal bronchioles to their related alveoli.

The lesions are initially focal, involving one or more lobules.

First red, then grey, they show a central bronchiole containing pus.

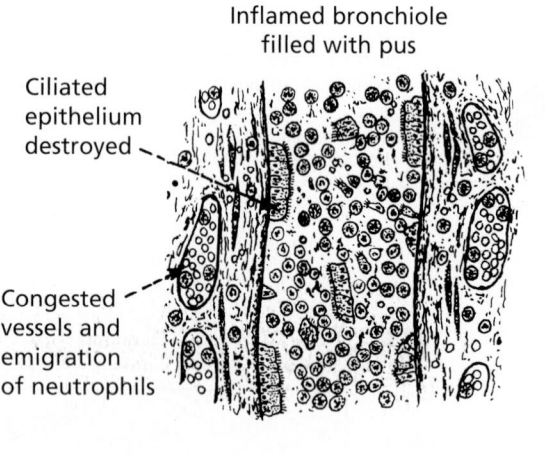

Inflamed bronchiole filled with pus

Ciliated epithelium destroyed

Congested vessels and emigration of neutrophils

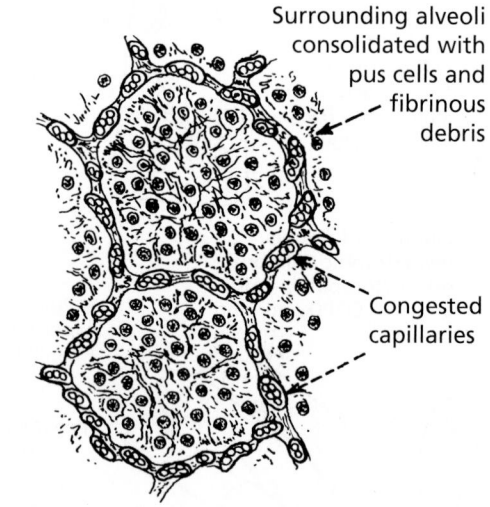

Surrounding alveoli consolidated with pus cells and fibrinous debris

Congested capillaries

## Possible sequels

1. Resolution – complete or partial (antibiotics and physiotherapy are important).
2. Patchy scarring.
3. Rarely, continuing sepsis with lung abscess formation.

# PNEUMONIA - LOBAR PNEUMONIA

## 2. LOBAR PNEUMONIA

As the name suggests, a complete lobe or even two lobes of a lung are affected, the most striking changes occurring in the alveoli. The disease is now rare in Western countries. It is seen typically in adults aged 20–50 years, with males predominating, and is caused by *S. pneumoniae*. Other organisms include *H. influenzae, Moraxella catarrhalis* and occasionally *Klebsiella pneumoniae*.

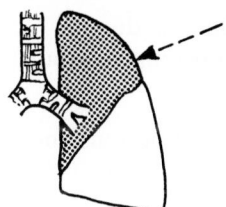 The whole affected lobe progresses uniformly through four distinct phases illustrating the classic progression of an acute inflammation: this has been so radically altered by antibiotic treatment that the following description is to some extent historical.

**Clinically**, the onset is acute with fever and often rigors. There is a dry cough and rusty sputum, dyspnoea and often chest pain due to pleurisy.

There are four distinct pathological phases illustrating the classic progression of an acute inflammation: this has been radically altered by the use of antibiotics.

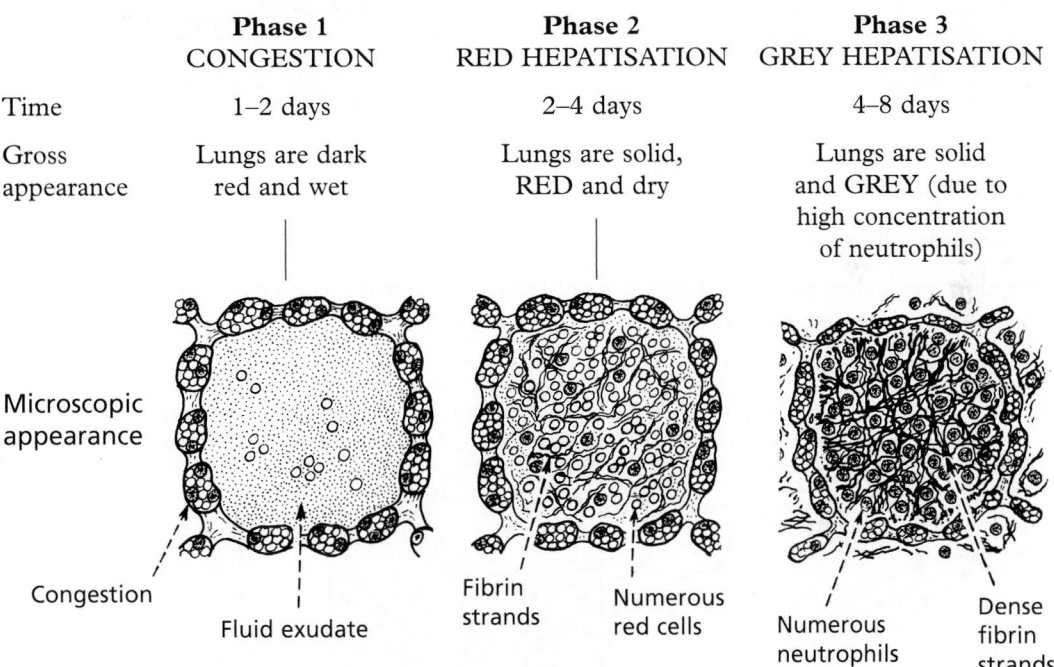

|  | **Phase 1**<br>CONGESTION | **Phase 2**<br>RED HEPATISATION | **Phase 3**<br>GREY HEPATISATION |
|---|---|---|---|
| Time | 1–2 days | 2–4 days | 4–8 days |
| Gross appearance | Lungs are dark red and wet | Lungs are solid, RED and dry | Lungs are solid and GREY (due to high concentration of neutrophils) |

Microscopic appearance

Congestion — Fluid exudate

Fibrin strands — Numerous red cells

Numerous neutrophils — Dense fibrin strands

**Phase 4** – RESOLUTION begins dramatically on day 8–10 and restoration to normal is rapid.

Complications include lung fibrosis, bacteraemia, lung abscesses, empyema, pleural effusion and death.

# ATYPICAL PNEUMONIAS

## 1. LEGIONNAIRE DISEASE

This is caused by a tiny Gram-negative bacillus – *Legionella pneumophila*. Infection is associated with inhalation of aerosol from contaminated water storage systems and may occur in small epidemics. It can cause lobar or bronchopneumonia. The elderly are particularly vulnerable with a death rate of up to 20%.

## 2. VIRAL PNEUMONIAS

This is common in early childhood but less common in adults. Viral pneumonia due to cytomegalovirus, measles or varicella is typically self-limiting in the immunocompetent but can cause fulminant infection in the immunocompromised.

**Influenza** is usually confined to the upper respiratory tract, but in debilitated persons and during epidemics, the whole respiratory tract is affected.

### Trachea and bronchi

Intense inflammation with haemorrhage develops.

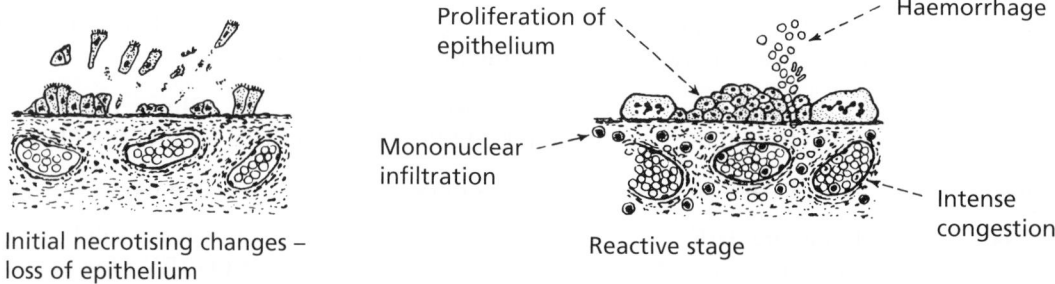

Initial necrotising changes – loss of epithelium

Reactive stage

Proliferation of epithelium — Haemorrhage

Mononuclear infiltration

Intense congestion

### Pneumonia changes

The lungs are bulky, purple-red and exude blood-stained froth when cut. The microscopic changes vary from one part to another.

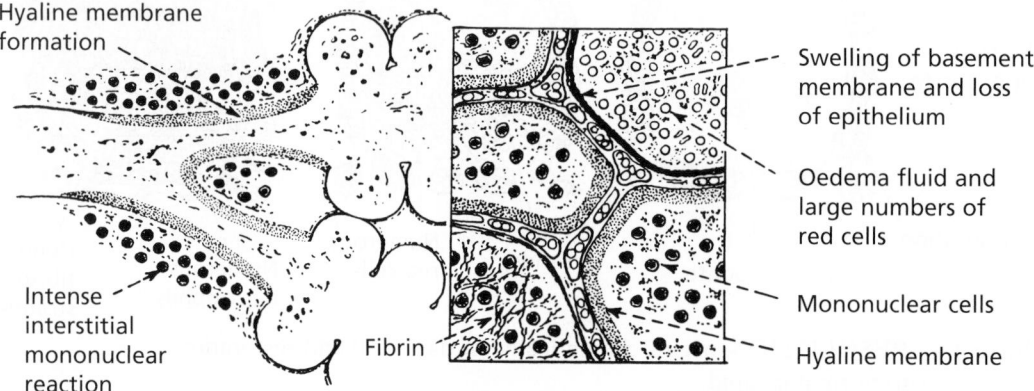

Hyaline membrane formation

Intense interstitial mononuclear reaction

Fibrin

Swelling of basement membrane and loss of epithelium

Oedema fluid and large numbers of red cells

Mononuclear cells

Hyaline membrane

# ATYPICAL PNEUMONIAS

## Infective agents

Of the three main types A, B and C, type A is the most virulent, and mutants of this type are responsible for most epidemics and the fatalities which occur. The 2009 pandemic was due to a swine influenza of type A known as H1N1. Severe disease and death were more common in children and pregnant women.

Secondary infection is common, the bacteria most frequently involved being *S. aureus*, *H. influenzae* and *S. pneumoniae*.

## Severe acute respiratory syndrome (SARS)

SARS is a recently recognised infectious atypical pneumonia caused by a novel corona virus, the SARS-associated corona virus. The disease was first recognised in Asia in February 2003 and caused a pandemic over the ensuing months.

## Myoplasmal pneumonia

Mycoplasma species account for 15–20% of community-acquired pneumonias. It most commonly occurs in children and young adults. It causes a low-grade chronic infection, often with organising pneumonia, which can lead onto pulmonary fibrosis.

## Chlamydia pneumonia

Psittacosis, also known as parrot fever as it is often contracted from infected birds, is caused by *Chlamydia psittaci*. It causes an atypical pneumonia often with fever, joint pains and conjunctivitis. *Chlamydia trachomatis* can cause pneumonia in infants infected during childbirth.

## PNEUMONIA IN THE IMMUNOCOMPROMISED

Infections caused by organisms that are usually non-pathogenic in the immunocompetent can cause severe pneumonia in the immunocompromised. With new immunosuppressive therapies and multidrug-resistant organisms, the number of potential pathogens is increasing.

Common opportunistic organisms include:

*Viruses* – Cytomegalovirus, influenza, Herpes simplex virus and varicella zoster virus. Inclusion bodies may be identified.
*Fungi* – *Pneumocystitis jirovecii*, *Candida albicans* and *Aspergillus fumagatus*.
*Bacteria* – non-tuberculosis mycobacteria, e.g. *Mycobacterium avium intracellulare*.

# PNEUMONIA – SPECIAL TYPES

### ASPIRATION PNEUMONIA

This is due to inhalation of food or infected material from the mouth or pharynx. It may occur during anaesthesia or coma or may complicate conditions associated with frequent regurgitation, e.g. oesophageal obstruction, pyloric stenosis or poor swallowing due to stroke or motor neurone disease.

In adult cases, the inhalation of acid gastric contents may cause an initial shock reaction; in other cases the onset is insidious.

Possible progression is as follows:

Inhalation of ⟶ Secondary ⟶ Bronchopneumonia
foreign material      infection          lung abscess

Histologically 'foreign material', usually vegetable matter, may be seen evoking a foreign body giant cell reaction. – – –

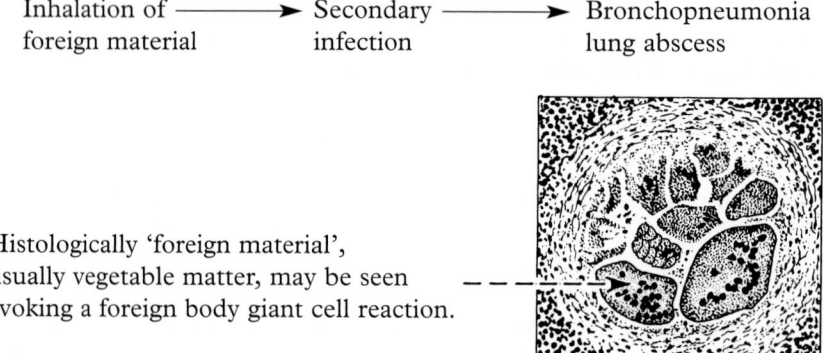

### Lipid pneumonia

– The exogenous form is due to long-continued inhalation of small quantities of oily material usually derived from nasal medicaments: it is often clinically silent. Oily vacuoles are seen in the lung tissue.
– The endogenous form is derived from tissue lipid debris distal to local bronchial obstruction. Foamy macrophages accumulate and the lung tissue is golden yellow in colour.

# LUNG ABSCESS

This is now an uncommon condition due to prompt treatment of preceding infection. The usual causes are:

1.  Inhalation of infected material from the larynx or pharynx.

2.  Obstruction of a bronchus by tumour growth or foreign body. Site depends on size of bronchus affected.

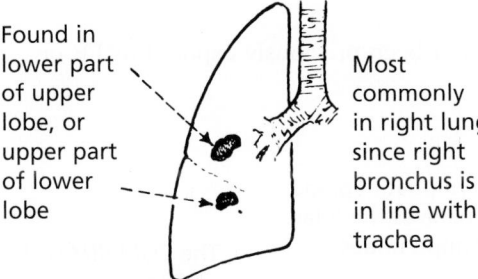

Found in lower part of upper lobe, or upper part of lower lobe

Most commonly in right lung since right bronchus is in line with trachea

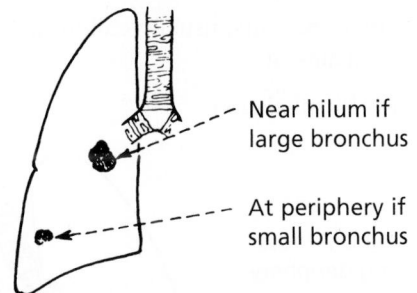

Near hilum if large bronchus

At periphery if small bronchus

3.  Infection of pre-existing cavities, e.g. in tuberculosis or bronchiectasis.
4.  Pneumonia. Abscess is most likely to occur in debilitated persons with bronchopneumonia.

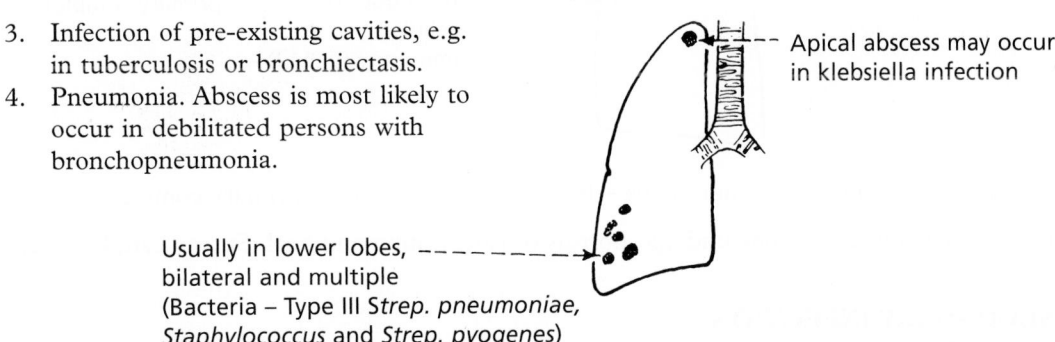

Apical abscess may occur in klebsiella infection

Usually in lower lobes, bilateral and multiple
(Bacteria – Type III *Strep. pneumoniae, Staphylococcus* and *Strep. pyogenes*)

Rarer causes of abscess are: pyaemia, trauma to lung, extension from suppuration in mediastinum, spinal column or sub phrenic region, and infection with *Entamoeba histolytica*.

## Sequelae of lung abscess

1.  Small abscesses may heal.
2.  Subpleural abscesses may extend to cause empyema.
3.  Bronchopleural fistula resulting in pyopneumothorax is a further complication following on (2).
4.  If a large pulmonary vessel is eroded, fatal haemorrhage can occur.
5.  Rarely, blood spread leads to meningitis or cerebral abscess.

# TUBERCULOSIS (TB)

The lungs are more commonly affected by TB than any other organ. The incidence of TB in developed countries is rising, partly due to AIDS. Drug resistant strains of mycobacteria are an increasing problem.

There are two patterns of pulmonary TB – primary and secondary.

## PRIMARY INFECTION

This occurs in patients, usually children, who have not been previously exposed to TB or vaccinated against it.

Infection is by inhalation.

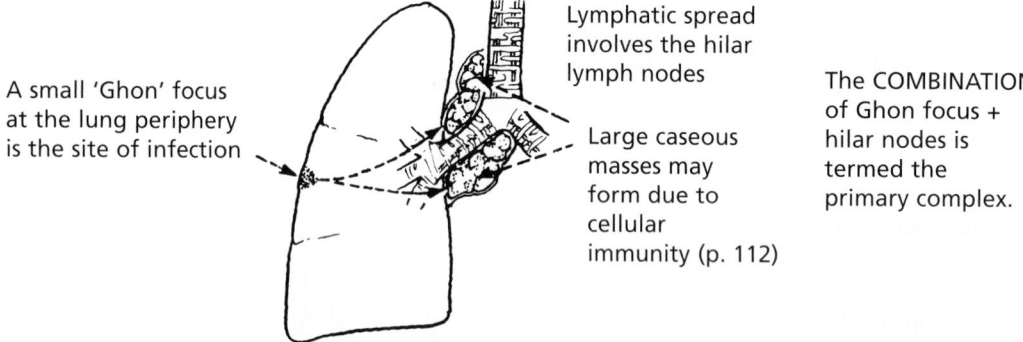

A small 'Ghon' focus at the lung periphery is the site of infection

Lymphatic spread involves the hilar lymph nodes

Large caseous masses may form due to cellular immunity (p. 112)

The COMBINATION of Ghon focus + hilar nodes is termed the primary complex.

The COMBINATION of Ghon focus + hilar nodes is termed the primary complex.

In most patients, the lesions undergo fibrosis or calcification and heal. Spread can, however, occur.

## SECONDARY INFECTION

This is a recurrence of TB in later life – either reactivation or reinfection. The patients have immunity to TB and develop a cellular response leading to CASEATION.

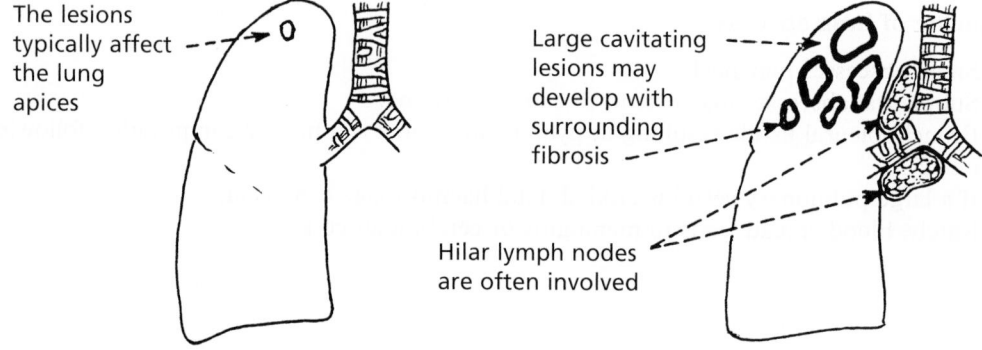

The lesions typically affect the lung apices

Large cavitating lesions may develop with surrounding fibrosis

Hilar lymph nodes are often involved

# SPREAD OF TUBERCULOSIS

## SPREAD OF TUBERCULOSIS

This is typically seen in secondary TB, but may also complicate primary infection.

The infection can spread by several pathways.

(a) **Direct spread** – e.g. to pleura and pericardium.

(b) **By the bronchi**.

Tubercle bacilli may spread to the larynx or by the bronchi to give tuberculous bronchopneumonia ('galloping consumption').

Consolidation is seen throughout large areas of lung parenchyma.

This occurs particularly in the immunosuppressed.

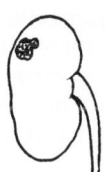

(c) **By the pulmonary veins**.
This may lead to isolated blood borne infection, e.g. tuberculous meningitis (p. 592), renal TB and bone TB, e.g. Pott disease of the spine, or to miliary spread throughout the body.

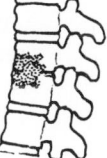

Kidney      Spine

(d) **By the pulmonary arteries** (probably by lymphatics draining into the inferior vena cava).

In this, miliary spread occurs throughout the lung fields alone.

The clinical course of TB is variable and depends on the immune status of the individual, the response of the bacteria to drugs, and intercurrent disease.

## COMPLICATIONS OF TB

Pulmonary fibrosis.
Obliteration of the pleural space by fibrosis.
Bronchiectasis (p. 291).

The **histological** features are as described on p. 112.

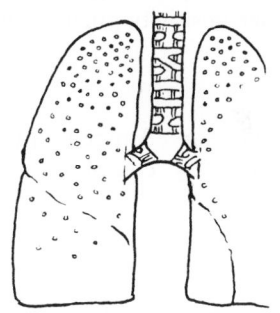

Miliary tubercles, approximately 1–2 mm, are seen throughout the lung fields.

# PNEUMOCONIOSES (DUST DISEASES)

The reaction to inhaled dust varies very considerably. Some dusts, e.g. pure carbon, are inert; others, e.g. silicates, cause severe lung disease.

## BASIC PATHOLOGY

1. *Inorganic dust* particles reaching the lungs are ingested by alveolar macrophages.

(a) Macrophage laden with inert dust.

**Inert dust**

Some ejected
in sputum

Migration to
lymphatics

To hilar
nodes

**Aggregation**
where there is least
respiratory movement,
e.g. around bronchioles –
but NO ILL EFFECTS

(b) Macrophage laden with damaging dust, e.g. silica.

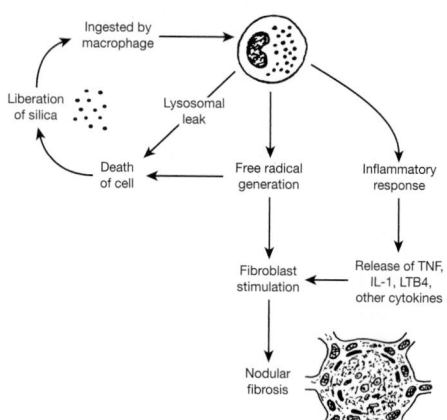

2. *Organic dust* particles which cause lung disease by a different mechanism include FUNGI encountered in many occupations, e.g. farmers, malt workers, bird fanciers.

The basic pathology is a Type III hypersensitivity reaction (p. 144) and the term 'hypersensitivity pneumonitis' (extrinsic allergic alveolitis) is used.

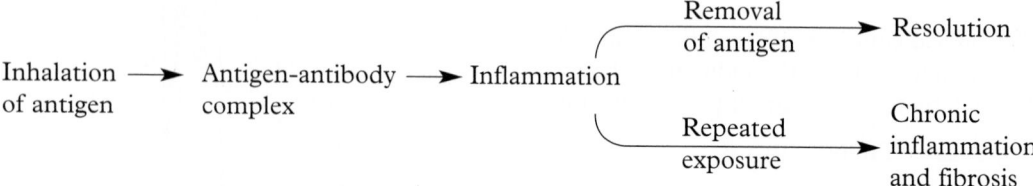

# PNEUMOCONIOSES (DUST DISEASES)

## COAL WORKER PNEUMOCONIOSIS

Pure carbon is biologically inert and is deposited as in (a) on page 300, with no ill effects. Damage to the lung seen in coal miners and in populations exposed to carbon-polluted atmosphere is potentiated by the content of silicates and other pollutants. There are three main types of pathology:

1. *Simple coal worker pneumoconiosis:* aggregation of coal dust particles may progress with the formation of small dust nodules and mild centrilobular emphysema (p. 289) with MINIMAL FUNCTION LOSS.
2. *Progressive massive fibrosis:* this supervenes in a few cases with SEVERE DISABILITY. The cause is unknown, theories include tuberculous infection as an initiator dust dose and composition, genetic factors and deviant immune responses.
3. *Caplan syndrome:* this occurs in coal workers with rheumatoid disease.

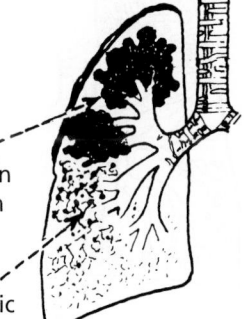

Irregular masses of black fibrous tissue in the upper lobes with cavities filled with black fluid

Simple anthracotic changes

The severe diseases caused by inorganic dust inhalation, usually occupationally, are described.

1. **Silicosis** – stone workers, sandblasters, miners.
2. **Asbestosis** – shipbuilding, insulation, electrical work.

The damage caused depends on:

(a) The type of dust, e.g. soluble/insoluble.

(b) The shape of the particle, e.g. 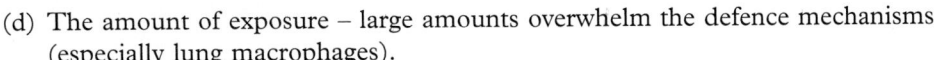 Fibres align in the long axis of the airways helping them to reach the lung.

(c) The size of the particle – particles longer than 5 µm are likely to be trapped in the nose and large airways.

(d) The amount of exposure – large amounts overwhelm the defence mechanisms (especially lung macrophages).

# PNEUMOCONIOSES (DUST DISEASES)

### SILICOSIS

The lung lesions are slowly progressive over many years. Silicates are particularly damaging to lung macrophages (see p. 300).

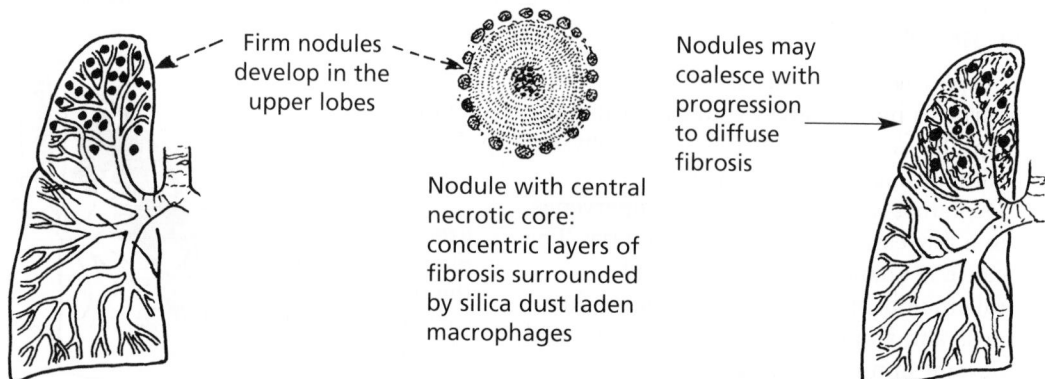

Firm nodules develop in the upper lobes

Nodule with central necrotic core: concentric layers of fibrosis surrounded by silica dust laden macrophages

Nodules may coalesce with progression to diffuse fibrosis

Patients develop increasing breathlessness and may die of respiratory failure and cor pulmonale.

The silicotic lung is particularly susceptible to **TB** (which may be due to the effects of silica on pulmonary macrophages). Historically, this was an important cause of death.

# ASBESTOSIS

**Asbestos** is the generic name for a group of fibrous silicates widely used in heavy industry for insulation (particularly in shipbuilding).

There are two distinct forms of asbestos – serpentine (curly and flexible) and amphibole (straight and stiff). Amphibole fibres (crocidolite and amosite) are more pathogenic than serpentine fibres (principally chrysotile).

**Asbestosis** results from chronic exposure.

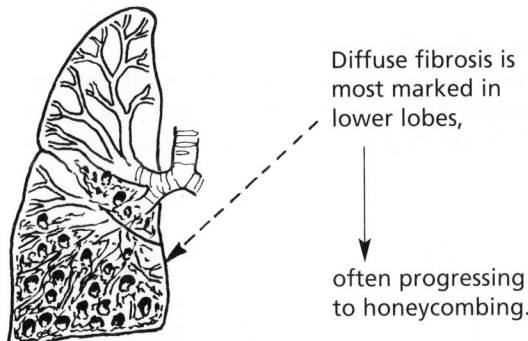

Diffuse fibrosis is most marked in lower lobes,

↓

often progressing to honeycombing.

Some asbestos fibres become encrusted with iron and protein.

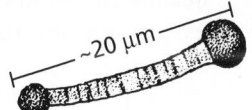

~20 µm

The ASBESTOS BODIES are markers of asbestos exposure and can be identified in SPUTUM or lung tissue.

Other important complications are:

1. **Lung cancer**
   Asbestos workers have an increased risk of lung cancer, especially if they also smoke.
   Risk of cancer = risk due to smoking × risk due to asbestos.
2. **Pleural pathology**

   (a) **Pleural plaques** – these are the most common manifestation of asbestos exposure.

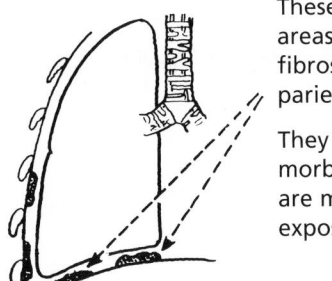

These are dense areas of hyaline fibrosis on the parietal pleura.

They cause no morbidity but are markers of exposure.

Rarely, there is diffuse pleural fibrosis.

   (b) **Mesothelioma** (malignant tumour of the pleura). This can occur up to 40 years after a brief exposure to asbestos (particularly crocidolite).

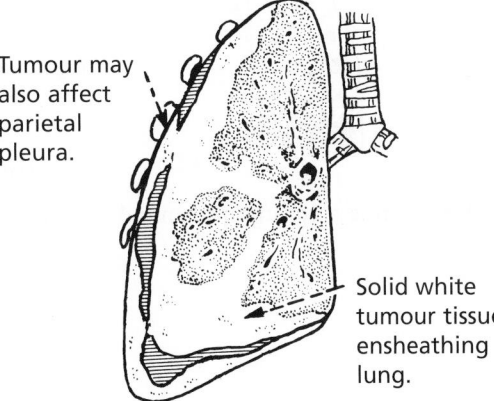

Tumour may also affect parietal pleura.

Solid white tumour tissue ensheathing lung.

*Note*: There are usually significantly fewer asbestos fibres/bodies in mesothelioma than in asbestosis.

*Note*: Mesothelioma may also affect the pericardium and peritoneum.

# DIFFUSE PARENCHYMAL LUNG DISEASE

### DIFFUSE PARENCHYMAL LUNG DISEASE

This encompasses a group of conditions in which the lung is altered by a combination of interstitial inflammation and fibrosis. Several histological patterns are recognised but it is thought that regardless of the type, the earliest manifestation is alveolitis and that this accumulation of leucocytes results in release of mediators that can injure parenchymal cells and stimulate fibrosis.

1. *Usual interstitial pneumonia (UIP) (idiopathic pulmonary fibrosis)*
   UIP is considered to be the caused by repeated cycles of alveolitis. After each cycle of alveolitis healing causes fibroblastic proliferation known as 'fibroblastic foci', such that as the disease progresses, the fibrosis is a different stages (temporal heterogeneity).

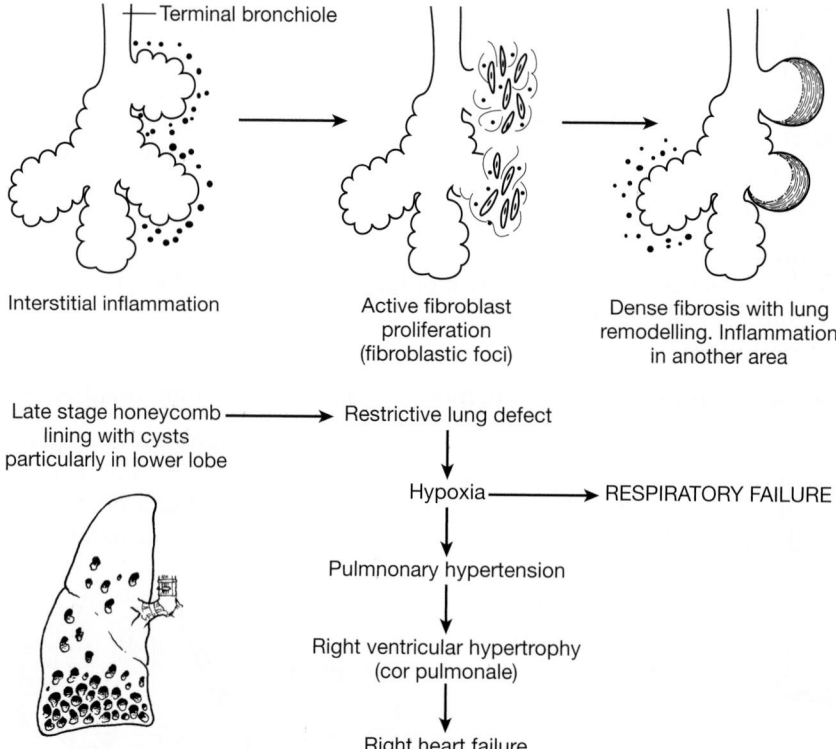

Infection is a common terminal event, and there is an increased risk of lung cancer.

# DIFFUSE PARENCHYMAL LUNG DISEASE

2. *Non-specific interstitial pneumonia (NSIP)*
   This form of fibrosis has a much better prognosis than UIP and is usually steroid responsive. The lung is uniformly affected by interstitial fibrosis and inflammation of variable severity. Fibroblastic foci are absent and progression to honeycombing is rare. This pattern is commonly seen in association with connective tissue diseases.

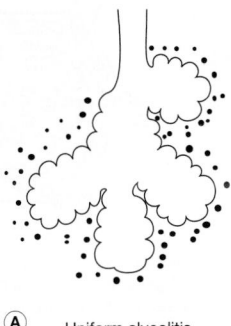

(A)  Uniform alveolitis

Uniform intestitial fibrosis
without loss of lung architecture

3. *Desquamative interstitial pneumonia (DIP) and respiratory bronchiolitis interstitial lung disease (RBILD)*
   These patterns are both seen almost exclusively in cigarette smokers. In RBILD, macrophages accumulate in a patchy distribution around respiratory bronchioles. In DIP there is diffuse distribution of macrophages.

4. *Cryptogenic organising pneumonia (COP) (bronchiolitis obliterans organising pneumonia)*
   This is characterised by a patchy distribution of polypoid plugs of fibroblastic tissue in alveoli, alveolar ducts and sometimes bronchioles. A similar pattern may be seen with certain infections, drugs or connective tissue diseases.

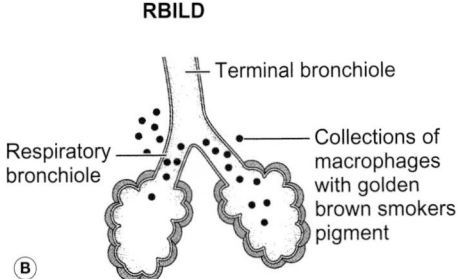

**RBILD**

Terminal bronchiole

Respiratory bronchiole

Collections of macrophages with golden brown smokers pigment

(B)

**DIP**

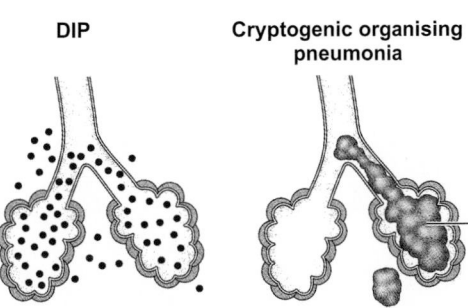

**Cryptogenic organising pneumonia**

Polypoid plugs of fibroblastic tissue

# DIFFUSE PARENCHYMAL LUNG DISEASE

### DIFFUSE ALVEOLAR DAMAGE

This is the pathological correlate of adult respiratory distress syndrome. It may be caused by sepsis, gastric aspiration, trauma and inhaled toxins. It may also be idiopathic – acute interstitial pneumonia (AIP; synonymous with Hamman–Rich syndrome).

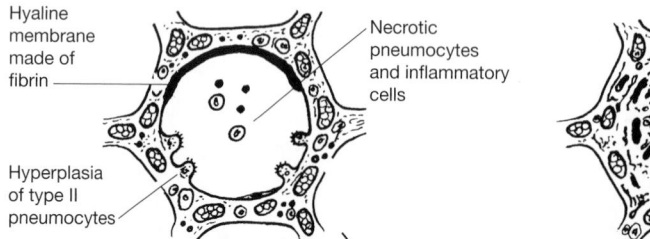

1. There is damage to capillaries and epithelium. Fibrin leak from capillaries leads to hyaline membranes. Type II pneumocytes replace damaged type I cells

2. If supportive treatment and steroids are not given early there is progressive fibrosis. Note: a similar pattern is seen in premature infants where the cause is lack of surfactant rather than capillary damage

### SARCOIDOSIS

This is a multisystem disease of unknown aetiology characterised by widespread non-caseating granulomas. The lungs are one of the most common sites affected.

# LUNG CANCER

Lung cancer (carcinoma of the bronchus) is the second-most common form of cancer in the United Kingdom and one which is largely preventable. Approximately 35 000 patients die of lung cancer in the United Kingdom each year.

## AETIOLOGY OF LUNG CANCER

The main factors are:

1. *Cigarette smoking* – this is by far the major cause, established by epidemiological and animal studies. Cigarette smoke contains carcinogens such as 3,4 benzpyrene and nitrosamines. Passive smoking is also significant.
2. *Industrial and atmospheric pollution* – there is a large number of pollutant industrial processes, e.g. asbestos workers, miners exposed to irradiation (e.g. radon, uranium) and metal smelters (e.g. chromium, nickel).

Lung cancer is more common in urban than in rural areas.

### Gross pathology

The tumour arises from the main bronchi or their large branches (central) or at the periphery of the lung (peripheral).

Most patients present with cough, haemoptysis or chest pain, but metastases may be the first sign.

The lung distal to the tumour may collapse or become consolidated (retention pneumonia).

Central tumours arise from the bronchial mucosa and form a friable mass which often partly obstructs the bronchial lumen.

307

# LUNG CANCER

**Tumour spread**

1. **LOCAL SPREAD**

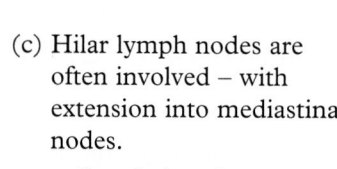

(b) Pleural involvement often results in a haemorrhagic effusion.

(c) Hilar lymph nodes are often involved – with extension into mediastinal nodes.

(a) The tumour directly invades adjacent lung tissue. Invasion of a large blood vessel may lead to severe haemorrhage (haemoptysis).

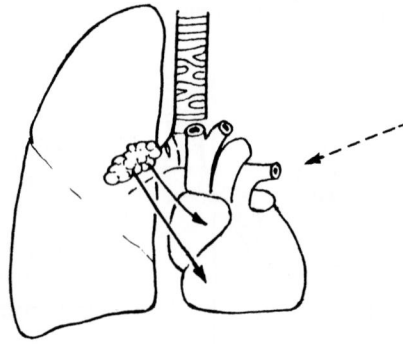

(d) Direct spread to the pericardium may cause pericardial effusion with subsequent involvement of the myocardium.

(e) Apical tumours (**Pancoast tumour**) can involve structures in the neck.

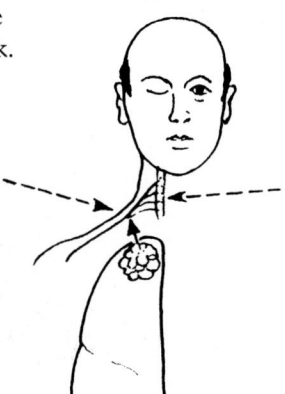

Involvement of the brachial plexus can give sensory and motor symptoms.

Involvement of cervical sympathetic chain causes Horn syndrome:
Ptosis – drooping eyelid.
Enophthalmos – sunken eye.
Miosis – small pupil.
Anhydrosis – loss of sweating.

(f) **Spread to the mediastinum**

  (i) The superior vena cava can be obstructed – venous congestion in head and neck.

  (ii) Nerves may be involved:
    Recurrent laryngeal ⟶ vocal cord paralysis.
    Phrenic ⟶ paralysis of diaphragm.

# LUNG CANCER

## 2. DISTANT SPREAD

*Haematogenous spread* is common, usually due to invasion of pulmonary veins. The common sites are: LIVER, BONE, BRAIN, ADRENAL (the last is usually asymptomatic but is found frequently at autopsy).

*Lymphatic spread* to cervical nodes and retrograde spread to the abdomen occurs.

## NON-METASTATIC EFFECTS

These include:

1. ACTH secretion → Adrenal hyperplasia → Raised blood cortisol → Cushing syndrome.

2. ADH secretion → Retention of water → Dilutional hyponatraemia.

3. Parathyroid hormone related peptide (PTHrP) secretion → Hypercalcaemia (p. 25).

Other syndromes include: encephalopathy, cerebellar degeneration, neuropathy, myopathy, Eaton–Lambert myasthenia-like syndrome, etc.

## HISTOLOGICAL TYPES

Four main types are recognised

| | | |
|---|---|---|
| 1. Small cell ......................................... | 20% | The |
| 2. Squamous carcinoma ........................... | 30% | proportions |
| 3. Adenocarcinoma ................................. | 40% | vary between |
| 4. Large cell carcinoma ........................... | 10% | series. |

The separation of small cell carcinoma from non-small cell variants is extremely important as the former tumour is treated by chemotherapy. Sub-classification of non-small cell variants is now important for certain targeted chemotherapies.

## SMALL CELL LUNG CARCINOMA

This is the most aggressive form of lung cancer and metastasises early and widely. It does respond well, at least initially, to cisplatin-based chemotherapy – some patients survive for up to 2 years.

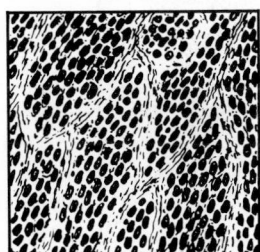

Almost no cytoplasm.

Spindle-shaped dark nuclei; may appear to be rounded or oval. May be arranged in sheets, cords or small round aggregates.

Clusters of hyperchromatic cells with nuclear moulding may be seen on sputum cytology.

The tumour arises from neuro-endocrine cells and expresses markers such as NCAM-1 (neural cell adhesion molecule-1). It is the form which most commonly has endocrine and other non-metastatic humoral effects.

# LUNG CANCER

### SQUAMOUS CARCINOMA

These tend to arise centrally from major bronchi, within dysplastic squamous epithelium following squamous metaplasia.

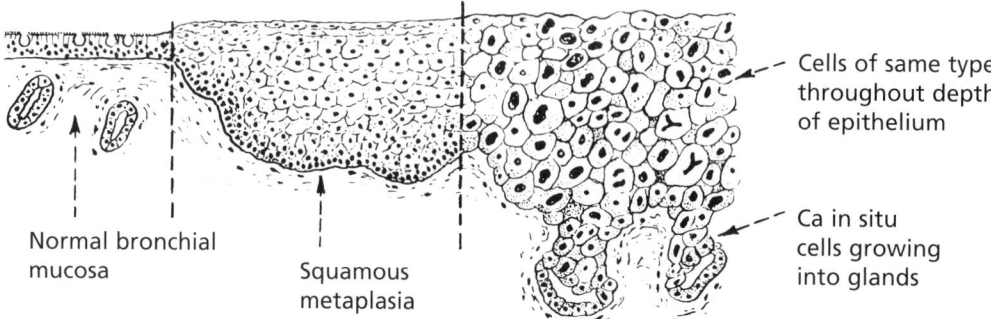

Cells of same type throughout depth of epithelium

Ca in situ cells growing into glands

Normal bronchial mucosa

Squamous metaplasia

Although squamous carcinoma is often slow growing, there is often extensive destruction of local tissues. The affected bronchi are often blocked, leading to retention pneumonia or collapse.

These tumours may produce keratin and often express markers such as p40, p63 and Cytokeratin 5.

### ADENOCARCINOMA

This tumour is a common tumour in women and is seen in non-smokers, but is increasingly associated with smoking. At least two-thirds arise in the periphery of the lung, sometimes in relation to scarring.

These tumours may be:

(a) Acinar: a well-defined mass of malignant cells arranged in acini with a fibrous stroma.

(b) Growth of tumour cells along the alveolar walls (so-called 'lepidic pattern').

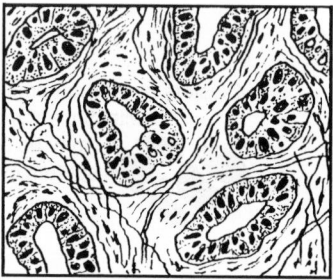

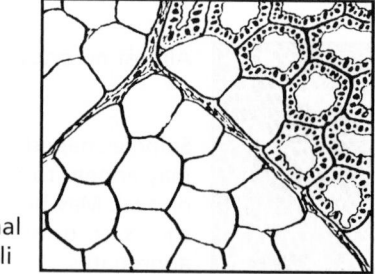

Tumour cells spreading along alveolar walls

Normal alveoli

Solid, papillary, micropapillary and clear cell patterns are also described.

The majority of these tumours express markers such as thyroid transcription factor (TTF-1) or Napsin.

# LUNG CANCER

## LARGE CELL CARCINOMA

As the name suggests, this tumour consists of large malignant cells without any specific differentiation. This is therefore a diagnosis of exclusion. The tumour usually arises centrally.

## TARGETED THERAPIES IN LUNG CANCER

In non-smoking women, particularly of East Asian origin, there is a high incidence of epidermal growth factor receptor (EGFR) mutations that confer responsiveness to specific tyrosine kinase inhibitors. The overall incidence of EGFR mutations in non-small cell lung cancer is 10–15%. Rearrangements also occur in anaplastic lymphoma kinase gene (*ALK-1*) and these too can be targeted with ALK-inhibitors. The incidence of ALK mutations is lower than EGFR mutations, about 4–5% of lung cancer patients. Other mutations, e.g. *ROS1* mutations, are continually being identified, predominantly in adenocarcinomas, and more targeted agents are continually becoming available. Alternative means of targeting lung tumours include blocking PD-1 (Programmed cell death protein – 1), thus allowing the immune system to attack tumour cells.

## SECONDARY LUNG TUMOURS

It must always be remembered that many other cancers spread to the lungs both by blood and lymphatic routes.

# OTHER TUMOURS OF THE BRONCHI AND LUNGS

Benign tumours of the bronchi and lung are unusual. There are two main types.

### 1. SQUAMOUS PAPILLOMA

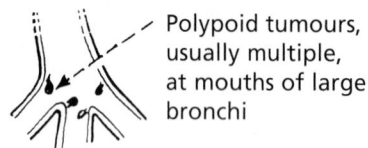
Polypoid tumours, usually multiple, at mouths of large bronchi

Papillomas are similar to the papillary tumours of the larynx. They occur in young people and on occasion may cause stridor due to partial bronchial obstruction. They are due to papilloma virus infection (types 6 and 11). Malignant change is exceptional.

### 2. CHONDROID HAMARTOMA

These are uncommon lesions of the lung which consist of lobules of cartilage and cleft-like spaces lined by bronchial epithelium. Their importance is that they appear as 'coin lesions' on chest X-ray and may simulate primary or secondary tumours. Current evidence suggests they are benign neoplasms rather than hamartomas.

## CARCINOID TUMOURS

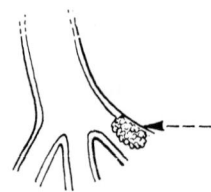

These tumours account for 1–2% of primary lung neoplasms. They often appear around the age of 50 years. Usually the tumour is situated in a primary bronchus or at the lung periphery. The tumour is a smooth-surfaced yellow nodule.

*Histologically* these resemble neuroendocrine tumours of the appendix (see p. 365). A small proportion of these tumours metastasise to regional lymph nodes – all are potentially malignant.

Central tumours tend to block the bronchus in which they arise.

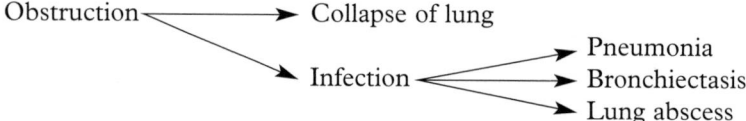

Obstruction → Collapse of lung
→ Infection → Pneumonia
→ Bronchiectasis
→ Lung abscess

**Atypical carcinoid tumours**: this subgroup of tumours shows nuclear pleomorphism, mitotic activity and necrosis. Over half eventually metastasise.

### Tumours of bronchial glands

Both benign and low-grade malignant tumours of the bronchial glands are occasionally seen and show histological similarity to salivary gland tumours. These may present as obstructing lesions.

# DISEASES OF THE PLEURA

## INFLAMMATION (PLEURISY)

There are several causes.

(a) *Infection* – usually due to spread from pneumonia or TB, or following penetrating injury, e.g. stab wound.
(b) *Autoimmunity* – e.g. rheumatoid arthritis, systemic lupus erythematosus.
(c) *Overlying a pulmonary infarct* (p. 81).

## FIBRINOUS PLEURISY

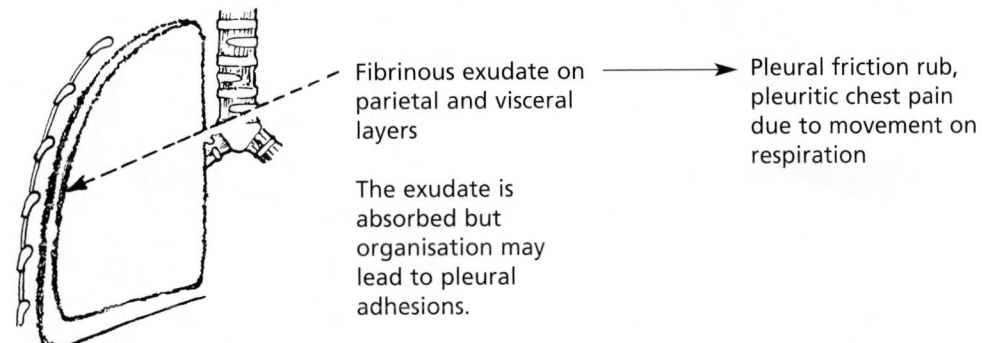

Fibrinous exudate on parietal and visceral layers $\longrightarrow$ Pleural friction rub, pleuritic chest pain due to movement on respiration

The exudate is absorbed but organisation may lead to pleural adhesions.

If fluid accumulates in excess, there is a pleural effusion – pain and friction rub disappear as the inflamed layers are separated.

If infection of the pleura proceeds, an empyema (a collection of pus in the pleura) may form. This is now unusual.

## PLEURAL EFFUSION

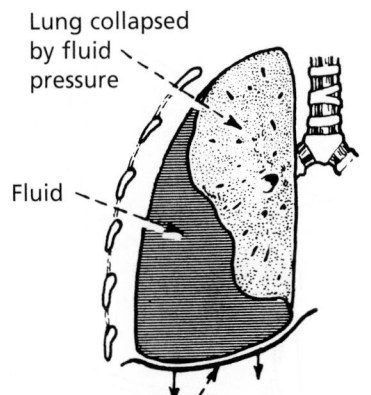

Lung collapsed by fluid pressure

Fluid

Diaphragm depressed

The accumulation of fluid within the pleura can be explained as a form of local oedema.

The composition of the fluid is related to the underlying cause.

| TRANSUDATE | EXUDATE |
| --- | --- |
| e.g. in heart failure | e.g. in fibrinous pleurisy |
| – low protein content | – high protein content |
| – few inflammatory cells | – numerous inflammatory cells |

Examination of the pleural fluid may show mesothelial cells, lymphocytes, macrophages, neutrophils and sometimes tumour cells.

# DISEASES OF THE PLEURA

### PNEUMOTHORAX

This is the accumulation of air in the pleural space. It may follow blunt trauma or penetrating wound, e.g. stabbing. Older patients with emphysema may develop spontaneous pneumothorax. In young people this is usually due to rupture of small bullae or excessive smoking of cannabis.

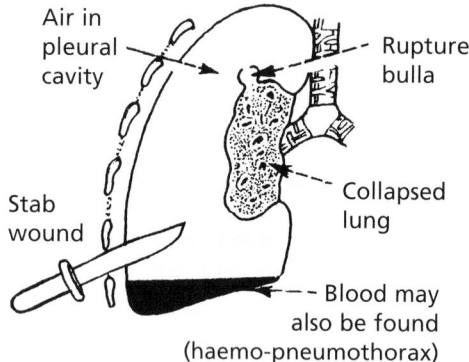

Air in pleural cavity

Ruptured bulla

Stab wound

Collapsed lung

Blood may also be found (haemo-pneumothorax)

In a TENSION PNEUMOTHORAX there is a valve effect – air continues to enter the pleura during inspiration but cannot exit during expiration.

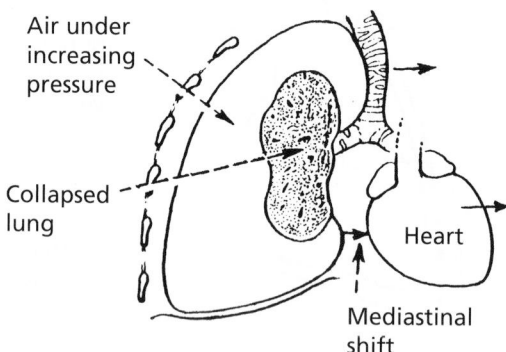

Air under increasing pressure

Collapsed lung

Heart

Mediastinal shift

Patients complain of chest pain and breathlessness.

### PLEURAL MALIGNANCY

Metastatic tumours affect the pleura in two ways.

(a) By LYMPHATIC spread – with numerous small nodules, e.g. breast carcinoma.
(b) By DIRECT spread, e.g. lung cancer.

There is usually a pleural effusion in which tumour cells can be found.

### Malignant mesothelioma

This primary pleural malignancy is usually due to asbestos exposure – often many years before.

The tumour may encase the entire lung and grow into the interlobar fissures

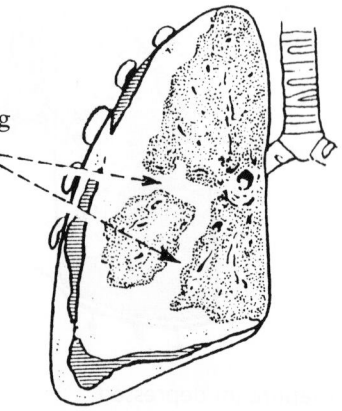

The tumour can metastasise to other sites, but most patients die due to the local respiratory effects.

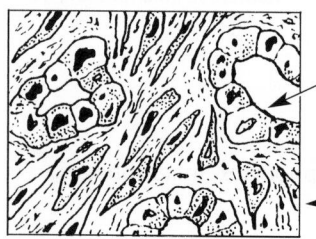

*Histologically*, the tumour consists of either epithelial or sarcomatous tissues, or may be mixed (biphasic).

There is often a malignant pleural effusion.

# GASTROINTESTINAL TRACT

## OBJECTIVES

1. To know the main pathologies that affect the oral cavity.
2. To have knowledge of the inflammatory and neoplastic disorders of the oesophagus.
3. To know the main forms of gastritis and their causes.
4. To understand the pathogenesis of gastric cancer.
5. To understand the pathology of malabsorption and its main causes.
6. To compare and contrast Crohn's disease and ulcerative colitis.
7. To know the main forms of gastrointestinal infection and their associated pathological features.
8. To understand colonic cancer and its pathogenesis.
9. To have a basic knowledge of neuroendocrine tumours of the gastrointestinal tract.

# THE MOUTH

### INFLAMMATION

A wide variety of inflammatory conditions can be seen.

### VIRAL INFECTIONS

*Herpes simplex* virus (usually Type I) infects the mouth in young children. This is often asymptomatic but in 10–20% of cases numerous vesicles and ulcers are seen. The virus can become latent in the trigeminal ganglion and repeated 'cold sores' occur on the lip in later life.

*Coxsackie viruses* can cause oral blistering (e.g. herpangina; hand, foot and mouth disease). Koplik spots are a feature of *measles*.

### FUNGAL INFECTION

*Candida albicans* is an oral commensal in 40% of the population.

Clinical infection is seen in infants, in patients on broad spectrum antibiotics, steroid or cytotoxic therapy and also in the immunosuppressed and diabetics. Extensive oral candida is common in patients with AIDS.

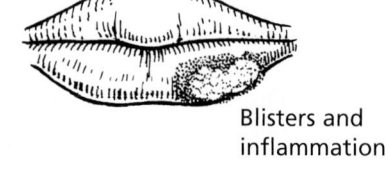

Blisters and inflammation

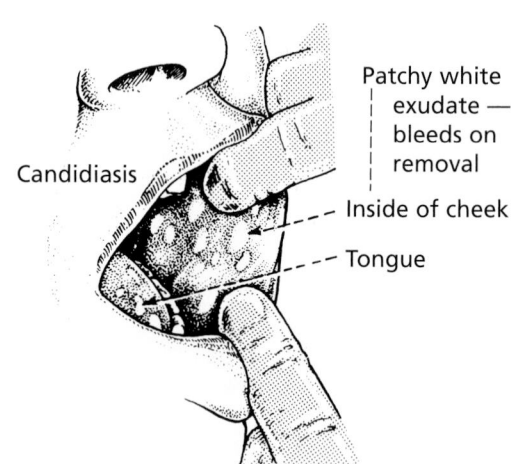

Candidiasis

Patchy white exudate — bleeds on removal

Inside of cheek

Tongue

# THE MOUTH

## BACTERIAL INFECTIONS

**Syphilis** is now uncommon in the West, but can involve the mouth. It can occur as a primary chancre or as irregular lines of ulceration, i.e. snail track ulcers of the secondary stage. It can also occur as small gummas (tertiary syphilis).

**Oral tuberculosis (TB)**, usually due to coughed up bacilli from pulmonary TB, is now very uncommon. Ulcers may occur on the tongue.

### Aphthous ulcers

Around 30% of the population are troubled by these painful, usually small, ulcers on the cheek, tongue and gums. The aetiology is unknown. In some individuals they are provoked by stress or local trauma.

**Dermatoses**, e.g. lichen planus – can affect the oral mucosa.

# ORAL CANCER

Oral cancer accounts for 2% of cancers in the United Kingdom. There is wide geographical variation. It is much commoner in South-East Asia. Men are at least twice as commonly affected as women. It is a disease of the elderly.

### Aetiology

The major causes are:

1. Tobacco – especially pipe and cigar smoking. Chewing tobacco, sometimes mixed with betel nuts (in Eastern countries) is also implicated.
2. Alcohol, especially spirits.
3. Exposure to ultraviolet light (cancer of the lip).
4. Human papilloma virus (type 16) may be involved.

### Pathology

Almost all cases are **squamous cell carcinomas**. The lip, tongue, floor of mouth and tonsil are affected in that order of frequency.

Ulcerated nodule often on the lower lip with raised edges.

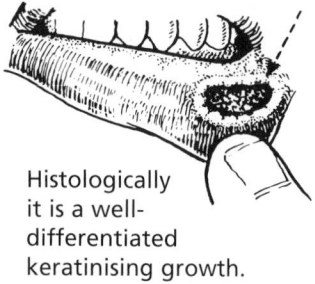

Histologically it is a well-differentiated keratinising growth.

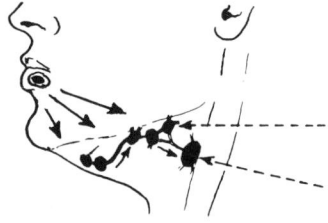

Growth is relatively slow but eventually spreads to the submandibular nodes and deeper cervical nodes.

### Tongue/floor of mouth

Carcinoma of the tongue and other sites within the mouth is a more aggressive growth than tumours of the lips. Starting as a nodule in the buccal sulcus adjacent to the tongue, it breaks down to form an irregular ulcer with ragged edges.

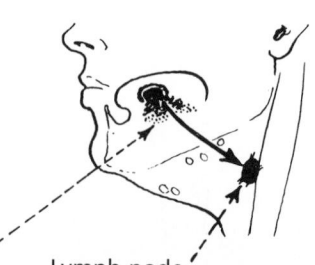

Local infiltration leads to fixation of the tongue. Spread may be extensive to floor of mouth, tonsils, pharynx and occasionally bone.

Lymph node involvement occurs early, usually to the deeper cervical nodes.

# MOUHT

# ERYTHROPLAKIA AND LEUKOPLAKIA

These terms describe velvety-red patches and white patches in the oral mucosa. These are important because they may represent dysplasia of the squamous epithelium and may lead to squamous cancer.

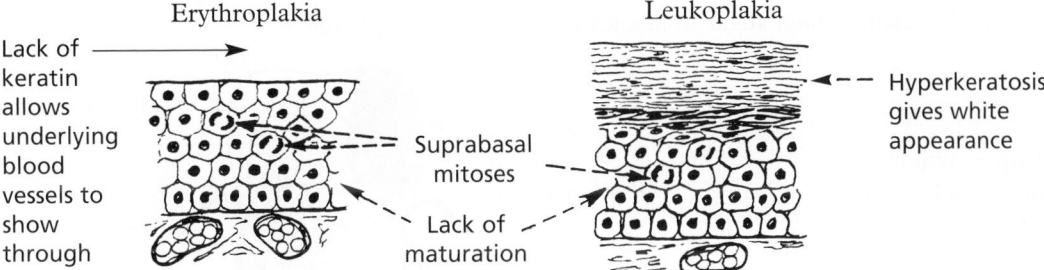

Erythroplakia — Leukoplakia

Lack of keratin allows underlying blood vessels to show through → Suprabasal mitoses → Lack of maturation — Hyperkeratosis gives white appearance

**Not all examples of leukoplakia are premalignant.** They may be due to:

– Chronic irritation (e.g. dentures)
– Pipe smoking
– Candida

A distinctive form – 'hairy leukoplakia' – occurs on the lateral border of the tongue in patients with AIDS. It is due to Epstein–Barr virus infection, often with superimposed candida.

## Pigmentations

Melanotic pigmentation of the mouth is seen in Addison disease, haemochromatosis and the Peutz–Jeghers syndrome.

## Benign tumours

A variety of benign tumours are seen, e.g. squamous papillomas and haemangiomas (often on the lips or tongue).

## Granular cell tumour

This is a rare tumour and its importance lies in the fact that it may be mistaken for carcinoma of the tongue.

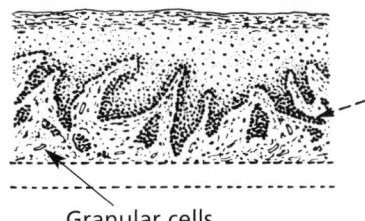

Granular cells

Overlying epithelium shows very irregular downgrowths – but it is not neoplastic (so-called 'pseudoepitheliomatous hyperplasia')

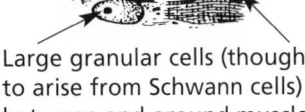

Large granular cells (thought to arise from Schwann cells) between and around muscle cells of tongue

*Note*: Epulis is a clinical term applied to swellings at the gum margin. Most of them are granulomas associated with chronic gingivitis. A few are true neoplasms.

# DENTAL CARIES AND PERIODONTAL DISEASE

These two very common processes are primarily of importance to dentists, but an understanding is also valuable for doctors.

## DENTAL CARIES

This is the commonest disease of teeth.

Poor oral hygiene + high sugar intake lead to formation of plaque.

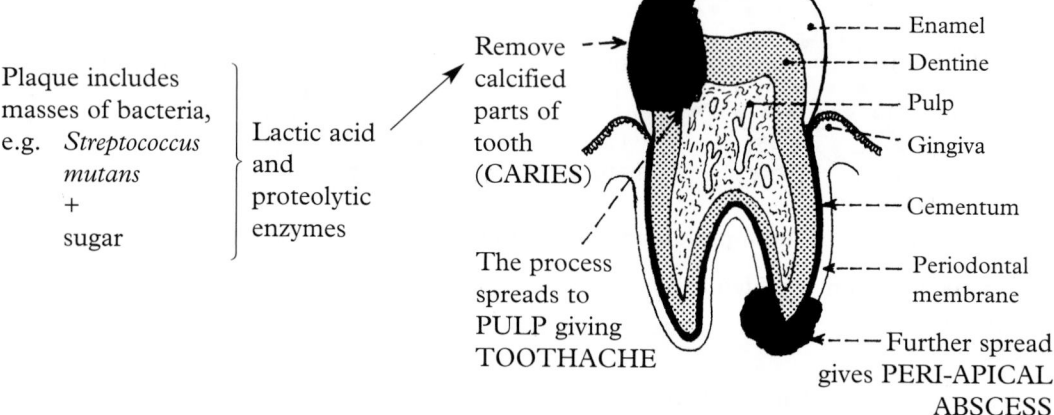

Plaque includes masses of bacteria, e.g. *Streptococcus mutans* + sugar

Lactic acid and proteolytic enzymes

Remove calcified parts of tooth (CARIES)

The process spreads to PULP giving TOOTHACHE

Enamel

Dentine

Pulp

Gingiva

Cementum

Periodontal membrane

Further spread gives PERI-APICAL ABSCESS

## PERIODONTAL DISEASE

This is the major cause of tooth loss in middle age. It is essentially due to gingivitis.

A pouch is formed between the gingiva and the neck of the tooth.

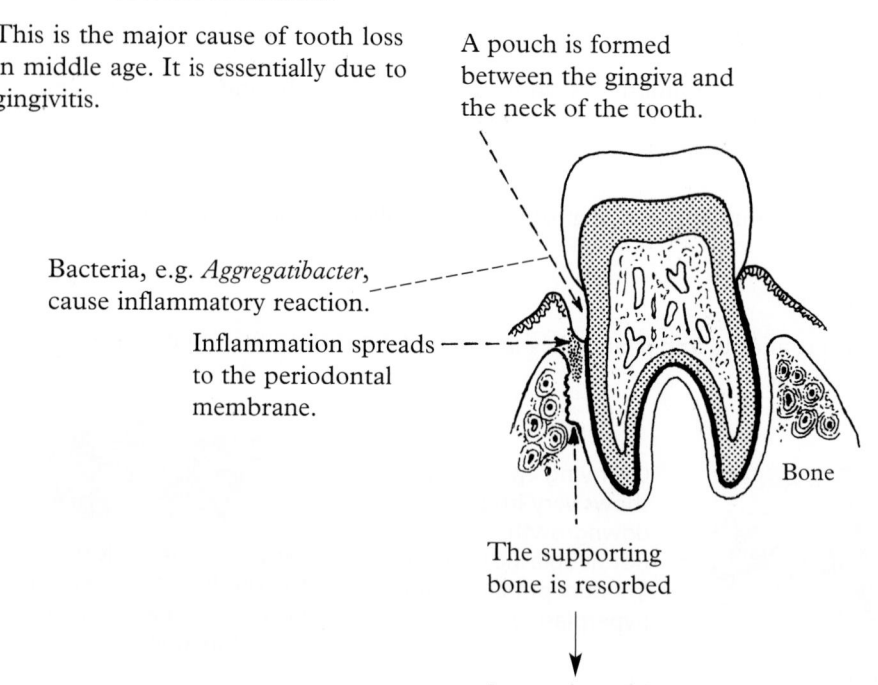

Bacteria, e.g. *Aggregatibacter*, cause inflammatory reaction.

Inflammation spreads to the periodontal membrane.

Bone

The supporting bone is resorbed

Loosening of tooth

# DISEASES OF THE SALIVARY GLANDS

## INFLAMMATION

The commonest acute inflammation is due to the mumps virus, which produces acute swelling, particularly of the parotid glands, with oedema and mononuclear infiltration of the interstitial tissue.

The testes and pancreas may also be inflamed and atrophy may follow.

Bacterial infection of these glands is uncommon and may occur during a prolonged illness, particularly if a calculus has formed in a duct.

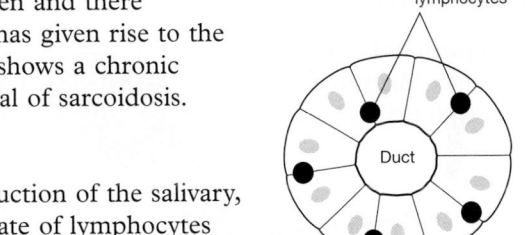

Chronic inflammation is rare. It may occur in sarcoidosis. The parotid gland becomes swollen and there may be an accompanying irido-cyclitis. This has given rise to the term 'uveo-parotid fever'. The parotid gland shows a chronic inflammatory reaction with granulomas typical of sarcoidosis.

### Sjögren syndrome

In this auto-immune condition there is destruction of the salivary, lacrimal and conjunctival glands by an infiltrate of lymphocytes (so-called 'lympho-epithelial lesions') and plasma cells. The duct epithelia often undergo reactive hyperplasia. It results in dryness of the mouth, caries due to lack of saliva, and ulceration of the conjunctiva caused by lack of secretion from the lacrimal and conjunctival glands. This is often associated with rheumatoid disease.

There is an increased risk of B cell lymphoma (p. 467).

### Calculi

Stones can form in the submandibular or, less often, the parotid duct. Blockage leads to episodes of swelling after food and eventually to atrophy of the gland. Acute inflammation may be superimposed.

## SALIVARY GLAND TUMOURS

The majority (80%) of tumours arise in the parotid gland and are usually benign.

The remainder occur in the submandibular and minor salivary glands where 30–40% are malignant.

# SALIVARY GLANDS – BENIGN TUMOURS

### PLEOMORPHIC ADENOMA

This is the commonest tumour of the salivary glands and most often occurs in the parotid. The term 'pleomorphic' applies not to the nuclei of the cells but to the different types of tissue found. These are derived from the epithelial and myoepithelial cells.

The tumour is lobulated and encapsulated but there are frequently small lobules which extend into the adjacent tissue.

If the tumour is 'shelled out' these lobules are left behind and cause local recurrence. For this reason superficial parotidectomy is usually performed, ensuring complete removal of the tumour.

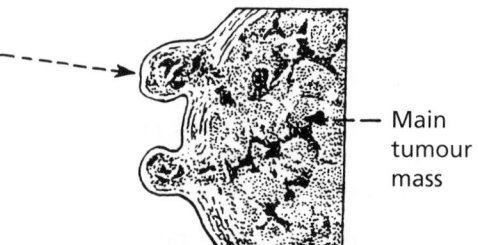

Main tumour mass

### HISTOLOGY

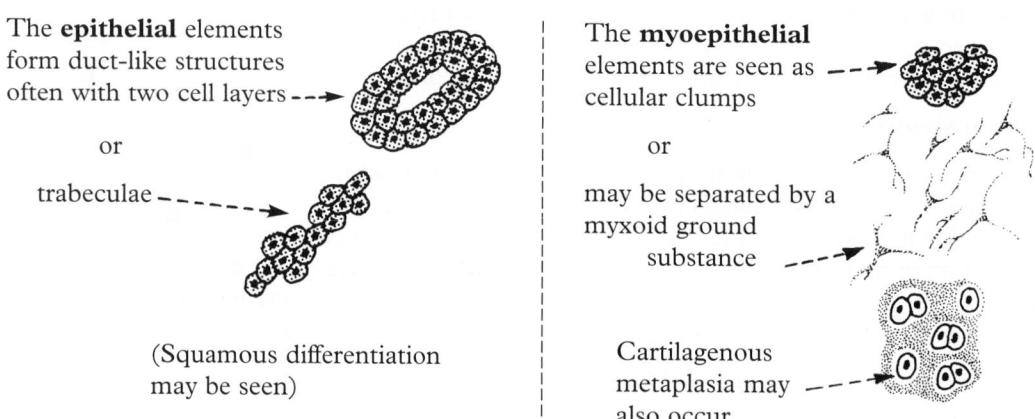

The **epithelial** elements form duct-like structures often with two cell layers

or

trabeculae

(Squamous differentiation may be seen)

The **myoepithelial** elements are seen as cellular clumps

or

may be separated by a myxoid ground substance

Cartilagenous metaplasia may also occur

### MALIGNANT CHANGE

Under 5% of these tumours become malignant, often after many years. Most of these are adenocarcinomas with a poor prognosis.

### WARTHIN TUMOUR

This is a benign lesion, mainly in the parotid of elderly men. It may be bilateral. It consists of tall epithelial cells with eosinophilic cytoplasm (oncocytes) and a reactive lymphoid infiltrate.

# SALIVARY GLANDS – CARCINOMAS

Almost all malignant tumours of the salivary glands are adenocarcinomas. They affect major and minor glands and arise de novo or from pre-existing pleomorphic adenoma. The prognosis is variable.

Three unusual subtypes are worth noting.

1.  **Acinic cell carcinoma**
    Approximately one-quarter of all malignant parotid tumours are of this type. It grows slowly, recurs after removal and sometimes there is late spread to the regional lymph nodes and distant organs.

2.  **Adenoid cystic carcinoma**
    This usually occurs in minor salivary glands. It extends by direct spread, especially along nerve sheaths, but metastases can occur to lymph nodes, lungs and bones.

3.  **Muco-epidermoid carcinoma**
    The behaviour of this type varies, but all tend to recur and infiltrate locally. More aggressive tumours metastasise to the lymph nodes and may invade the blood stream. They are generally found in the major salivary glands.

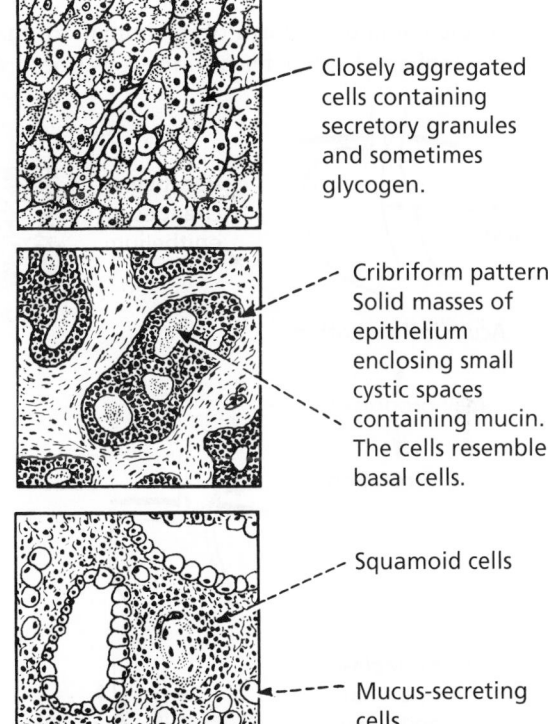

Closely aggregated cells containing secretory granules and sometimes glycogen.

Cribriform pattern. Solid masses of epithelium enclosing small cystic spaces containing mucin. The cells resemble basal cells.

Squamoid cells

Mucus-secreting cells

# OESOPHAGUS

The oesophagus is a muscular tube 25 cm long lined by stratified squamous epithelium which is resistant to damage by heat, cold and mechanical trauma.

## INFLAMMATION

### Reflux oesophagitis

This is the commonest form of inflammation due to reflux of gastric acid through a relaxed lower oesophageal sphincter into the lower oesophagus, often associated with hiatus hernia.

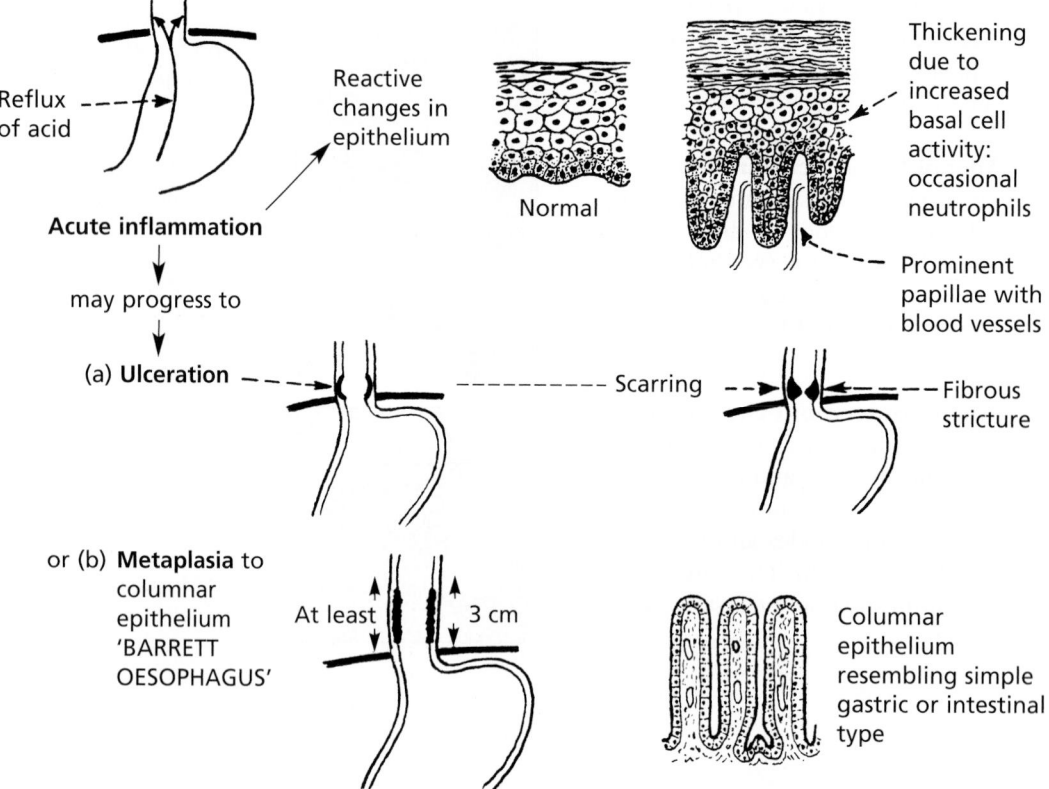

Reflux of acid

Reactive changes in epithelium

Normal

Thickening due to increased basal cell activity: occasional neutrophils

Prominent papillae with blood vessels

**Acute inflammation**

may progress to

(a) **Ulceration** — — — Scarring — — Fibrous stricture

or (b) **Metaplasia** to columnar epithelium 'BARRETT OESOPHAGUS'

At least 3 cm

Columnar epithelium resembling simple gastric or intestinal type

Barrett oesophagus is an important premalignant lesion with a 30–40-fold increased risk of CANCER.

METAPLASIA ⟶ DYSPLASIA (detected ⟶ ADENOCARCINOMA
by endoscopy and biopsy)

### Other forms of oesophagitis

1. Eosinophilic oesophagitis. Some patients, often atopic, develop dysphagia and biopsy shows numerous eosinophils within the squamous epithelium.
2. Infection by *Herpes simplex virus*, cytomegalovirus and *C. albicans* occurs particularly in the immunosuppressed and AIDS.
3. Ingestion of drugs, e.g. non-steroidal anti-inflammatory drugs, may cause ulceration of the distal oesophagus.

# OESOPHAGUS

## HIATUS HERNIA

In hiatus hernia, part of the stomach herniates into the thorax. This is common, particularly in the elderly, though often asymptomatic. Two forms are seen:

1. **Sliding hernia**
   - the distal oesophagus and proximal stomach slide proximally so the latter lies in the thorax. Most cases are of this type.

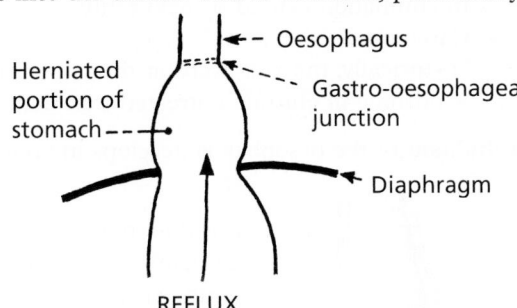

2. **Rolling hernia**
   - a loop of stomach rolls upwards and passes through the diaphragm alongside the oesophagogastric junction. Since the junction is preserved reflux is unusual.

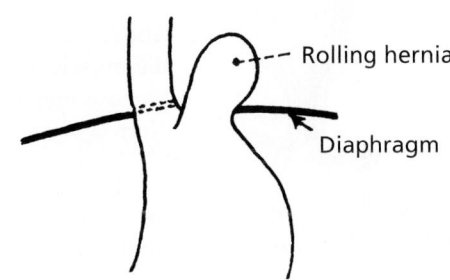

## DIVERTICULA

These are relatively rare and are of two varieties.

1. **Pulsion type**
   Involves pharynx (pharyngeal pouch). Sac is distended during swallowing of food. By pushing down behind oesophagus, it may compress this structure. Abnormal function of the upper oesophageal sphincter is an aetiological factor.

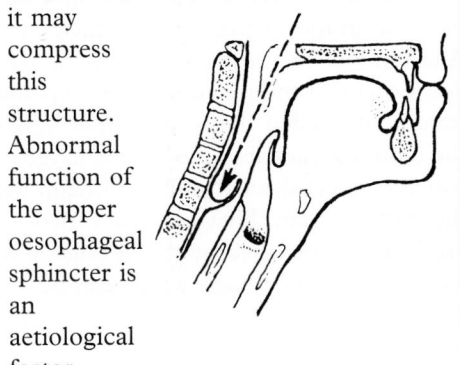

2. **Traction type**
   This is due to traction of fibrous tissue produced by mediastinal inflammation, e.g. TB of lymph nodes.

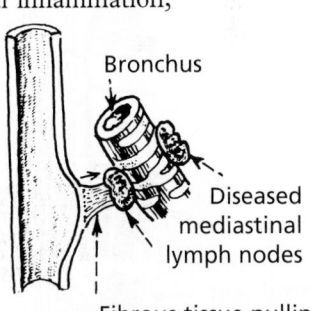

Rarely, there may be a congenital diverticulum at the level of the bifurcation of the trachea.

# OESOPHAGUS

**Obstruction** usually leads to dysphagia – difficulty in swallowing. The causes include:
**Strictures** of the oesophageal wall due to:
- Inflammation caused by acid reflux.
- Carcinoma.
- Historically, mucosal webs at the upper end were a feature of the Plummer–Vinson syndrome in chronic untreated iron deficiency anaemia.

**Achalasia** of the oesophagus develops in young adults and may cause severe obstruction.

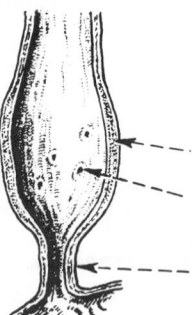

It is due to a conduction failure in the peristaltic mechanism preventing relaxation of the cardiac sphincter. Reduced numbers of ganglion cells are found in the myenteric plexus.

Above the obstruction the oesophagus is dilated, the muscle is hypertrophied and the mucosa may be ulcerated.

Narrowing occurs at the lower end.

(In South American trypanosomiasis, the myenteric plexus may be destroyed [CHAGAS DISEASE]). Long-standing diabetic autonomic neuropathy may cause a similar problem.

In **systemic sclerosis**, replacement of muscle by fibrous tissue converts the oesophagus into a rigid tube.

## OESOPHAGEAL VARICES

These dilated veins occur secondarily to portal hypertension caused mainly by cirrhosis of the liver (see p. 381).

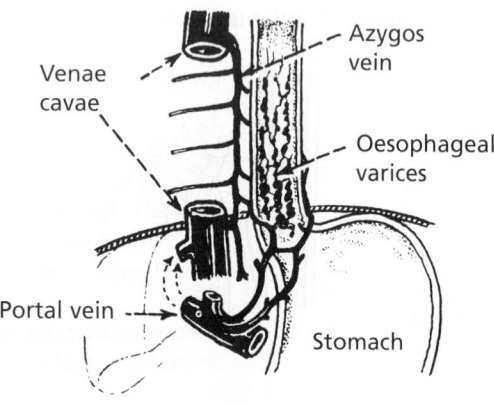

Fibrosis in the liver obstructs the flow of blood from the gastrointestinal tract. Anastomotic channels connecting the portal and systemic venous systems open up and become distended. The most important are the oesophageal tributaries of the azygos vein which connect through the diaphragm with the portal system. They become varicose, and are easily traumatised by the passage of food, leading to haemorrhage, which can be severe.

**Spontaneous rupture** of the oesophagus is rare. Mucosal tears causing haemorrhage may occur (Mallory–Weiss syndrome). This tends to occur due to severe vomiting.

**Congenital abnormalities** include stenosis and atresia with fistula formation.

# OESOPHAGUS – TUMOURS

Benign tumours of the oesophagus are rare. They are almost always of connective tissue origin (usually leiomyomas) and form polyps within the lumen, causing obstruction.

## Carcinoma

Carcinoma of the oesophagus occurs in two main forms:

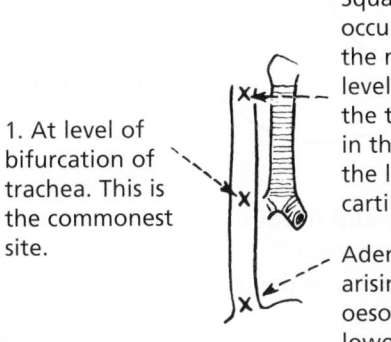

1. At level of bifurcation of trachea. This is the commonest site.

Squamous carcinomas occur most commonly in the mid oesophagus at the level of the bifurcation of the trachea and less often in the upper oesophagus at the level of the cricoid cartilage.

Adenocarcinomas, often arising in Barrett oesophagus, affect the lower one-third.

The disease is more common in men by a ratio of at least 4:1.

The tumours may narrow the lumen or cause a polypoid mass.

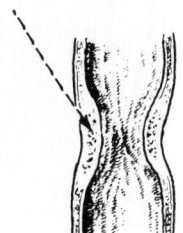

2. Soft polypoidal growth filling lumen

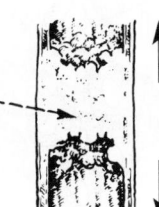

In both, the tumour grows longitudinally in the submucosal lymphatics. This means that the surgeon has to remove the tumour with wide margins.

## Spread

Middle-third tumours may involve the trachea with fistula formation leading to aspiration pneumonia. Tumours of the lower third may invade the mediastinum. Lymph node involvement is common and blood borne metastases to liver occur late.

## Aetiology

There is geographical variation, tumours being common in China and Africa. Smoking and diet, including alcohol consumption, are important in squamous carcinoma. Post-cricoid carcinoma in women is a rare late complication of the dysphagia, complicating iron deficiency anaemia. Adenocarcinoma is largely due to Barrett oesophagus and reflux.

# STOMACH

The stomach is divided into
five anatomical regions:

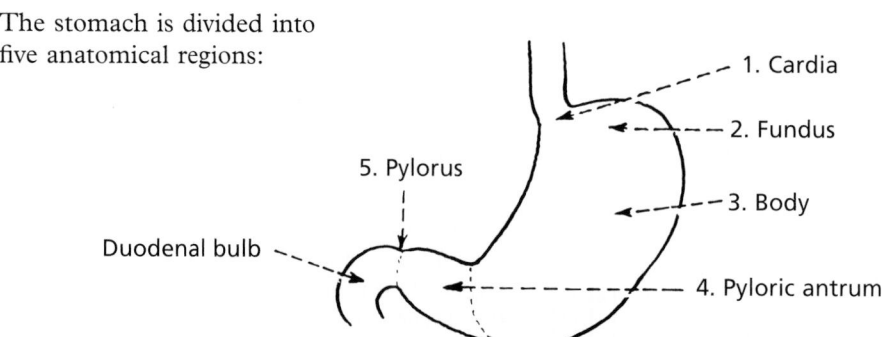

1. Cardia
2. Fundus
3. Body
4. Pyloric antrum
5. Pylorus

Duodenal bulb

Three forms of mucosa are seen:

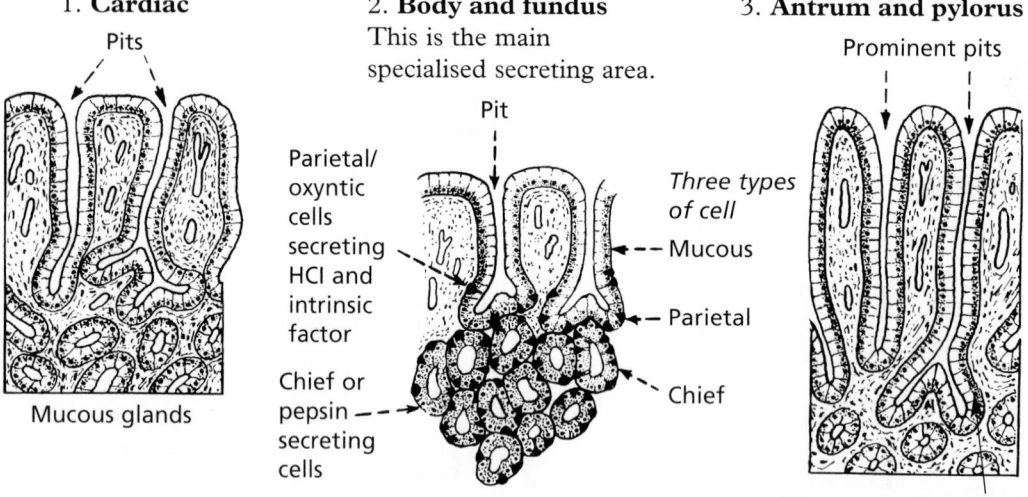

### 1. Cardiac

Pits

Mucous glands

### 2. Body and fundus

This is the main
specialised secreting area.

Pit

Parietal/
oxyntic
cells
secreting
HCl and
intrinsic
factor

Chief or
pepsin
secreting
cells

Three types
of cell

Mucous

Parietal

Chief

### 3. Antrum and pylorus

Prominent pits

Mucus secreting glands
including endocrine cells

## ACUTE GASTRITIS

Mild acute gastritis with neutrophils in the mucosa may be
caused by alcohol and non-steroidal anti-inflammatory drugs
(NSAIDs), and is seldom biopsied. Acute haemorrhagic or
erosive gastritis is a more severe form, also associated with
aspirin and NSAIDs, and is also a complication of shock.

Tiny ulcers affect all parts of the stomach, occurring on the
apex of mucosal folds, and can heal rapidly.

Naked eye appearance

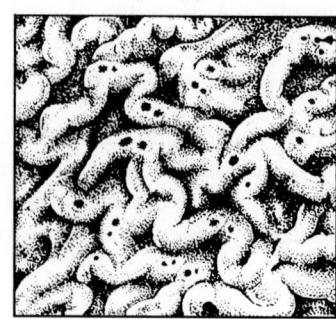

# GASTRITIS

## ACUTE INFLAMMATION

Mild acute gastritis is an acute inflammation with neutrophil reaction in the superficial layers of the mucosa. Pain and sickness have a multitude of causes varying from hot fluids, alcohol and aspirin, which act as direct irritants to infections such as childhood fevers, viral infections and bacterial food poisoning.

### Stress ulcers

Occasionally, particularly in severe shock, there is deeper acute ulceration with considerable haemorrhage and even perforation.

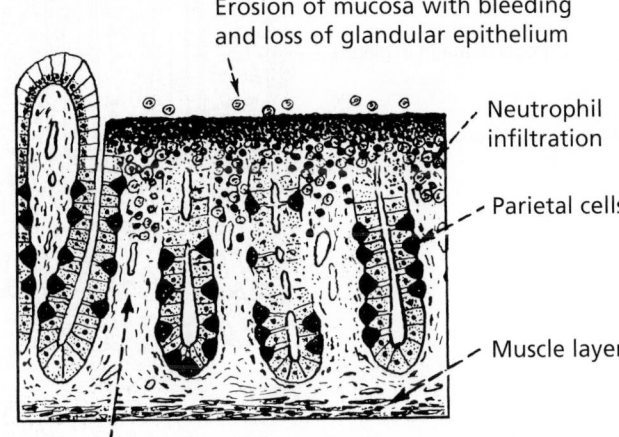

Erosion of mucosa with bleeding and loss of glandular epithelium

Neutrophil infiltration

Parietal cells

Muscle layer

Oedema resulting in swelling of mucosa and separation of glands

## CHRONIC GASTRITIS

There are three main causes of chronic gastritis:
- *Helicobacter pylori.*
- Chemical.
- Auto-immune.

## 1. *H. pylori* ASSOCIATED CHRONIC GASTRITIS

*Prevalence*: 80% of chronic gastritis cases are of this type. The organism has a worldwide distribution. In Western countries the prevalence of *Helicobacter* is over 30% by 30 years of age. In developing countries it is even higher.

*Aetiology*: *H. pylori* is a Gram-negative spiral bacterium which is specifically adapted to colonise the gastric mucosa.

*Site affected*: the antrum and pyloric canal particularly.

*Morphological changes* are of mucosal inflammation.

# GASTRITIS

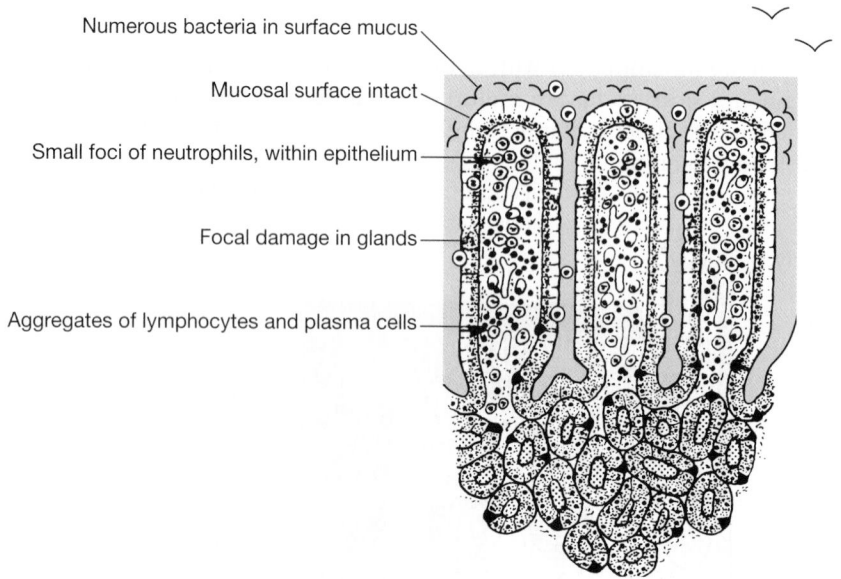

Numerous bacteria in surface mucus

Mucosal surface intact

Small foci of neutrophils, within epithelium

Focal damage in glands

Aggregates of lymphocytes and plasma cells

***Complications***:

    (a) GASTRIC and DUODENAL ulcer (see p. 334).

    (b) Progression to CARCINOMA, often preceded by INTESTINAL METAPLASIA.

    (c) Association with LYMPHOMAS OF B CELL TYPE.

## 2. CHEMICAL (REFLUX) GASTRITIS

***Prevalence***: this is the second-most common cause of chronic gastritis, accounting for approximately 10% of cases.

***Aetiology***: due to reflux of bile from duodenum, and to drugs.

***Site affected***: antrum and pylorus.

***Morphology***: there is foveolar hyperplasia and oedema with little inflammation.

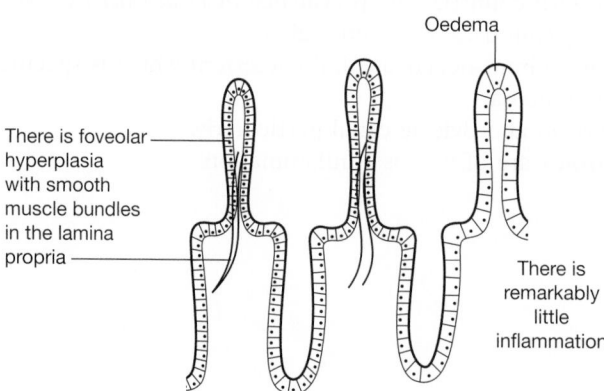

Oedema

There is foveolar hyperplasia with smooth muscle bundles in the lamina propria

There is remarkably little inflammation

# GASTRITIS

## 3. AUTO-IMMUNE ASSOCIATED GASTRITIS

*Prevalence*: 5% of chronic gastritis cases are of this type.

*Aetiology*:

    (a) Presence of antibodies to parietal cells and intrinsic factor.

    (b) Associated with other auto-immune disorders, e.g. thyroiditis.

*Sites affected*: The fundus and body predominantly.

*Morphological changes* are progressive over several years with gradual thinning of the mucosa.

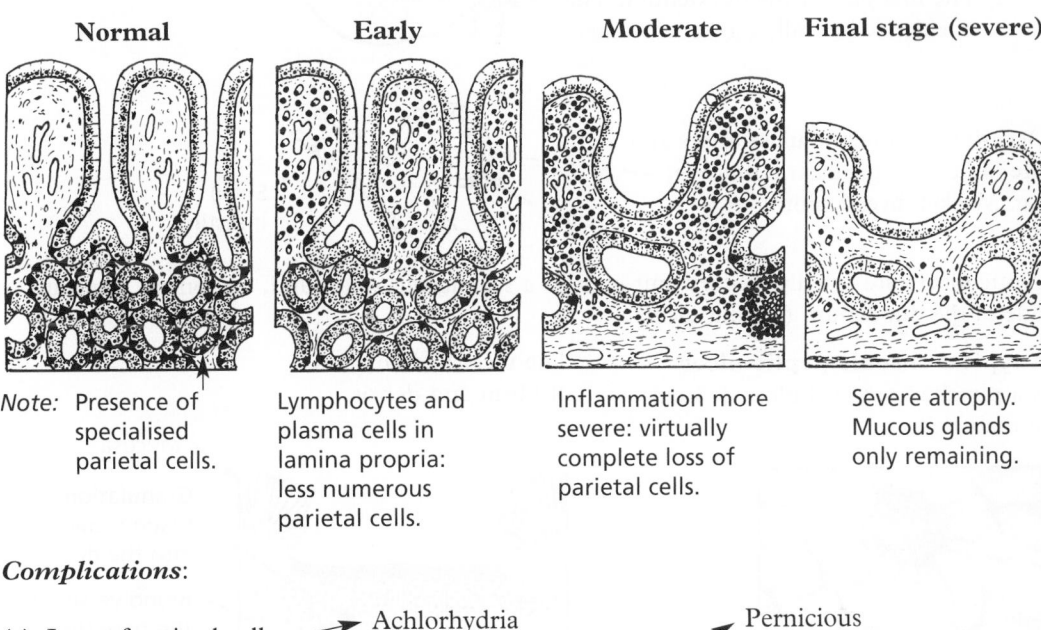

| Normal | Early | Moderate | Final stage (severe) |
|---|---|---|---|
| *Note:* Presence of specialised parietal cells. | Lymphocytes and plasma cells in lamina propria: less numerous parietal cells. | Inflammation more severe: virtually complete loss of parietal cells. | Severe atrophy. Mucous glands only remaining. |

*Complications*:

    (a) Loss of parietal cells → Achlorhydria / Absence of intrinsic factor → Pernicious anaemia (see p. 424)

    (b) There is an association with the development of GASTRIC CARCINOMA often preceded by INTESTINAL METAPLASIA.

## OTHER FORMS OF GASTRITIS

These include eosinophilic gastritis associated with food allergy, collagen diseases and parasites.

Granulomatous gastritis has many causes including Crohn's disease, TB and sarcoidosis.

Lymphocytic gastritis shows an increase in intraepithelial lymphocytes and is often associated with coeliac disease (p. 338).

# PEPTIC ULCERATION

Peptic ulcers occur when acid-containing gastric juices breach the mucosa of the gut.

**Chronic peptic ulcers** are found in three main sites.

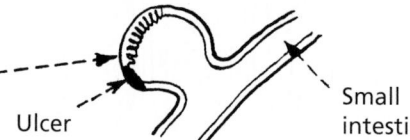

2. Gastric ulcers usually affect the antrum on the lesser curve.

3. Reflux of acid may lead to oesophageal ulcers.

1. The first part of the duodenum. The incidence has fallen in recent years.

Occasionally a peptic ulcer arises at a site of heterotopic gastric mucosa, e.g. Meckel diverticulum.

Ulcer

Small intestine

Peptic ulcers are usually solitary, but in 10% a second ulcer is found, e.g. on the opposite side of the duodenum (kissing ulcer).

A **typical chronic peptic ulcer** is a punched out oval ulcer 2–3 cm in diameter.

The ulcer bed consists of fibrin and debris.

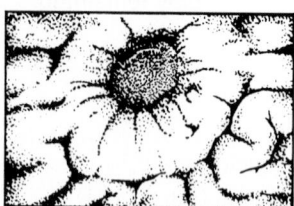

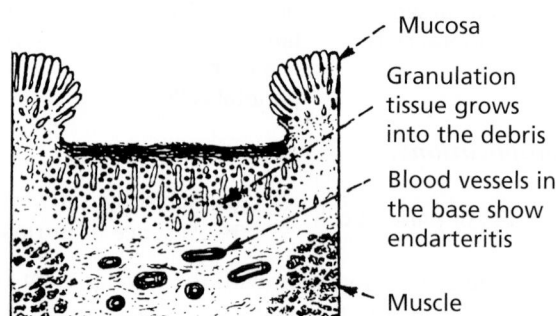

Mucosa

Granulation tissue grows into the debris

Blood vessels in the base show endarteritis

Muscle

The surrounding mucosa often shows stellate folds due to scarring.

In long-standing lesions fibrous tissue replaces muscle.

**Acute gastric ulcers** (often called stress ulcers) may be seen in patients with severe burns, after major trauma or with raised intracranial pressure. These may cause bleeding, but usually heal completely. Acute ulcers may also be due to treatment with NSAIDs.

# PEPTIC ULCERATION

## SEQUELS AND COMPLICATIONS

1. **Healing** is common, particularly when treated.

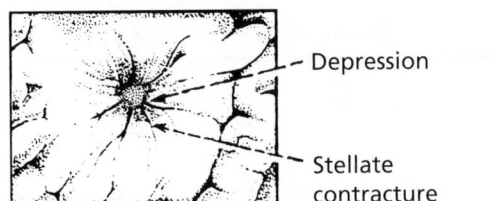

- Depression
- Stellate contracture

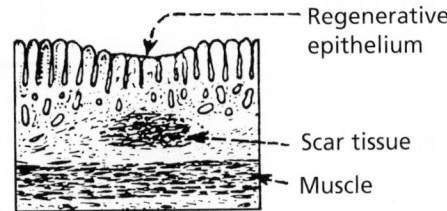

- Regenerative epithelium
- Scar tissue
- Muscle

2. **Scarring** may lead to stricture formation.

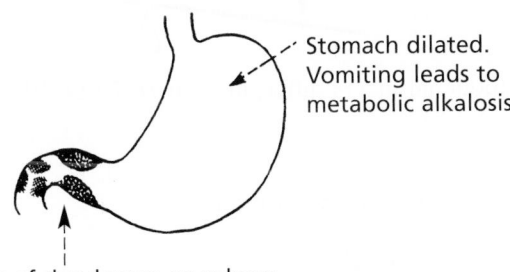

Stomach dilated. Vomiting leads to metabolic alkalosis.

Lesions of duodenum or pylorus lead to gastric outlet obstruction.

Lesions of the lesser curvature produce an 'hour glass' stomach.

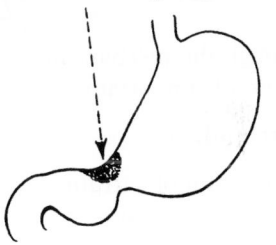

3. **Perforation** of an ulcer causes **acute peritonitis**. This may be:

**Generalised**  or  **Localised**

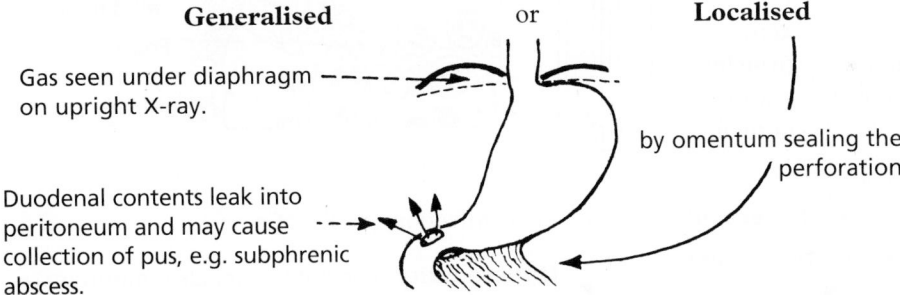

Gas seen under diaphragm on upright X-ray.

by omentum sealing the perforation

Duodenal contents leak into peritoneum and may cause collection of pus, e.g. subphrenic abscess.

4. **Haemorrhage.**

Minor bleeding is common and can lead to anaemia.

Major haemorrhage can lead to haematemesis, to 'coffee ground' vomit or to melaena (tarry black stools).

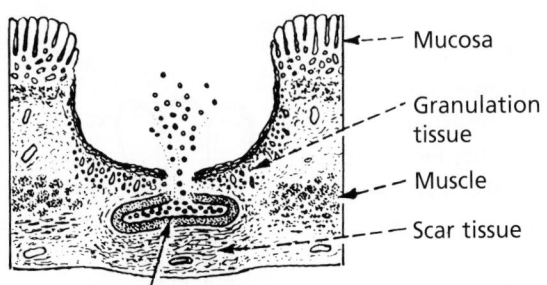

- Mucosa
- Granulation tissue
- Muscle
- Scar tissue

Eroded artery in ulcer base

# PEPTIC ULCER – AETIOLOGY

Normally gastric mucosal
damage is prevented by a
balance between the
damaging agents and the
mucosal defences.

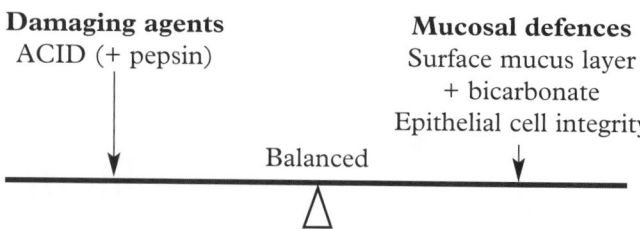

**Damaging agents**
ACID (+ pepsin)

**Mucosal defences**
Surface mucus layer
+ bicarbonate
Epithelial cell integrity

Balanced

**Peptic ulceration** results from imbalance.

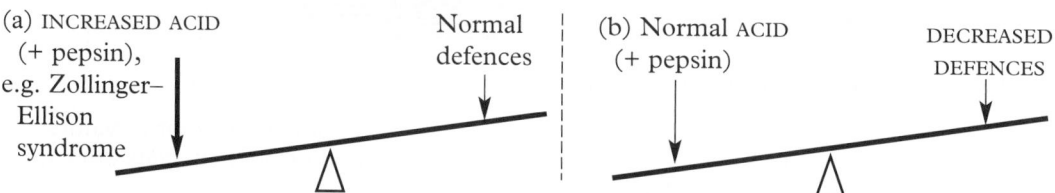

(a) INCREASED ACID
(+ pepsin),
e.g. Zollinger–
Ellison
syndrome

Normal
defences

(b) Normal ACID
(+ pepsin)

DECREASED
DEFENCES

Although the mechanisms in gastric and duodenal ulcers differ, in both *H. PYLORI*
infection is important.

**Gastric ulcer**

Colonisation of antrum
by *H. pylori* (70%).

NSAIDS ⟶ REDUCED MUCOSAL
DEFENCES

DUODENO-GASTRIC
REFLUX (including
bile; aggravated by
smoking)

ACID
(usually
low or
normal)

*High magnification*

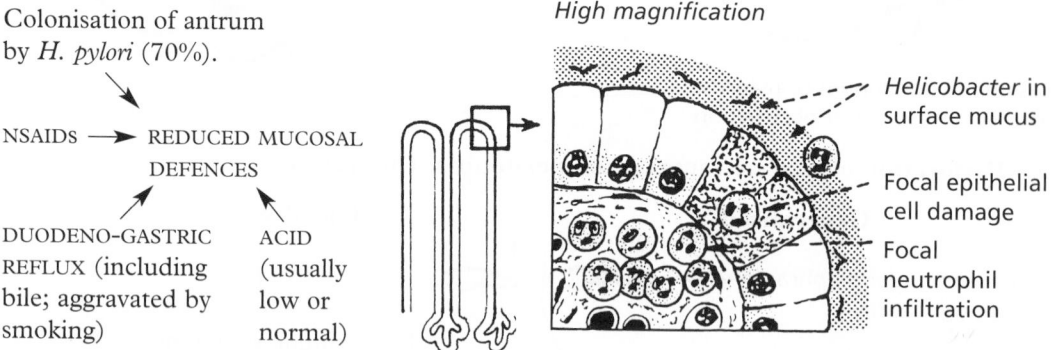

*Helicobacter* in
surface mucus

Focal epithelial
cell damage

Focal
neutrophil
infiltration

**Duodenal ulcer**

The main factors are **hyperacidity** and *H. pylori* infection (>90% of cases).

*H. pylori* ⟶ Gastric infection

Increased gastrin

**Hyperacidity** (genetic factors also important)

*H. pylori* infection
of duodenum
+ other factors, e.g.
stress, smoking

ACID

DUODENITIS ⟶ ULCER

METAPLASIA

Focal
metaplasia
of tips of
duodenal
villi

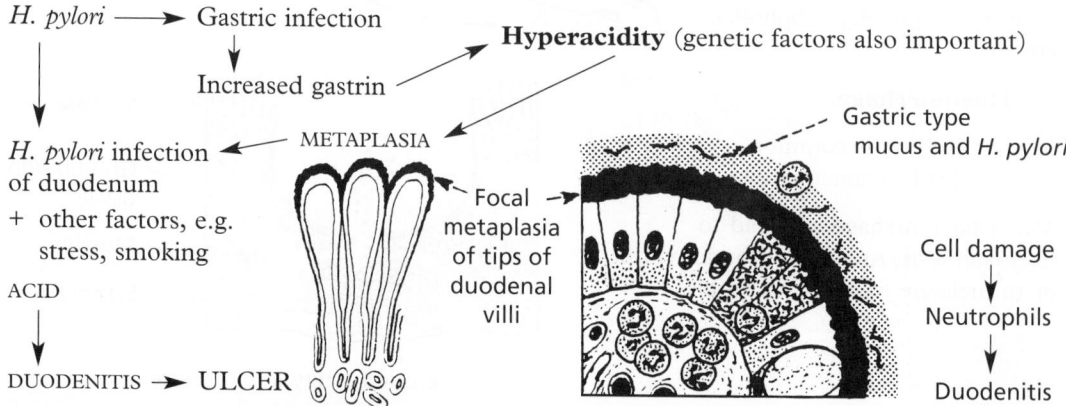

Gastric type
mucus and *H. pylori*

Cell damage

Neutrophils

Duodenitis

334   *Note*: Duodenal ulcer is cured when *H. pylori* is eliminated and acid reduced.

# GASTRIC CARCINOMA

This important tumour has an especially high incidence in Japan, Chile and Eastern Europe. Its incidence has fallen in the United Kingdom and the USA since the 1930s.

*Morphologically*, there are several types.

### 1. EXOPHYTIC

These exophytic tumours are commonly seen in the fundus.

Eventually the tumour spreads through the stomach wall to the serosa and is often ulcerated on the surface.

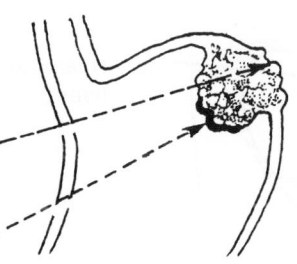

Tumours may occur at the cardia or distal stomach. Different aetiologies apply.

### 2. ULCERATIVE

These tumours, often in the antrum, produce large irregular ulcers with a rolled edge. The rolled edge, rather than the ulcer base, should be biopsied.

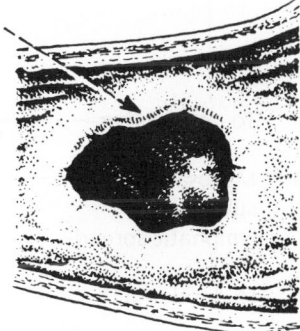

### 3. DIFFUSE PATTERN

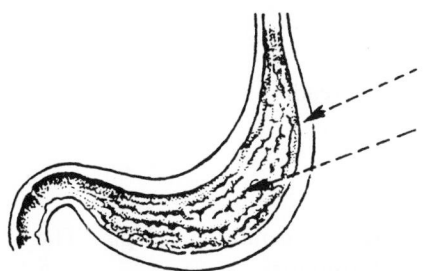

In this form of tumour the entire gastric wall is thickened. Ulceration is usually minimal, but the mucosal folds are prominent.
This is sometimes known as 'leather-bottle stomach' (linitis plastica).

*Histologically*, gastric cancers tend to fall into one of two types:

### (a) Intestinal

Malignant cells arranged in **acini** invade through the muscle of the stomach wall.

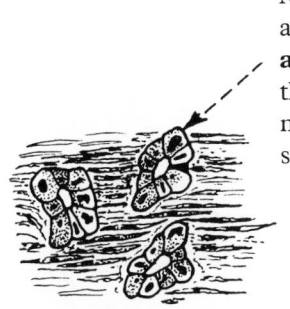

### (b) Diffuse

Typically seen in linitis plastica. These tumours consist of **signet ring cells.**

Extracellular mucin may also be present.

Globules of mucin push the nucleus to one side.

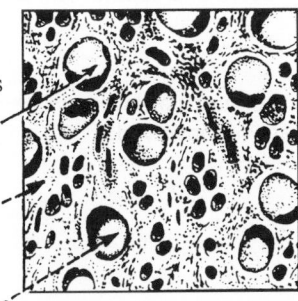

# GASTRIC CARCINOMA

Gastric carcinomas are aggressive tumours with both local and distant spread.

**LOCAL** spread

**DISTANT** spread

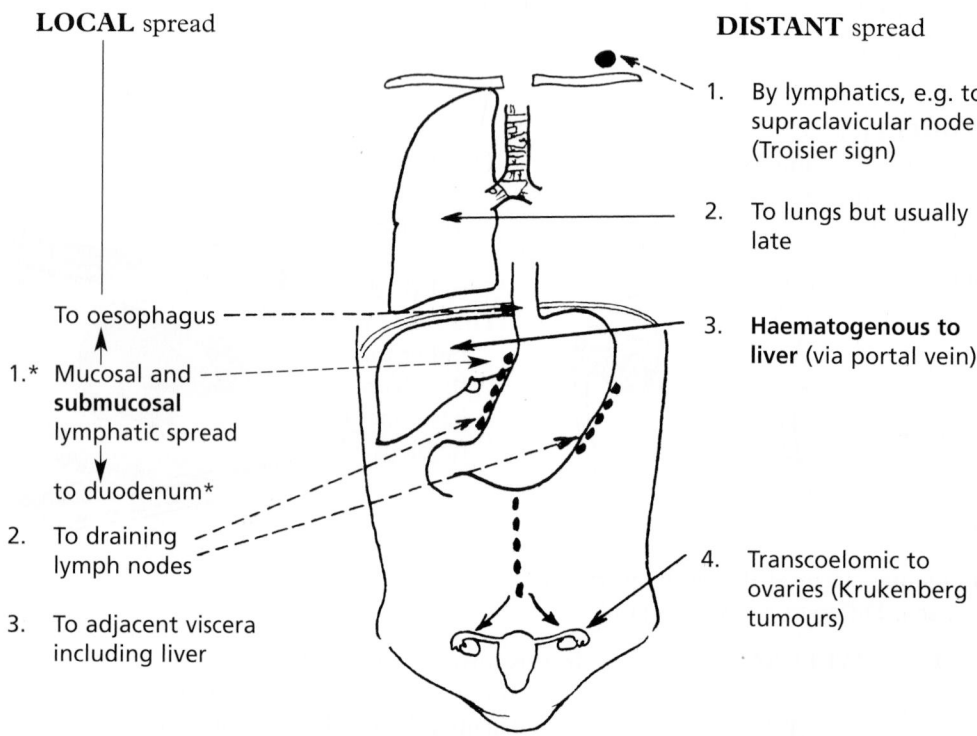

1.  By lymphatics, e.g. to supraclavicular node (Troisier sign)

2.  To lungs but usually late

3.  **Haematogenous to liver** (via portal vein)

4.  Transcoelomic to ovaries (Krukenberg tumours)

To oesophagus

1.* Mucosal and **submucosal** lymphatic spread

to duodenum*

2.  To draining lymph nodes

3.  To adjacent viscera including liver

*Note*: The duodenal mucosa is resistant to direct mucosal spread.
Staging is by the TNM system (Tumour: Nodes: Metastases).

## EARLY GASTRIC CANCER

Early gastric cancers are common in populations where there is screening, e.g. Japan. The prognosis is far better than for deeply penetrating 'advanced' tumours.

By definition, the tumour is confined to the mucosa or mucosa and submucosa.

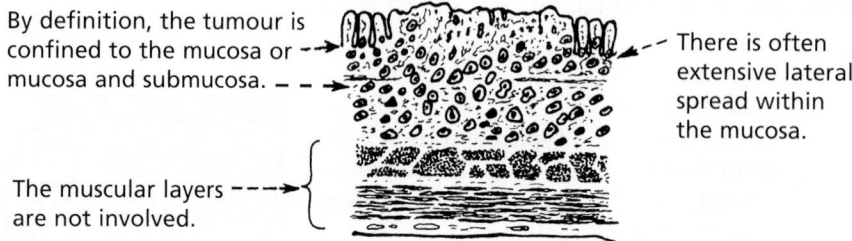

There is often extensive lateral spread within the mucosa.

The muscular layers are not involved.

# GASTRIC CARCINOMA

**Aetiology**

It has long been recognised that gastric cancer occurs in achlorhydric states, especially with chronic atrophic gastritis.

It is now clear that *H. pylori* is a major carcinogenic factor for these tumours arising in the distal stomach. Acid reflux is responsible for those in the proximal stomach.

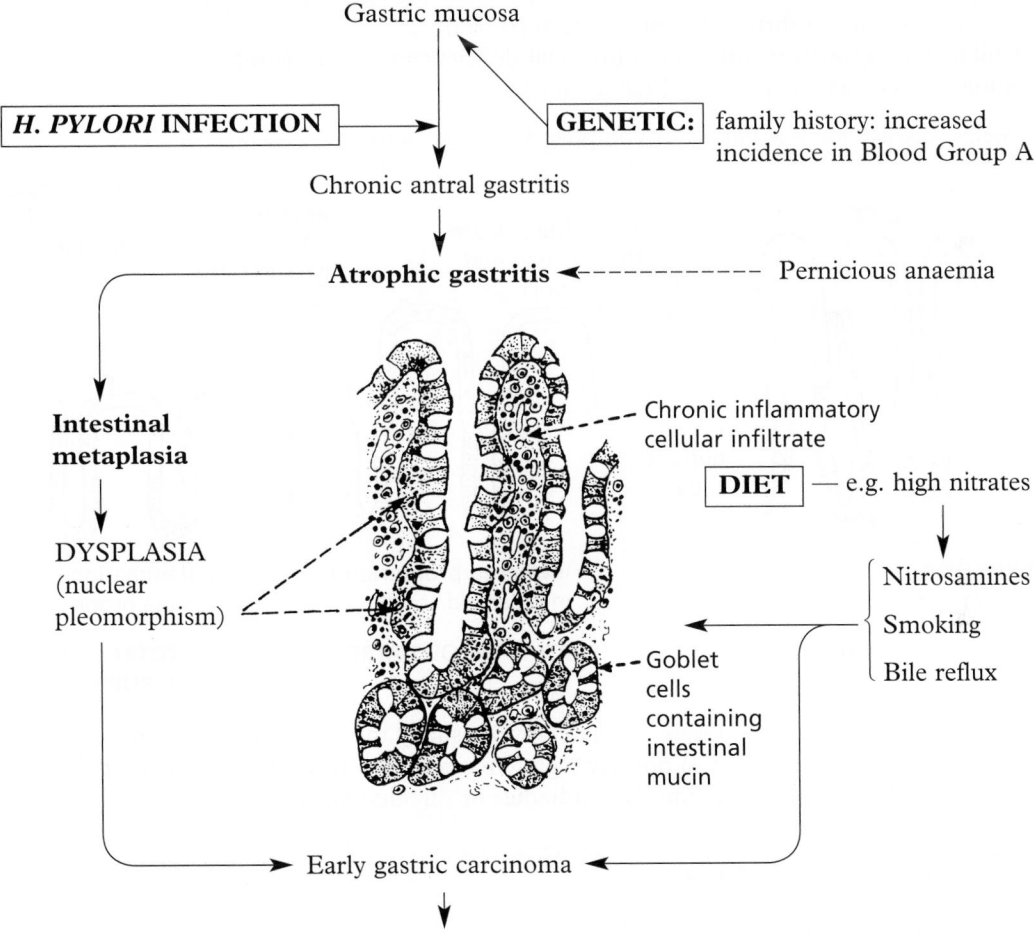

## OTHER GASTRIC TUMOURS

Benign gastric polyps are often seen at endoscopy. Fundic gland polyps are found in patients on proton pump inhibitors.

Gastrointestinal stromal tumours (GISTs) arise from within the stomach wall and may cause haemorrhage. (see p. 364) All are potentially malignant. In advanced cases they can be treated with selective tyrosine kinase inhibitors, e.g. imatinib.

GASTRIC LYMPHOMAS account for 5% of gastric malignancy. They are usually 'B' cell lymphomas of MALT type. They are strongly associated with *H. pylori* infection and some lymphomas respond to eradication of *H. pylori*.

# SMALL INTESTINE – MALABSORPTION

The main function of the small intestine is digestion and absorption of food.

**Malabsorption** may be due to disorders of the small bowel, pancreas or biliary tract.

## COELIAC DISEASE

This important cause of malabsorption is due to sensitivity to gliadin, a component of the wheat protein **gluten**. The clinical features depend on the age at presentation.

Infancy – failure to thrive, diarrhoea (steatorrhoea).
Childhood – growth retardation, nutritional deficiencies, e.g. anaemia.
Adults – anaemia, altered bowel habit, weight loss.

In coeliac disease there is partial or complete villous atrophy.

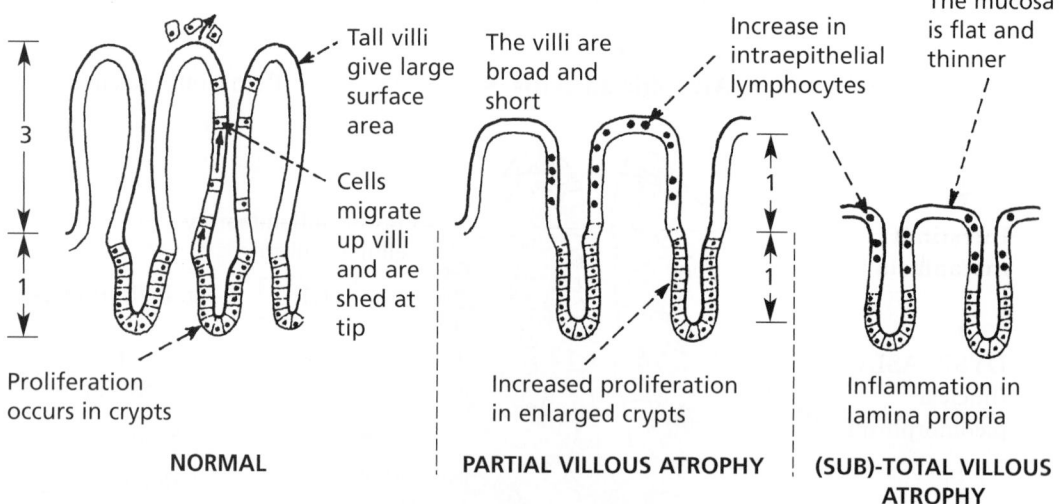

These changes are seen in biopsies of small bowel, usually the distal duodenum by endoscope. The changes revert to normal if gluten is removed from the diet. Serological tests are available with anti-endomysial antibodies or directed against tissue transglutaminase (tTG).

The basic mechanism is as follows:
Genetic predisposition
(e.g. HLA DQ2 or HLA DQ8 +ve)

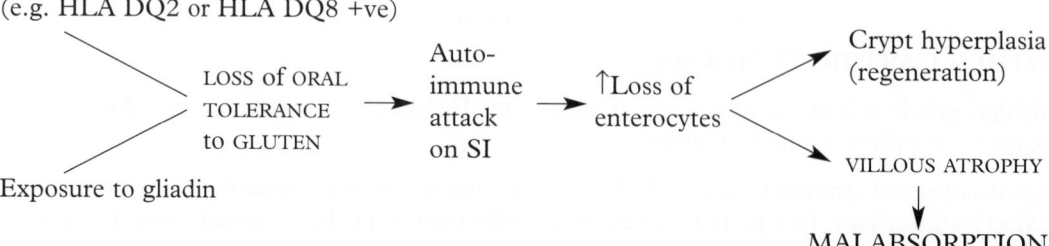

Patients with coeliac disease also have increased prevalence of auto-immune diseases, e.g. diabetes, auto-immune thyroiditis, and of lymphocytic colitis, a cause of diarrhoea (see p. 343). They are at increased risk of developing small bowel **lymphoma** which is of T cell type.

# MALABSORPTION

Other causes of malabsorption in the small bowel include:

1.  **TROPICAL SPRUE**

    This is a disease of unknown aetiology occurring in the tropics. Villous atrophy is seen and patients develop steatorrhoea, weight loss and deficiency of vitamin $B_{12}$ and folate, leading to megaloblastic anaemia. Treatment with folic acid and antibiotics causes the disease to remit.

2.  **GIARDIASIS**

    An infection with the protozoan *Giardia lamblia*, giardiasis is associated with diarrhoea and malabsorption. Patients with hypogammaglobulinaemia are especially at risk.

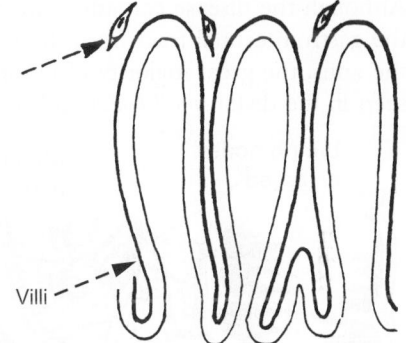

Villi

3.  **WHIPPLE DISEASE**

    In this rare condition, mainly of middle-aged men, malabsorption, arthritis, lymphadenopathy and skin pigmentation are seen.

    Large macrophages fill the lamina propria. They contain mucopolysaccharides (are periodic acid-Schiff [PAS] positive). Electron microscopy shows numerous intracellular bacteria – now thought to be a Gram-positive organism *Tropheryma whippelii*. Antibiotics are curative.

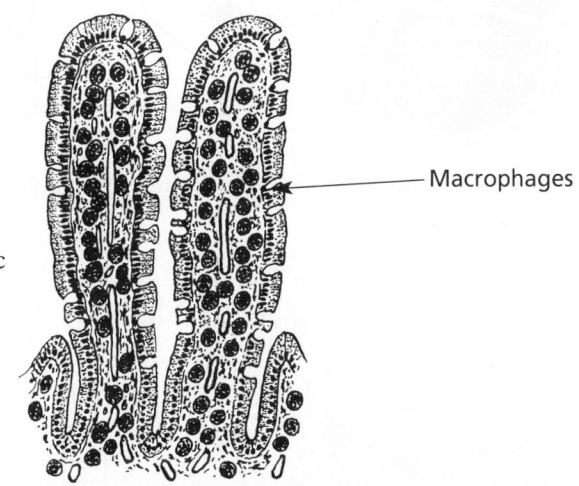

Macrophages

4.  **CROHN'S DISEASE** (p. 340).
5.  After **SMALL BOWEL RESECTION.**
6.  **BIOCHEMICAL DISORDERS,** e.g. disaccharidase deficiency, abetalipoproteinaemia.
7.  **BACTERIAL COLONISATION** of the small bowel, e.g. blind loop syndrome.

    Pancreatic diseases, e.g. cystic fibrosis (p. 407) and obstructive jaundice (p. 372), also cause malabsorption.

# CROHN'S DISEASE

Crohn's disease and ulcerative colitis are two forms of **non-infective inflammatory bowel disease**. They have similarities and striking contrasts (p. 342).

## CROHN'S DISEASE

Patients, usually young adults, present with diarrhoea, abdominal pain and weight loss. Although the disease can affect any part of the gastrointestinal tract from the mouth to the anus, the great majority of lesions are seen in the distal *small bowel* and *colon*.

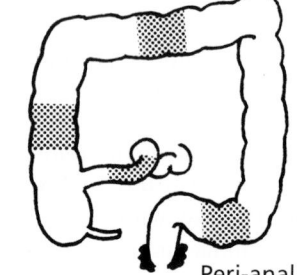

The disease is discontinuous, with 'skip' lesions and normal intervening bowel.

Peri-anal lesions are common.

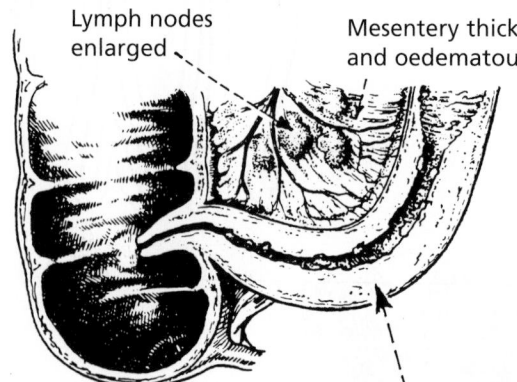

Lymph nodes enlarged

Mesentery thick and oedematous

Mucosal 'cobblestone' appearance.

Linear 'fissured' ulcers

Surviving mucosa forming 'cobbles'

In its classic form, 'regional ileitis', the terminal ileum is thickened and the lumen narrowed and ulcerated.

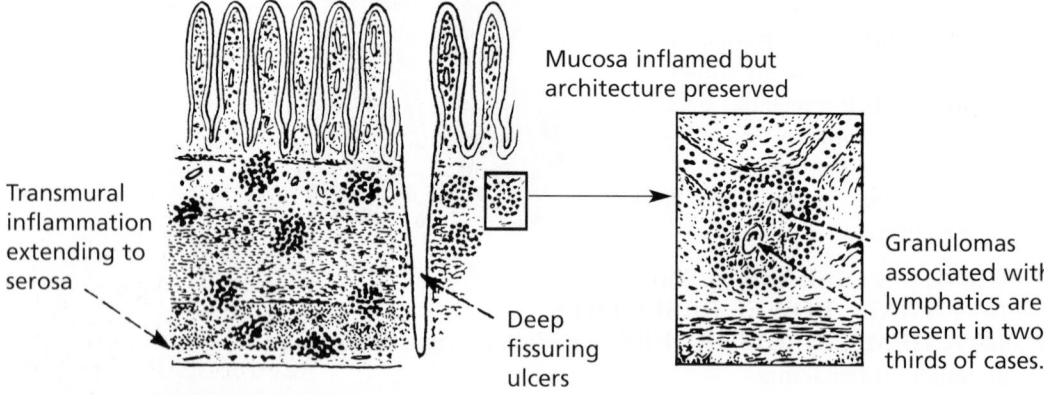

Mucosa inflamed but architecture preserved

Transmural inflammation extending to serosa

Deep fissuring ulcers

Granulomas associated with lymphatics are present in two-thirds of cases.

## LOCAL COMPLICATIONS

**Transmural inflammation** ⟶ adhesions between viscera; fistulae to bowel, bladder, vagina.

**Lumenal narrowing** ⟶ intestinal obstruction.

**Ileal involvement** ⟶ malabsorption, especially of vitamin $B_{12}$.

**Cancer** ⟶ increased risk of colonic and **small intestinal** cancer, but not so great as the risk of colonic cancer in ulcerative colitis.

# ULCERATIVE COLITIS

## Clinical features

Patients, usually young adults, present with diarrhoea, often bloody. The disease has a remitting/relapsing course.

In severe cases weight loss and anaemia occur.

The disease begins in the rectum and shows continuous spread proximally.

The whole colon is affected in 20% of cases.

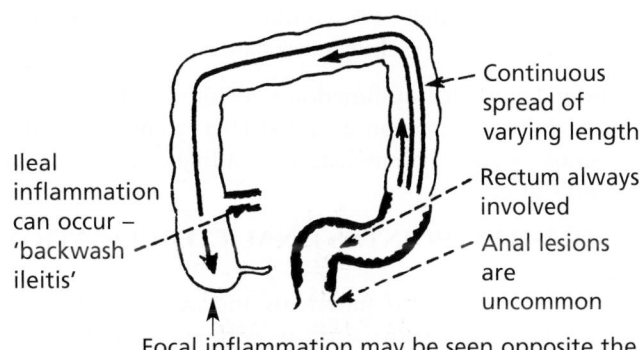

Continuous spread of varying length

Ileal inflammation can occur – 'backwash ileitis'

Rectum always involved

Anal lesions are uncommon

Focal inflammation may be seen opposite the appendix – 'caecal patch'

In the established disease the **gross appearances** are striking.

**Microscopy** shows the evolution.

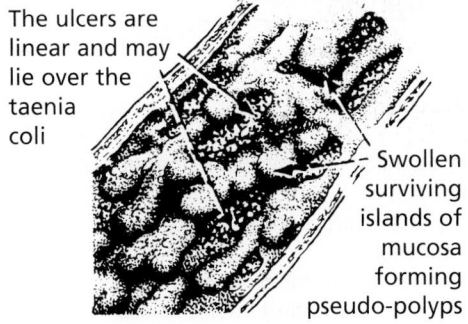

The ulcers are linear and may lie over the taenia coli

Swollen surviving islands of mucosa forming pseudo-polyps

**Early phase**

Mucosa acutely congested especially over the tips of mucosal folds

Neutrophils in the crypts form 'crypt abscesses'

Muscularis mucosae

**Established phase**

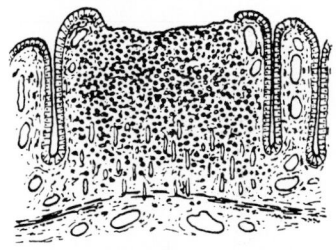

Epithelium lost with ulceration

The inflammation is usually **confined to the mucosa**

**Periods of remission** occur when many of the ulcerated areas heal.

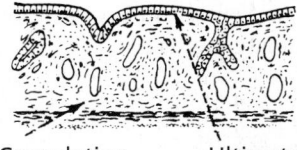

The glands do not reform completely

Granulation tissue

Ultimately the surface may be covered by a simple layer of mucus-secreting epithelium without glands

## LOCAL COMPLICATIONS

**Toxic megacolon**: In a small number of patients, inflammation is very severe and the colon becomes greatly dilated and thinned. There is a high risk of perforation with peritonitis.

**Dysplasia and colonic cancer**: Patients with (a) early onset, (b) total colonic involvement and (c) long-lasting (10–20 years) disease have a greatly increased risk. These patients require colonoscopic surveillance with biopsy to look for dysplasia and cancer.

# CROHN'S DISEASE AND ULCERATIVE COLITIS

The aetiology of these two conditions is uncertain. Both have mild familial tendency (approximately 10%). Infectious causes have been suggested but never proven.

Intestinal epithelial dysfunction may allow entry of bacterial components stimulating mucosal immune responses. Food allergy and stress may be involved in ulcerative colitis. Ex-smokers and non-smokers have a higher risk of ulcerative colitis; the converse is true for Crohn's disease.

## EXTRA-GASTROINTESTINAL COMPLICATIONS – BOTH DISEASES

1. Eye disorders – conjunctivitis and uveitis in <5%.
2. Joints – seronegative arthritis with spinal and peripheral joint involvement approximately 15% (p. 655).
3. Liver – sclerosing cholangitis and cholangiocarcinoma may be seen in ulcerative colitis, but very rarely in Crohn's disease.
4. Erythema nodosum and pyoderma gangrenosum may be found in both.

**Macroscopic differences** in the pathology of ulcerative colitis and Crohn's disease:

| ULCERATIVE COLITIS | CROHN'S DISEASE |
|---|---|
| 1. Lesions continuous – mucosal | Skip lesions – transmural |
| 2. Rectum always involved | Rectum normal in 50% |
| 3. Terminal ileum involved in <10% (backwash ileitis – mild); caecal patch | Terminal ileum involved in 30% |
| 4. Granular, ulcerated mucosa; no fissuring | Discretely ulcerated mucosa; cobblestone appearance; fissuring |
| 5. Often intensely vascular | Vascularity seldom pronounced |
| 6. Normal serosa | Serositis common |
| 7. Muscular shortening of colon | Fibrous shortening; strictures common |
| 8. Fistulae rare | Enterocutaneous or intestinal fistulae in 10% |
| 9. Malignant change – well recognised | Malignant change – less common |
| 10. Anal lesions uncommon | Anal lesions in 75%; anal fistulae; ulceration or chronic fissure |

It may be impossible to distinguish between ulcerative colitis and Crohn's disease. This is classified as 'indeterminate colitis'.

# MICROSCOPIC COLITIS

This term describes two forms of colitis which are often overlooked because the colon appears normal on colonoscopy. Both tend to occur in middle-aged women who present with chronic watery diarrhoea. The diagnoses depend on identification of characteristic histological findings.

## COLLAGENOUS COLITIS

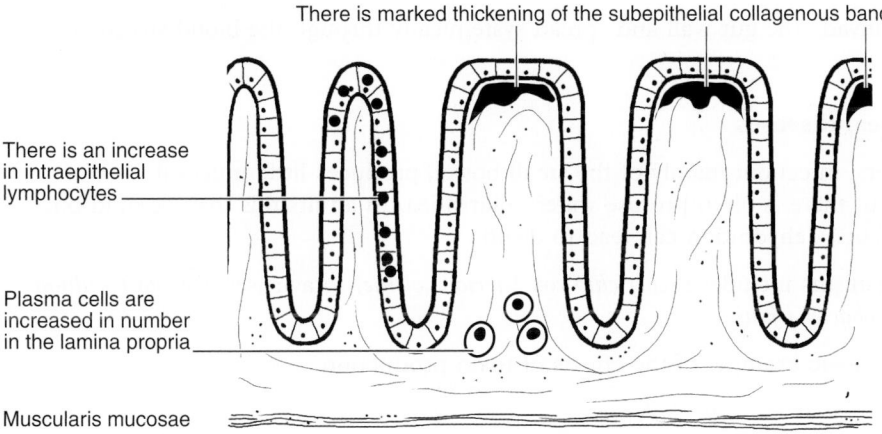

There is marked thickening of the subepithelial collagenous band

There is an increase in intraepithelial lymphocytes

Plasma cells are increased in number in the lamina propria

Muscularis mucosae

Patients often have co-existing diseases, typically auto-immune, such as rheumatoid arthritis, coeliac disease and diabetes.

## LYMPHOCYTIC COLITIS

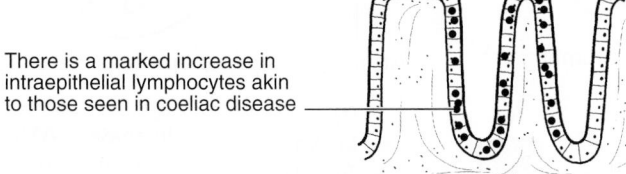

There is a marked increase in intraepithelial lymphocytes akin to those seen in coeliac disease

It is likely that collagenous and lymphocytic colitis are part of the spectrum of the same disease. A relapsing and remitting course is often seen.

# INTESTINAL INFECTIONS

Viruses, bacteria, protozoa and worms can all infect the gastrointestinal tract. There are three main patterns of infection:

1. Organisms remain within the lumen of the gut and release toxins which damage the surface epithelium, e.g. cholera.
2. Organisms invade the wall of the gut, but remain localised to the gut wall, e.g. bacillary dysentery.
3. Organisms invade the gut wall and spread systemically through the blood stream, e.g. typhoid.

**Acute diarrhoeal diseases**

In these disorders, infection, mainly of the small bowel, produces little mucosal inflammation, but there is often profuse watery diarrhoea. In adults this may be mild but, especially in infants, dehydration can lead to death.

Responsible organisms include: *Escherichia coli, Vibrio cholerae,* rotaviruses, *Cryptosporidium parvum, Campylobacter jejuni.*

**Cholera** is the classic example of the effects of toxin production.

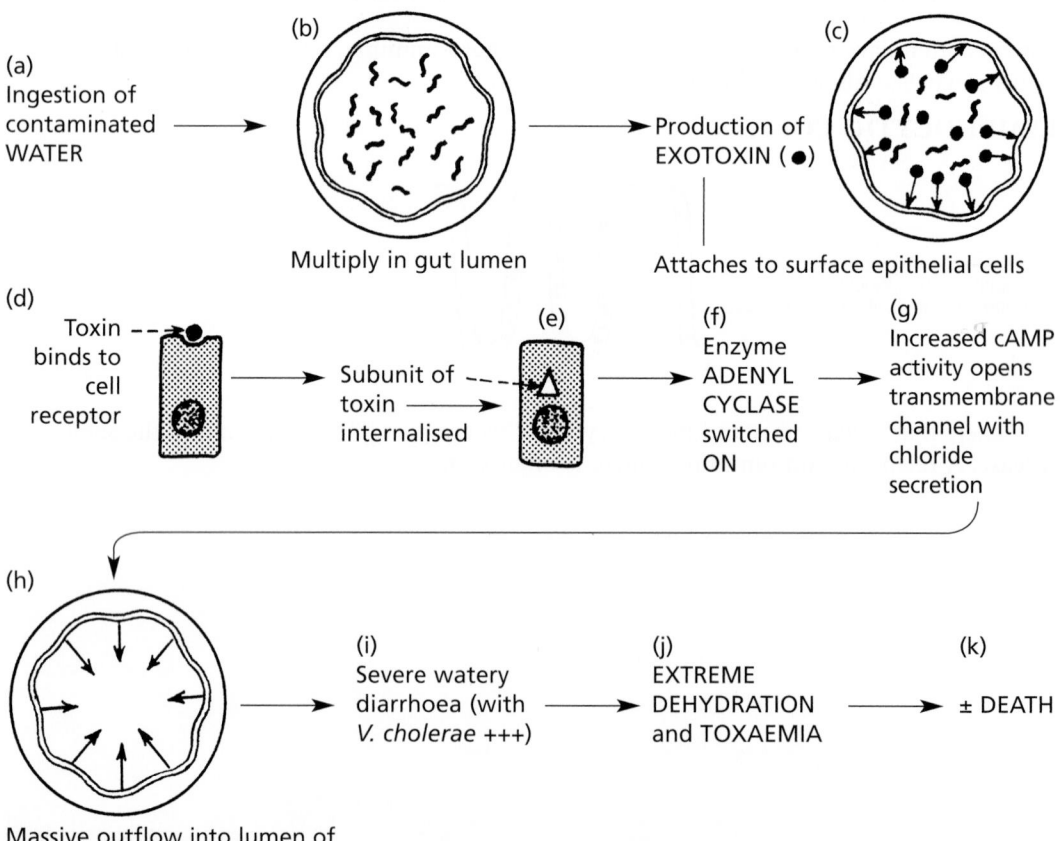

# INTESTINAL INFECTIONS

***E. coli*** 0157 is a strain which produces exotoxin causing haemorrhagic colitis, often complicated by renal failure in the elderly or the haemolytic uraemic syndrome in children. The contamination is on meat or meat products. Outbreaks and sporadic cases occur worldwide.

**Toxic enteritis** (food poisoning)

Many bacteria release enterotoxins into food before it is consumed: although cooking kills the bacteria, the preformed toxin may be heat resistant. *Staphylococcus aureus* and *Bacillus cereus* (in rice particularly) are good examples.

In **ROTAVIRUS infection**, seen especially in children under 5 years, the mechanism is different.

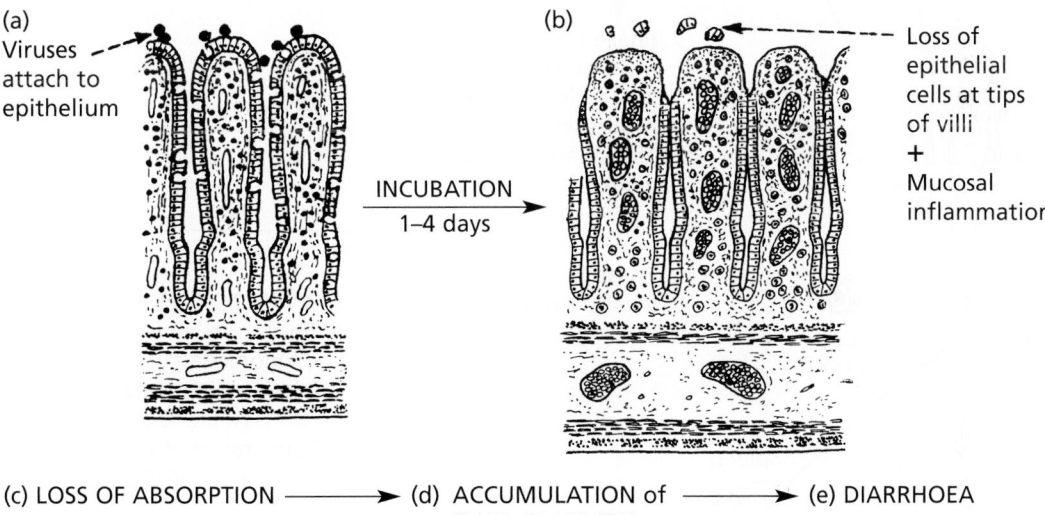

(a) Viruses attach to epithelium

INCUBATION 1–4 days

(b) Loss of epithelial cells at tips of villi

\+

Mucosal inflammation

(c) LOSS OF ABSORPTION ⟶ (d) ACCUMULATION of ⟶ (e) DIARRHOEA
FLUID IN LUMEN

*Note*: Recovery is usually rapid and complete, providing dehydration is treated. Vaccination against rotavirus is now given routinely to babies.

# TYPHOID

### Salmonella infections

Salmonella infections vary from food poisoning, usually a mild inflammation with diarrhoea, to typhoid fever which if untreated is often fatal.

### TYPHOID FEVER

Following ingestion of *Salmonella typhi*, the disease process falls into three distinct phases.

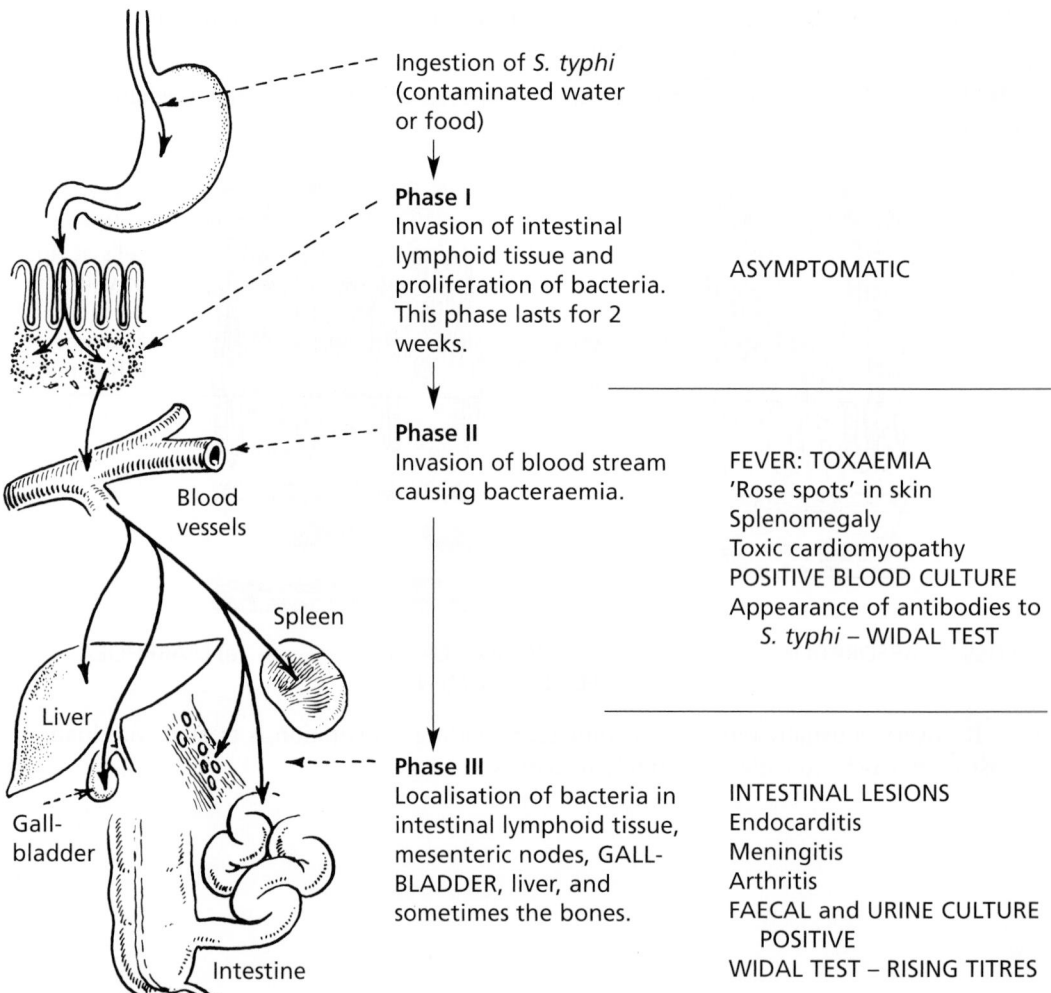

Ingestion of *S. typhi* (contaminated water or food)

**Phase I**
Invasion of intestinal lymphoid tissue and proliferation of bacteria. This phase lasts for 2 weeks.

ASYMPTOMATIC

**Phase II**
Invasion of blood stream causing bacteraemia.

FEVER: TOXAEMIA
'Rose spots' in skin
Splenomegaly
Toxic cardiomyopathy
POSITIVE BLOOD CULTURE
Appearance of antibodies to
   *S. typhi* – WIDAL TEST

Blood vessels

Spleen

Liver

Gall-bladder

Intestine

**Phase III**
Localisation of bacteria in intestinal lymphoid tissue, mesenteric nodes, GALL-BLADDER, liver, and sometimes the bones.

INTESTINAL LESIONS
Endocarditis
Meningitis
Arthritis
FAECAL and URINE CULTURE
   POSITIVE
WIDAL TEST – RISING TITRES

# TYPHOID

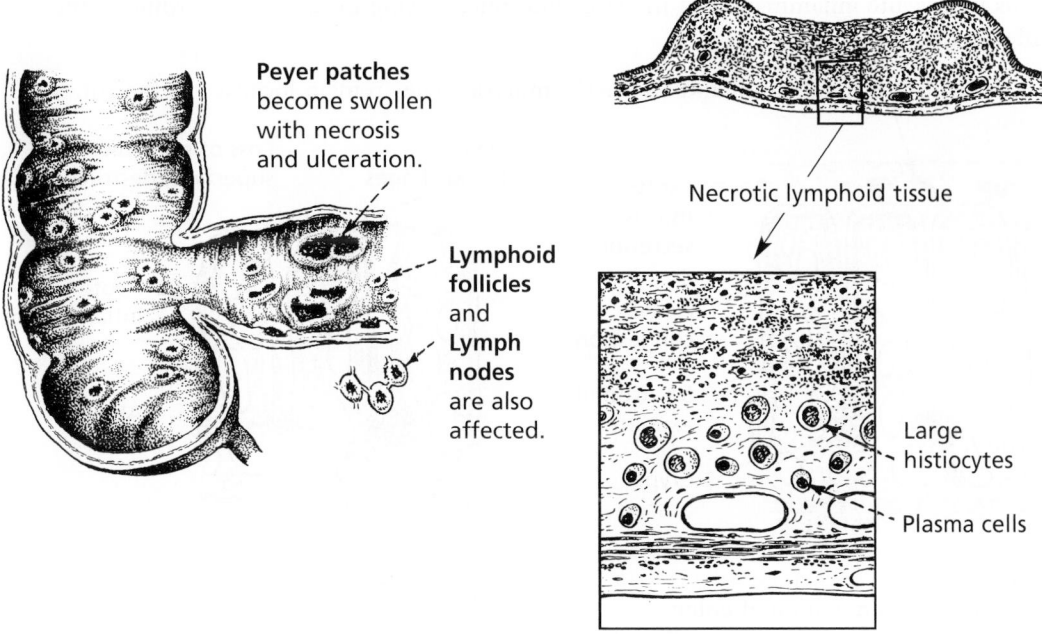

Peyer patches become swollen with necrosis and ulceration.

Lymphoid follicles and Lymph nodes are also affected.

Necrotic lymphoid tissue

Large histiocytes

Plasma cells

## Sequelae

1.  Healing is the usual outcome.

2.  Deep intestinal ulceration — haemorrhage.
    — perforation and peritonitis (usually fatal).

3.  Persistent infection (1–3%) – usually GALLBLADDER or urinary tract.

These carriers appear healthy but are an important source of outbreaks.

## PARATYPHOID FEVER

This disease is clinically indistinguishable from typhoid fever but is usually much less severe.

The pathological changes resemble those of typhoid fever but are commonly limited to a small portion of the bowel. Frequently there is an absence of ulceration.

Two serological types of the paratyphoid organism are recognised, A and B. Type B is a common cause of enteric fever in Europe. As in typhoid, patients often become 'carriers'.

*Note*: TAB vaccination, using antigens derived from *S. typhi* and *Salmonella paratyphi A and B*, produces a very effective active immunity.

# BACILLARY DYSENTERY

This is an acute inflammation of the large intestine, varying in severity according to the infecting agent.

The bacteria adhere to and *invade* the mucosa. They remain localised to the gut.

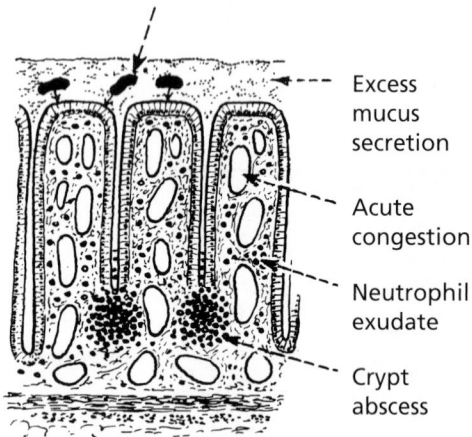

Excess mucus secretion

Acute congestion

Neutrophil exudate

Crypt abscess

*Shigella sonnei*
Mild acute inflammation of colon.
Commonest form in the United Kingdom.

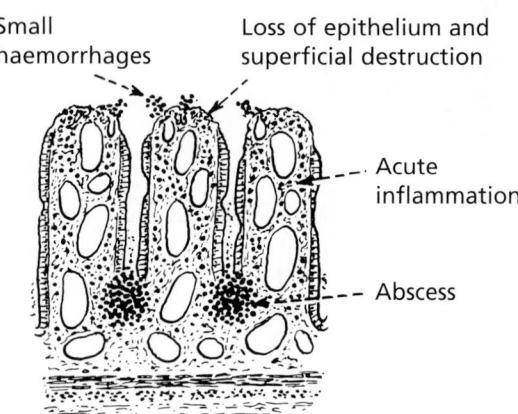

Small haemorrhages

Loss of epithelium and superficial destruction

Acute inflammation

Abscess

*Shigella flexneri*
Severe acute inflammation.

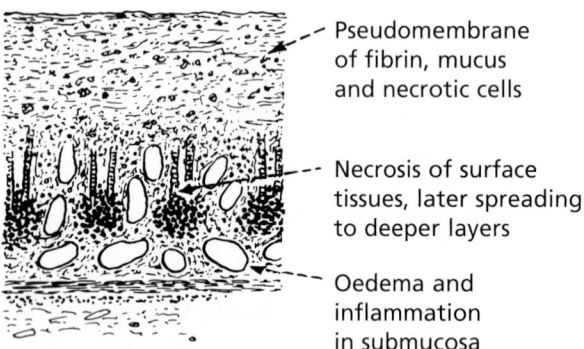

Pseudomembrane of fibrin, mucus and necrotic cells

Necrosis of surface tissues, later spreading to deeper layers

Oedema and inflammation in submucosa

*Shigella dysenteriae*
Most severe type, occurs in tropics.

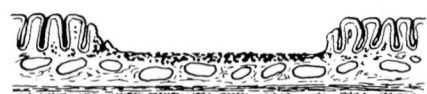

Irregular spreading ulcers with thin shredded margins are formed by shedding of necrotic material.

### Clinical manifestations

There is acute diarrhoea with abdominal pain, tenesmus and the passage of blood-stained mucus. *S. dysenteriae* infections are often associated with severe toxaemia and sometimes a shock-like condition. Blood, mucus and neutrophils are found in the faeces, and in the early stages the bacilli can be isolated.

Healing by resolution with complete restoration of the mucosa is usual. Only in exceptional cases does relapse occur with consequent scarring.

# AMOEBIC DYSENTERY

This is due to infection by *Entamoeba histolytica* in food and water. It is most often seen in tropical and subtropical countries.

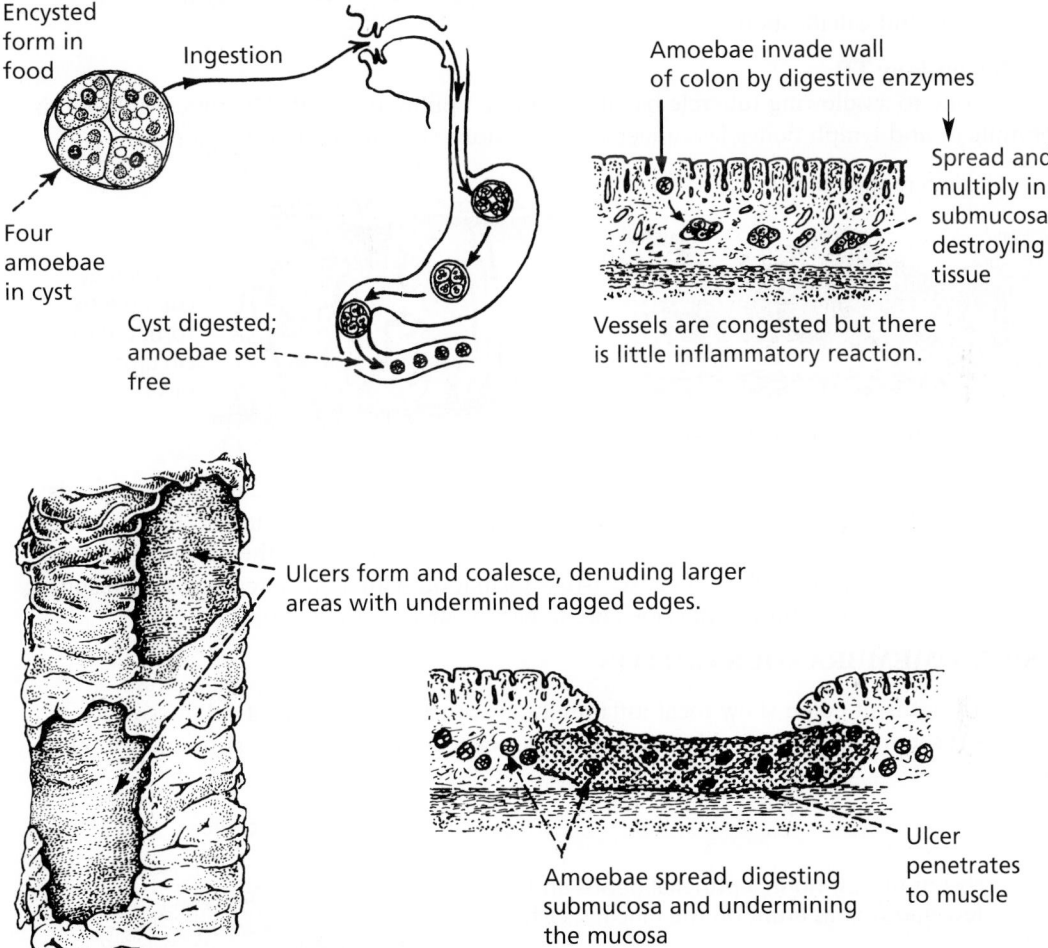

Encysted form in food

Ingestion

Four amoebae in cyst

Cyst digested; amoebae set free

Amoebae invade wall of colon by digestive enzymes

Spread and multiply in submucosa, destroying tissue

Vessels are congested but there is little inflammatory reaction.

Ulcers form and coalesce, denuding larger areas with undermined ragged edges.

Amoebae spread, digesting submucosa and undermining the mucosa

Ulcer penetrates to muscle

Healing of the ulcers with fibrosis occurs. The disease persists with overgrowth of fibrous tissue, adhesions to various structures. Fistulae may occur. Occasionally the amoebae may invade portal venous tributaries and cause amoebic abscess of the liver (p. 391).

Large numbers of motile amoebae can be found in the faeces during the acute phase of the disease. Later, in the chronic state, they are frequently in an encysted form. Mucus and blood are abundant.

*Note*: Non-pathogenic amoebae can be found in the colon of healthy individuals.

# TUBERCULOUS ENTERITIS AND PSEUDOMEMBRANOUS COLITIS

1. **Primary TB infection** usually follows ingestion of infected milk containing bovine tubercle bacilli. It affects the small bowel. It is similar to primary TB of the lung – a small mucosal lesion and enlarged caseous lymph nodes. These usually heal with fibrosis and calcification.

2. **Secondary TB**

This is due to swallowing tubercle bacilli from open pulmonary TB. The mucosal lesion is prominent and lymph nodes less affected. The lesions start in the Peyer's patches.

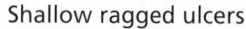

Shallow ragged ulcers

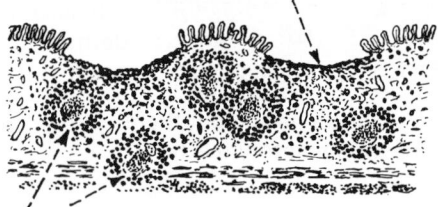

Caseating granulomas in all layers.

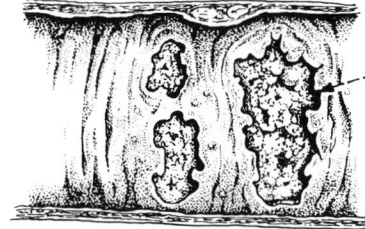

Ulcers may coalesce to form a large circumferential ulcer.

As in the lung, there is a good deal of fibrous granulation tissue surrounding the caseous lesions and the vessels undergo obliteration. For this reason, perforation and haemorrhage are uncommon. Adhesions to other loops of bowel are common and the caseating process may erode through the walls and cause fistula formation with short circuiting and resulting malabsorption. If the fibrous adhesions are dense, obstruction may arise.

## PSEUDOMEMBRANOUS COLITIS

Varying lengths of colon show focal inflammation with the formation of yellow surface plaques (pseudomembranes). Most cases are associated with the use of antibiotics in elderly patients.

**Microscopic**

Foci of mucus, fibrin, epithelial debris and a few neutrophils erupt on the mucous surface

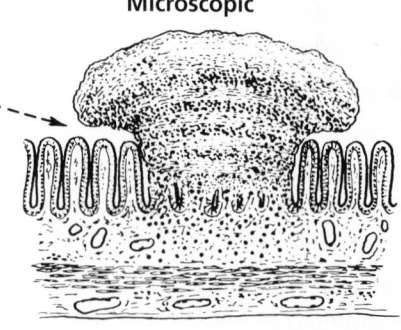

**Naked eye appearance**

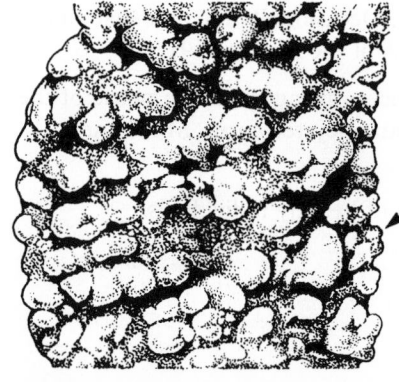

The lesions may coalesce forming typical adherent plaques over large areas, resulting in death. The lesions are caused by toxins from *Clostridium difficile* – an anaerobe normally present in small numbers which proliferate due to elimination of competing bacteria by the antibiotic. The toxin can be found in the stools.

# APPENDICITIS

**Acute appendicitis** is a common cause of abdominal pain requiring surgery, particularly in the West where there is a low roughage diet.

Appendicitis usually follows obstruction of the lumen with distal infection and ulceration. The usual causes are:

(a) Viral infection → reactive hyperplasia of lymphoid follicles. (Infection by *Yersinia enterocolitica* can have similar effects.)

(b) Inspissated faeces (faecoliths).

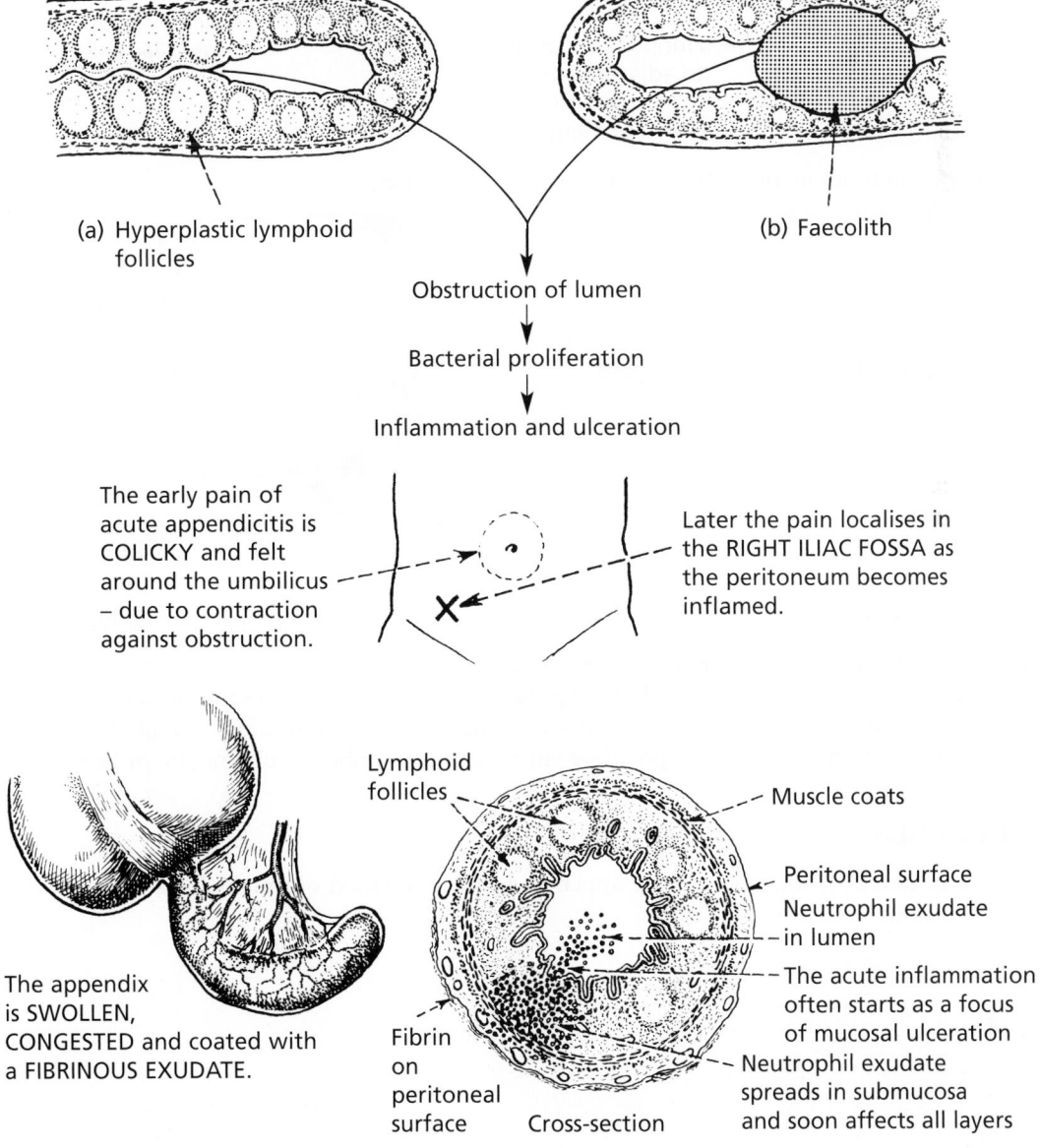

(a) Hyperplastic lymphoid follicles

(b) Faecolith

Obstruction of lumen

Bacterial proliferation

Inflammation and ulceration

The early pain of acute appendicitis is COLICKY and felt around the umbilicus – due to contraction against obstruction.

Later the pain localises in the RIGHT ILIAC FOSSA as the peritoneum becomes inflamed.

The appendix is SWOLLEN, CONGESTED and coated with a FIBRINOUS EXUDATE.

Lymphoid follicles

Muscle coats

Peritoneal surface

Neutrophil exudate in lumen

The acute inflammation often starts as a focus of mucosal ulceration

Fibrin on peritoneal surface

Cross-section

Neutrophil exudate spreads in submucosa and soon affects all layers

# APPENDICITIS – SEQUELS

If untreated the appendicitis may become suppurative or gangrenous. The following complications are fortunately very rare.

1. **General peritonitis** is the most important complication since it results in toxaemia and may be fatal. It is especially associated with gangrenous appendicitis but may complicate any type of acute appendicitis.

2. **Appendix abscess**

This arises in the following way:

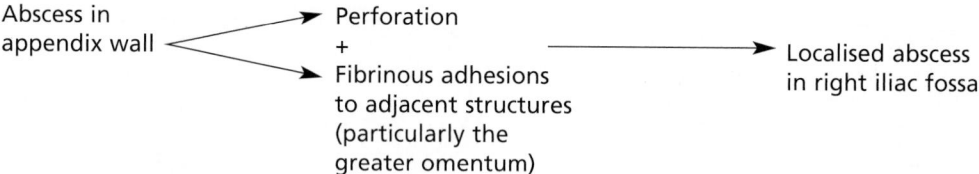

Further complications may arise due to spread of infection:
(a) Along the right paracolic gutter to produce a subphrenic abscess between the diaphragm and liver.
(b) Into the pelvis to form abscesses around bladder and rectum. In the female the uterus and fallopian tube may be involved.

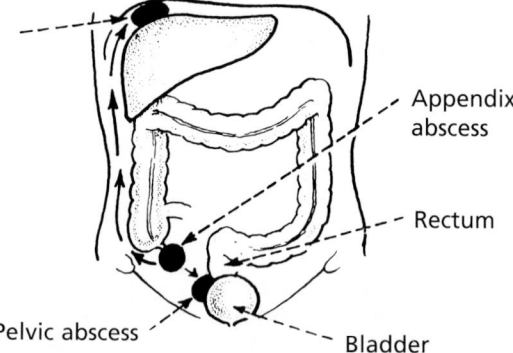

3. **Adhesions**
Intestinal obstruction may result from constricting bands, or volvulus may be induced.

4. **Liver abscesses and portal pylephlebitis**
These are now rare. They are due to spread of infection to the mesenteric veins resulting in septic embolism. Liver abscesses usually arise from infective emboli, but occasionally there may be a spreading suppurating thrombosis culminating in hepatic sepsis.

## MUCOCELE

This term describes dilatation of the appendix by accumulation of mucus. This may be due to a mucinous cystadenoma.

# DIVERTICULAR DISEASE

**Diverticula** are common in the **sigmoid colon,** affecting at least 50% of adults over 60 years in societies where the diet lacks fibre (low residue).

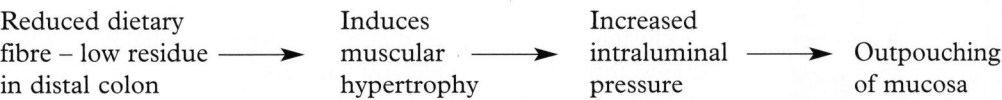

Reduced dietary fibre – low residue in distal colon ⟶ Induces muscular hypertrophy ⟶ Increased intraluminal pressure ⟶ Outpouching of mucosa

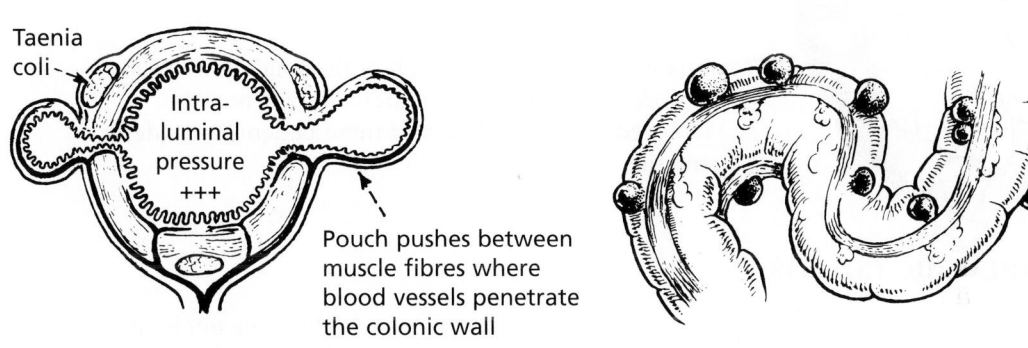

Pouch pushes between muscle fibres where blood vessels penetrate the colonic wall

## COMPLICATIONS

Diverticulitis is common.

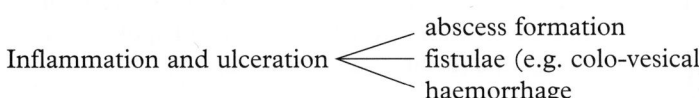

Inflammation and ulceration ⟨— abscess formation
— fistulae (e.g. colo-vesical)
— haemorrhage

Repeated attacks
↓
Fibro-muscular thickening
↓
Stenosis

*Note*: This may simulate carcinoma.

**Other diverticula** are also found in the caecum and small intestine: in the latter, colonisation by bacteria which utilise vitamin $B_{12}$ may lead to macrocytic anaemia.

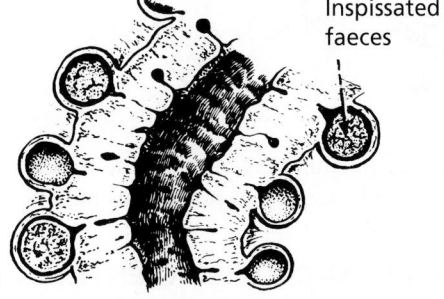

Inspissated faeces

Inflammatory fibromuscular thickening

**Meckel diverticulum** of the small intestine is present in 2% of the population.

It is a remnant of the **vitello-intestinal duct** about 60 cm proximal to the ileo-caecal valve.

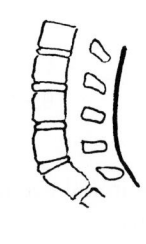

Complications are rare:

(1) The wide communication with the bowel precludes stasis and inflammation.
(2) Rarely ectopic gastric or pancreatic tissue cause local damage (p. 332).

353

# ISCHAEMIA AND THE INTESTINES

### ACUTE VASCULAR OCCLUSION

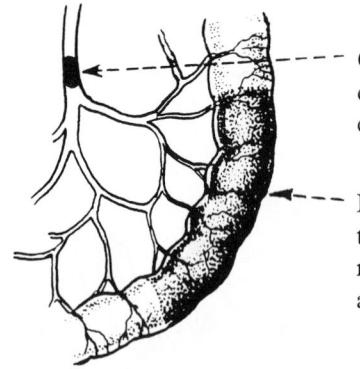

Occlusion of the superior mesenteric artery is usually due to thrombosis complicating atheroma, or embolism from the left side of the heart or aorta.

Infarction of a loop or much of the small bowel leads to abdominal pain. The infarcted bowel must be removed surgically. Many of these patients are elderly and die.

### ISCHAEMIC COLITIS

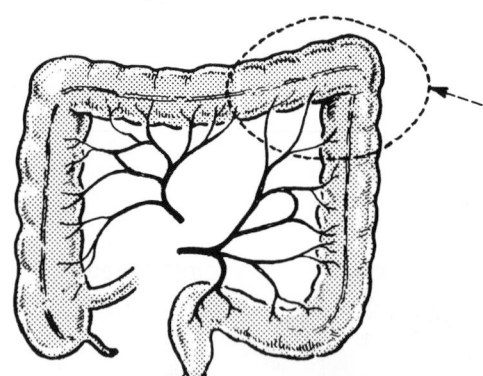

The colon is more vulnerable to chronic ischaemia than the small bowel.

Ischaemic colitis commonly affects the splenic flexure – the watershed zone. It often occurs in patients with arterial disease with hypotension, e.g. due to shock or cardiac failure.

Milder ischaemia ⟶ mucosal ulceration
↓
healing with stricture

Severe ischaemia ⟶ gangrene of bowel

Intestinal ischaemia may also be due to arteritis, as a side effect of radiation therapy. Drug-induced ulcers, e.g. potassium tablets and NSAIDs, appear to be due to local ischaemia.

### NEONATAL NECROTISING ENTEROCOLITIS

This lesion occurs in premature babies in their first week.

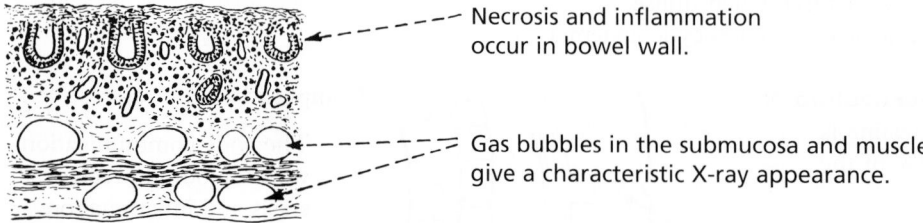

Necrosis and inflammation occur in bowel wall.

Gas bubbles in the submucosa and muscle give a characteristic X-ray appearance.

Bowel ischaemia appears to be the initial event, but there is then bacterial superinfection, especially by gas-forming organisms.

# INTESTINAL OBSTRUCTION

Intestinal obstruction can be caused by:

(a) External compression – e.g. hernias, volvulus.
(b) Lesions of the bowel wall – e.g. tumours, inflammatory strictures, intussusception.
(c) Intraluminal blockage – e.g. gallstone ileus (p. 399).

The patient may present with colicky abdominal pain, vomiting and failure to pass flatus or faeces.

### Acute obstruction

Immediately following the obstruction there is a period of very active peristalsis

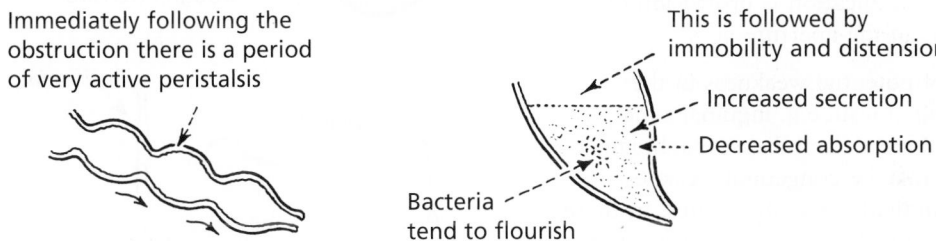

This is followed by immobility and distension

Increased secretion

Decreased absorption

Bacteria tend to flourish

### Subacute obstruction

As the condition develops gradually, hypertrophy of the muscle is seen proximal to the obstruction.

Later, obstruction increases and muscle hypertrophy cannot compensate.

Dilatation of the bowel follows with accumulation of gas and fluid.

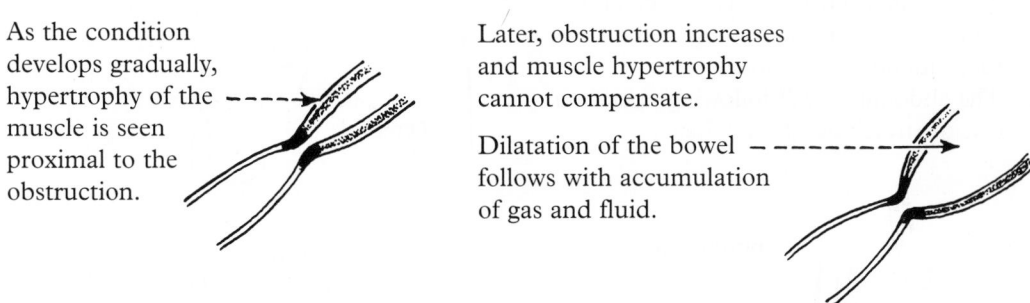

This gross distension has several effects:

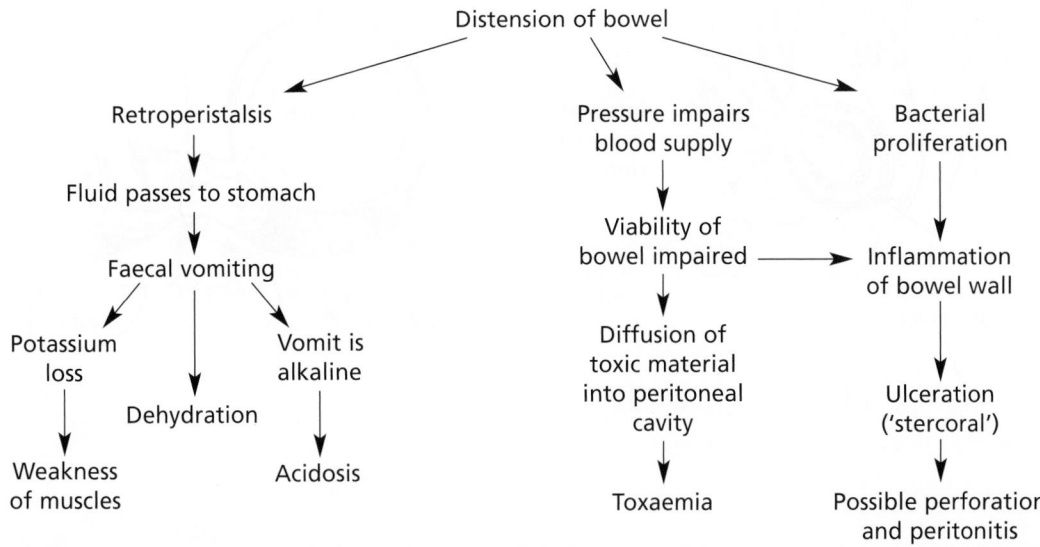

Distension of bowel

Retroperistalsis → Fluid passes to stomach → Faecal vomiting → Potassium loss → Weakness of muscles; Dehydration; Vomit is alkaline → Acidosis

Pressure impairs blood supply → Viability of bowel impaired → Diffusion of toxic material into peritoneal cavity → Toxaemia

Bacterial proliferation → Inflammation of bowel wall → Ulceration ('stercoral') → Possible perforation and peritonitis

355

# HERNIA

### HERNIA

This means the protrusion of peritoneum through an aperture.

When the hernial swelling appears on the surface of the body, it is termed 'external'; those which do not present on the body surface are 'internal'.

The main complication is protrusion of bowel through the aperture at:

1. Sites of potential weakness in the abdominal wall, e.g. inguinal canal, femoral canal, umbilicus, diaphragm. There may be congenital weakness in some individuals at these sites. In these cases a pouch of peritoneum protrudes through the aperture.
2. Normal peritoneal extensions, e.g. the foramen of Winslow leading to the lesser sac, jejunoduodenal fossa.
3. The abdominal wall following operation due to stretching of scar tissue.

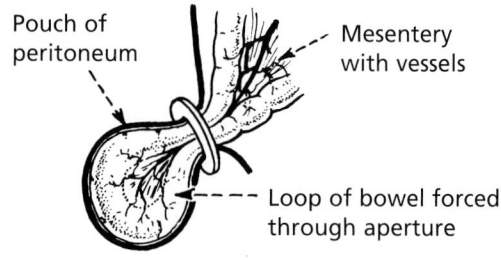

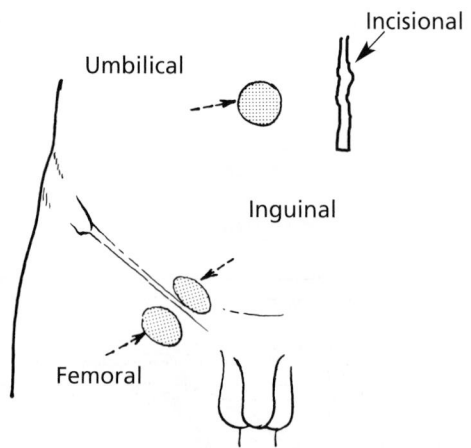

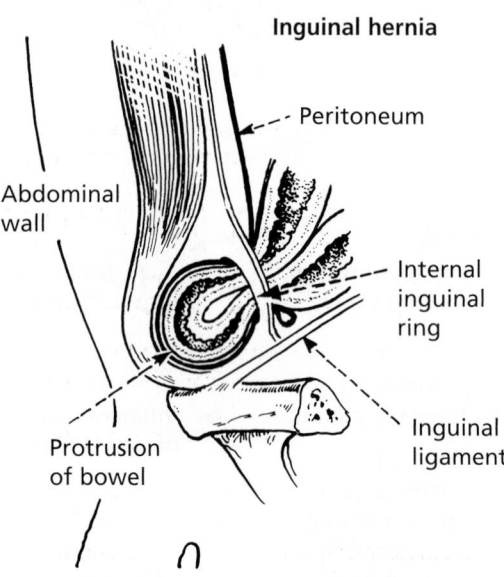

**Inguinal hernia**

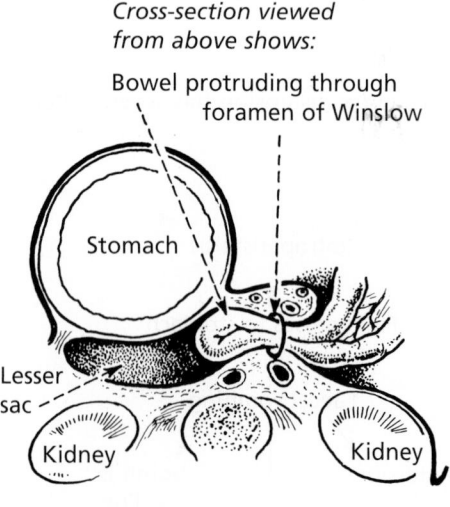

*Cross-section viewed from above shows:*

# HERNIA – COMPLICATIONS

## Complications of hernia

Initially, when the herniated portion of bowel is small it can be pushed back into the abdominal cavity – *reducible*.

Increased intra-abdominal pressure, e.g. during muscular exertion, coughing or straining due to constipation, helps to induce the herniation. With time the hernia increases in size. Secondary changes may occur.

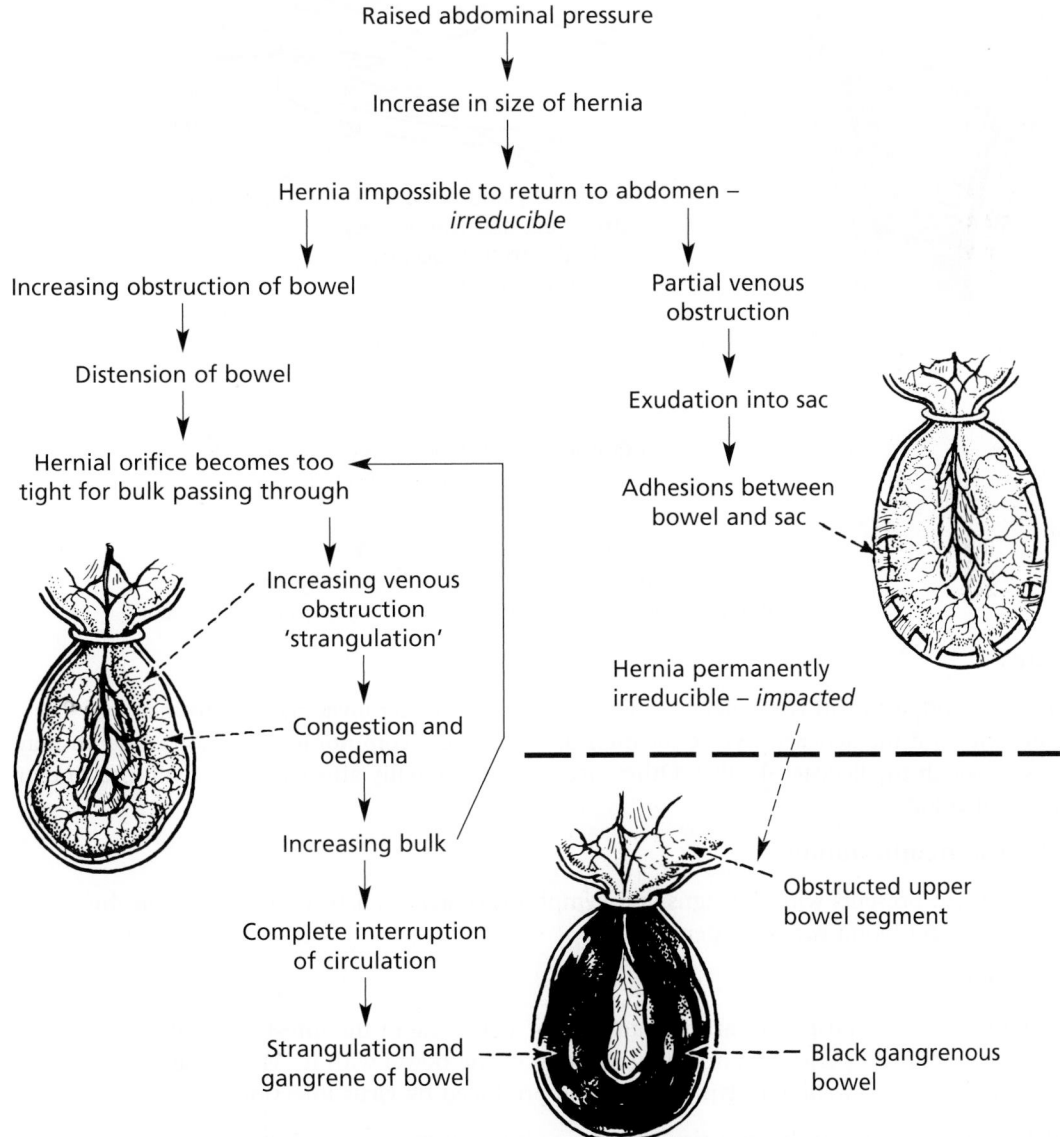

Raised abdominal pressure

↓

Increase in size of hernia

↓

Hernia impossible to return to abdomen – *irreducible*

Increasing obstruction of bowel

↓

Distension of bowel

↓

Hernial orifice becomes too tight for bulk passing through

↓

Increasing venous obstruction 'strangulation'

↓

Congestion and oedema

↓

Increasing bulk

↓

Complete interruption of circulation

↓

Strangulation and gangrene of bowel

Partial venous obstruction

↓

Exudation into sac

↓

Adhesions between bowel and sac

Hernia permanently irreducible – *impacted*

Obstructed upper bowel segment

Black gangrenous bowel

# INTUSSUSCEPTION

## INTUSSUSCEPTION

This is a condition in which the bowel is invaginated into itself.

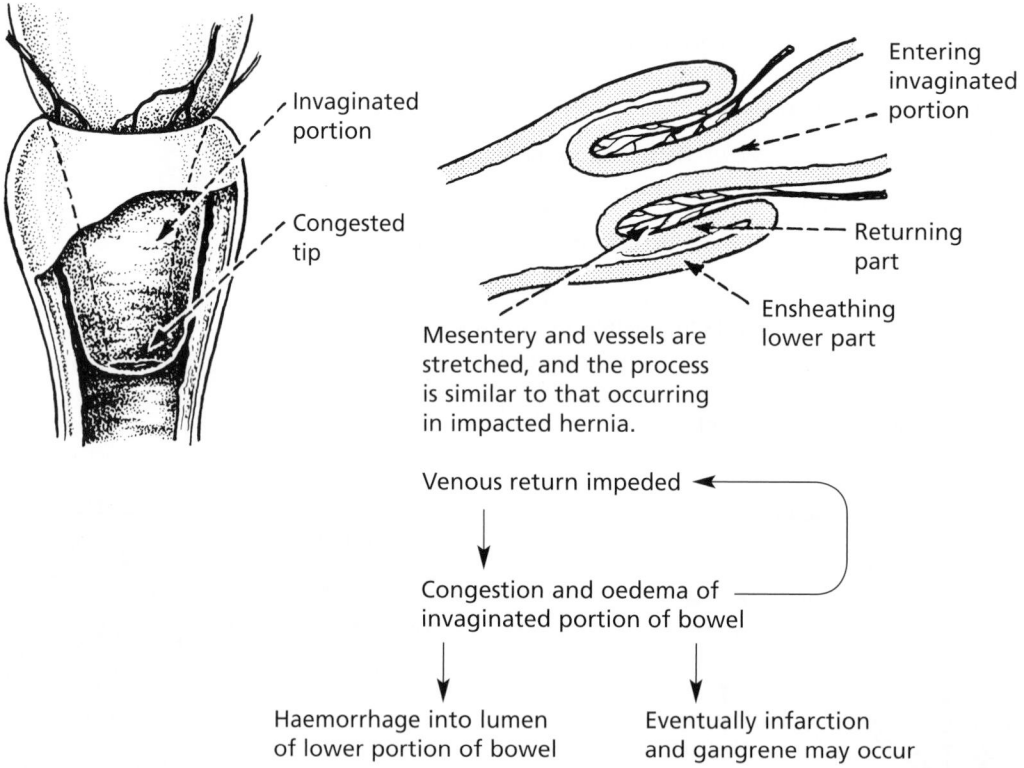

### Sites

The commonest form is the ileocaecal type, the ileum being invaginated into the large intestine with the ileocaecal valve forming the apex. Less commonly, a portion of ileum may pass through the ileocaecal valve. Other sites are occasionally affected, e.g. small intestine or parts of colon.

### Clinical manifestations

The patient presents with the signs and symptoms of acute obstruction, a mass in the abdomen and blood is passed per rectum.

### Aetiology

It is thought that most cases arise as a result of a swelling in the intestinal wall which is pushed distally by peristalsis, dragging the wall of the bowel with it. Most cases arise in childhood due to swelling of lymphoid tissue produced by virus infection.

Polypoidal tumours of the intestine may cause intussusception in adults.

# VOLVULUS AND HIRSCHSPRUNG DISEASE

## VOLVULUS

As the name suggests, this is a rotation or revolving of the bowel. It affects bowel with a long mesentery. Another factor is the closeness of the ends of the affected loop.

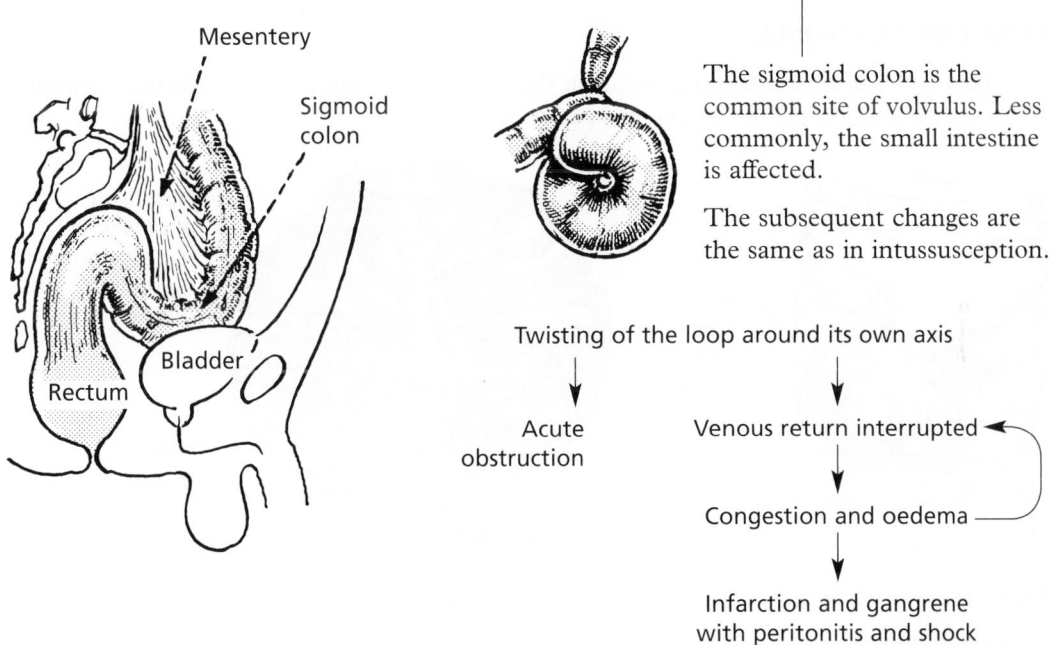

The sigmoid colon is the common site of volvulus. Less commonly, the small intestine is affected.

The subsequent changes are the same as in intussusception.

Twisting of the loop around its own axis

Acute obstruction

Venous return interrupted

Congestion and oedema

Infarction and gangrene with peritonitis and shock

## HIRSCHSPRUNG DISEASE

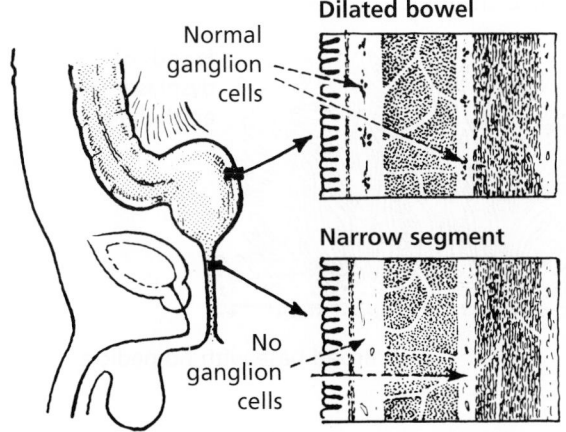

Hirschsprung disease is a rare cause of chronic intestinal obstruction. It is due to a congenital absence of ganglion cells in the parasympathetic Auerbach and Meissner complexes of the rectum. Mutations in genes, including the RET gene, are often responsible.

The aganglionic rectal segment and anus cannot relax and the bowel above becomes grossly distended and hypertrophied.

# TUMOURS OF THE COLON

The main tumours of the colon are epithelial – adenomas and carcinomas.

**Adenomas** – These are important because they may lead on to carcinoma, and for this reason bowel screening has been introduced to the United Kingdom to detect polyps and early cancers. (Adenoma–carcinoma sequence, p. 189)

## TUBULAR ADENOMA

The majority of tubular adenomas occur in the rectum and sigmoid colon. In the beginning it is a sessile swelling but soon becomes pedunculated.

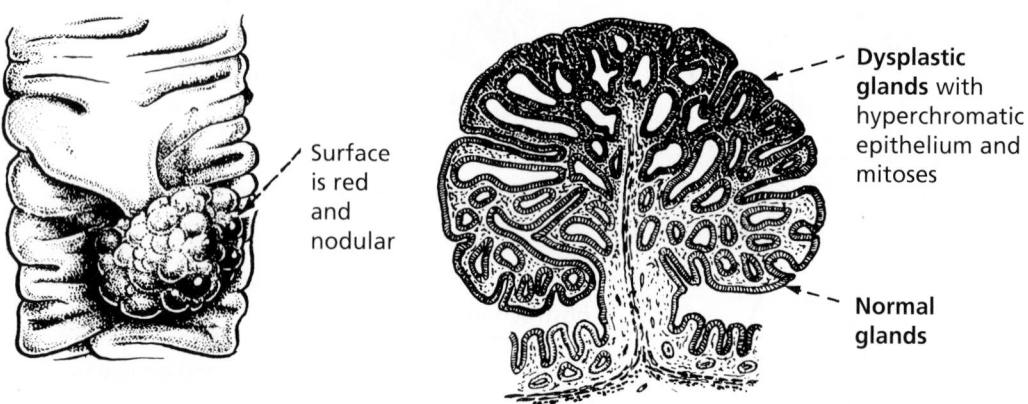

Surface is red and nodular

Dysplastic **glands** with hyperchromatic epithelium and mitoses

**Normal glands**

They are common in the older age groups and are frequently multiple.

## VILLOUS ADENOMA

Villous adenomas are most commonly found in the rectum. They form a sessile mass which may be quite large and have a delicate frond-like structure.

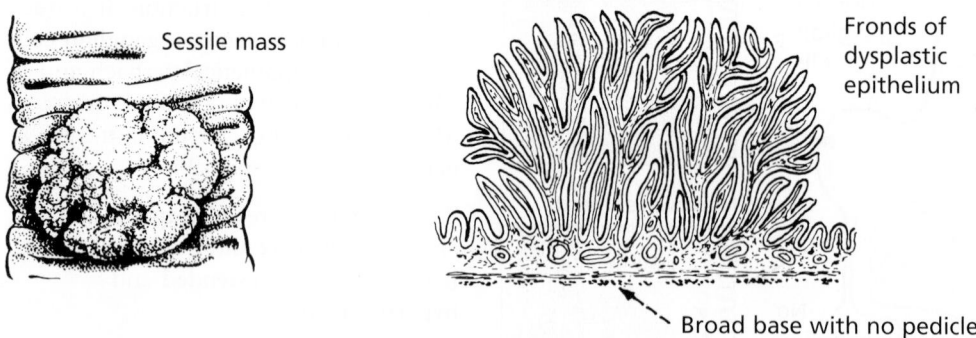

Sessile mass

Fronds of dysplastic epithelium

Broad base with no pedicle

These often present with rectal bleeding.

Very rarely, there is an excessive production of mucus and fluid which may lead to marked loss of potassium, causing muscular weakness and metabolic alkalosis.

Many polyps are of mixed variety – tubulo-villous. In pedunculated polyps, the stalk is invaded before the intestinal wall itself.

# TUMOURS OF THE COLON

## ADENOMATOSIS COLI

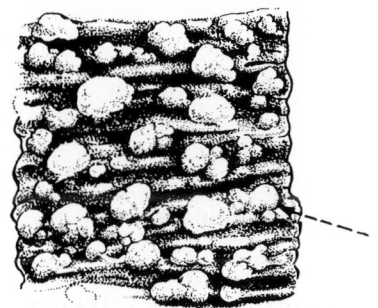

This is an inherited condition (autosomal dominant: 50% of children affected) due to mutation of the APC (adenomatous polyposis coli) gene, a tumour suppressor gene on chromosome 5.

Adenomatous polyps are found throughout the entire colon, appearing in late childhood. Carcinoma almost always occurs by the third or fourth decade if colectomy is not carried out.

Polyps may also be seen in the stomach and small bowel.

### Other colonic polyps

1. **HYPERPLASTIC POLYPS**

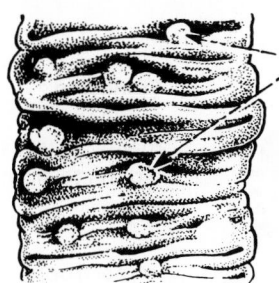

These are usually multiple and present as a small sessile nodule showing hyperplastic change in the epithelium. They are found in later life and do not become malignant. Some polyps, known as serrated adenomas, have a similar saw-toothed outline but have dysplastic glands and carry the same risk of malignant change as adenomas.

2. **JUVENILE POLYPS** are globular protrusions of the rectal mucosa in children who present with rectal bleeding. They are usually ulcerated and inflamed but probably represent a developmental abnormality. They are occasionally multiple, when there is a small risk of malignancy.

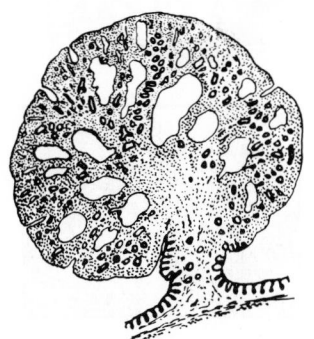

3. **INFLAMMATORY POLYPS** associated with chronic inflammatory bowel disease are described on page 341.

# CARCINOMA OF THE COLON

This malignancy is the third commonest cancer worldwide. Tumours in the right and left side tend to present differently.

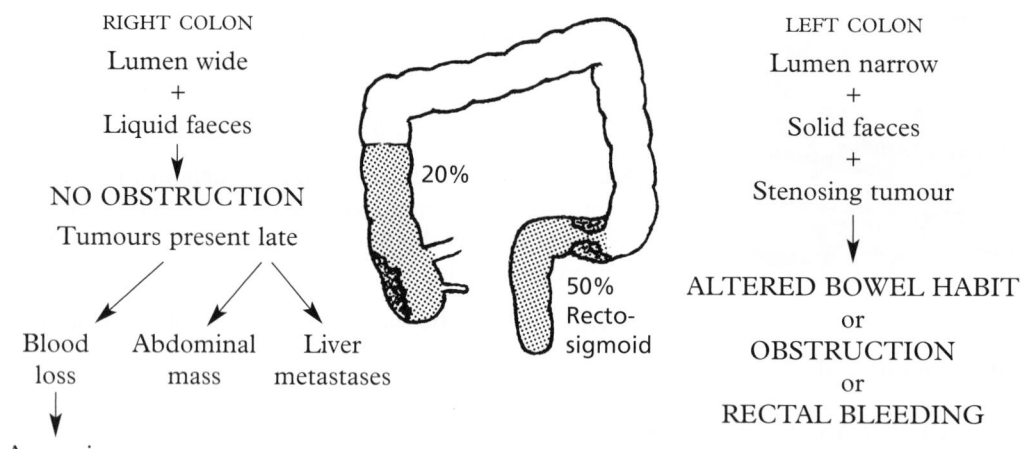

RIGHT COLON

Lumen wide
+
Liquid faeces
↓
NO OBSTRUCTION

Tumours present late

Blood loss — Abdominal mass — Liver metastases

↓
Anaemia

20%

50%
Recto-sigmoid

LEFT COLON

Lumen narrow
+
Solid faeces
+
Stenosing tumour
↓
ALTERED BOWEL HABIT
or
OBSTRUCTION
or
RECTAL BLEEDING

**Types of growth**

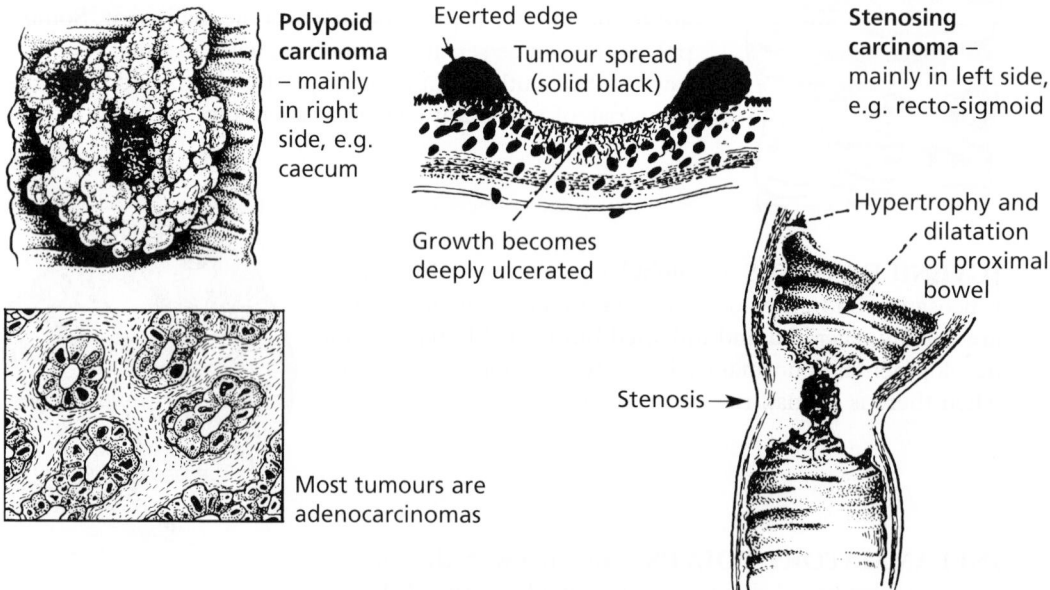

**Polypoid carcinoma** – mainly in right side, e.g. caecum

Everted edge
Tumour spread (solid black)

Growth becomes deeply ulcerated

Most tumours are adenocarcinomas

**Stenosing carcinoma** – mainly in left side, e.g. recto-sigmoid

Hypertrophy and dilatation of proximal bowel

Stenosis →

**Aetiology**

There are genetic and environmental factors.

(a) **Environmental**: diets rich in animal fat and protein, especially low residue diets.

(b) **Genetic**: e.g. adenomatosis coli (APC gene); hereditary non-polyposis colorectal cancer syndrome (HNPCC) due to mutation of mismatch repair genes. MOST CASES ARE SPORADIC.

(c) **Pre-existing lesions**:
  i. Adenomatous polyps including familial adenomatosis coli.
  ii. Inflammatory bowel disease (especially ulcerative colitis).

# CARCINOMA OF THE COLON

## SPREAD AND STAGING (DUKES STAGING)

Both Dukes staging and the TNM classification are used in routine practice. They correlate very well with prognosis. Both systems take into account extent of local invasion, lymph node involvement and distal metastases.

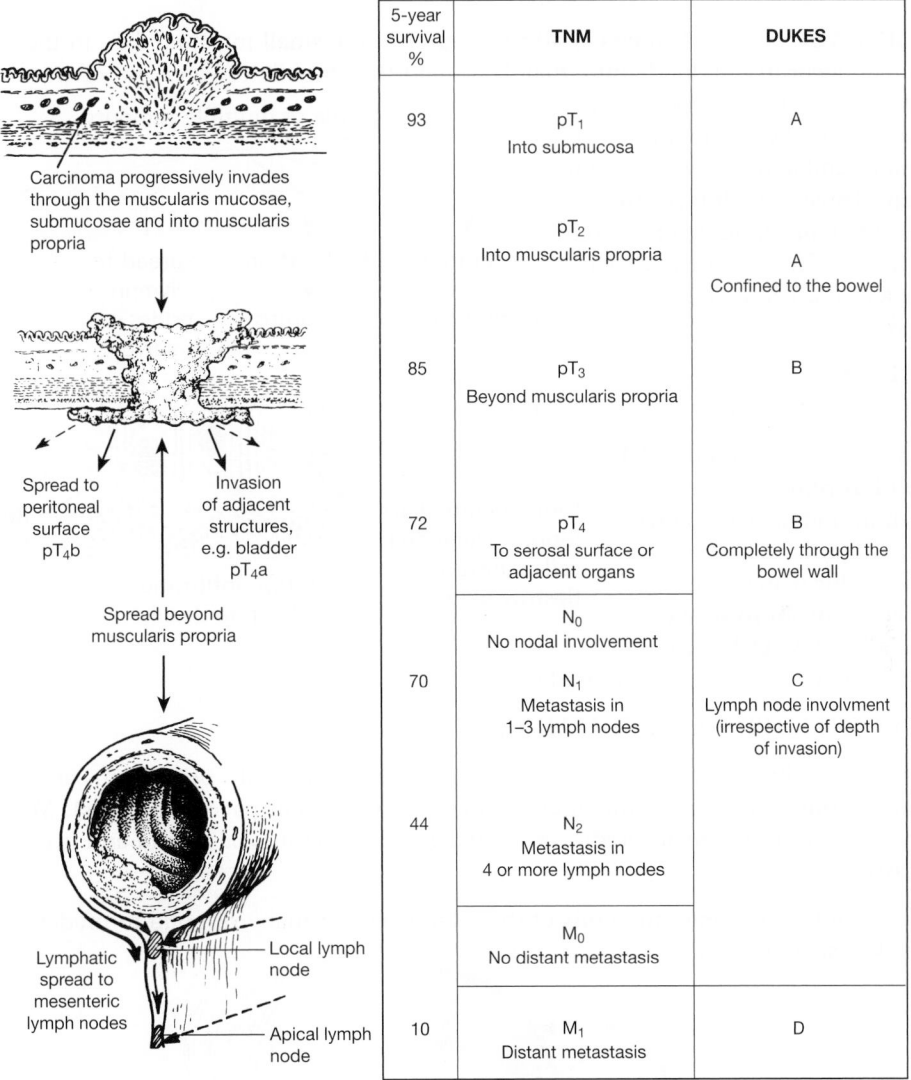

| 5-year survival % | TNM | DUKES |
|---|---|---|
| 93 | $pT_1$ Into submucosa | A |
| | $pT_2$ Into muscularis propria | A Confined to the bowel |
| 85 | $pT_3$ Beyond muscularis propria | B |
| 72 | $pT_4$ To serosal surface or adjacent organs | B Completely through the bowel wall |
| | $N_0$ No nodal involvement | |
| 70 | $N_1$ Metastasis in 1–3 lymph nodes | C Lymph node involvment (irrespective of depth of invasion) |
| 44 | $N_2$ Metastasis in 4 or more lymph nodes | |
| | $M_0$ No distant metastasis | |
| 10 | $M_1$ Distant metastasis | D |

Diagram labels:

Carcinoma progressively invades through the muscularis mucosae, submucosae and into muscularis propria

Spread to peritoneal surface $pT_4b$

Invasion of adjacent structures, e.g. bladder $pT_4a$

Spread beyond muscularis propria

Lymphatic spread to mesenteric lymph nodes

Local lymph node

Apical lymph node

Blood borne metastases to the liver usually occur later. Extramural vascular invasion is a poor prognostic factor.

### Other tumours

Carcinoid tumour (p. 365), lymphoma and connective tissue tumours, e.g. GISTs, are occasionally found.

# TUMOURS OF SMALL INTESTINE

**BENIGN TUMOURS**: adenomas, leiomyomas and lipomas are rare, but may cause intussusception (p. 358).

**Hamartomatous polyps**, consisting of glands and muscle, occur in the Peutz–Jeghers syndrome, an autosomal-dominant condition. Melanotic pigmentation of the lips and mouth is also seen.

**CARCINOMA**: adenocarcinoma is 50 times rarer in the small intestine than in the colon. About half occur in the duodenum, mainly around the ampulla of Vater and often arise from adenomas. These present with obstructive jaundice. Tumours in the jejunum resemble those of the colon and may obstruct the lumen. An increased risk of carcinoma is seen in patients with Crohn's disease, coeliac disease and the Peutz–Jeghers syndrome.

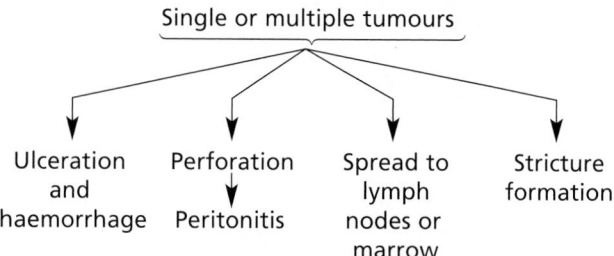

Single or multiple tumours

Ulceration and haemorrhage · Perforation → Peritonitis · Spread to lymph nodes or marrow · Stricture formation

**LYMPHOMA**: these are non-Hodgkin lymphomas of 'B' or 'T' cell type.

(a) **Enteropathy-associated T cell lymphoma**. These are seen in middle-aged patients who often have had coeliac disease for many years.

(b) **B cell lymphomas are usually of MALT type**. These may be of low or high grade.

Lymphoepithelial lesions – lymphoid cells infiltrate and destroy glands.

Diffuse infiltration of lymphoid cells

Reactive lymphoid follicle

## GASTROINTESTINAL STROMAL TUMOURS

GISTs occur within the stomach, small bowel and, less commonly, oesophagus and colon. They arise from precursors of the interstitial cells of Cajal (gut pacemaker cells). Mitotic activity and size are the main predictors of malignancy – peritoneal spread and liver metastasis.

Most are due to activating mutations of the c-kit gene and many respond to modern tyrosine kinase inhibitors.

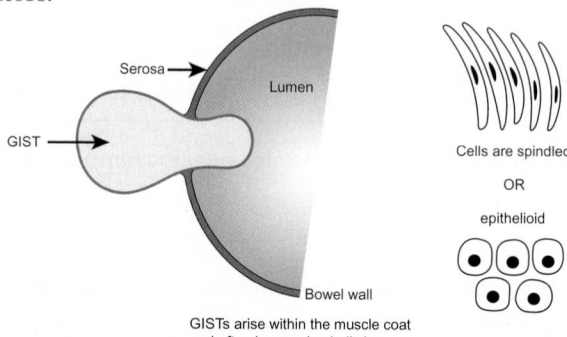

Serosa
Lumen
GIST
Bowel wall

GISTs arise within the muscle coat and often have a dumbbell shape

Cells are spindled

OR

epithelioid

GISTs arise within the muscle coat and often have a dumbbell shape.

# CARCINOID TUMOURS

These tumours, now classified as neuroendocrine tumours, arise from endocrine cells and can occur in the gut and lung. They are commonest in the appendix and small bowel.

## APPENDICEAL CARCINOIDS

These may be incidental findings at appendicectomy or may cause appendicitis.

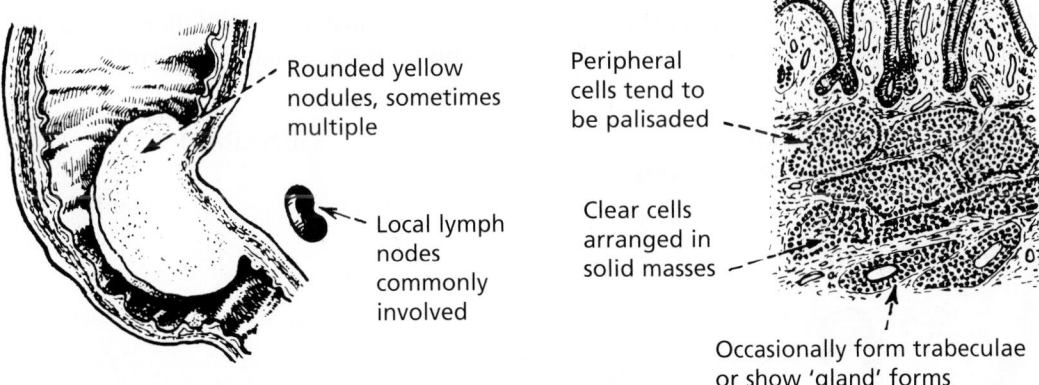

Yellow nodule

10% occur at base          70% occur at tip

## SMALL BOWEL CARCINOIDS

These are commonest in the ileum.

Rounded yellow nodules, sometimes multiple

Local lymph nodes commonly involved

Peripheral cells tend to be palisaded

Clear cells arranged in solid masses

Occasionally form trabeculae or show 'gland' forms

They contain neurosecretory granules (electron microscope) and express endocrine markers, e.g. chromogranin, synaptophysin. The cells can bind and reduce silver compounds and are known as 'ARGENTAFFIN CELLS'.

## CARCINOID SYNDROME

These tumours may secrete a variety of neuroendocrine and paraendocrine substances, in many cases without any apparent clinical functional effects.

However, ileal carcinoids tend to produce peptides such as 5-hydroxytryptamine (5HT; serotonin). This is normally destroyed in the liver and lungs. When metastatic deposits are present in the liver the active agents enter the general circulation and produce the CARCINOID SYNDROME, characterised by episodic flushing, diarrhoea and right heart failure.

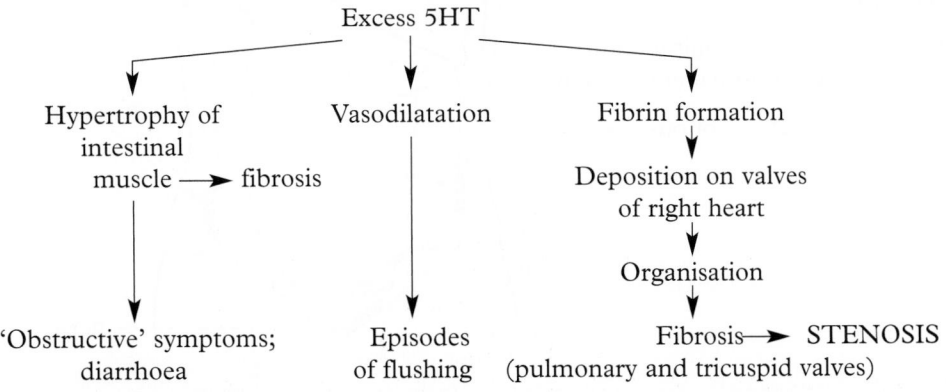

Excess 5HT

Hypertrophy of intestinal muscle ⟶ fibrosis

Vasodilatation

Fibrin formation

Deposition on valves of right heart

Organisation

'Obstructive' symptoms; diarrhoea

Episodes of flushing

Fibrosis ⟶ STENOSIS (pulmonary and tricuspid valves)

# THE PERITONEAL CAVITY

### PERITONITIS

Acute peritonitis usually follows inflammation of a viscus,

e.g. 1. Appendicitis, cholecystitis, pancreatitis.
    2. Perforation, e.g. duodenal ulcer, ruptured diverticulum.
    3. Ischaemia – vascular occlusion, volvulus, intussusception.

Patients on chronic ambulatory peritoneal dialysis (CAPD) are prone to episodes of peritonitis.

### Primary peritonitis

In the absence of visceral inflammation, primary peritonitis may occur in children with the nephrotic syndrome (pneumococcus) or in adults with cirrhosis (usually coliforms).

Peritonitis can be:

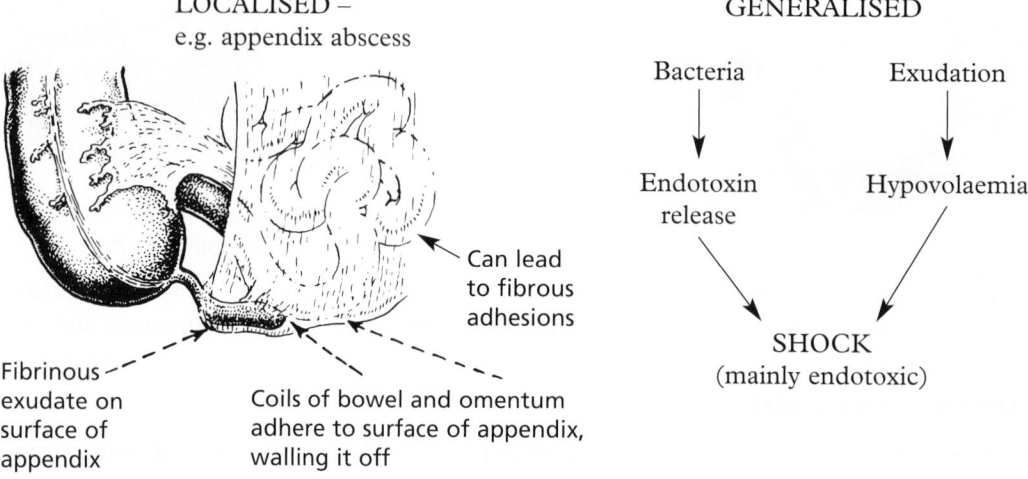

LOCALISED –
e.g. appendix abscess

Can lead to fibrous adhesions

Fibrinous exudate on surface of appendix

Coils of bowel and omentum adhere to surface of appendix, walling it off

GENERALISED

Bacteria → Endotoxin release

Exudation → Hypovolaemia

SHOCK
(mainly endotoxic)

### Consequences of peritonitis

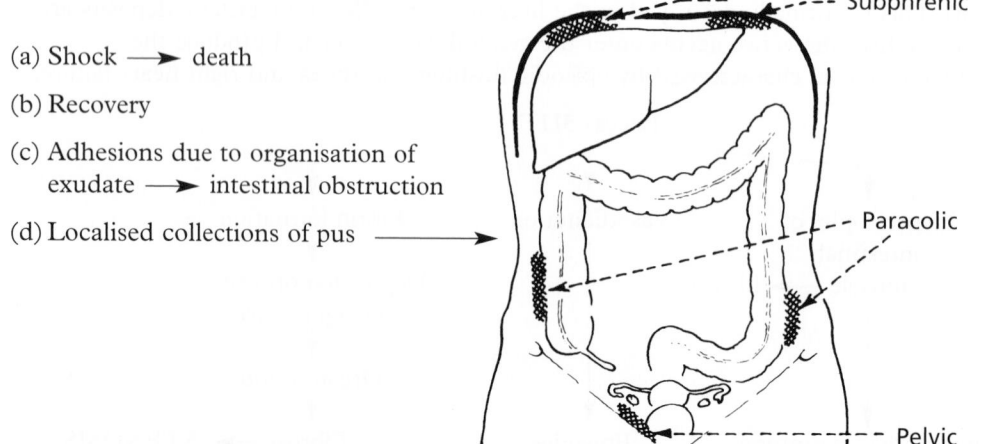

(a) Shock ⟶ death

(b) Recovery

(c) Adhesions due to organisation of exudate ⟶ intestinal obstruction

(d) Localised collections of pus ⟶

Subphrenic

Paracolic

Pelvic

# THE PERITONEAL CAVITY

## Chronic peritonitis

The most common type of chronic inflammation involving the peritoneum is that resulting from non-resolution of acute peritonitis.

A form of sclerosing peritonitis may complicate long-term peritoneal dialysis.

TB of the peritoneum is uncommon in Western countries, but frequent in developing countries. It commonly takes one of the following forms:

1. **Serous effusion**. Small grey nodules (tubercles) are usually scattered over the peritoneal surface. In addition, the omentum is more extensively involved with the formation of a large fibrous mass in the upper abdomen.
2. **Caseation**. This can vary in extent, from isolated small masses to diffuse caseation involving most of the cavity.
3. **Adhesive peritonitis**. The cavity may be reduced to small pockets containing serous fluid. The source of infection may be caseous lymph nodes, tuberculous salpingitis or tuberculous ulcer of the intestine.

## Ascites

Accumulation of serous fluid can occur:

1. As part of a general oedema from any cause such as cardiac or renal failure.
2. Portal venous obstruction as in hepatic cirrhosis, portal thrombosis or compression of the portal vein by tumour growth.
3. Tumours of the ovary.
4. Tumours of the peritoneum.

## Tumours

Secondary tumours are common, due to spread of carcinoma from the stomach, ovary and large intestine.

Eventually loops of bowel are stuck together by tumour and adhesions resulting in 'frozen abdomen'.

Pseudomyxoma peritonei is seen when mucin secreting tumours, typically arising in the appendix, spread widely throughout the peritoneum.

Primary tumours are rare. Mesothelioma is the most important. It is related to the inhalation of asbestos and the pathology is similar to that of mesothelioma of the pleura; large white plaques of solid tumour. Primary carcinomas of the peritoneum are very similar to serous carcinomas of the ovary (p. 549).

# CHAPTER 10

# LIVER, GALL BLADDER AND PANCREAS

## OBJECTIVES

1. To know the main hepatitis viruses and pathological consequences of their infection.
2. To have knowledge of the pathology of alcoholic liver disease.
3. To know about cirrhosis and its complications.
4. To have a knowledge of metabolic disorders of the liver and infections of the liver.
5. To know the main tumour types to affect the liver.
6. To know the main pathologies to involve the gallbladder and biliary tree.
7. To have a basic understanding of the pathogenesis of both acute and chronic pancreatitis.
8. To have knowledge of the main tumour types arising in the pancreas.

# LIVER – ANATOMY

**Conventionally** the liver was considered to be composed of regular lobules, each arranged around a 'central vein' with portal tracts at the periphery.

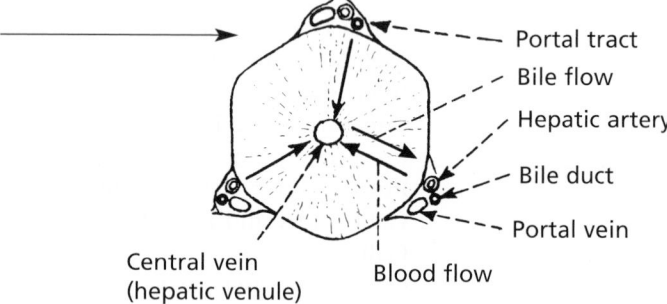

Portal tract
Bile flow
Hepatic artery
Bile duct
Portal vein

Central vein
(hepatic venule)
Blood flow

The acinar concept is now used.

The smallest unit is the simple acinus.

The portal venule and hepatic arteriole both send terminal branches into the acinus (two-thirds of the blood supply is portal and one-third is arterial). They join to form a common trunk which will then contain partially oxygenated blood, and this percolates through the sinusoids to several 'terminal hepatic venules' (as in diagram).

In terms of oxygen supply and other nutrients, three zones exist.

  Zone 1 – with the best supply;
  Zone 2 – with a reasonable supply;
  Zone 3 – with the poorest supply, which makes it most vulnerable to hypoxia.

In zone 1, glycogen synthesis and glycogenolysis take place. It is also the main area of protein metabolism and formation of plasma proteins. Conjugation of certain drugs takes place.

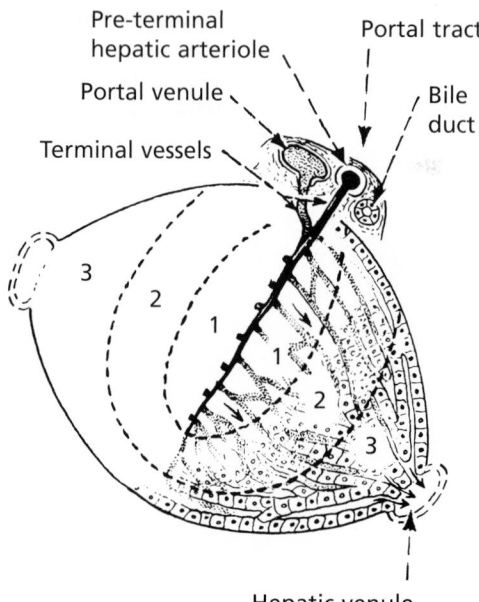

Pre-terminal hepatic arteriole
Portal tract
Portal venule
Bile duct
Terminal vessels
Hepatic venule

Zone 3 is associated with glycogen storage, lipid and pigment formation and metabolism of certain drugs and chemicals. Zone 2 shares functions with the other zones.

# ANATOMY – HEPATIC LESIONS

Adjacent liver acini form a complex architecture best appreciated when diseases affect the varying zones. Factors involved in this include the $pO_2$ of blood and enzyme function of the zones.

## LIVER NECROSIS

### Perivenular necrosis

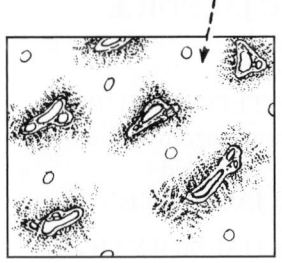

This form is a feature of many apparently unrelated conditions. It is brought about by damage in zone 3 (*A* in diagram). Thus it is a feature of shock due to circulatory collapse reducing the oxygen supply to zone 3. It also occurs in poisoning with chlorinated hydrocarbons (e.g. chloroform) and drugs (e.g. paracetamol) metabolised in zone 3.

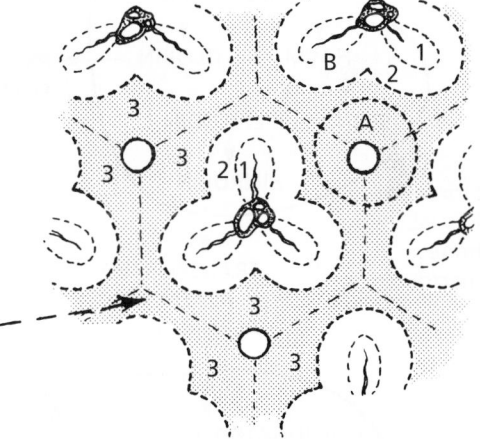

It is important to realise that zone 3, particularly, is continuous from one acinus to another, and in severe cases the hepatic venules are linked together by necrotic tissues.

### Mid-zonal necrosis

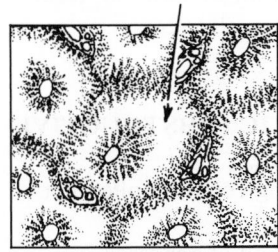

This is uncommon. It is seen in yellow fever and injury affecting zones 2 and 1 (*B* in diagram).

### Periportal necrosis

Rarely, necrosis in zone 1 is due to its metabolism of drugs and chemicals, e.g. phosphorus poisoning causes marked fatty change in the periportal parenchyma, followed by necrosis.

### Massive necrosis

This is an unusual lesion which can follow poisoning due to drugs, industrial chemicals or mushrooms. Rarely it is a complication of viral hepatitis.

# JAUNDICE

If the serum bilirubin level exceeds 50 μmol/L, the patient becomes jaundiced.

Bilirubin is derived from the breakdown of aged red cells by the macrophage system, mainly in the spleen. It is conjugated to glucuronic acid in the liver and secreted in the bile.

There are three main forms of jaundice:

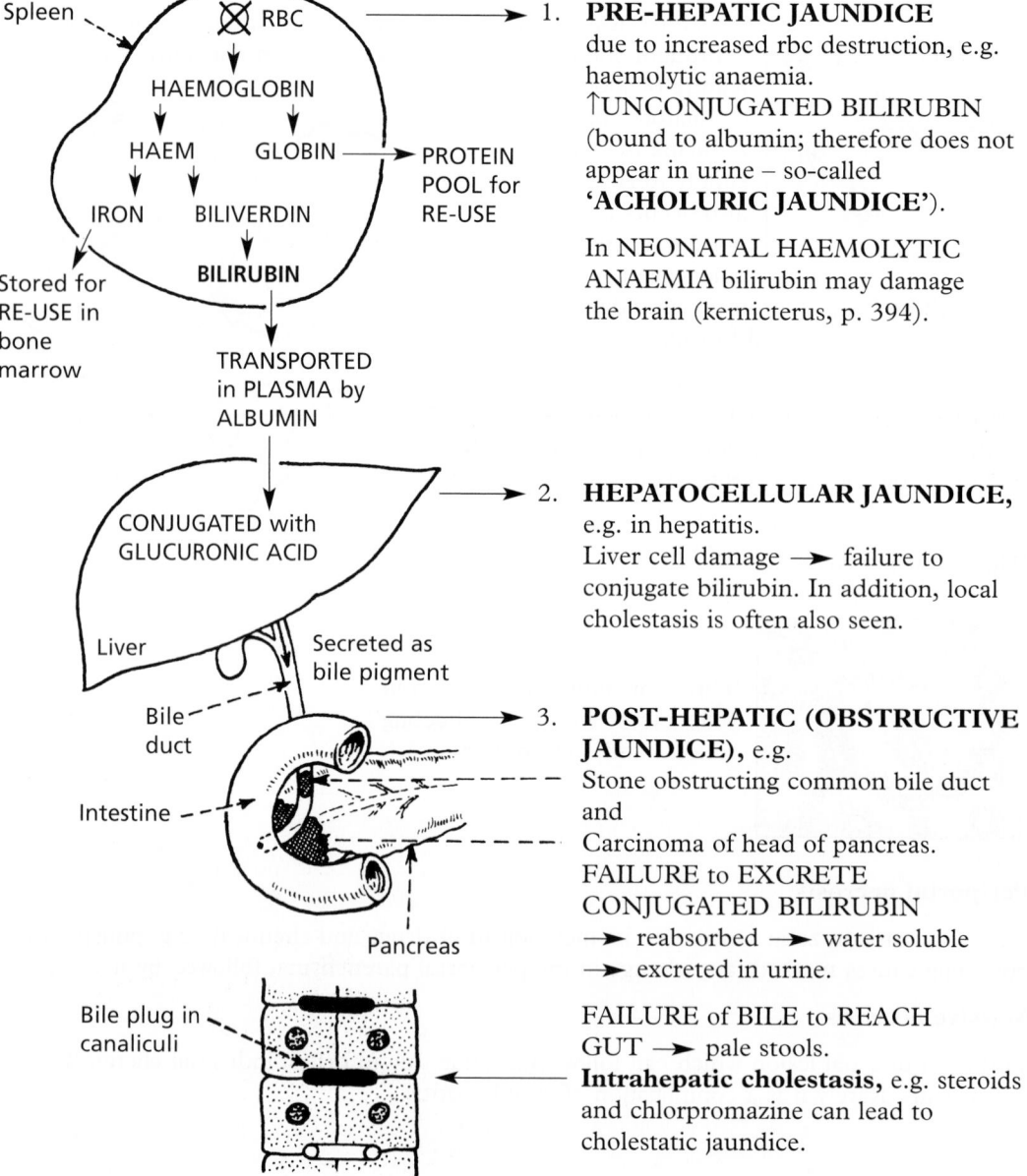

1. **PRE-HEPATIC JAUNDICE**
due to increased rbc destruction, e.g. haemolytic anaemia.
↑UNCONJUGATED BILIRUBIN (bound to albumin; therefore does not appear in urine – so-called **'ACHOLURIC JAUNDICE'**).

In NEONATAL HAEMOLYTIC ANAEMIA bilirubin may damage the brain (kernicterus, p. 394).

2. **HEPATOCELLULAR JAUNDICE,** e.g. in hepatitis.
Liver cell damage ➤ failure to conjugate bilirubin. In addition, local cholestasis is often also seen.

3. **POST-HEPATIC (OBSTRUCTIVE JAUNDICE),** e.g.
Stone obstructing common bile duct and
Carcinoma of head of pancreas.
FAILURE to EXCRETE CONJUGATED BILIRUBIN
➤ reabsorbed ➤ water soluble
➤ excreted in urine.

FAILURE of BILE to REACH GUT ➤ pale stools.
**Intrahepatic cholestasis,** e.g. steroids and chlorpromazine can lead to cholestatic jaundice.

# VIRAL HEPATITIS

## ACUTE VIRAL HEPATITIS

Viral hepatitis is the most important form of hepatitis. It is seen worldwide. Viral hepatitis may be sporadic or epidemic and, depending on the responsible virus, transmitted by the faeco-oral or parenteral route.

### Clinical features

Many episodes of viral hepatitis are subclinical; mild symptomatic cases are characterised by nausea, fever and anorexia. Severe attacks are characterised by jaundice and hepatic failure, and may be fatal.

### Pathological features

**EARLY** stage

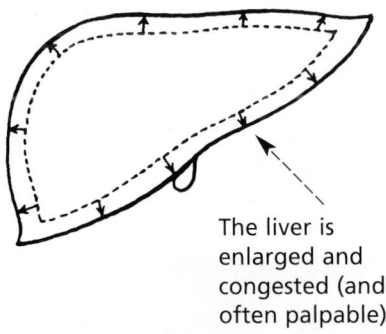

The liver is enlarged and congested (and often palpable)

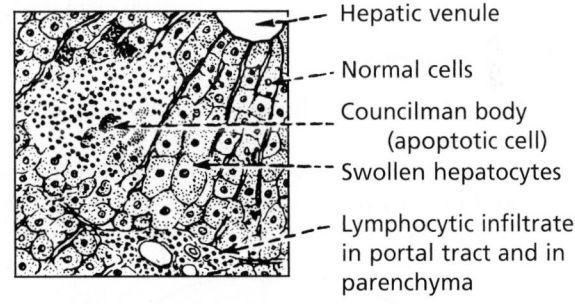

Hepatic venule

Normal cells

Councilman body (apoptotic cell)

Swollen hepatocytes

Lymphocytic infiltrate in portal tract and in parenchyma

Liver cell necrosis is always present. It is most marked in zone 3 (p. 370).

Necrosis may be:

(a) focal (spotty) – scattered as single cells, or

(b) more severe – forming areas of bridging between vessels (portal to hepatic venule), or

(c) panacinar – necrosis of complete acini up to massive necrosis of a large part of the liver occasionally occurs. When it does, it is most marked in the left lobe.

**LATER** stage

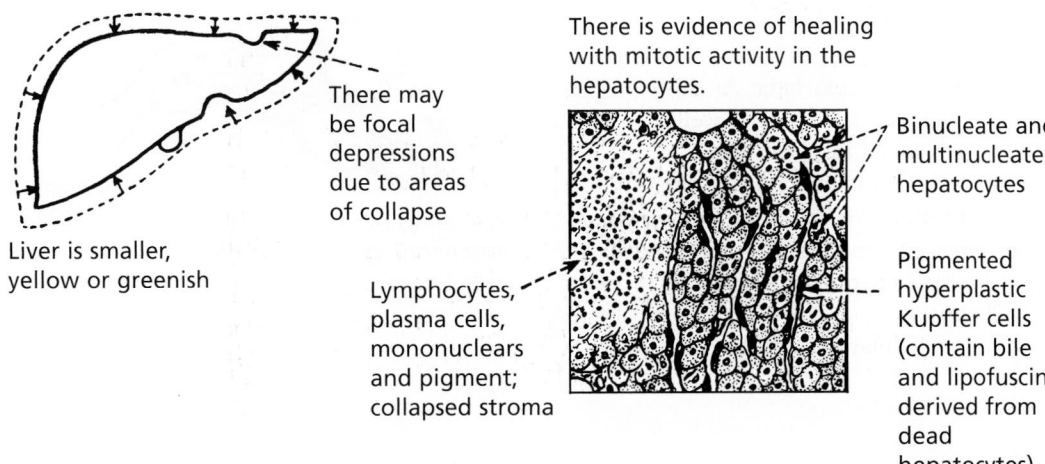

There may be focal depressions due to areas of collapse

Liver is smaller, yellow or greenish

Lymphocytes, plasma cells, mononuclears and pigment; collapsed stroma

There is evidence of healing with mitotic activity in the hepatocytes.

Binucleate and multinucleate hepatocytes

Pigmented hyperplastic Kupffer cells (contain bile and lipofuscin derived from dead hepatocytes)

# VIRAL HEPATITIS

### Biochemical changes

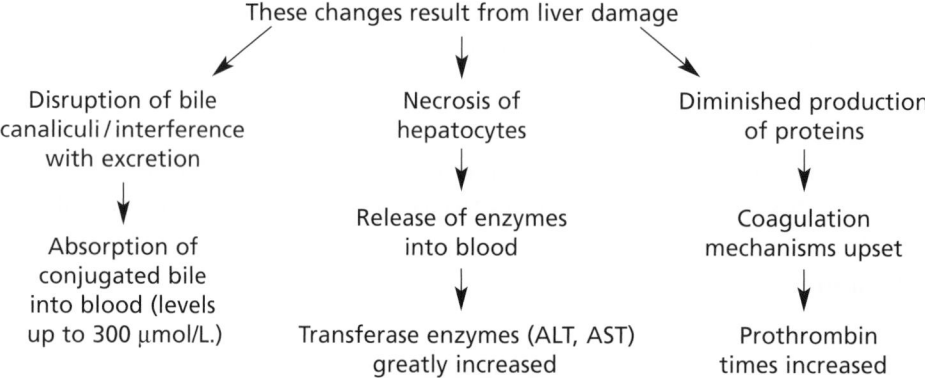

These changes result from liver damage

Disruption of bile canaliculi / interference with excretion

↓

Absorption of conjugated bile into blood (levels up to 300 μmol/L.)

Necrosis of hepatocytes

↓

Release of enzymes into blood

↓

Transferase enzymes (ALT, AST) greatly increased

Diminished production of proteins

↓

Coagulation mechanisms upset

↓

Prothrombin times increased

### Clinical progress

1. In most cases, the disease is self-limiting and complete recovery occurs within 4–6 weeks.
2. Rarely, death may occur due to massive (panacinar) liver necrosis.
   (a) In the early pre-icteric stage within 10 days – fulminant hepatic failure.
   (b) In 2–3 weeks. The liver is reduced in size.

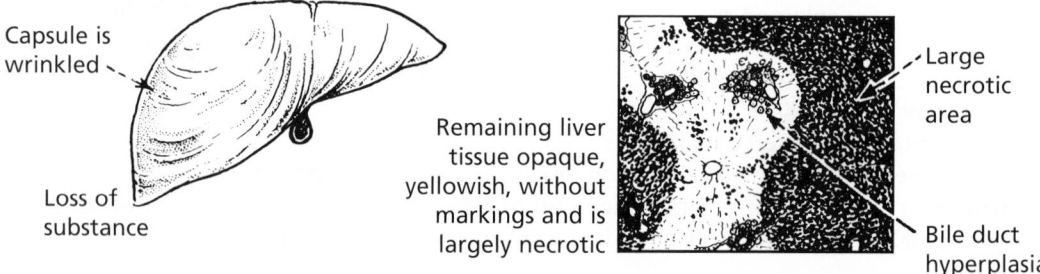

Capsule is wrinkled

Loss of substance

Remaining liver tissue opaque, yellowish, without markings and is largely necrotic

Large necrotic area

Bile duct hyperplasia

This condition was often termed 'acute yellow atrophy'.

(c) Several weeks later. At this stage, regeneration is well advanced in places but function is inadequate and progressive failure occurs.

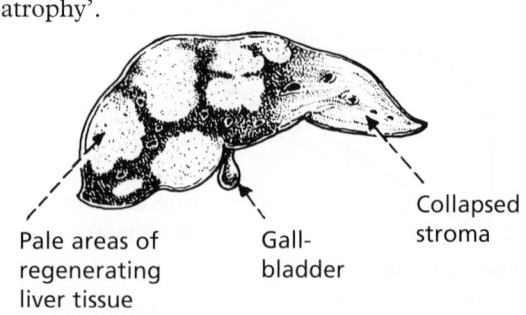

Some types of hepatitis may progress to

3. Chronic hepatitis (p. 378)
4. Cirrhosis
5. Hepatocellular carcinoma

Pale areas of regenerating liver tissue

Gall-bladder

Collapsed stroma

# VIRAL HEPATITIS

At least five viruses cause liver damage without significantly damaging other tissues (hepatitis A, B, C, D and E). The features are summarised and then discussed individually.

| VIRUS | HAV | HBV | HCV | HDV | HEV |
|---|---|---|---|---|---|
| Type | Picorna Virus | Hepadna Virus | RNA Flavivirus | Defective RNA Virus | RNA Calicivirus |
| Spread | Faeco-oral | Parenteral | Parenteral | Parenteral | Faeco-oral |
| Incubation period (weeks) | 2–4 | 4–26 | 7–8 | 4–16 | 4–5 |
| Severity of hepatitis | Usually mild | Often severe | Usually mild | Severe | Often mild Severe in pregnancy |
| Chronicity | No | Approx. 5% of adults, 90% of children | Approx. 50% | Coinfection 5% Superinfection 95% | No |
| Carrier state | No | Yes | Yes | Yes | No |
| Vaccine | Yes | Yes | No | Protected by HBV vaccine if HBV −ve | No |

Other viruses which can affect the liver, but also affect other tissues include:

Yellow fever.
Herpes viruses – Epstein–Barr, cytomegalovirus, herpes simplex.
Coxsackie A and B.
Lassa fever.

# HEPATITIS B INFECTION

The **hepatitis B virus** is a member of the HEPA DNA virus group. Infection is by the parenteral route – mainly intravenous drug abuse, blood products and sexual transmission, and in childbirth in high prevalence areas.

The virus has several components:

**A core** containing

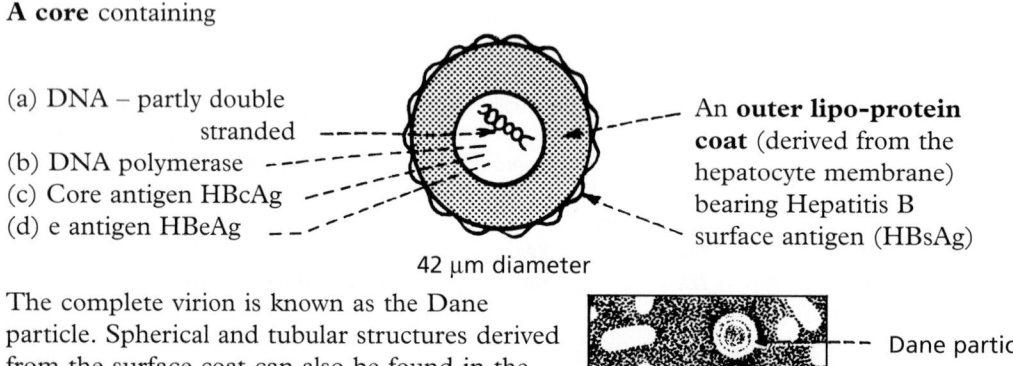

(a) DNA – partly double stranded
(b) DNA polymerase
(c) Core antigen HBcAg
(d) e antigen HBeAg

An **outer lipo-protein coat** (derived from the hepatocyte membrane) bearing Hepatitis B surface antigen (HBsAg)

42 µm diameter

The complete virion is known as the Dane particle. Spherical and tubular structures derived from the surface coat can also be found in the peripheral blood.

These antigens and antibodies to them are the basis for diagnosis of hepatitis B infection.

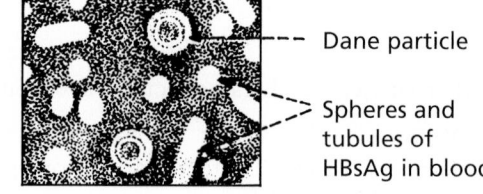

Dane particle

Spheres and tubules of HBsAg in blood

In **histological preparations**

HBsAg accumulates in the cytoplasm of cells – giving a 'ground glass' appearance.

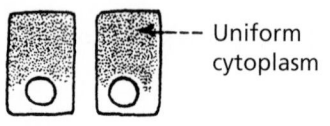

Uniform cytoplasm

HBcAg is found in the nuclei

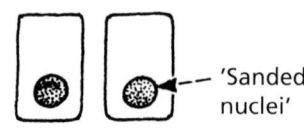

'Sanded nuclei'

or can be stained by immunocytochemistry.

Positive staining with Anti-HBs

Positive staining with Anti-HBc

**Serology**: antibodies to the various antigens appear in the blood.

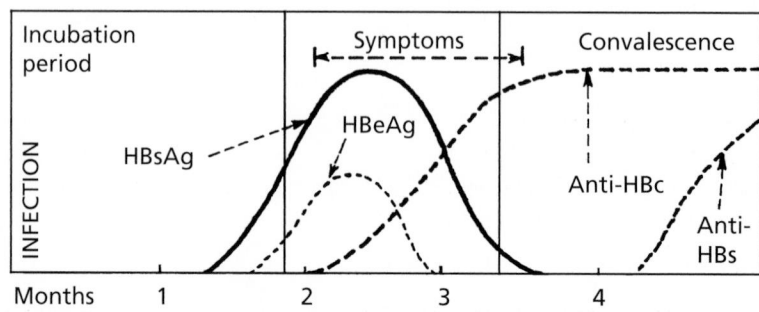

Six weeks after infection the surface antigen (HBsAg) appears in the blood, followed 2 weeks later by the e antigen (HBeAg), at the time of maximal viral replication.

# VIRAL HEPATITIS

## Outcome of hepatitis B infection

In >90% of cases there is a vigorous immune reaction (cell-mediated and humoral) to the virus resulting in its elimination. In the remaining patients, the illness pursues one of several courses:

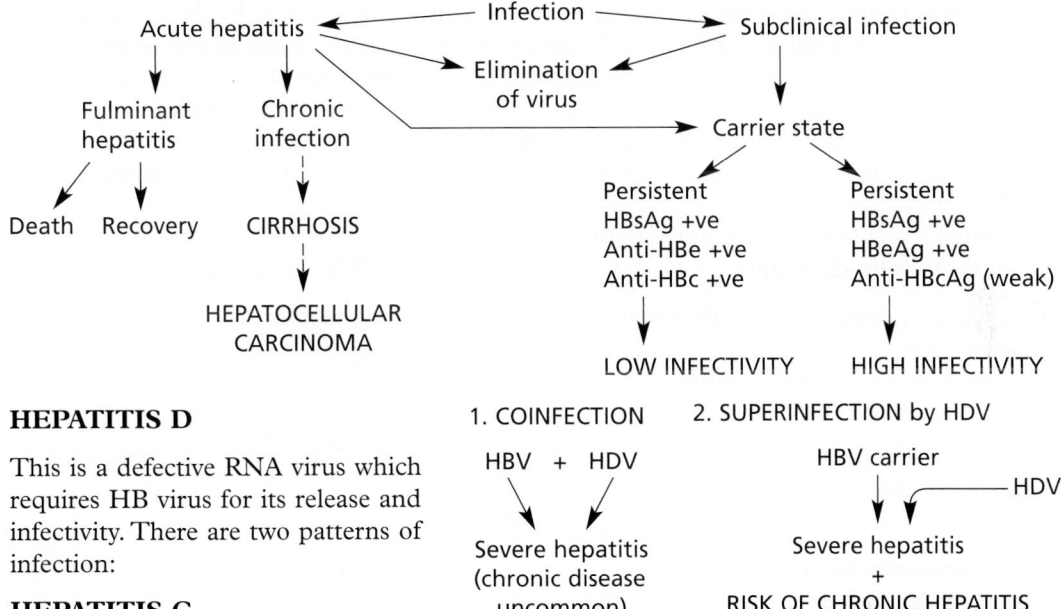

## HEPATITIS D

This is a defective RNA virus which requires HB virus for its release and infectivity. There are two patterns of infection:

## HEPATITIS C

**1. COINFECTION**

HBV + HDV

Severe hepatitis
(chronic disease
uncommon)

**2. SUPERINFECTION by HDV**

HBV carrier
⎯⎯ HDV

Severe hepatitis
+
RISK OF CHRONIC HEPATITIS

This small RNA virus is transmitted parenterally and is seen in intravenous drug users or following infected blood transfusion. Acute hepatitis is mild and patients are rarely jaundiced. It is important because of the high risk of chronicity.

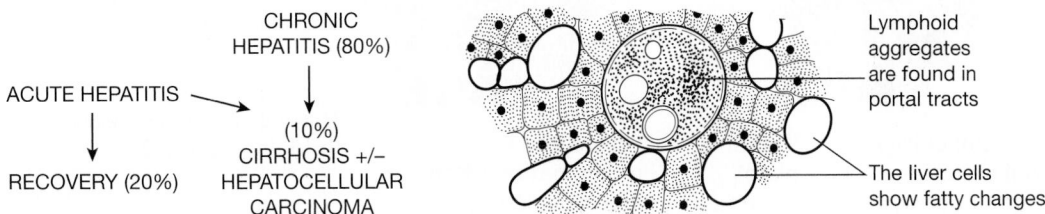

## HEPATITIS A

This picornavirus is transmitted by the faeco-oral route, especially where hygiene is poor. Hepatitis is usually mild in children, but more severe in adults. IgM immunoglobulin M and immunoglobulin G antibodies appear in the blood in the acute phase, and IgG during convalescence, thus conferring lifelong immunity. Chronic liver disease does not occur.

## HEPATITIS E

This is most commonly seen in Africa and Asia. Although usually mild, it is particularly severe in pregnant women, with a mortality of approximately 20%.

# CHRONIC HEPATITIS

Inflammation of the liver which lasts for more than 6 months is regarded as chronic. (This definition excludes disorders such as alcoholic hepatitis.)

There are four main **causes**:

1. **Persistent viral infection** – hepatitis B, D and C.
2. **Auto-immune hepatitis**. This occurs especially in young women. In classic (type I) disease, anti-nuclear and anti-smooth muscle antibodies are present in the serum. Liver specific autoantibodies, e.g. to a sialoglycoprotein receptor (ASGP-R), on periportal hepatocyte cell surfaces can also be found. These patients often have other auto-immune diseases, e.g. thyroiditis. A smaller subgroup, type II, is defined by anti-liver kidney microsomal antibodies (anti-LKM-1) and has a more aggressive disease.
3. **Drugs** – e.g. methyldopa, nitrofurantoin.
4. **In metabolic disorders** – e.g. $\alpha_1$-antitrypsin deficiency, Wilson disease (p. 388).

Histologically, three areas of inflammation are seen to varying degrees.
- Portal tract
- Parenchymal (within the acinus)
- At the interface (limiting plate)

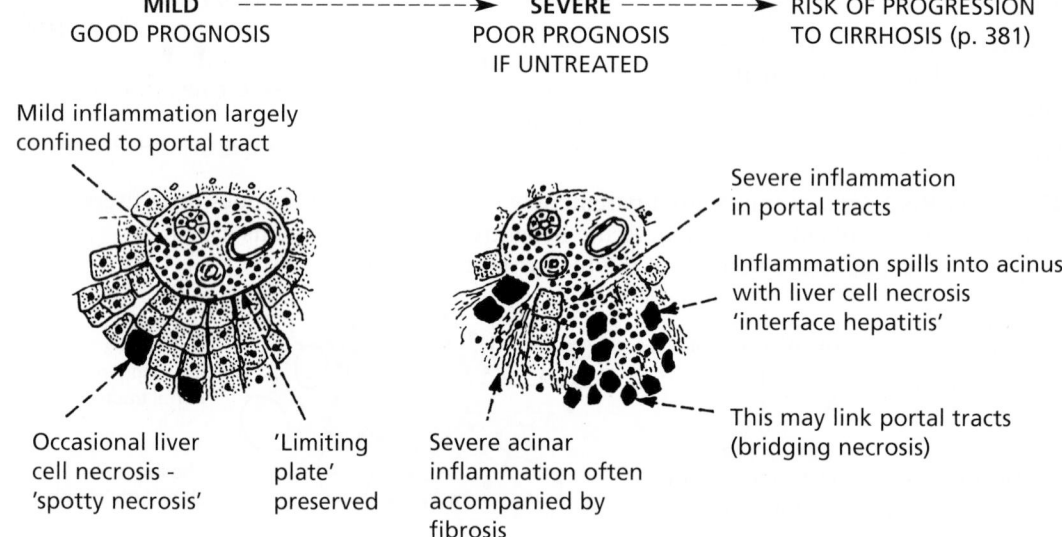

MILD - - - - - - - - - - - - - - -→ SEVERE - - - - - - - - -→ RISK OF PROGRESSION
GOOD PROGNOSIS                    POOR PROGNOSIS              TO CIRRHOSIS (p. 381)
                                 IF UNTREATED

Mild inflammation largely confined to portal tract

Severe inflammation in portal tracts

Inflammation spills into acinus with liver cell necrosis 'interface hepatitis'

This may link portal tracts (bridging necrosis)

Occasional liver cell necrosis - 'spotty necrosis'

'Limiting plate' preserved

Severe acinar inflammation often accompanied by fibrosis

# ALCOHOLIC LIVER DISEASE

Excess consumption of alcohol is associated with liver disease in three main forms.

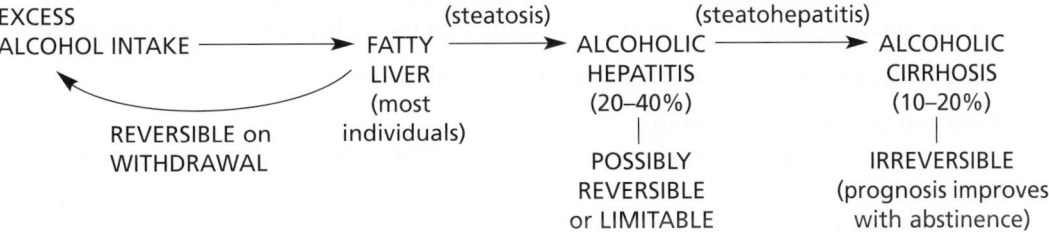

EXCESS ALCOHOL INTAKE ⟶ FATTY LIVER (most individuals) ⟵ REVERSIBLE on WITHDRAWAL

(steatosis) ⟶ ALCOHOLIC HEPATITIS (20–40%) | POSSIBLY REVERSIBLE or LIMITABLE

(steatohepatitis) ⟶ ALCOHOLIC CIRRHOSIS (10–20%) | IRREVERSIBLE (prognosis improves with abstinence)

The progression from left to right does not occur in all patients: genetic predisposition, co-existent nutritional deficiencies, amount and duration of drinking and other factors determine the risk.

## FATTY LIVER

This occurs in most heavy drinkers, even after a single episode of heavy intake. Fat accumulates in the hepatocytes due to abnormalities in the intermediate metabolism of lipids and carbohydrates.

*Note*: Fatty liver usually resolves within 2–4 weeks of abstinence.

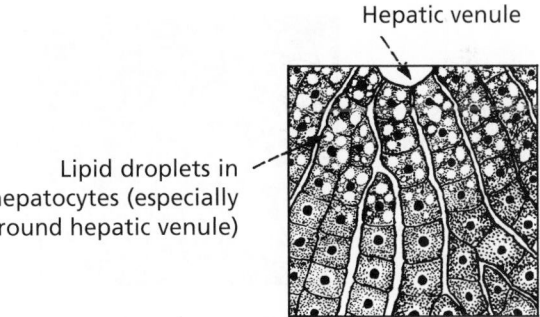

Hepatic venule

Lipid droplets in hepatocytes (especially around hepatic venule)

### Alcohol metabolism

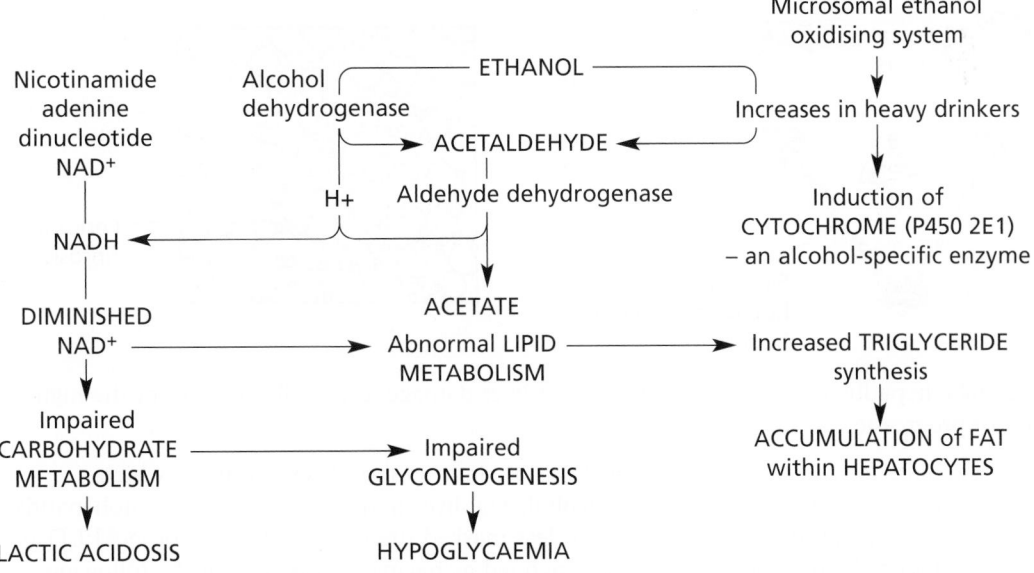

Microsomal ethanol oxidising system

Nicotinamide adenine dinucleotide NAD$^+$

Alcohol dehydrogenase ⟶ ETHANOL

ACETALDEHYDE ⟵ Increases in heavy drinkers

H+ Aldehyde dehydrogenase

NADH

Induction of CYTOCHROME (P450 2E1) – an alcohol-specific enzyme

DIMINISHED NAD$^+$ ⟶ ACETATE

Abnormal LIPID METABOLISM ⟶ Increased TRIGLYCERIDE synthesis

Impaired CARBOHYDRATE METABOLISM ⟶ Impaired GLYCONEOGENESIS

ACCUMULATION of FAT within HEPATOCYTES

LACTIC ACIDOSIS

HYPOGLYCAEMIA

# ALCOHOLIC HEPATITIS

In 20–40% of heavy drinkers, alcoholic hepatitis is superimposed on fatty change. This varies from asymptomatic hepatitis to a life threatening condition with nausea, vomiting, abdominal pain and jaundice. Signs of liver failure and portal hypertension may be found.

**Histologically**, the main features are seen around hepatic venules:

1. Liver cell swelling – ballooning.
2. Accumulation of Mallory hyaline – protein derived from intermediate filaments (mainly cytokeratin).
3. Liver cell necrosis.
4. Neutrophil polymorph infiltration.
5. Pericellular fibrosis.

**Acute phase**

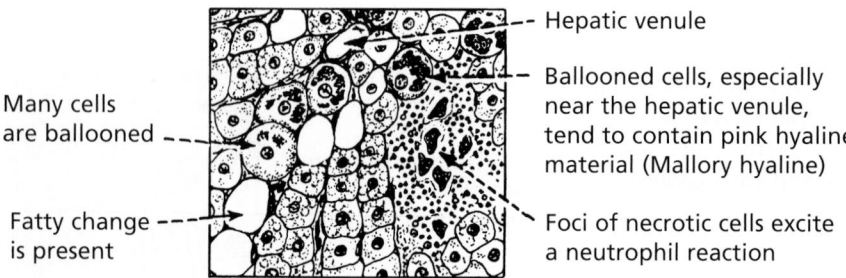

Many cells are ballooned

Fatty change is present

Hepatic venule

Ballooned cells, especially near the hepatic venule, tend to contain pink hyaline material (Mallory hyaline)

Foci of necrotic cells excite a neutrophil reaction

**Progressing to pericellular fibrosis**

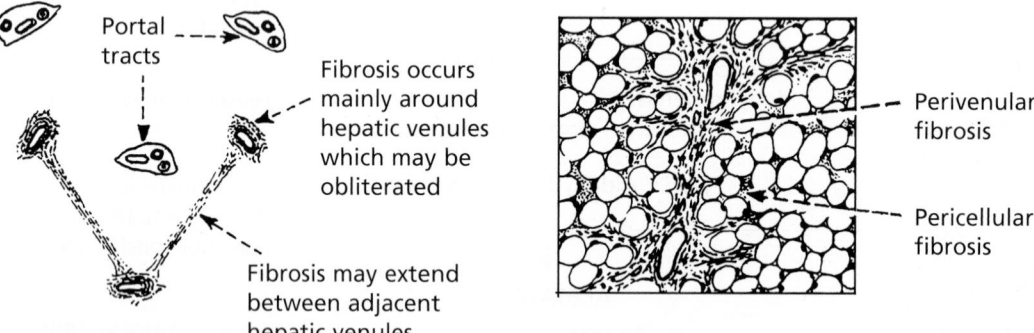

Portal tracts

Fibrosis occurs mainly around hepatic venules which may be obliterated

Fibrosis may extend between adjacent hepatic venules

Perivenular fibrosis

Pericellular fibrosis

Alcoholic hepatitis is important as a cause of liver damage, especially because of the high risk of progression to cirrhosis.

Non-alcoholic fatty liver disease (NAFLD) is a common fatty liver condition which develops in patients who do not drink alcohol. The liver may show steatosis, steatohepatitis or cirrhosis although the changes are often less marked than seen with alcohol. NAFLD is associated with the metabolic syndrome – defined as having at least two of the following, obesity, insulin resistance, dyslipidaemia or hypertension.

# CIRRHOSIS

**Cirrhosis** is the end stage of many liver diseases. It is defined as:

A DIFFUSE process (i.e. the whole liver is affected) characterised by FIBROSIS and conversion of the liver architecture into abnormal NODULES.

## Aetiology

There are many causes including:

(i) Drugs and toxins, e.g. alcohol, methotrexate, methyldopa.
(ii) Infections, e.g. hepatitis B and C.
(iii) Auto-immune diseases – chronic active hepatitis, primary biliary cirrhosis.
(iv) Metabolic conditions, e.g. haemochromatosis, $\alpha_1$-antitrypsin deficiency, Wilson disease (excess accumulation of copper).
(v) Biliary obstruction, e.g. gallstones, strictures, sclerosing cholangitis, cystic fibrosis.
(vi) Cryptogenic, i.e. cause unknown.

The **mechanism** common to all cirrhosis is:

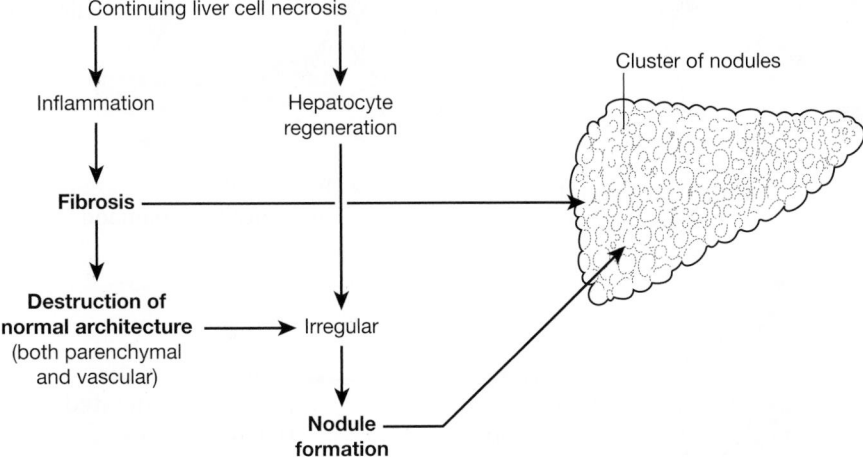

Hepatic stellate (fat-storing) cells found in the space of Disse are activated and transformed into myofibroblast-like cells under the influence of cytokines such as TGF-$\alpha$, PDGF and TGF-$\beta$. The activated cells synthesise collagen leading to fibrosis.

The **major complications** of cirrhosis are:

1. Hepatocellular failure.
2. Portal hypertension.
3. Hepatocellular carcinoma.

# CIRRHOSIS

The initiating factor in the progression to cirrhosis is continuing hepatocellular damage. Its location within the acinus (p. 338) and also its cause are reflected in the progression to irreversible damage.

The following contrasting diagrams illustrate the differing patterns in cirrhosis depending on the cause.

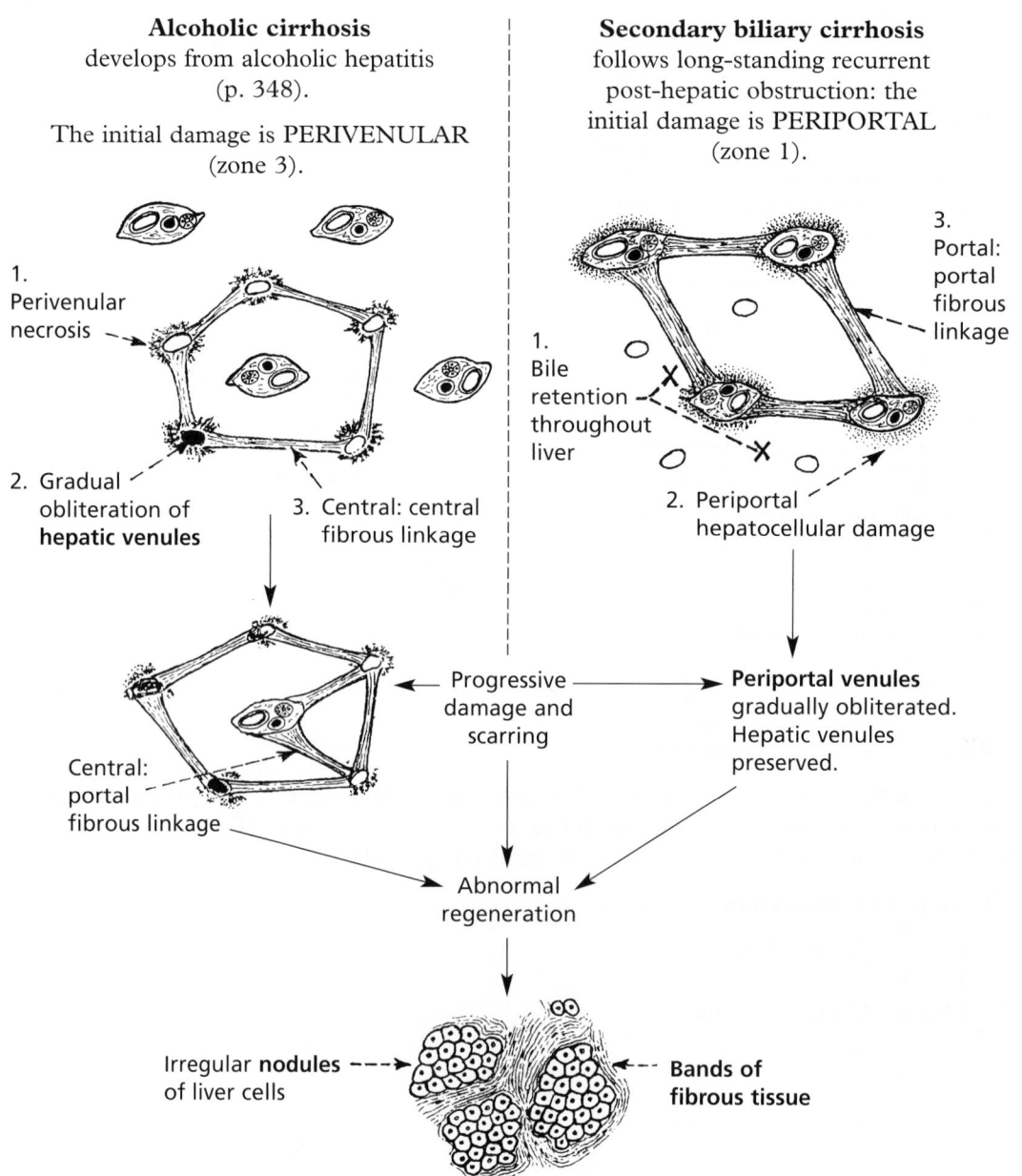

**Alcoholic cirrhosis**
develops from alcoholic hepatitis (p. 348).

The initial damage is PERIVENULAR (zone 3).

1. Perivenular necrosis

2. Gradual obliteration of **hepatic venules**

3. Central: central fibrous linkage

Central: portal fibrous linkage

**Secondary biliary cirrhosis**
follows long-standing recurrent post-hepatic obstruction: the initial damage is PERIPORTAL (zone 1).

3. Portal: portal fibrous linkage

1. Bile retention throughout liver

2. Periportal hepatocellular damage

Progressive damage and scarring

**Periportal venules** gradually obliterated. Hepatic venules preserved.

Abnormal regeneration

Irregular **nodules** of liver cells

**Bands of fibrous tissue**

# BILIARY DISEASE

## PRIMARY BILIARY CIRRHOSIS (PBC)

This is a chronic disorder mainly affecting middle-aged women. Destruction of intra-hepatic bile ducts leads to scarring and eventually to cirrhosis. Patients typically present with fatigue, itching (from bile salt retention) or jaundice. Hyperlipidaemia is common.

### Aetiology

This is an auto-immune disorder. Over 95% of patients have anti-mitochondrial antibodies in their serum. An overlap may be seen with auto-immune chronic hepatitis.

### Pathology

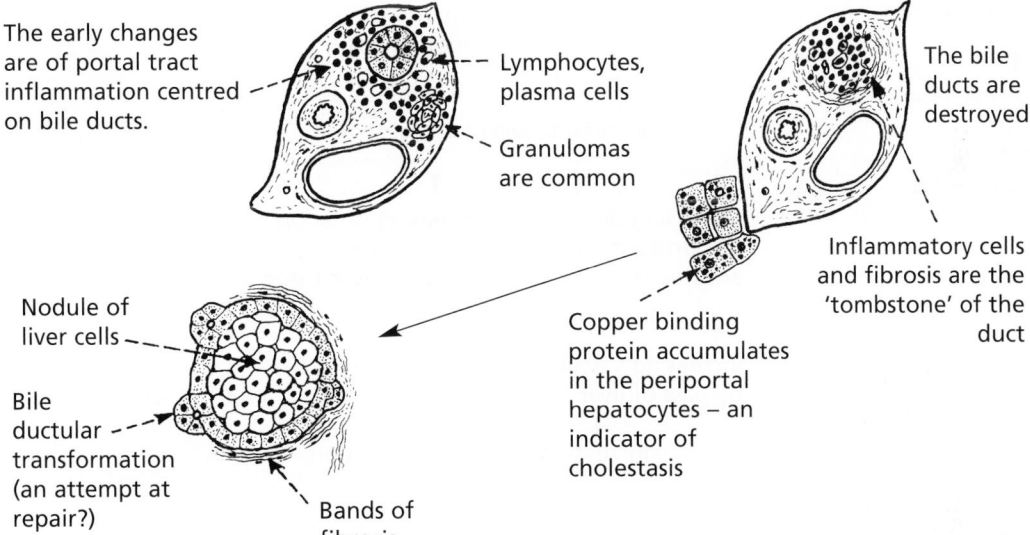

The early changes are of portal tract inflammation centred on bile ducts.

Lymphocytes, plasma cells

Granulomas are common

The bile ducts are destroyed

Inflammatory cells and fibrosis are the 'tombstone' of the duct

Copper binding protein accumulates in the periportal hepatocytes – an indicator of cholestasis

Nodule of liver cells

Bile ductular transformation (an attempt at repair?)

Bands of fibrosis

*Note*: Long-standing biliary obstruction can give rise to secondary biliary cirrhosis if untreated.

## PRIMARY SCLEROSING CHOLANGITIS

This disease also attacks bile ducts, both intra- and extrahepatic. Men are usually affected and there is a strong association with ulcerative colitis.

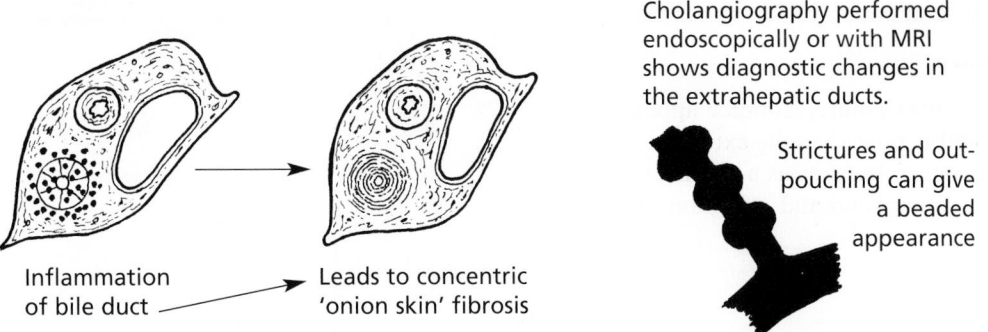

Cholangiography performed endoscopically or with MRI shows diagnostic changes in the extrahepatic ducts.

Strictures and out-pouching can give a beaded appearance

Inflammation of bile duct → Leads to concentric 'onion skin' fibrosis

The late effects are similar to PBC. Liver failure and bile duct carcinoma are frequent complications.

# HEPATOCELLULAR FAILURE

**Failure of liver function can be:**

1. Acute, with rapid onset (<8 weeks from onset of liver disease), e.g. in cases of massive necrosis due to poisoning, e.g. paracetamol (or, less commonly, acute hepatitis).
2. Chronic and sometimes recurring, of slow onset, e.g. in cirrhosis or chronic hepatitis, representing decompensation.

The mechanism is different in the two types.

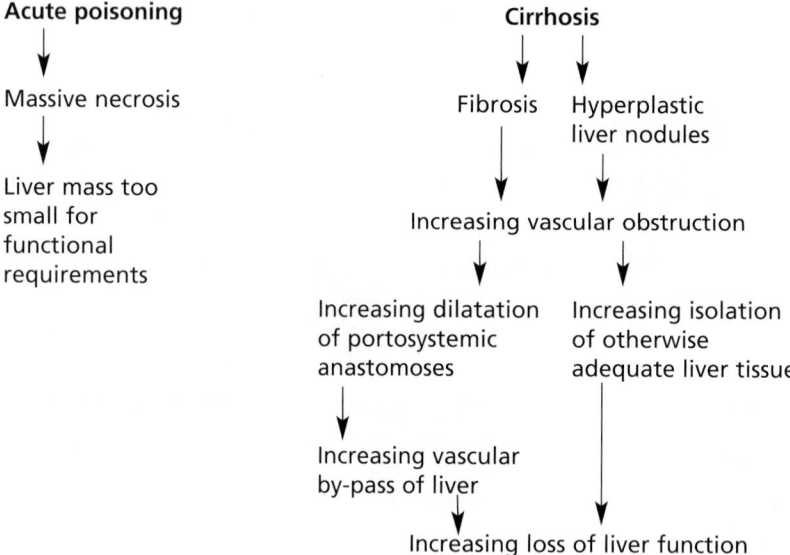

**Acute poisoning**

↓

Massive necrosis

↓

Liver mass too small for functional requirements

**Cirrhosis**

↓ ↓

Fibrosis    Hyperplastic liver nodules

↓ ↓

Increasing vascular obstruction

↓ ↓

Increasing dilatation of portosystemic anastomoses    Increasing isolation of otherwise adequate liver tissue

↓

Increasing vascular by-pass of liver

↓ ↓

Increasing loss of liver function

The **cardinal signs of hepatocellular failure are:**

1. Jaundice.
2. Hepatic encephalopathy.
3. Ascites.
4. Bleeding diathesis.

Other features include hypoglycaemia, acidosis and endocrine disturbances.

## Jaundice

In acute liver failure, jaundice appears early and is related to the extent of liver damage. It arises as a result of lack of conjugation and excretion of bilirubin.

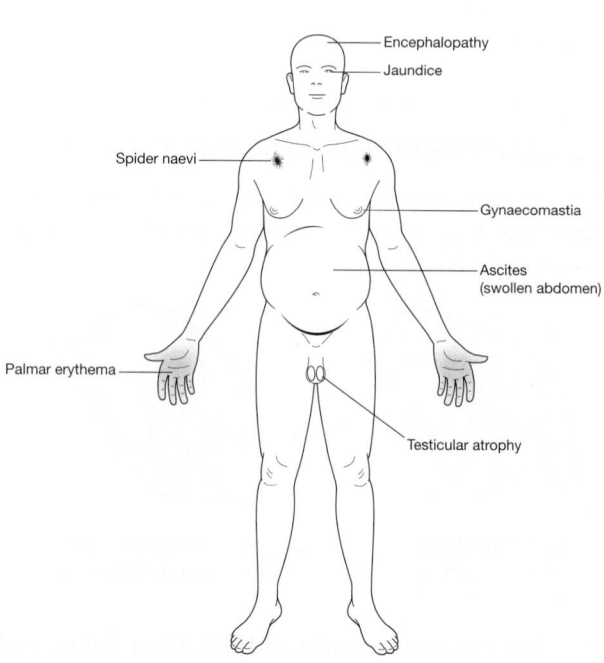

Encephalopathy

Jaundice

Spider naevi

Gynaecomastia

Ascites (swollen abdomen)

Palmar erythema

Testicular atrophy

# HEPATOCELLULAR FAILURE

## HEPATIC ENCEPHALOPATHY

This term refers to the impaired mental state and neurological function due to liver failure. It takes the form of tremors, behavioural changes, convulsions, delirium, drowsiness and coma. In the acute form, severe symptoms such as convulsions, delirium and coma develop rapidly, while in chronic conditions milder changes are seen and coma is a late feature, unless a complication arises.

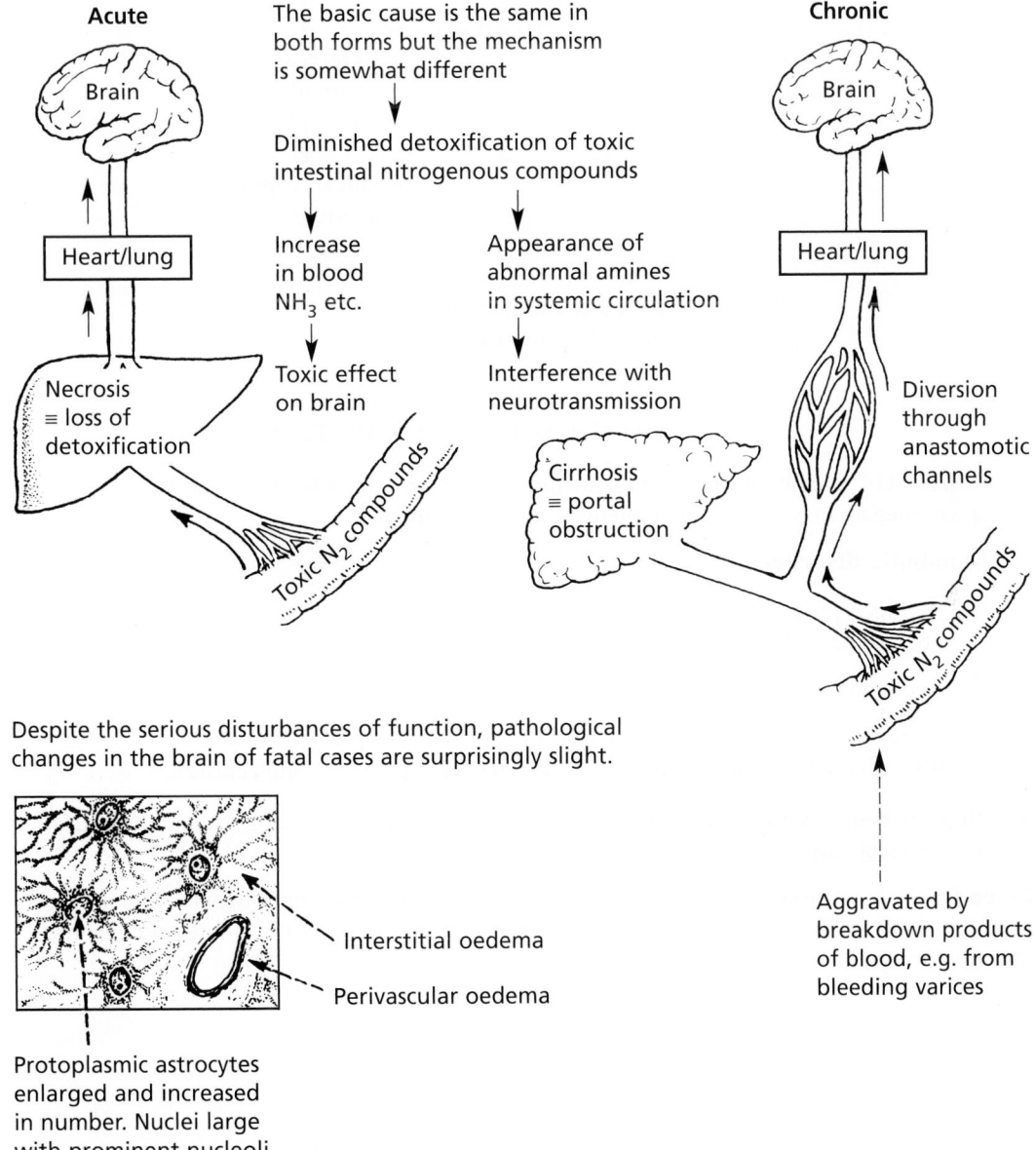

**Acute**

Brain

Heart/lung

Necrosis ≡ loss of detoxification

Toxic N₂ compounds

The basic cause is the same in both forms but the mechanism is somewhat different

Diminished detoxification of toxic intestinal nitrogenous compounds

Increase in blood $NH_3$ etc.

Toxic effect on brain

Appearance of abnormal amines in systemic circulation

Interference with neurotransmission

Cirrhosis ≡ portal obstruction

**Chronic**

Brain

Heart/lung

Diversion through anastomotic channels

Toxic N₂ compounds

Despite the serious disturbances of function, pathological changes in the brain of fatal cases are surprisingly slight.

Interstitial oedema

Perivascular oedema

Protoplasmic astrocytes enlarged and increased in number. Nuclei large with prominent nucleoli.

Aggravated by breakdown products of blood, e.g. from bleeding varices

# HEPATOCELLULAR FAILURE

1.  **ASCITES** is usually due to a combination of **portal hypertension** and **hepatocellular failure**.

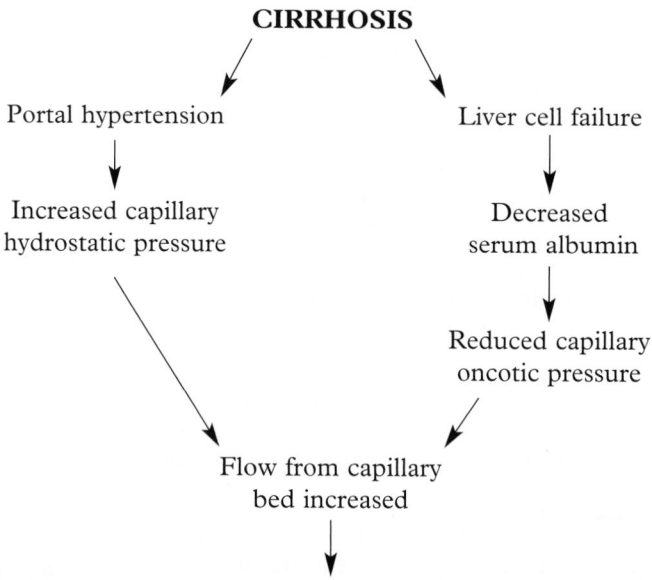

**CIRRHOSIS**

Portal hypertension → Increased capillary hydrostatic pressure

Liver cell failure → Decreased serum albumin → Reduced capillary oncotic pressure

Flow from capillary bed increased

Accumulation of peritoneal fluid = **ASCITES**

2.  **ANAEMIA** usually of normocytic/normochromic type (p. 440) is common splenomegaly may cause hypersplenism and pancytopenia.

3.  **Metabolic disorders**

    (a) Reduced protein synthesis, e.g. fibrinogen, prothrombin, factors V, VII, IX, X ⟶ bleeding diathesis.

    (b) Reduced liver glycogen storage ⟶ hypoglycaemia.

    (c) Reduced elimination of endogenous oestrogen ⟶ gynaecomastia, testicular atrophy and spider naevi (small skin capillary telangiectasia).

4.  **Hepato-renal syndrome** is an important complication of a major haemorrhage from oesophageal varices.

**Liver transplantation** is increasingly used to treat acute and chronic hepatocellular failure, as well as hepatocellular carcinoma. As with other transplanted organs, acute and chronic rejection are seen.

# PORTAL HYPERTENSION

In cirrhosis of the liver, **portal hypertension** is also important.

## Causes

By far, the most important cause is cirrhosis, but there are many others broadly classified as (1) pre-sinusoidal, (2) intra-sinusoidal and (3) post-sinusoidal.

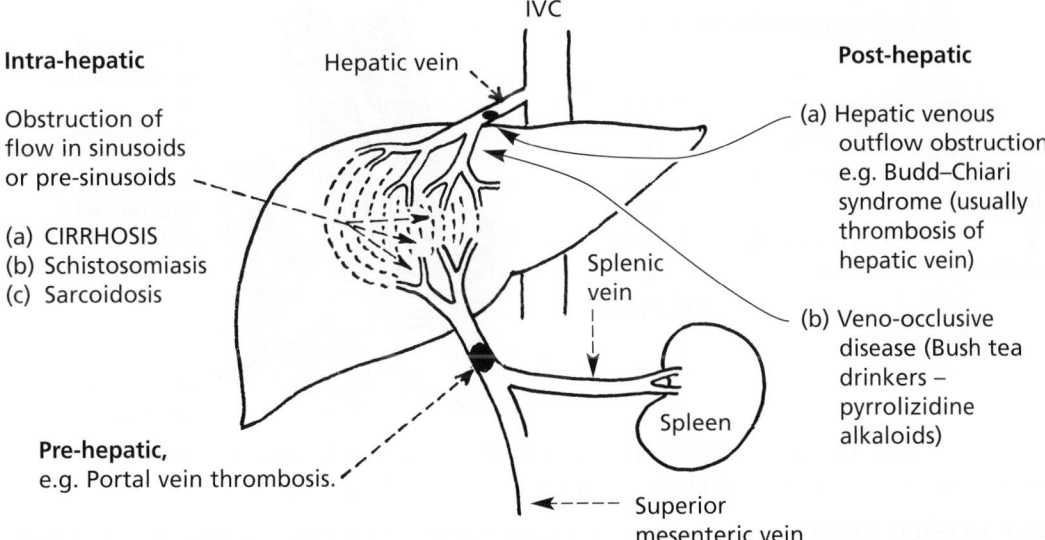

**Intra-hepatic**

Obstruction of flow in sinusoids or pre-sinusoids

(a) CIRRHOSIS
(b) Schistosomiasis
(c) Sarcoidosis

IVC

Hepatic vein

Splenic vein

Spleen

**Post-hepatic**

(a) Hepatic venous outflow obstruction, e.g. Budd–Chiari syndrome (usually thrombosis of hepatic vein)

(b) Veno-occlusive disease (Bush tea drinkers – pyrrolizidine alkaloids)

**Pre-hepatic,**
e.g. Portal vein thrombosis.

Superior mesenteric vein

## Effects

The main consequences are:

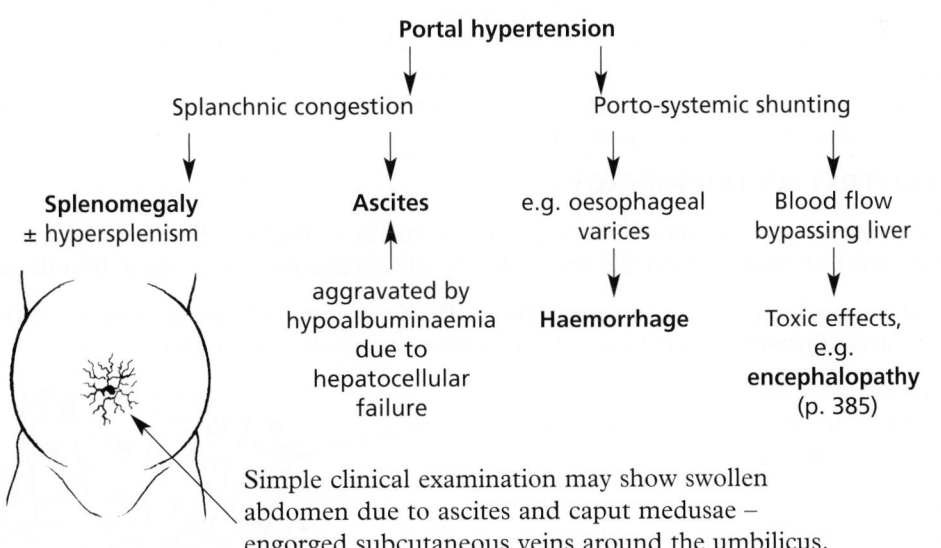

**Portal hypertension**

Splanchnic congestion

Porto-systemic shunting

**Splenomegaly**
± hypersplenism

**Ascites**

e.g. oesophageal varices

Blood flow bypassing liver

aggravated by hypoalbuminaemia due to hepatocellular failure

**Haemorrhage**

Toxic effects, e.g. **encephalopathy** (p. 385)

Simple clinical examination may show swollen abdomen due to ascites and caput medusae – engorged subcutaneous veins around the umbilicus.

# METABOLIC DISORDERS OF THE LIVER

### HAEMOCHROMATOSIS

This is an autosomal recessive disorder characterised by excessive accumulation of body iron. It is due to a mutation on chromosome 6, encoding the HFE protein which regulates iron absorption. Whilst heterozygotes absorb excess iron, only homozygotes develop the disease.

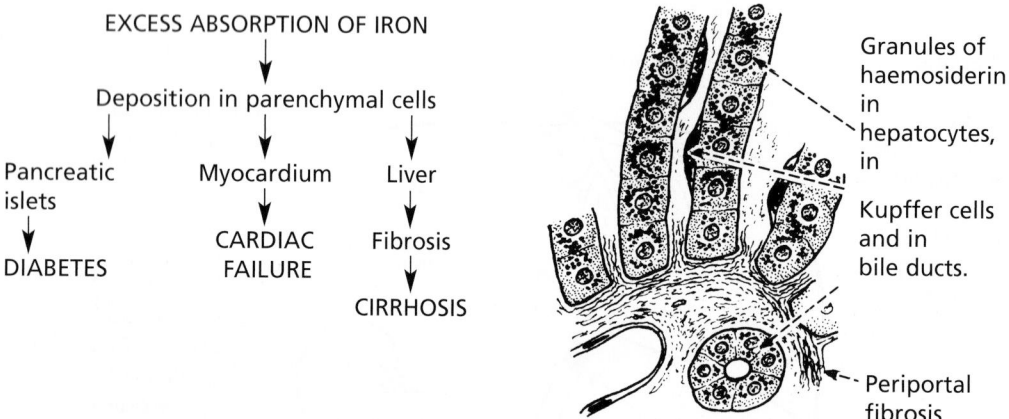

EXCESS ABSORPTION OF IRON

Deposition in parenchymal cells

Pancreatic islets → DIABETES

Myocardium → CARDIAC FAILURE

Liver → Fibrosis → CIRRHOSIS

Granules of haemosiderin in hepatocytes, in Kupffer cells and in bile ducts.

Periportal fibrosis

*Note*: In the skin, the iron is deposited mainly in the sweat glands: excessive melanin production in the epidermis explains the term 'bronzed diabetes' for these cases.

**HAEMOSIDEROSIS** – excess dietary iron and repeated blood transfusions may overload the body iron stores but cause less liver damage.

### WILSON DISEASE (HEPATO-LENTICULAR DEGENERATION)

A rare autosomal recessive condition (due to mutation of the ATP7B gene on chromosome 13 which encodes a copper transporting enzyme). This is characterised by accumulation of copper in the liver, brain (basal ganglia) and cornea (Kayser–Fleischer rings). Serum levels of caeruloplasmin (a copper-binding protein) are reduced. The liver can show steatosis, an acute hepatitis, chronic hepatitis or cirrhosis.

### $\alpha_1$-ANTITRYPSIN DEFICIENCY

This enzyme is a protease inhibitor (Pi) produced mainly by the liver. Reduced levels or activity of the enzyme (abnormal forms coded by allelic variants) may result in liver damage.

Liver disease is found in most **homozygotes** (PiZZ) and presents as neonatal hepatitis, chronic active hepatitis or cirrhosis. Heterozygotes are rarely badly affected.

The abnormal enzyme is not secreted by liver cells and accumulates as globules in the periportal hepatocytes.

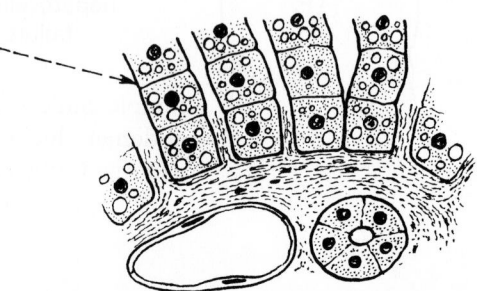

*Note*: $\alpha_1$-antitrypsin deficiency is an important factor in the development of emphysema (p. 289).

# INFECTIONS

## PYOGENIC INFECTIONS

These are now much less common due to the use of antibiotics. Abscess of the liver, usually due to coliforms, occurs mainly in two conditions:

1. **Ascending cholangitis**

2. **Suppurative pylephlebitis**

This arises from suppurative lesions in the abdominal cavity such as:

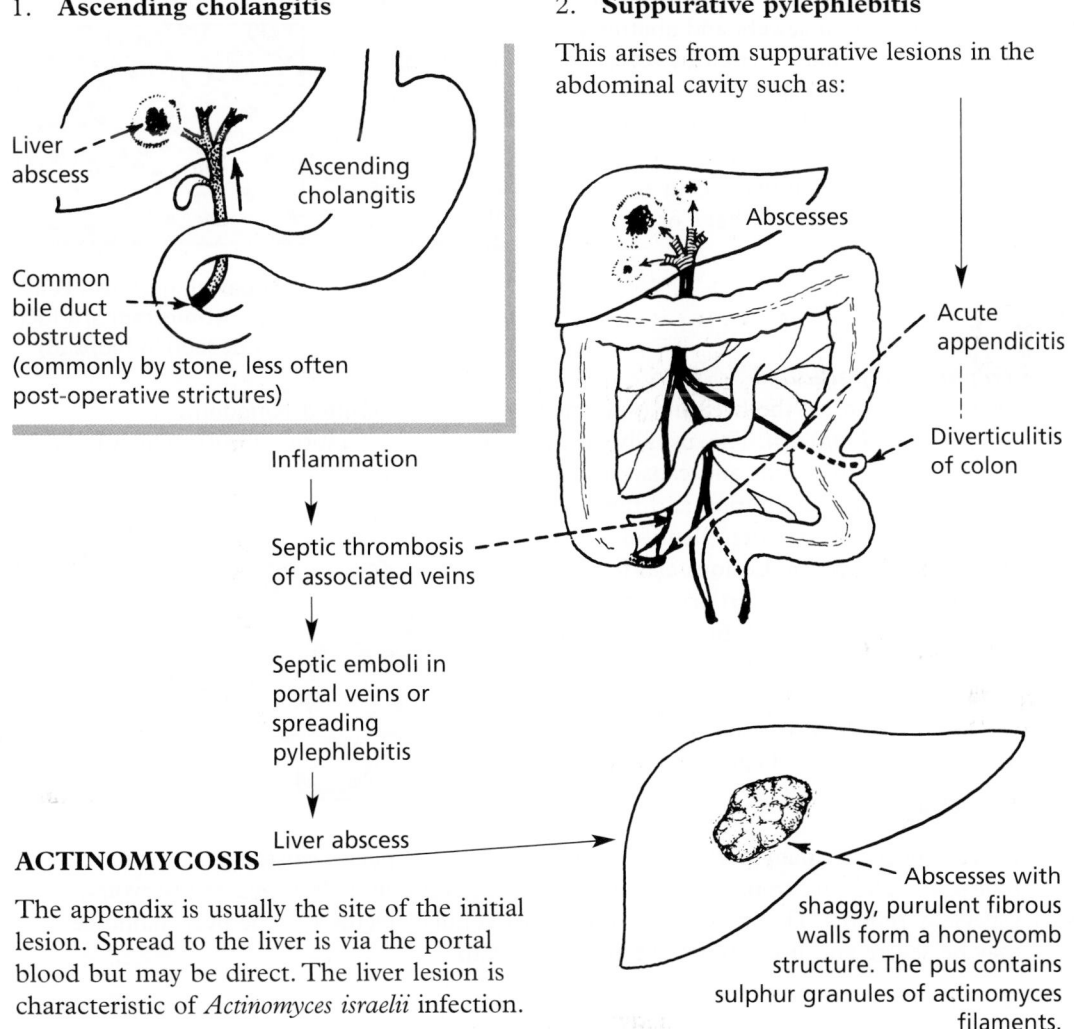

Inflammation

↓

Septic thrombosis of associated veins

↓

Septic emboli in portal veins or spreading pylephlebitis

↓

Liver abscess

## ACTINOMYCOSIS

The appendix is usually the site of the initial lesion. Spread to the liver is via the portal blood but may be direct. The liver lesion is characteristic of *Actinomyces israelii* infection.

Abscesses with shaggy, purulent fibrous walls form a honeycomb structure. The pus contains sulphur granules of actinomyces filaments.

## TUBERCULOSIS

This is rare. Miliary tubercles may be seen in generalised infection.

## HEPATIC GRANULOMAS

Granulomas are also common in sarcoidosis and may also occur in brucellosis, histoplasmosis and PBC, among many other causes.

# INFECTIONS

### SPIROCHAETAL INFECTIONS

Three spirochaetal infections can involve the liver.

1. *Leptospira icterohaemorrhagica* **(Weil disease)**

   This organism is transmitted from rats to man, especially these working in wet conditions, e.g. in sewers and abattoirs.
   The disease is characterised by fever, jaundice, haemorrhage into various organs, e.g. lungs, kidneys, and renal damage. The liver lesion is characteristic. Death may occur from intrapulmonary haemorrhage or renal failure.

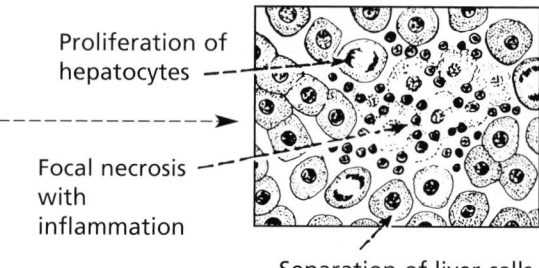

Proliferation of hepatocytes

Focal necrosis with inflammation

Separation of liver cells (a post-mortem artefact – not seen in biopsies)

2. *Treponema pallidum*

   Syphilitic lesions of the liver are now uncommon in the United Kingdom.

   (a) *Congenital infection.* This usually produces a diffuse interstitial fibrosis which isolates individual liver cells and causes ischaemic atrophy. It is accompanied by a striking mononuclear infiltration and tiny areas of coagulative necrosis – miliary gummas. Spirochaetes are often plentiful.

   (b) *Acquired infection.* Lesions can occur in the secondary and tertiary stages. In the secondary stage, a diffuse, inflammatory reaction with miliary gummas can occur. Large gummas may be seen in tertiary syphilis. Gross scarring with distortion follows healing – hepar lobatum.

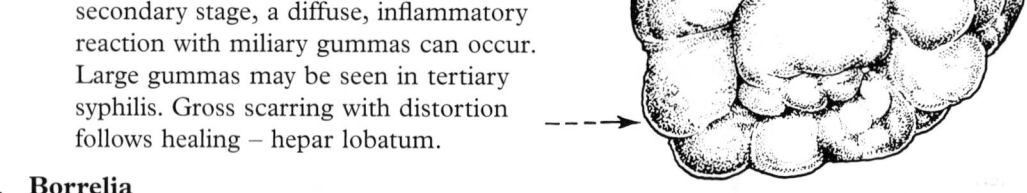

3. **Borrelia**

Borrelia occur in many parts of the world and several species exist, e.g. *Borrelia recurrentis.* They are transmitted by lice and ticks from animals acting as reservoirs, especially rodents. The infections produce perivenular necrosis of the liver. Jaundice may be severe and liver failure can result in death.

# INFECTIONS

## PROTOZOAL DISEASES

### Amoebic 'abscess'

This is a complication of amoebic dysentery due to *Entamoeba histolytica*. The 'abscess' is usually single, in the upper right lobe of liver. An irregular fibrous wall encloses off necrotic liver cells, debris and red cells. Amoebae may be found in the inner wall. It may remain localised or track through the diaphragm into the lung, pleural or pericardial cavities.

### Malaria

On initial infection, the parasites develop within the hepatocytes but produce little damage. In chronic malaria, red cells containing parasites are engulfed by Kupffer cells which become hyperplastic and contain brown malarial pigment.

### Kala-azar (visceral leishmaniasis)

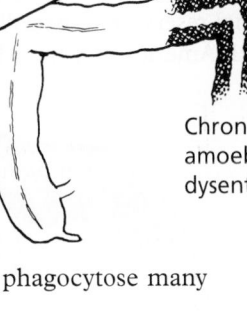

Venous drainage

Chronic amoebic dysentry

The liver is enlarged due to hyperplasia of the Kupffer cells which phagocytose many Leishman–Donovan bodies, the protozoan responsible.

## METAZOAL DISEASES TREMATODES (FLUKES)

### Schistosomiasis (bilharzia)

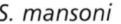

*S. mansoni*

*Schistosoma mansoni* is common in Egypt and other parts of Africa. *Schistosoma japonicum* is found in China, Japan and the Philippines. Both infections involve the liver.

The schistosomes colonise the intestinal tract. They invade the intestinal veins; ova are released into the blood stream and embolise the portal venules of the liver. There is a focal granulomatous reaction which may lead to extensive portal fibrosis without cirrhosis. Portal hypertension can result with its associated complications.

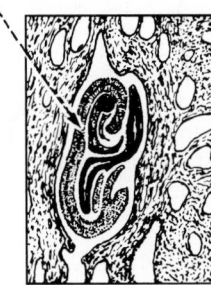

# INFECTIONS

Two other varieties of fluke disease exist –
clonorchiasis (Chinese fish fluke) and fascioliasis
(sheep fluke). Both produce an ascending
cholangitis. Clonorchiasis can cause biliary
obstruction and marked proliferation of bile ducts.
Cholangiocarcinoma may develop. Infestation in
both cases is due to eating raw or undercooked
food.

Flukes

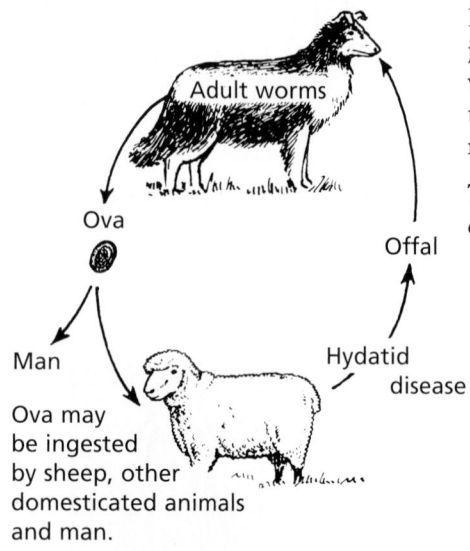

### Hydatid disease

This condition is caused by the embryos of
*Echinococcus granulosus*, a small tapeworm. The disease is caught by close contact with
animal reservoirs especially sheep and dogs. It is commonest in Australia, New Zealand,
South America and the Middle East.

Adult worms

Ova

Man

Ova may
be ingested
by sheep, other
domesticated animals
and man.

Offal

Hydatid
disease

Digestion of the chitinous membrane by gastric
juice releases the ova which invade the intestinal
veins and reach the liver. Sometimes they pass into
the systemic circulation and cysts form in the lungs,
muscles, kidneys, spleen or brain.

The cyst may be very large, usually multilocular,
due to budding of daughter cysts.

Serological tests are
positive in half of cases.

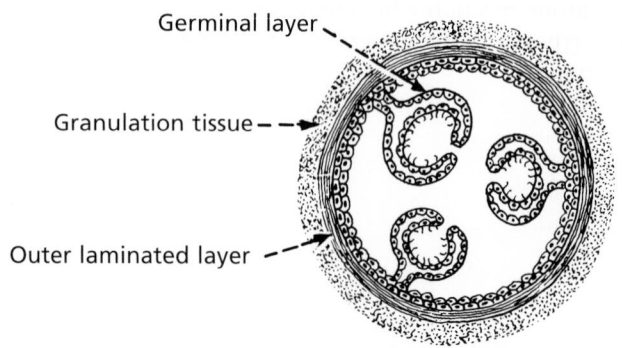

Germinal layer

Granulation tissue

Outer laminated layer

# TUMOURS OF THE LIVER

## PRIMARY BENIGN TUMOURS

1. **Cavernous haemangioma.** This is the commonest type. It forms a dark purple, sharply demarcated geometric patch on the liver surface and consists of dilated blood vessels.
2. **Liver cell adenoma.** These small tumours are rare and are associated with the use of the contraceptive pill and anabolic steroids. They consist of normal liver trabeculae without normal portal tracts. Intraperitoneal bleeding may occur.
3. **Bile duct adenoma.** These small tumours are usually incidental findings at laparotomy. They consist of tiny bile duct structures set in loose connective tissue. Occasionally bile duct cystadenomas form large tumours.

## SECONDARY TUMOURS (METASTASES)

The liver is by far the most frequent site of secondary tumour deposits and these are far commoner than primary liver tumours. The common primary sites are the gastrointestinal tract, lung and breast. Melanoma, leukaemic infiltration and involvement by lymphoma are also often seen.

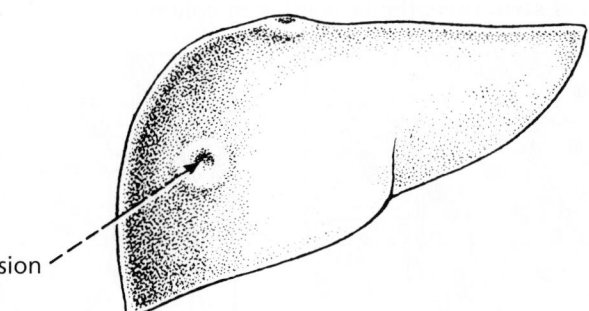

Umbilication, i.e. central depression due to necrosis, is common.

The metastases often grow rapidly and are frequently the main cause of death. An exception is metastatic carcinoid tumour which grows slowly over a period of years (p. 365).

Increasingly, metastases, e.g. from colorectal cancers, are treated by radio frequency ablation or surgical resection.

# PRIMARY CARCINOMA OF LIVER

### HEPATOCELLULAR CARCINOMA (HCC)

This is the commonest primary malignancy of the liver. It is unusual in Western Europe, but is very common in Africa and South-East Asia due to the high levels of hepatitis B infection. Males are particularly affected. There is a strong association with cirrhosis, especially in Western countries.

Three main types of growth are described:

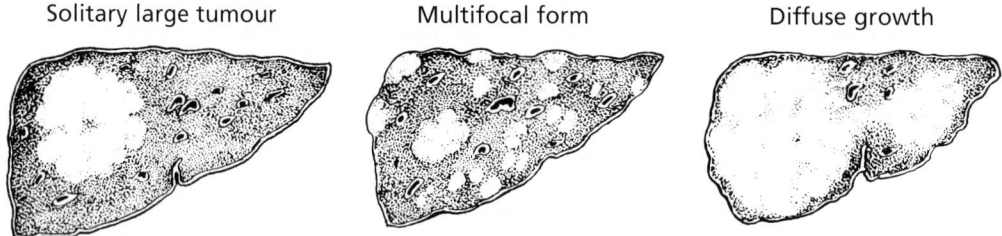

Solitary large tumour       Multifocal form       Diffuse growth

In all three forms the liver is often cirrhotic (80%), particularly in the West.

**Histological structure**: the cells grow in columns resembling normal liver.

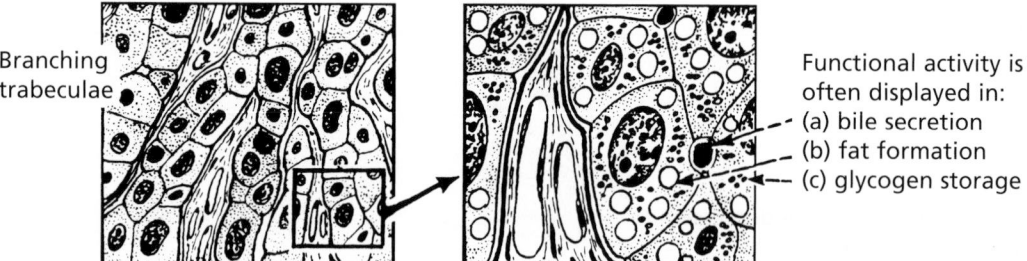

Branching trabeculae

Functional activity is often displayed in:
(a) bile secretion
(b) fat formation
(c) glycogen storage

### Spread

In addition to diffuse growth within the liver, **invasion of hepatic veins** occurs early. There may be metastases to lung, bone and also the draining lymph nodes.

The **cause of death** may be (i) liver failure, (ii) the complications of portal hypertension (especially in cirrhotic patients) and (iii) massive intraperitoneal haemorrhage.

Systemic manifestations include hypoglycaemia, hypercalcaemia and polycythaemia (due to production of erythropoietin).

# PRIMARY CARCINOMA OF LIVER

## Diagnosis

Liver biopsy is usually required. High levels of alpha-fetoprotein (normally produced in the fetal liver) >500 μg/L are strong supportive evidence (not all tumours produce this protein). This can be demonstrated in tumour cells by immunostaining. In situ hybridisation can show mRNA for albumin in alpha-fetoprotein–negative tumours.

## Aetiology

The aetiological agents vary in low and high incidence areas.

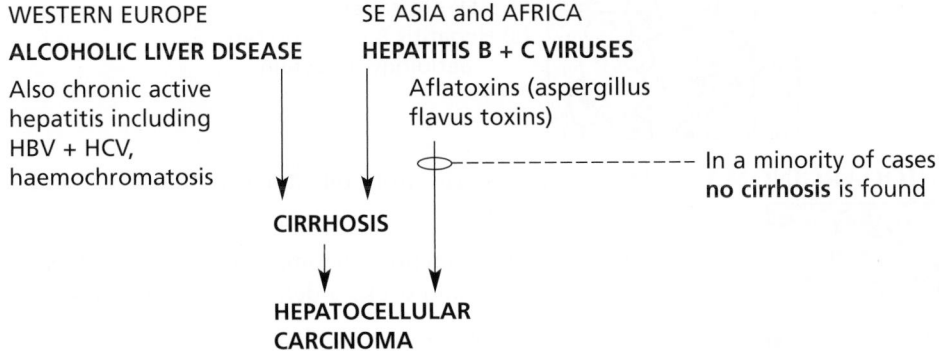

WESTERN EUROPE
**ALCOHOLIC LIVER DISEASE**

Also chronic active hepatitis including HBV + HCV, haemochromatosis

SE ASIA and AFRICA
**HEPATITIS B + C VIRUSES**

Aflatoxins (aspergillus flavus toxins)

In a minority of cases **no cirrhosis** is found

**CIRRHOSIS**

**HEPATOCELLULAR CARCINOMA**

# PRIMARY LIVER CELL TUMOURS

### FIBROLAMELLAR CARCINOMA

This uncommon variant (<5%) occurs especially in young adults. It is important because the prognosis is much better following surgical resection.

Histologically

Large polygonal tumour cells form trabeculae separated by fibrous stroma

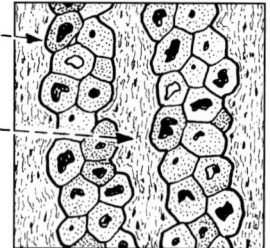

Other differences from conventional HCC are
(1) Usually no cirrhosis
(2) AFP not raised
(3) Hepatitis B infection rare
    – aetiology uncertain

### CHOLANGIOCARCINOMA

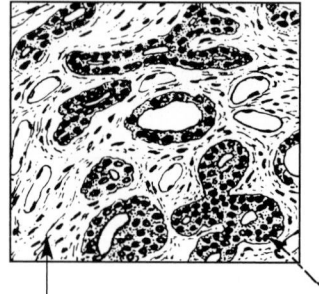

Fibrous stroma

Cells resemble bile duct epithelium

These tumours arise from bile ducts at both intra- and extrahepatic sites.

They are usually adenocarcinomas: some show excess mucus secretion and evoke a dense fibrous response.

Cirrhosis is rarely present.

There is an increased incidence in association with ulcerative colitis and primary sclerosing cholangitis, and in the Far East there is a clear association with liver fluke (clonorchis) infestation.

# GALLBLADDER AND BILE DUCT – ANATOMY

**Anatomy**

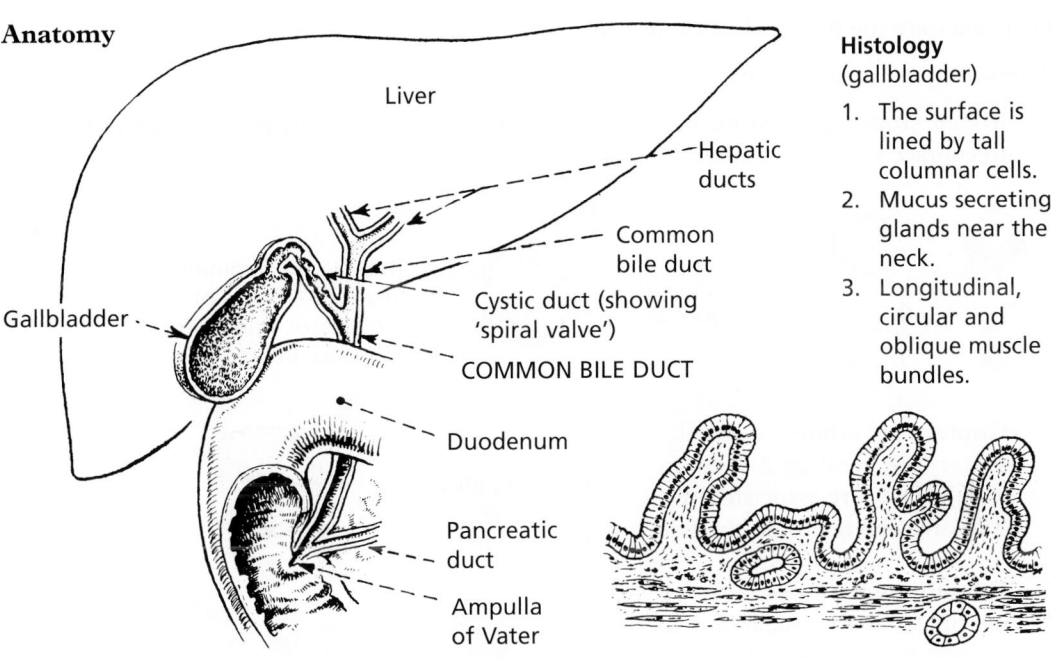

**Histology**
(gallbladder)

1. The surface is lined by tall columnar cells.
2. Mucus secreting glands near the neck.
3. Longitudinal, circular and oblique muscle bundles.

# GALLSTONES

Gallstones are the principal cause of gallbladder disease and its consequences.

There are three main types:

1. **Mixed stones** account for 80% of all gallstones. They are **multiple** and **faceted** due to contact with one another.

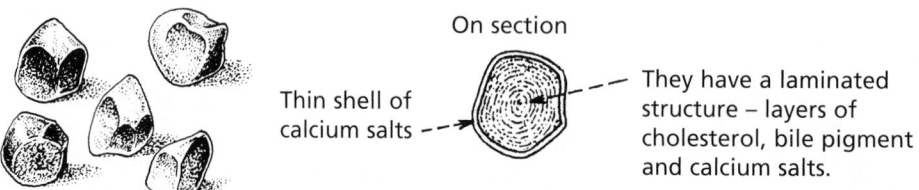

On section

Thin shell of calcium salts

They have a laminated structure – layers of cholesterol, bile pigment and calcium salts.

2. **Cholesterol stone** – is usually solitary, oval and up 2–3 cm in length. They are associated with excessive cholesterol in the bile.

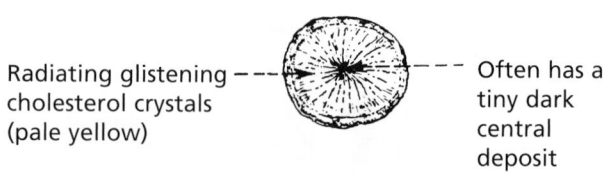

Radiating glistening cholesterol crystals (pale yellow)

Often has a tiny dark central deposit

3. **Bile pigment stones** – are multiple and are usually due to chronic haemolysis with excess bilirubin production.

Rarely more than 1 cm in diameter, black and irregular.

## GALLSTONES

### Clinical manifestations and complications

Many patients are asymptomatic or have only mild dyspepsia; others develop symptomatic complications.

### 1. ACUTE CHOLECYSTITIS

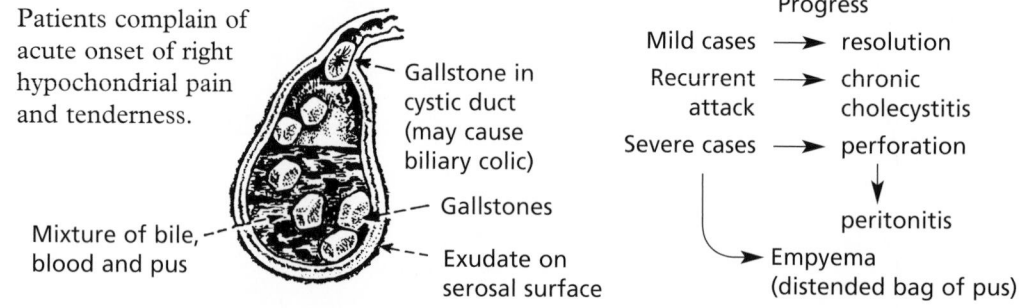

Patients complain of acute onset of right hypochondrial pain and tenderness.

Gallstone in cystic duct (may cause biliary colic)

Gallstones

Mixture of bile, blood and pus

Exudate on serosal surface

Progress

Mild cases → resolution

Recurrent attack → chronic cholecystitis

Severe cases → perforation → peritonitis

Empyema (distended bag of pus)

# GALLSTONES

## 2. CHRONIC CHOLECYSTITIS

In the majority of cases the symptoms are of vague 'indigestion', intolerance of fatty foods and vague right hypochondrial pain: in some cases there is a history of acute attacks.

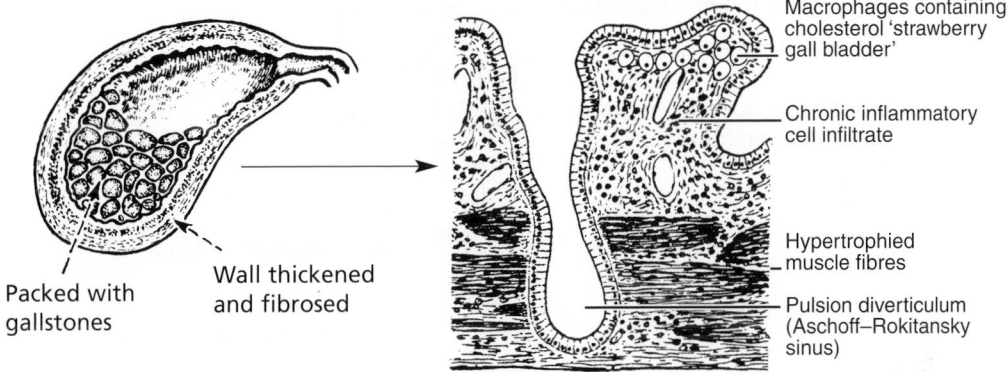

Packed with gallstones

Wall thickened and fibrosed

Macrophages containing cholesterol 'strawberry gall bladder'

Chronic inflammatory cell infiltrate

Hypertrophied muscle fibres

Pulsion diverticulum (Aschoff–Rokitansky sinus)

## 3. MUCOCELE – can occur when the cystic duct is blocked.

This occurs when there has been long-standing obstruction of the cystic duct.

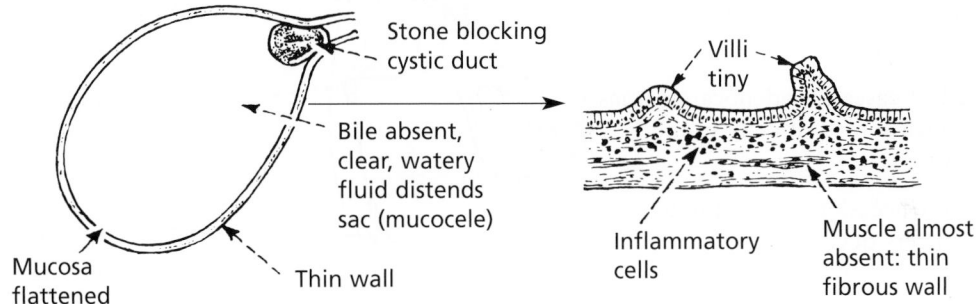

Stone blocking cystic duct

Bile absent, clear, watery fluid distends sac (mucocele)

Mucosa flattened

Thin wall

Villi tiny

Inflammatory cells

Muscle almost absent: thin fibrous wall

## 4. COMMON BILE DUCT GALLSTONES

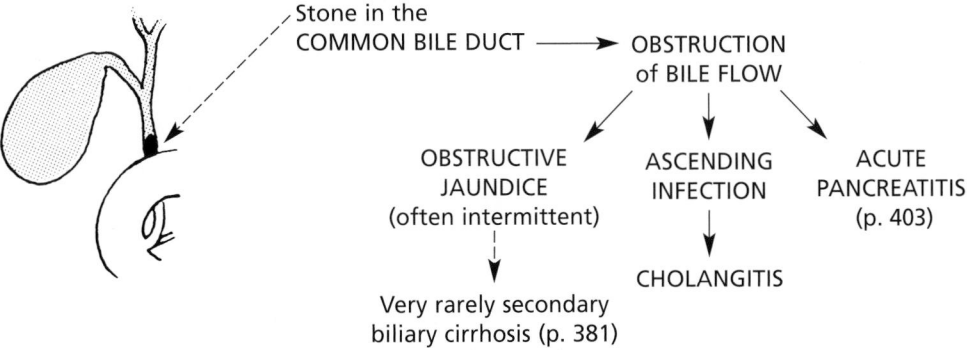

Stone in the COMMON BILE DUCT ⟶ OBSTRUCTION of BILE FLOW

OBSTRUCTIVE JAUNDICE (often intermittent)

ASCENDING INFECTION

ACUTE PANCREATITIS (p. 403)

CHOLANGITIS

Very rarely secondary biliary cirrhosis (p. 381)

*Note*: In addition to jaundice, persistent skin itching, due to retention of bile salts, may occur.

# GALLSTONES

### 5. GALLSTONE ILEUS

Very rarely a stone may ulcerate through the gallbladder into the intestine and cause obstruction.

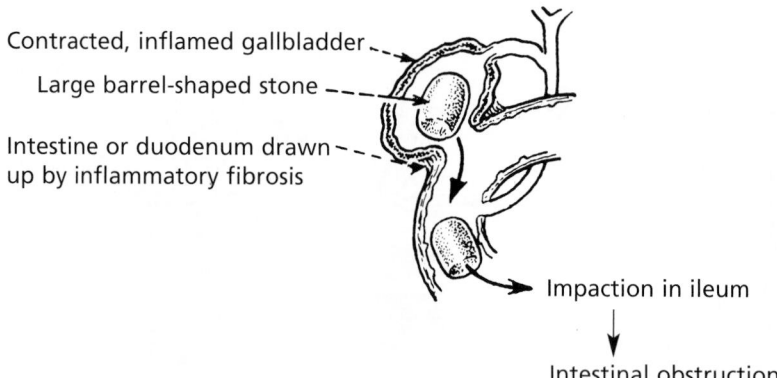

Contracted, inflamed gallbladder

Large barrel-shaped stone

Intestine or duodenum drawn up by inflammatory fibrosis

Impaction in ileum

Intestinal obstruction

### 6. CARCINOMA OF THE GALLBLADDER

This is uncommon, but almost always associated with gallstones.

Most cases are adenocarcinomas which spread directly to the liver.

Very occasionally squamous cancers develop.

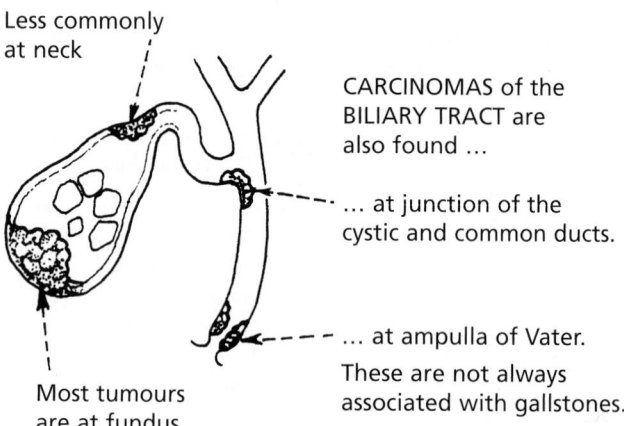

Less commonly at neck

CARCINOMAS of the BILIARY TRACT are also found …

… at junction of the cystic and common ducts.

… at ampulla of Vater. These are not always associated with gallstones.

Most tumours are at fundus

# GALLSTONES – AETIOLOGY

Although gallstones are found in 10–20% of the population, the prevalence increasing with age, the exact mechanisms of their formation remain incompletely understood. Risk factors include (a) female gender, (b) obesity, (c) pregnancy, (d) drugs such as the cholesterol-lowering drug clofibrate, now seldom used and (e) gastrointestinal disease, e.g. Crohn's disease.

The principal constituents of bile are **cholesterol, phospholipids** and **bile acids** (cholic acid and chenodeoxycholic acid).

The **stability of cholesterol** depends on adequate amounts of bile acids. Micelles are formed.

Their **enterohepatic circulation** is essential to maintain adequate concentrations of bile salts.

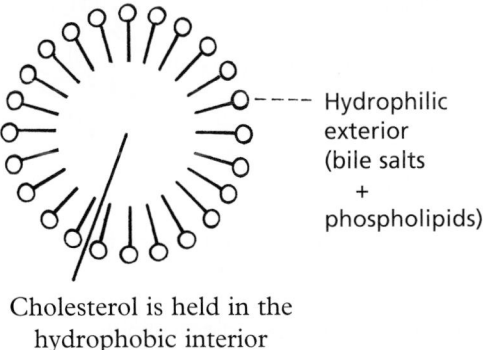

Hydrophilic exterior (bile salts + phospholipids)

Cholesterol is held in the hydrophobic interior

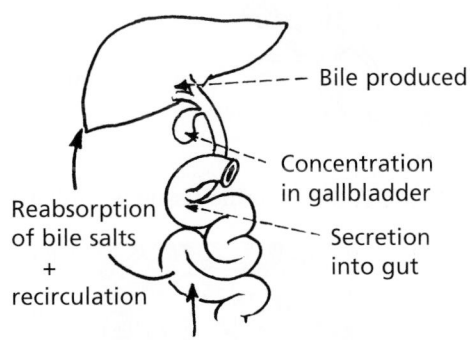

Bile produced

Concentration in gallbladder

Reabsorption of bile salts + recirculation

Secretion into gut

This can be interrupted by mucosal disease, e.g. Crohn's disease

The ratio of cholesterol to bile salts is very important.

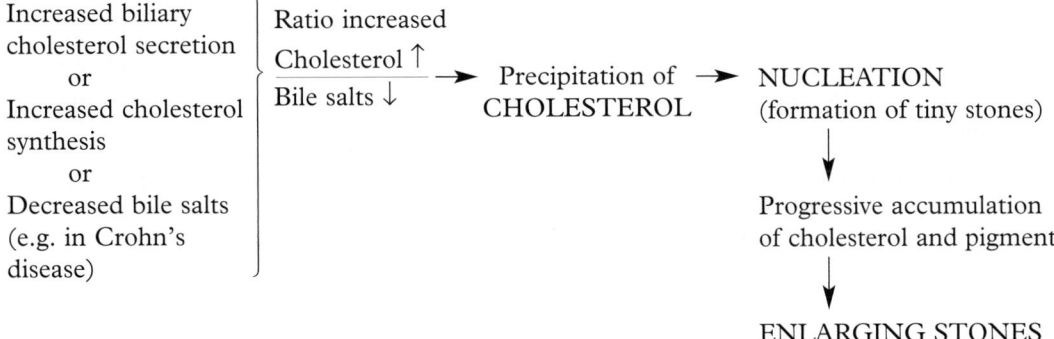

Increased biliary cholesterol secretion
or
Increased cholesterol synthesis
or
Decreased bile salts (e.g. in Crohn's disease)

Ratio increased
$\dfrac{\text{Cholesterol} \uparrow}{\text{Bile salts} \downarrow}$ → Precipitation of CHOLESTEROL → NUCLEATION (formation of tiny stones)

Progressive accumulation of cholesterol and pigment

ENLARGING STONES

Stones often lead to infection: it is likely that infection promotes further stone production.

These mechanisms are responsible for cholesterol and mixed stones. Pigment stones are seen in haemolytic anaemia, but also in relation to infection, e.g. of *Escherichia coli*. The mechanisms are poorly understood.

# PANCREAS

The exocrine glandular portion of the pancreas produces digestive secretions which are released into the second part of the duodenum.

Anatomical variations occur in this region.

Commonly the pancreatic and bile ducts fuse as they enter the ampulla of Vater …

Bile duct

Pancreas

Pancreatic duct

Duodenum

…but sometimes they enter the duodenum separately.

*Microscopically*, the exocrine tissue is similar to salivary glands.

In addition, foci of endocrine islet tissue occur throughout the pancreas (islets of Langerhans)

Exocrine secretory granules

*Function:* the exocrine pancreas produces an alkaline secretion containing digestive enzymes.
Sodium bicarbonate – gives a pH 7.5–8.0
Amylase – splits starches. Lipase – digests lipids.
Trypsinogen ⎱ converted to active proteolytic
Chymotrypsinogen ⎰ enzymes, trypsin, chymotrypsin.
The islet tissue produces insulin and glucagon (and other neuropeptides). Disorders of the islets, e.g. diabetes, are discussed on page 685.

There is evidence that mild pancreatitis is not uncommon but, in a significant number of cases, progression to a severe fatal disease occurs. Clinically, there is an acute abdominal emergency with pain and shock.

The essential pathological changes are due to tissue necrosis caused by the action of liberated enzymes on the pancreatic tissues. The severity of the lesion depends on the amount of enzyme set free, the distance it diffuses, anti-proteolytic factors and the structures affected.

# ACUTE PANCREATITIS

Early changes are seen in the centre of the lobules.

**Periductal necrosis** – in the centre of each affected lobule.

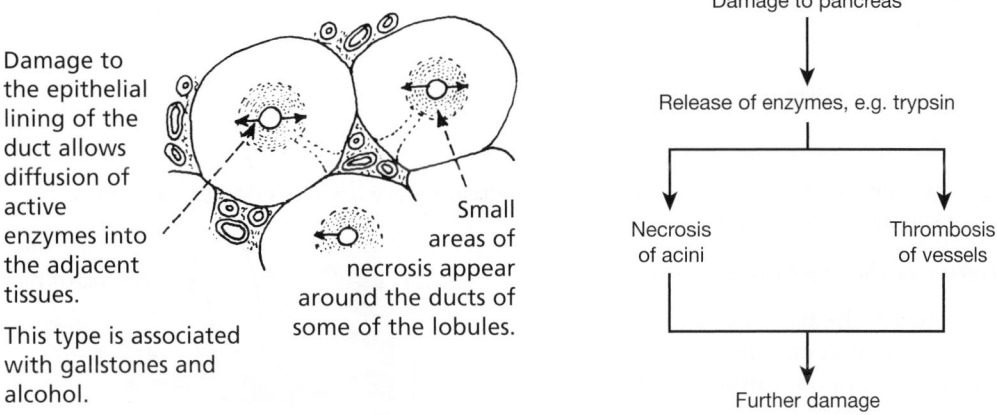

Damage to the epithelial lining of the duct allows diffusion of active enzymes into the adjacent tissues.

This type is associated with gallstones and alcohol.

Small areas of necrosis appear around the ducts of some of the lobules.

Damage to pancreas

↓

Release of enzymes, e.g. trypsin

↓

Necrosis of acini          Thrombosis of vessels

↓

Further damage

Unless this damage is inhibited by $\alpha_1$ antitrypsin and $\alpha_2$ macroglobulins from the blood and pancreatic secretory trypsin inhibitor, inflammation progresses to:

## PANLOBULAR PANCREATITIS

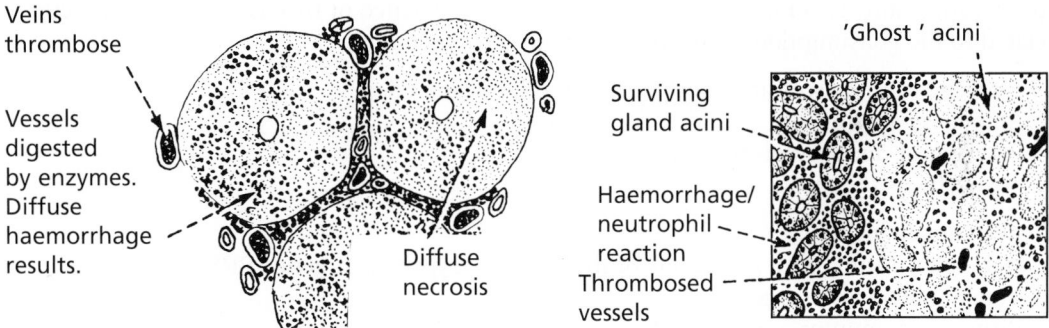

Veins thrombose

Vessels digested by enzymes. Diffuse haemorrhage results.

Diffuse necrosis

'Ghost' acini

Surviving gland acini

Haemorrhage/ neutrophil reaction

Thrombosed vessels

Release of enzymes beyond the pancreas leads to fat necrosis of the omentum.

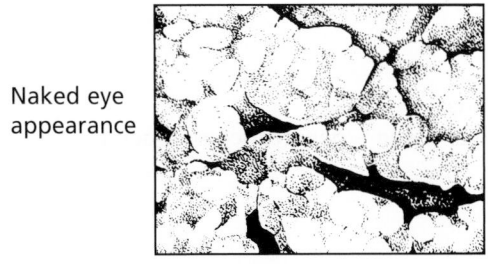

Naked eye appearance

Opaque white patches of necrotic fatty tissue containing free fatty acids – due to action of phospholipase and proteolytic enzymes – lipase splits fat.

In acute pancreatitis, acute inflammation is associated with necrosis of pancreatic acini and fat.

# ACUTE PANCREATITIS

Patients present with abdominal pain and vomiting with a differential diagnosis of perforated duodenal ulcer. A serum level of amylase >1200 IU/L and serum lipase >160 IU/L confirms the diagnosis. Many cases are mild, but one-third of severe cases have a mortality of 50%.

### Aetiology

Two factors are important: (1) gallstones and (2) alcohol.

### Gallstones

Between 40% and 60% of all cases of severe pancreatitis are associated with gallstones. Recurrent attacks are common.

#### *Bile reflux is the initiating event*

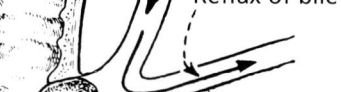

In most patients, the bile duct and pancreatic duct have a common entrance to the ampulla of Vater. Stones around 3 mm in diameter passing down the bile duct can, by blocking the ampulla, cause reflux of bile along the pancreatic duct.

#### *Alcohol*

Acute pancreatitis is common in alcoholics and the incidence of this association is directly related to the consumption of alcohol by the local population.

The precise mechanisms are poorly understood, but include:
• Ampullary spasm.
• Plugging of ducts by inspissated secretion.
• Toxic effects on acinar cells.

**Other causes** include:
• Hereditary forms, with mutations of the cationic trypsinogen gene (PRSS-1).
• Trauma, including surgery.
• Viruses, e.g. mumps, coxsackie B.
• Hypercalcaemia, e.g. in hyperparathyroidism.
• Drugs, e.g. steroids.

### Complications

(i)   Shock is the major cause of death.
(ii)  Recurrent attacks may lead to chronic pancreatitis.
(iii) Collections of fluid may be surrounded by fibrous tissue – pancreatic pseudocyst
       (p. 406).

# CHRONIC PANCREATITIS

Chronic pancreatitis predominantly affects alcoholics.

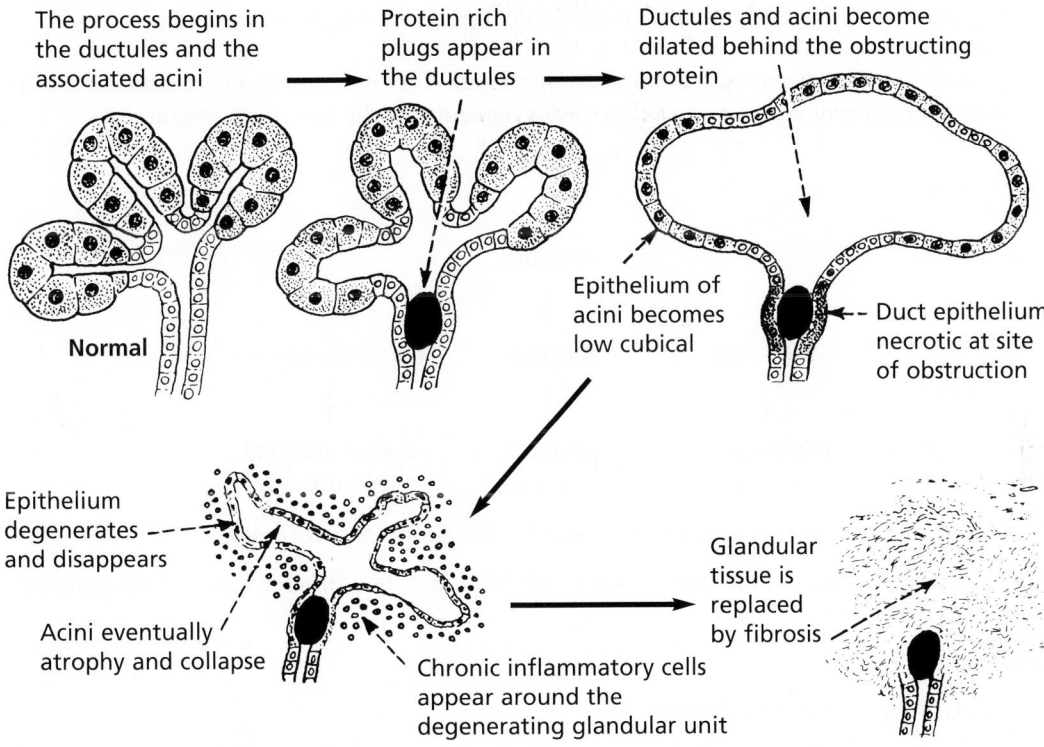

The process begins in the ductules and the associated acini → Protein rich plugs appear in the ductules → Ductules and acini become dilated behind the obstructing protein

Normal

Epithelium of acini becomes low cubical

Duct epithelium necrotic at site of obstruction

Epithelium degenerates and disappears

Acini eventually atrophy and collapse

Chronic inflammatory cells appear around the degenerating glandular unit

Glandular tissue is replaced by fibrosis

The change is focal. More and more protein plugs form, some in larger ducts. Obstruction of these may lead to production of cysts.

Ultimately, a large proportion of the exocrine tissue is destroyed.

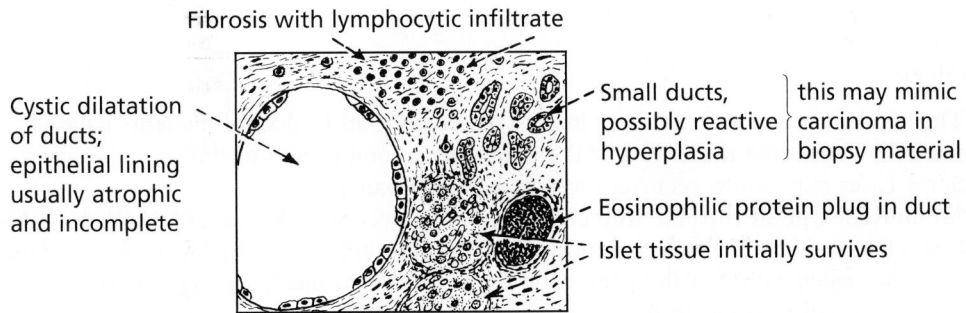

Fibrosis with lymphocytic infiltrate

Cystic dilatation of ducts; epithelial lining usually atrophic and incomplete

Small ducts, possibly reactive hyperplasia } this may mimic carcinoma in biopsy material

Eosinophilic protein plug in duct

Islet tissue initially survives

# CHRONIC PANCREATITIS

With progress of the disease, two other developments take place:

1. *Calcification.* This occurs mainly in the protein plugs in the ducts, resulting in the formation of calculi.
2. *Rupture of the duct cysts into the surrounding tissues.* A granulation tissue reaction is set up with formation of a pseudocyst. The result depends on the site of the pseudocyst.

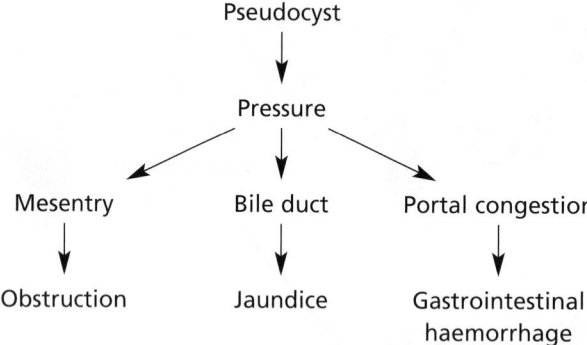

Rupture into the peritoneal cavity causes ascites, frequently haemorrhagic.

Progressive destruction of the parenchyma with fibrosis may ultimately convert the pancreas into a thin hard cord.

### Effects

Patients typically complain of abdominal pain.

Apart from the complications due to cyst rupture, destruction of pancreatic tissue may lead to:

1. Insufficiency of exocrine secretion → steatorrhoea and wasting.
2. Diabetes mellitus. Thirty percent of patients eventually develop this due to destruction of islet tissue.

### Aetiology

1. The main factor in 75% of cases in Western civilisation is alcohol. Patients have generally consumed more than 150 g daily over a long period of time.
2. Some cases may follow recurrent attacks of acute pancreatitis.
3. An unusual type of chronic 'tropical' pancreatitis occurs in Africa and South-East Asia. It is related to chronic malnutrition with particular deficiency of protein, from infancy. Extensive calcification of the pancreatic tissue occurs. It has been suggested that there is a genetic predisposition to the disease.
4. Genetic causes are increasingly recognised as in acute pancreatitis.
5. Auto-immune pancreatitis is a distinct form of chronic pancreatitis characterised by a striking infiltrate of lymphoplasmacytic cells positive for IgG4, accompanied by distinctive fibrosis. This may mimic carcinoma and can respond to steroid therapy.

# CYSTIC FIBROSIS (MUCOVISCIDOSIS)

This is a common autosomal recessive inherited disease due to genetic mutation on chromosome 7. A high percentage (about 4%) of the population are carriers.

The gene involved is called cystic fibrosis transmembrane conductance regulator (CFTR). Its essential function is the control of the transfer of chloride across cell membranes. Many mutations of the gene have been recorded, each being responsible for subtle variations in the evolution of the disorder.

All the exocrine secretory tissues are affected to some extent. The clinical features vary according to which organs are severely affected – pancreas, bronchi, bowel, biliary tree, testis.

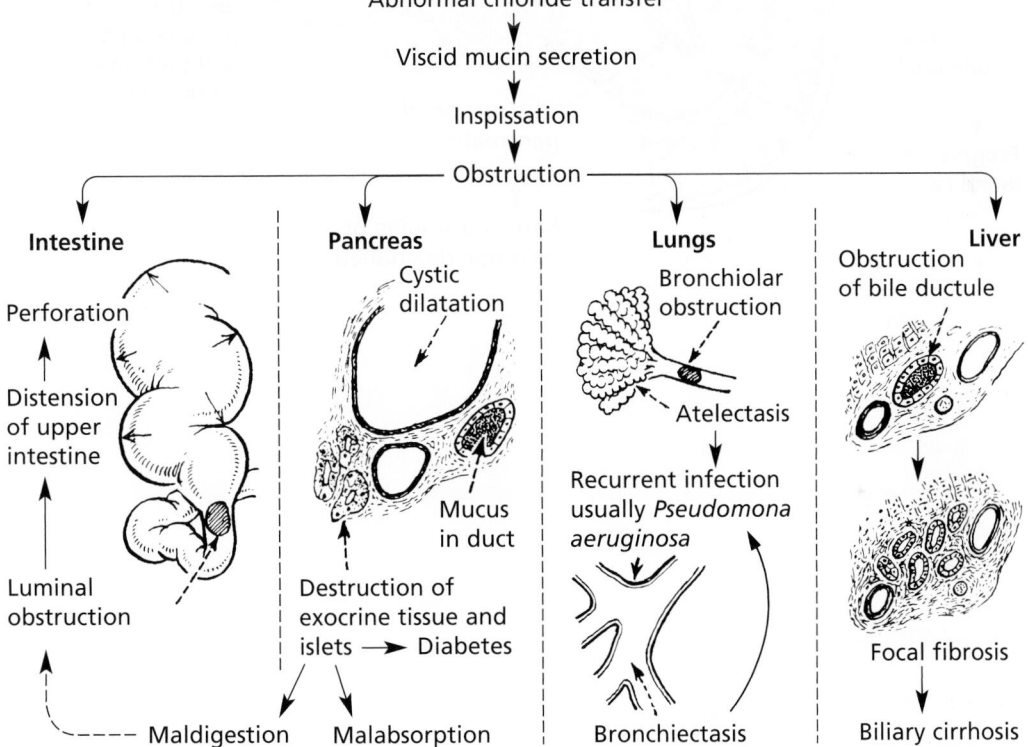

Abnormal chloride transfer → Viscid mucin secretion → Inspissation → Obstruction

**Intestine**
Perforation ← Distension of upper intestine ← Luminal obstruction ← Maldigestion

**Pancreas**
Cystic dilatation
Mucus in duct
Destruction of exocrine tissue and islets → Diabetes
Malabsorption

**Lungs**
Bronchiolar obstruction
Atelectasis
Recurrent infection usually *Pseudomona aeruginosa*
Bronchiectasis

**Liver**
Obstruction of bile ductule
Focal fibrosis
Biliary cirrhosis

## Clinical features

### Neonatal
Intestinal obstruction (meconium ileus) may lead to intestinal perforation and fatal peritonitis.

### Childhood
There is failure to thrive due to maldigestion and malabsorption, and steatorrhea is common – all features of pancreatic insufficiency. Recurrent episodes of pneumonia often lead to death in early adult life. Lung transplantation and gene therapy offer hope of improved survival. Liver lesions develop later.

Sodium chloride levels are raised in sweat detected in the 'sweat test'. Genetic screening is now available.

# TUMOURS OF PANCREAS

Benign tumours of the pancreas such as cystadenomas are rare. They may produce symptoms due to pressure on other structures.

## CARCINOMA

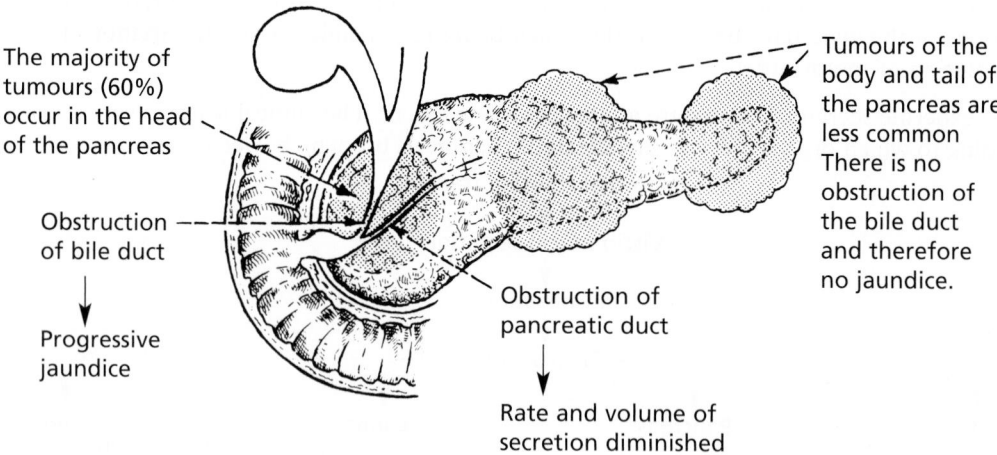

The majority of tumours (60%) occur in the head of the pancreas

Obstruction of bile duct

↓

Progressive jaundice

Obstruction of pancreatic duct

↓

Rate and volume of secretion diminished

Tumours of the body and tail of the pancreas are less common There is no obstruction of the bile duct and therefore no jaundice.

# TUMOURS OF PANCREAS

Local spread and/or distant metastases are found in 85% of cases at the time of diagnosis and the 5-year survival rate is 3–5%.

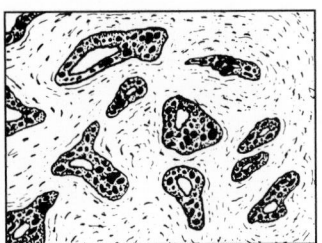

The tumour arises from the duct epithelium and in almost all cases it is an adenocarcinoma. Papillary cystadenocarcinoma, adenosquamous carcinoma and giant cell carcinoma are forms occasionally encountered.

Tumours in the body and tail are commonly larger than tumours of the head, probably due to later diagnosis in the relative absence of symptoms.

Thrombosis of unknown cause and at distant sites (thrombophlebitis migrans, p. 260), e.g. femoral vein, may occur.

### Aetiology

1. Pancreatic carcinoma is most frequent in males in the fifth to seventh decades.
2. There is a statistical association with alcohol, cigarette smoking, a diet high in fat and carbohydrate, and chronic pancreatitis.
3. In the United States, the incidence is higher in the black population and a similar situation is true of the Maoris in New Zealand.

**Endocrine tumours** are described on page 689.

# HAEMOPOIETIC AND LYMPHO-RETICULAR TISSUES

## OBJECTIVES

1. To classify the different types of anaemia and understand their pathogenesis and pathological features.
2. To have knowledge of polycythaemia and its pathology.
3. To know the coagulation cascade and the pathologies associated with it.
4. To have knowledge of the causes of lymphadenopathy and their pathological features.
5. To know about the spleen and the causes of splenomegaly.
6. To have an understanding of the disorders which affect the thymus.
7. To have a basic understanding of the different types of lymphoma and their pathological consequences.
8. To have a basic understanding of leukaemias and their classification.
9. To have a basic knowledge of the main myeloproliferative disorders.

## HAEMOPOIESIS

**The derivation of blood cells**

In the **bone marrow** a '**pluripotent**' **stem cell** gives rise to **all blood cells.**

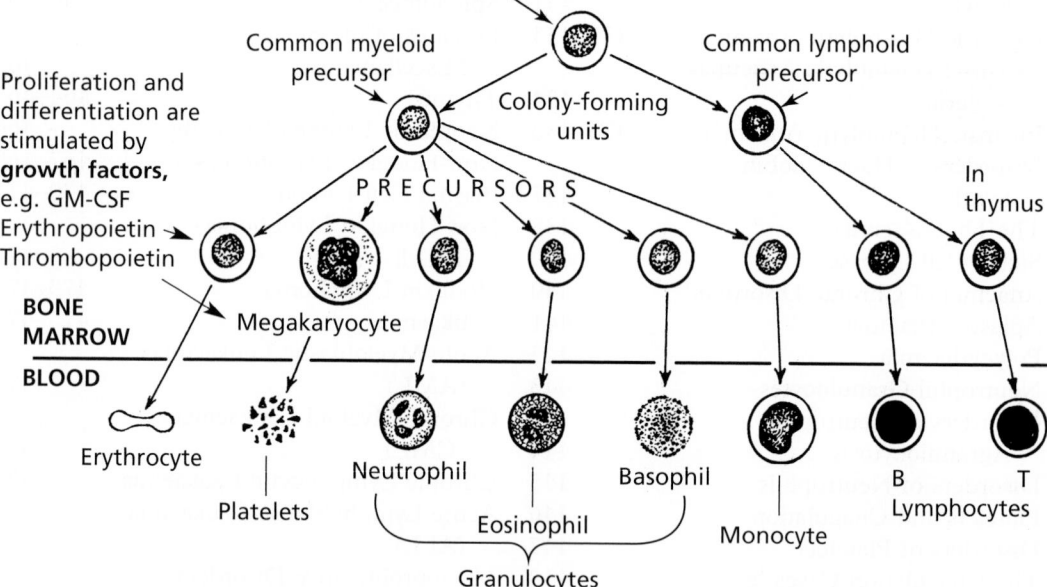

# HAEMOPOIESIS

## Haemopoiesis in bone marrow

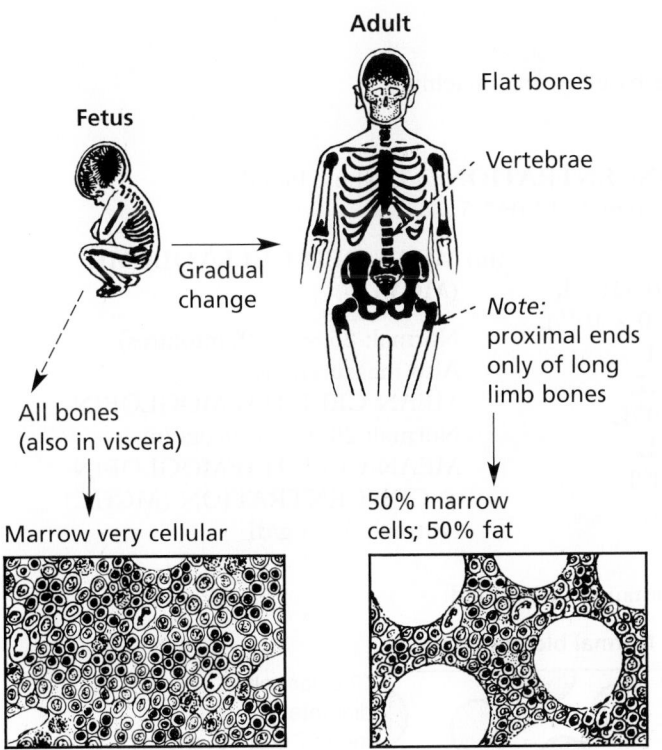

**Fetus**

Gradual change

All bones (also in viscera)

Marrow very cellular

**Adult**

Flat bones

Vertebrae

*Note:* proximal ends only of long limb bones

50% marrow cells; 50% fat

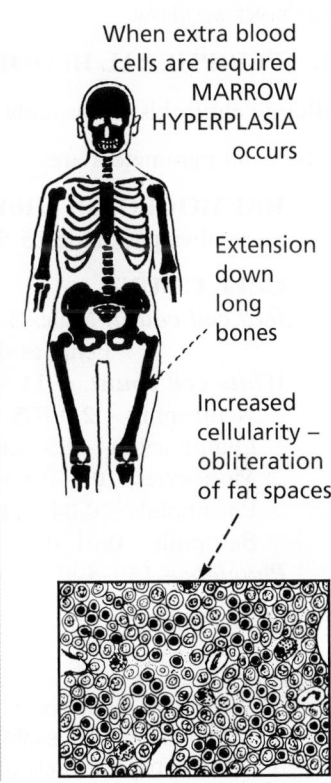

When extra blood cells are required MARROW HYPERPLASIA occurs

Extension down long bones

Increased cellularity – obliteration of fat spaces

# HAEMATOLOGY – LABORATORY TESTS

Investigation of blood diseases depends on examination of (1) PERIPHERAL BLOOD and (2) BONE MARROW.

## 1. PERIPHERAL BLOOD

Blood count: this is normally done by electronic machines.

The main parameters are:

(i) **HAEMOGLOBIN (Hb) CONCENTRATION** (g/L whole blood)
Normal values: male 15.5±2.5, female 14.0±2.5

(ii) **CELL COUNT**
   *Red cell count*: Males 5.5±1.0 ×$10^{12}$/l,
                  Females 4.8±1.0 × $10^{12}$/l.
   *White cell count*: 4–11 × $10^{9}$/L
     Neutrophils – 2.0–7.5 × $10^{9}$/L
     Lymphocytes – 1.5–4.0 × $10^{9}$/L
     Monocytes – 0.2–0.8 × $10^{9}$/L
     Eosinophils – 0.04–0.4 × $10^{9}$/L
     Basophils – 0.01–0.1 × $10^{9}$/L
   *Platelets* – 150–400 × $10^{9}$/L

(iii) **MEAN RED CELL VOLUME (MCV)**

Normal: 85±8 fL (femtolitres)
Also measured are:
MEAN CELL HAEMOGLOBIN
Normal: 29.5±2.5 picograms
MEAN CELL HAEMOGLOBIN
  CONCENTRATION (MCHC)
Normal: 33±3 g/dL

**BLOOD FILM** – stained by a Romanowski method.

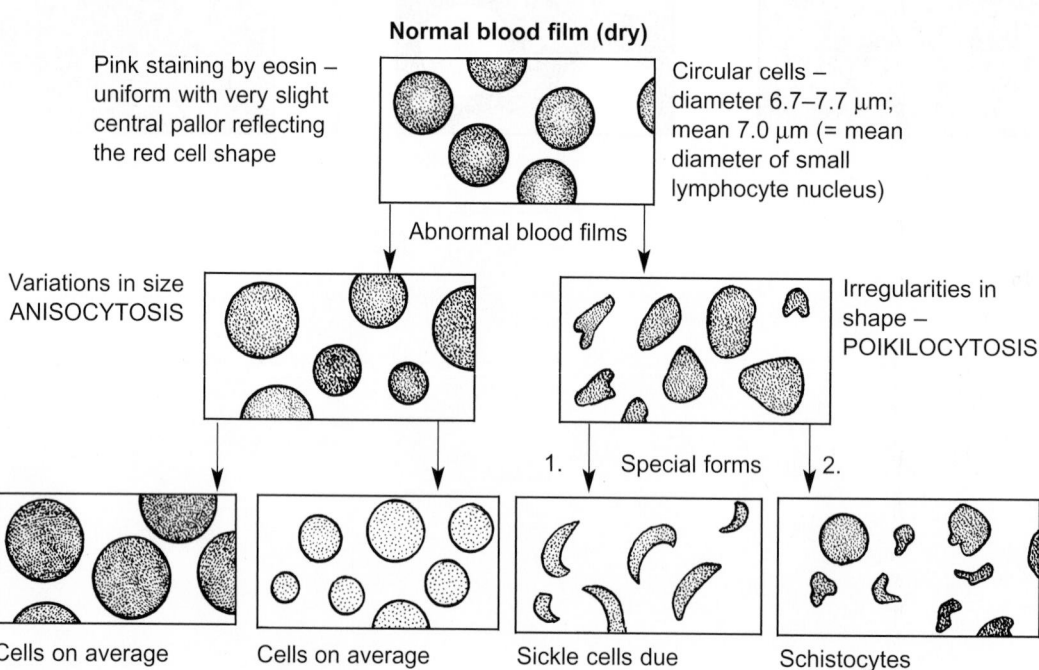

**Normal blood film (dry)**

Pink staining by eosin – uniform with very slight central pallor reflecting the red cell shape

Circular cells – diameter 6.7–7.7 μm; mean 7.0 μm (= mean diameter of small lymphocyte nucleus)

Abnormal blood films

Variations in size ANISOCYTOSIS

Irregularities in shape – POIKILOCYTOSIS

1.    Special forms    2.

Cells on average LARGER – MACROCYTIC

Cells on average SMALLER – MICROCYTIC and often paler staining (hypochromic)

Sickle cells due to abnormal haemoglobin (p. 439)

Schistocytes (fragments of red cells damaged in the flowing blood, e.g. through abnormal vessels or cardiac prostheses)

# HAEMATOLOGY – LABORATORY TESTS

Another useful test is the measurement of the **PACKED CELL VOLUME (PCV)** or haematocrit.

This is obtained by centrifuging anticoagulated whole blood in a haematocrit tube.

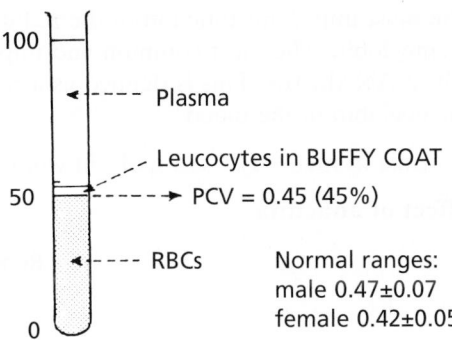

100

Plasma

Leucocytes in BUFFY COAT

50 — PCV = 0.45 (45%)

RBCs

Normal ranges:
male 0.47±0.07
female 0.42±0.05

0

## 2. BONE MARROW EXAMINATION

Examination of bone marrow is important in explaining abnormalities of the peripheral blood.

In the past, aspiration of marrow from the sternum was commonly performed. Now the posterior iliac crest is used – it is safer and allows marrow to be **aspirated** and a **trephine biopsy** to be taken.

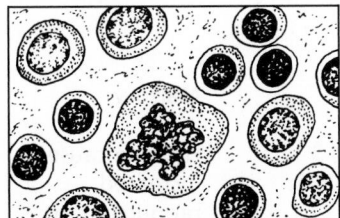

Film of aspirate allows detailed observation of **cell morphology**.

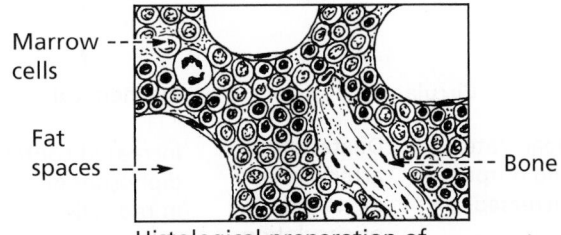

Marrow cells

Fat spaces

Bone

Histological preparation of trephine material allows assessment of **architecture**.

## ERYTHROPOIESIS

Normal marrow erythropoiesis is said to be NORMOBLASTIC.

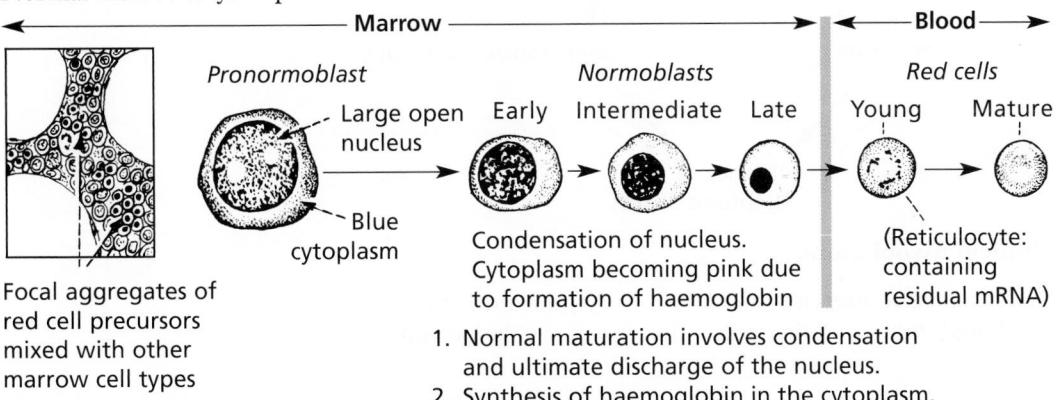

◄——————— Marrow ——————————► ◄— Blood —►

*Pronormoblast*  *Normoblasts*  *Red cells*

Large open nucleus  Early  Intermediate  Late  Young  Mature

Blue cytoplasm

Focal aggregates of red cell precursors mixed with other marrow cell types

Condensation of nucleus. Cytoplasm becoming pink due to formation of haemoglobin

(Reticulocyte: containing residual mRNA)

1. Normal maturation involves condensation and ultimate discharge of the nucleus.
2. Synthesis of haemoglobin in the cytoplasm.
3. Diminution in cell size.

When the essential factors vitamin $B_{12}$ or folic acid are deficient, the red cell precursors show morphological changes – erythropoiesis is said to be MEGALOBLASTIC (p. 423).

# ANAEMIA

The most important function of the red cell is the transport of oxygen bound to haemoglobin. The most common and important disorder associated with disease of the red cells is ANAEMIA. This is defined as a reduction below normal of the concentration of haemoglobin in the blood.

Anaemia in men – Hb <13 g/dL; in women – <11.5 g/dL.

**Effect of anaemia**

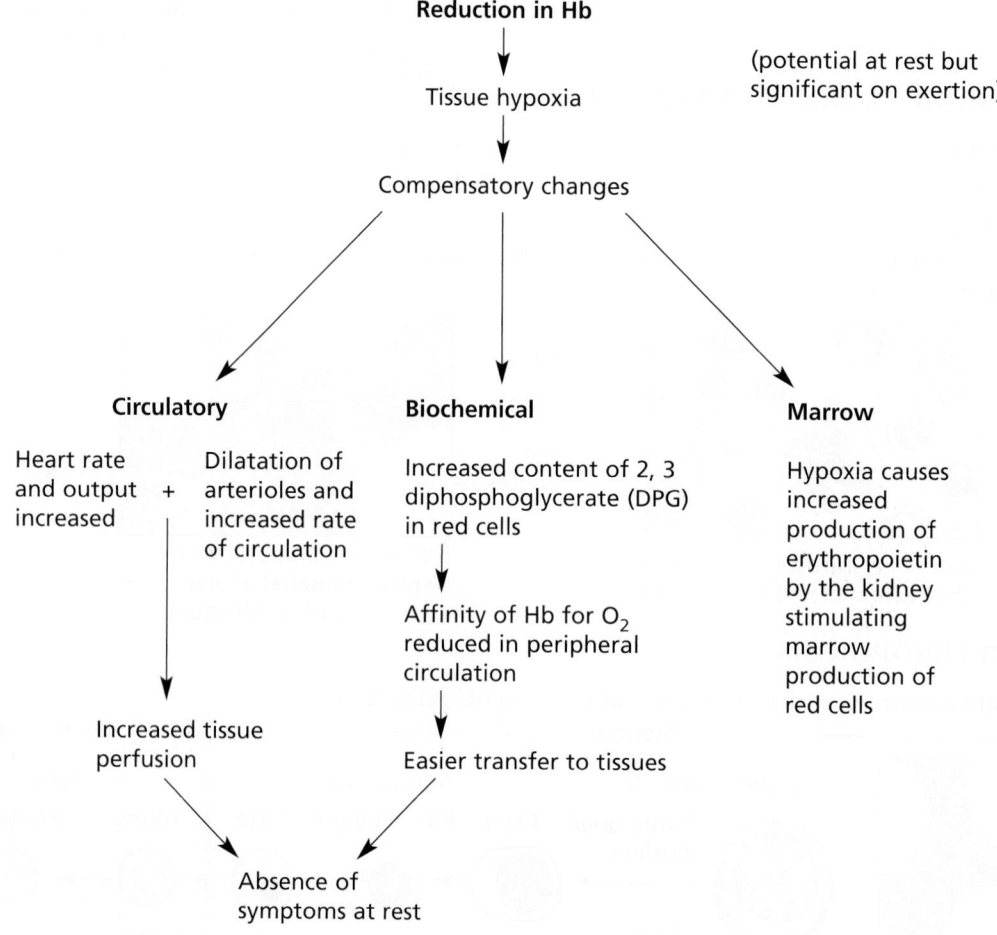

**Reduction in Hb**
↓
Tissue hypoxia     (potential at rest but significant on exertion)
↓
Compensatory changes

**Circulatory**

Heart rate and output increased  +  Dilatation of arterioles and increased rate of circulation
↓
Increased tissue perfusion

**Biochemical**

Increased content of 2, 3 diphosphoglycerate (DPG) in red cells
↓
Affinity of Hb for $O_2$ reduced in peripheral circulation
↓
Easier transfer to tissues

**Marrow**

Hypoxia causes increased production of erythropoietin by the kidney stimulating marrow production of red cells

Absence of symptoms at rest

**Clinical associations**

1.  Diminished exercise tolerance, i.e. dyspnoea on exertion.
2.  Rapid, full, bounding pulse: decreased circulation time.

# ANAEMIA

The effects of anaemia depend on its severity, rate of development and duration.

In slowly developing moderate anaemias, symptoms such as dyspnoea only appear on exertion, and even when the haemoglobin falls as low as 6–7 g/dL, clinical features may be slight.

**Pathological complications of anaemia**

1. Effects of degenerative arterial disease are aggravated, e.g. symptoms of ANGINA PECTORIS and lower limb CLAUDICATION are increased.
2. In severe anaemias effects are seen in organs.

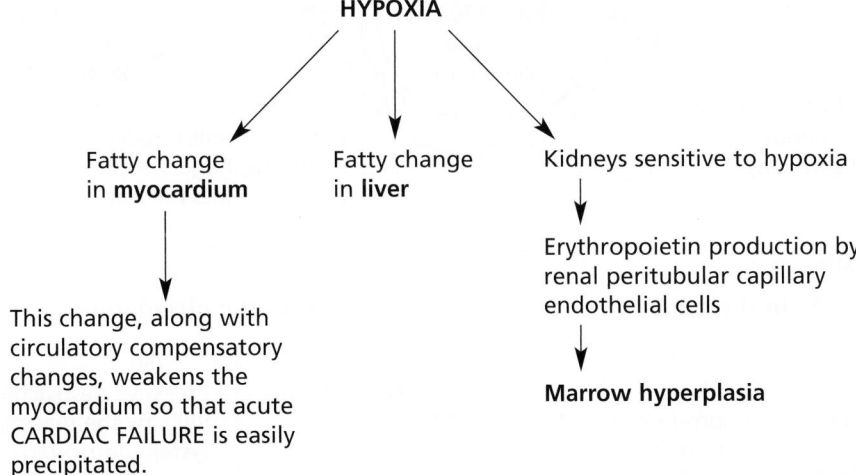

*Note*: Blood transfusion used in the treatment of anaemia is given *slowly* and as *packed cells* to avoid fluid overload.

In very rapidly developing anaemias, the compensatory mechanisms cannot adjust adequately – the condition merges into SHOCK.

# ANAEMIA

**Causes of anaemia**

To understand the **four main mechanisms** by which anaemia develops it is important to have a knowledge of the lifecycle of red blood cells (RBCs).

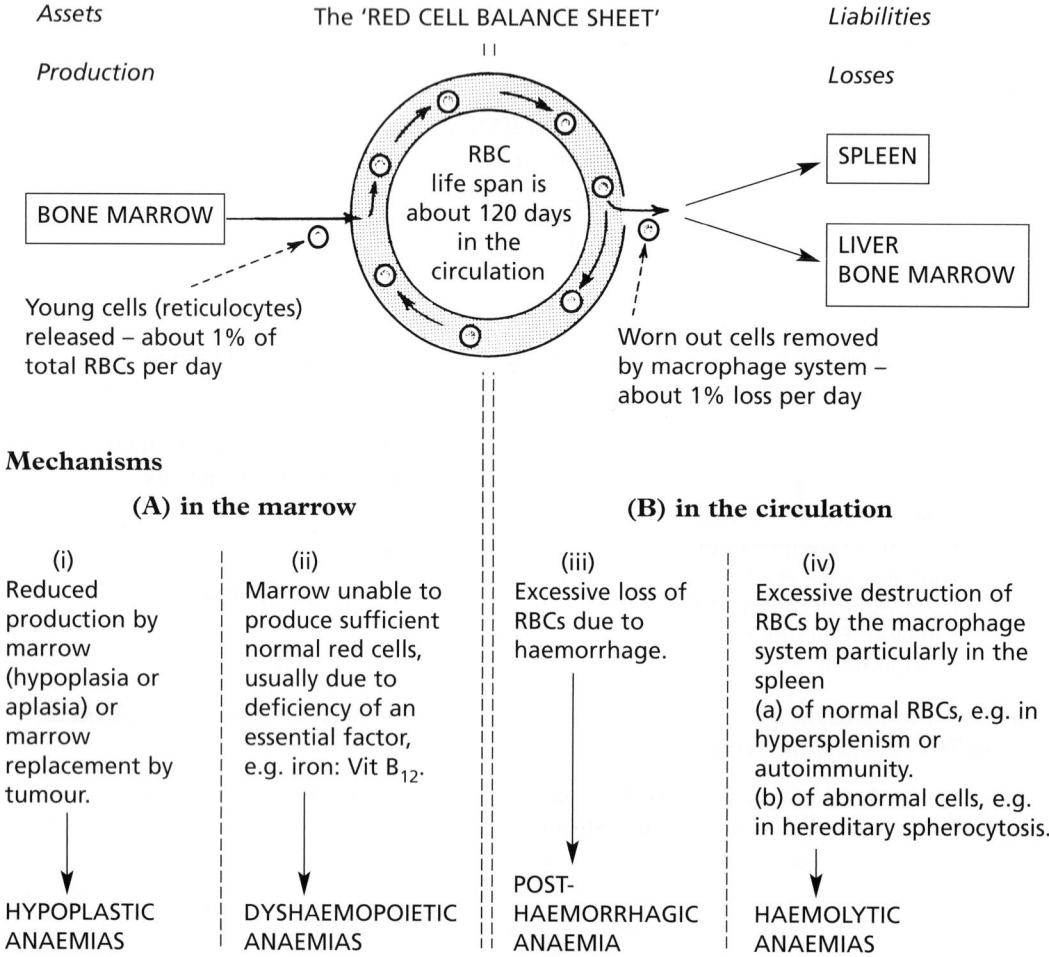

*Assets*  The 'RED CELL BALANCE SHEET'  *Liabilities*

*Production*  *Losses*

BONE MARROW

RBC life span is about 120 days in the circulation

SPLEEN

LIVER
BONE MARROW

Young cells (reticulocytes) released – about 1% of total RBCs per day

Worn out cells removed by macrophage system – about 1% loss per day

**Mechanisms**

| **(A) in the marrow** | | **(B) in the circulation** | |
|---|---|---|---|
| (i)<br>Reduced production by marrow (hypoplasia or aplasia) or marrow replacement by tumour.<br><br>↓<br><br>HYPOPLASTIC ANAEMIAS | (ii)<br>Marrow unable to produce sufficient normal red cells, usually due to deficiency of an essential factor, e.g. iron: Vit $B_{12}$.<br><br>↓<br><br>DYSHAEMOPOIETIC ANAEMIAS | (iii)<br>Excessive loss of RBCs due to haemorrhage.<br><br><br><br>↓<br>POST-HAEMORRHAGIC ANAEMIA | (iv)<br>Excessive destruction of RBCs by the macrophage system particularly in the spleen<br>(a) of normal RBCs, e.g. in hypersplenism or autoimmunity.<br>(b) of abnormal cells, e.g. in hereditary spherocytosis.<br><br>↓<br>HAEMOLYTIC ANAEMIAS |

*Note*: Many forms of anaemia have more than one component,

e.g. 1. The abnormal cells produced in hypoplastic and dyshaemopoietic anaemias have a shortened life span so that a haemolytic element is superimposed.
2. The anaemia of chronic blood loss is almost wholly dyshaemopoietic due to the loss of iron.

# ANAEMIA

## HYPOPLASTIC AND APLASTIC ANAEMIAS

These are rare conditions and, as the names imply, are due to marrow failure with diminished numbers or absence of haemopoietic cells. Usually all three marrow cell lines are affected, resulting in pancytopenia in the peripheral blood.

Marrow failure of this type is dealt with in detail on page 441.

Marrow failure due to extensive tumour infiltration or fibrosis may also occur.

The anaemias associated with miscellaneous chronic diseases ('secondary' anaemias) are dealt with on page 440.

## DYSHAEMOPOIETIC ANAEMIAS

The usual cause of these anaemias is deficiency of an essential factor required for proper haemoglobin synthesis or erythroblast maturation and development. They are associated with a hypercellular marrow. They are divided into two main groups:

(1) normoblastic and (2) megaloblastic, depending on the type of erythroblastic maturation in the marrow.

### Deficiency of essential factor

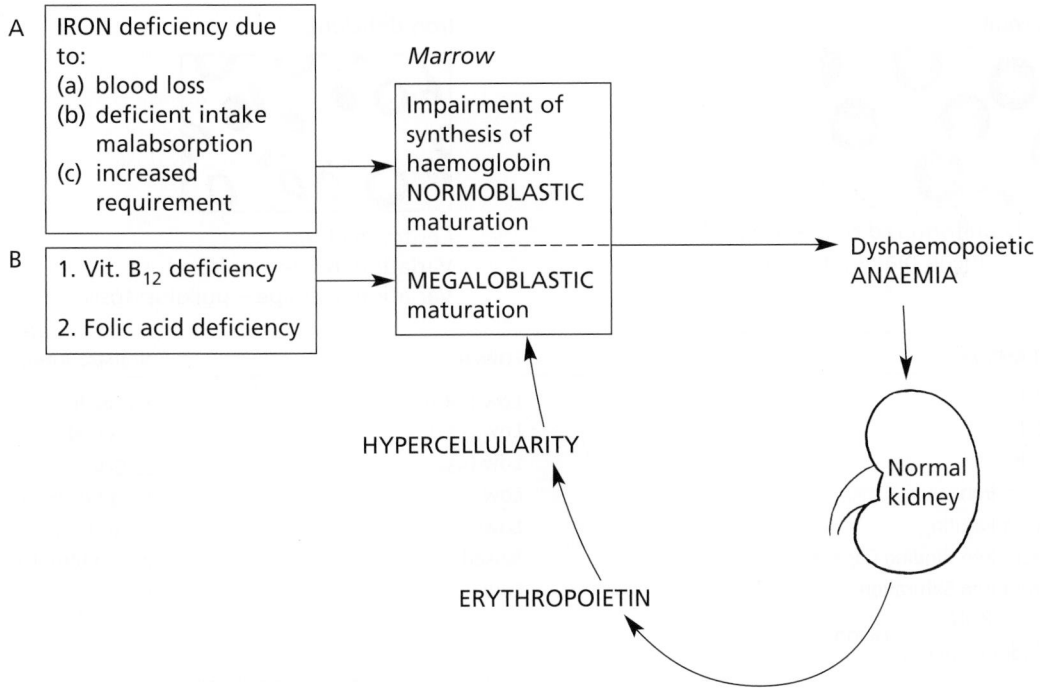

# IRON DEFICIENCY ANAEMIA

**IRON DEFICIENCY ANAEMIA** is the commonest anaemia worldwide due to (a) poor nutrition, (b) intestinal parasites (esp. hookworm) causing bleeding and (c) multiple pregnancies.

In Western countries, in the adult male and post-menopausal women, iron deficiency anaemia is nearly always due to gastrointestinal blood loss from cancer, peptic ulceration, aspirin and non-steroidal ingestion, etc.

Without IRON the haem component of the haemoglobin molecule cannot be synthesised.

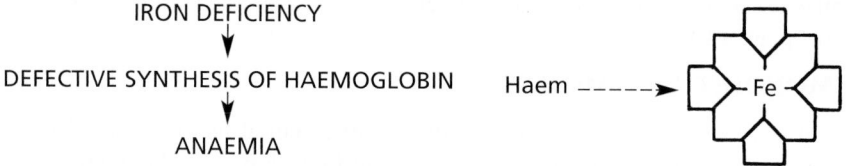

IRON DEFICIENCY
↓
DEFECTIVE SYNTHESIS OF HAEMOGLOBIN         Haem ------→ Fe
↓
ANAEMIA

**Changes in the blood**: the red cells which show:

MICROCYTOSIS (cells smaller – mean diameter <6.7 μm).
HYPOCHROMASIA (contain less haemoglobin ∴ less well stained).
ANISOCYTOSIS – variation in size.
POIKILOCYTOSIS – variation in shape.

**Normal**

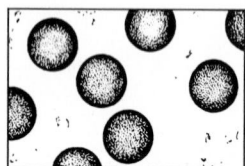

Fairly uniform red cells – size and shape (mean diameter 7 μm)

**Iron deficient**

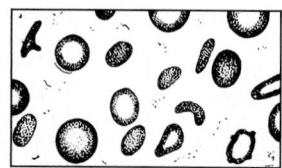

Central pallor
Variation in size – anisocytosis
Variation in shape – poikilocytosis

| PARAMETER | LOW/HIGH | NORMAL RANGE |
|---|---|---|
| MCV | Low (<80) | 80–92 fL |
| MCH | Low (<27) | 27–32 pg |
| MCHC | Low (<30) | 33 g/dL |
| Serum Iron | Low | 10–30 mmol/L |
| Serum Ferritin | Low | 15–300 mg/L |
| Serum Iron Binding Capacity | Raised | 45–70 mmol/L |
| Serum Iron Saturation | Low | 16–60% |

$$\left[\frac{\text{IRON}}{\text{Binding capacity}}\right] \times 100$$

The **reticulocyte count** is NORMAL except following episodes of haemorrhage. Usually there are no changes in the leucocytes and platelets.

The **bone marrow** is hypercellular and contains small, poorly haemoglobinised normoblasts; iron stores are reduced.

# IRON DEFICIENCY ANAEMIA

## IRON METABOLISM

Iron is absorbed mainly in the duodenum and upper jejunum. Only small amounts are normally required to replace iron losses. Since the average diet contains more iron than is required, its absorption is controlled by the *mucosal apoferritin mechanism*.

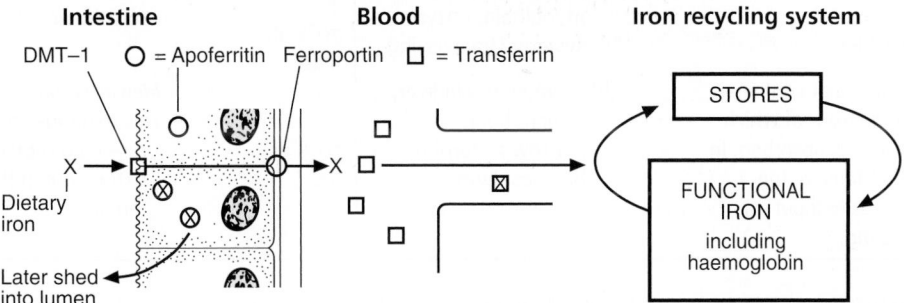

The iron *(X)* in the diet enters the mucosal cell through an apical uptake transporter *(DMT-1)* and having combined with apoferritin *(O)* is retained in the cell as ferritin *(⊗)*.

**Note: This bound iron is subsequently shed along with the cell into the lumen.**

**Iron unbound by apoferritin passes through the cell** through a basolateral transporter (ferroportin) and is transported in the blood to join the iron recycling system.

*Note:* New haemoglobin formed in the bone marrow contains 95% iron from recycling system, 5% from diet.

The state of the iron stores controls the apoferritin (a form of intracellular transferrin) content of the intestinal mucosal cell by a feed-back mechanism.

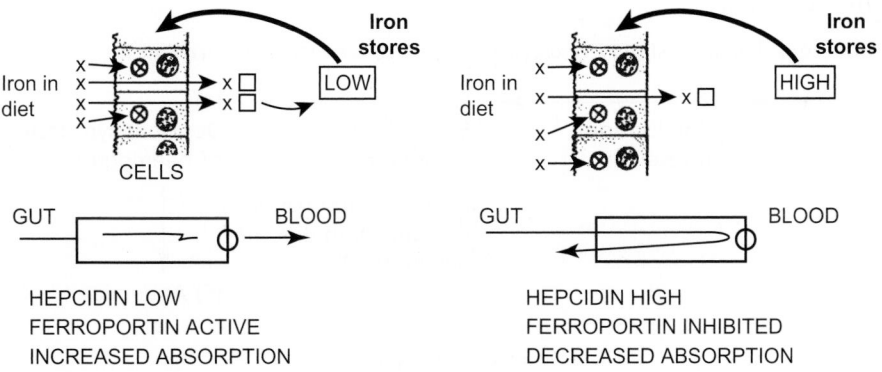

HEPCIDIN LOW
FERROPORTIN ACTIVE
INCREASED ABSORPTION

HEPCIDIN HIGH
FERROPORTIN INHIBITED
DECREASED ABSORPTION

## ACUTE IRON OVERLOAD

If a large dose of medicinal iron preparations is taken (particularly by children in error), the absorption and transport mechanisms are overwhelmed and free iron radicals exert very toxic effects.

# IRON DEFICIENCY ANAEMIA

The iron balance may be summarised as follows.

| INPUT (Adult male) | BODY IRON TOTAL 3–6 g | | OUTPUT |
|---|---|---|---|
| Average: 1 mg/day derived from foods<br>(a) animal muscle<br>(b) vegetables | (a) *Functional iron* in haemoglobin, myoglobin, enzyme systems, transferring | } 70% at least | Average: 1 mg/day<br>Skin desquamation and miscellaneous secretions |
| The average diet contains 10–20 mg iron, of which about 10% is absorbed. In the adult female, the average daily input is about 2 mg. | (b) *Storage iron* in liver, spleen, bone marrow as ferritin, haemosiderin | } 30% or less | *Menstruation*<br>This extra loss of about 0.5–1 mg requires extra input in the female |

Anaemia results when this balance is upset in:

1. *Increased output*
   This almost always is caused by blood loss – often small in amount and chronic (1 mL blood = 0.5 mg iron). In the female, uterine bleeding is a common cause, and in both sexes bleeding from the gastrointestinal tract is important.
2. *Decreased input*
   (a) Poor diet (including diets containing substances antagonistic to iron absorption, e.g. phytates, phosphates).
   (b) Malabsorption – due to bowel disease, e.g. coeliac disease, or post-surgical, e.g. post-gastrectomy.
3. *Increased body requirement*
   (a) During rapid growth in childhood.
   (b) In pregnancy.

Usually anaemia develops slowly (except in cases of serious haemorrhage).

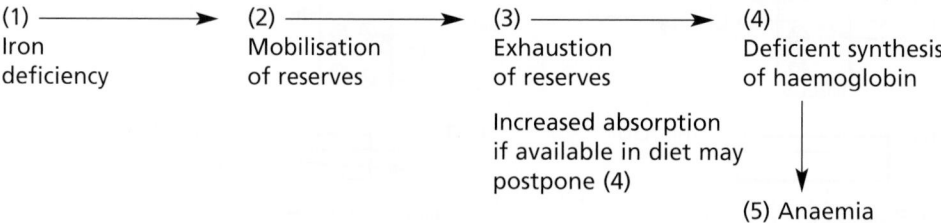

# THE MEGALOBLASTIC ANAEMIAS

These dyshaemopoietic anaemias are almost always caused by deficiency of either vitamin $B_{12}$ or folic acid which are intracellular co-enzymes important for the synthesis of DNA.

The effects of deficiency occur in most organs of the body but are prominent where cell turnover is rapid, e.g. in the **marrow**.

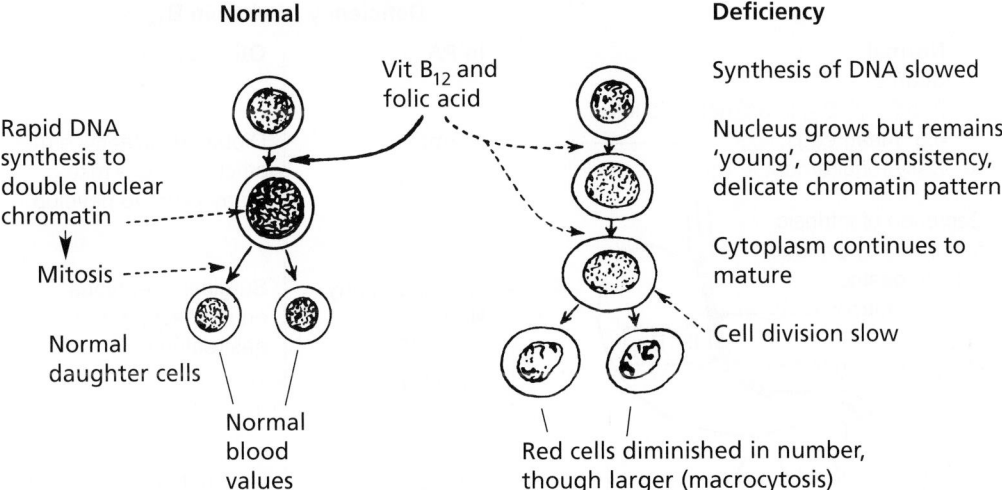

**Normal**

Vit $B_{12}$ and folic acid

Rapid DNA synthesis to double nuclear chromatin

Mitosis

Normal daughter cells

Normal blood values

**Deficiency**

Synthesis of DNA slowed

Nucleus grows but remains 'young', open consistency, delicate chromatin pattern

Cytoplasm continues to mature

Cell division slow

Red cells diminished in number, though larger (macrocytosis)

**Results in organs particularly affected**

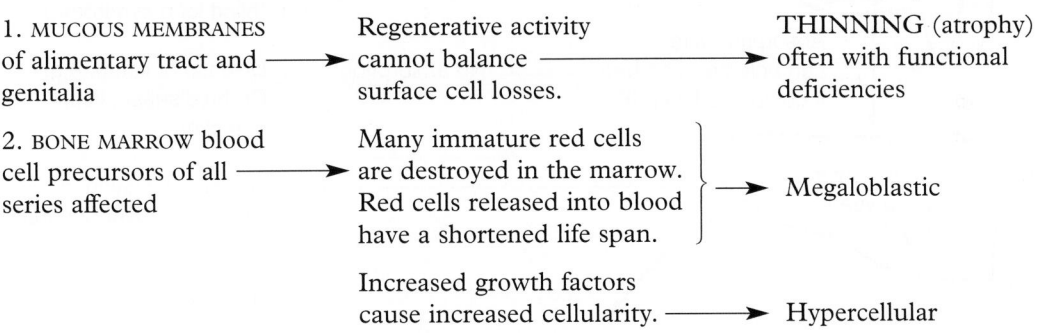

1. MUCOUS MEMBRANES of alimentary tract and genitalia → Regenerative activity cannot balance surface cell losses. → THINNING (atrophy) often with functional deficiencies

2. BONE MARROW blood cell precursors of all series affected → Many immature red cells are destroyed in the marrow. Red cells released into blood have a shortened life span. } → Megaloblastic

Increased growth factors cause increased cellularity. → Hypercellular

*Note:*

(a) Vitamin $B_{12}$ (but not folic acid) has a separate function in the maintenance of the integrity of myelin. Therefore deficiency leads to neuropathies – particularly **subacute combined degeneration of the spinal cord** (p. 425).

(b) The marrow and blood appearances are similar in deficiency of vitamin $B_{12}$ and folic acid from any cause. The classic disease of this type is **pernicious anaemia.**

# PERNICIOUS ANAEMIA (PA)

This anaemia was first described by the English physician Addison in the mid-19th century. It is due to vitamin $B_{12}$ deficiency and is always associated with achlorhydria and gastric mucosal atrophy, due to auto-immune gastritis.

**Vitamin $B_{12}$ metabolism and causes of deficiency:**

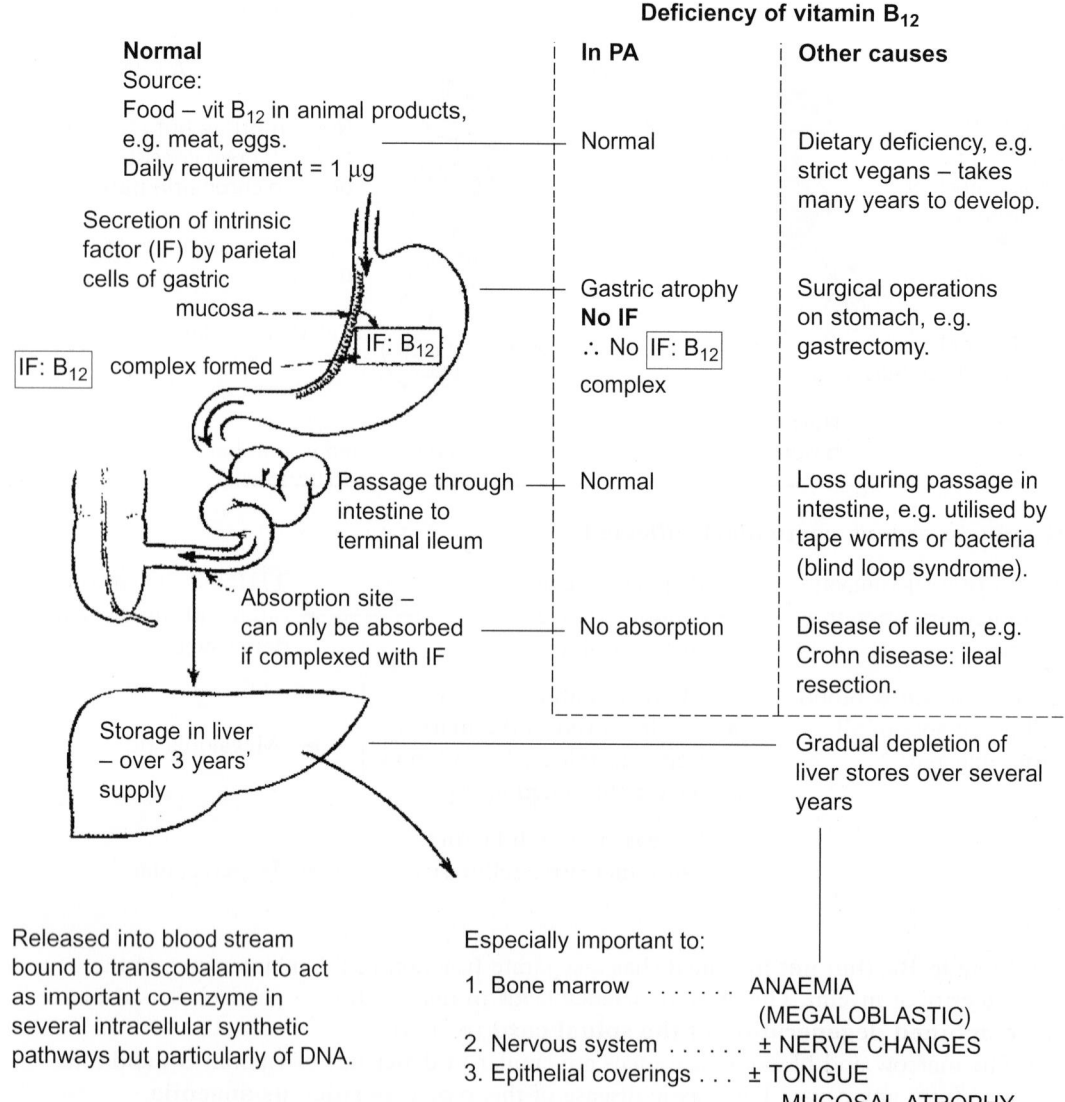

**Deficiency of vitamin $B_{12}$**

| **Normal** | **In PA** | **Other causes** |
|---|---|---|
| Source:<br>Food – vit $B_{12}$ in animal products, e.g. meat, eggs.<br>Daily requirement = 1 μg | Normal | Dietary deficiency, e.g. strict vegans – takes many years to develop. |
| Secretion of intrinsic factor (IF) by parietal cells of gastric mucosa<br>IF: $B_{12}$ complex formed | Gastric atrophy<br>**No IF**<br>∴ No IF: $B_{12}$ complex | Surgical operations on stomach, e.g. gastrectomy. |
| Passage through intestine to terminal ileum | Normal | Loss during passage in intestine, e.g. utilised by tape worms or bacteria (blind loop syndrome). |
| Absorption site – can only be absorbed if complexed with IF | No absorption | Disease of ileum, e.g. Crohn disease: ileal resection. |
| Storage in liver – over 3 years' supply | | Gradual depletion of liver stores over several years |

Released into blood stream bound to transcobalamin to act as important co-enzyme in several intracellular synthetic pathways but particularly of DNA.

Especially important to:

1. Bone marrow ....... ANAEMIA (MEGALOBLASTIC)
2. Nervous system ...... ± NERVE CHANGES
3. Epithelial coverings ... ± TONGUE MUCOSAL ATROPHY

# PERNICIOUS ANAEMIA (PA)

## Mechanism of production of gastritis

PA is an auto-immune disease. The gastric atrophy is caused by an immune reaction against parietal cell cytoplasmic constituents and specifically by antibodies to intrinsic factor (IF).

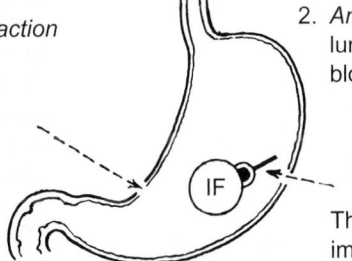

1. *Anti-parietal cell immune reaction* gradually causes complete mucosal atrophy including destruction of parietal cells. These antibodies occur in 90% of patients with PA.

2. *Anti-IF antibody* secreted in stomach lumen as well as blood. Specifically blocks any residual IF activity.
    (a) Receptor sites for B$_{12}$ complex are blocked.
    (b) Receptor sites for ileal absorption are blocked.
    There is also cell mediated immunity to IF.

There is an increased familial incidence of PA and other organ specific auto-immune diseases, e.g. Hashimoto thyroiditis.

## Blood changes

There is a pancytopenia, i.e. reduction in RBCs, granulocytes and platelets but the red cells are larger (macrocytosis).

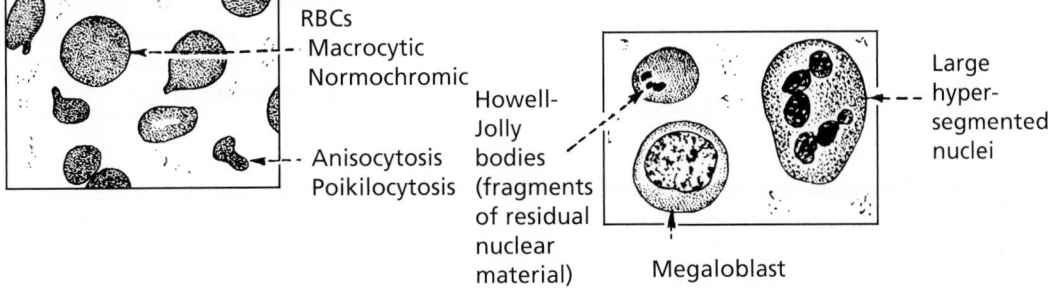

RBCs
Macrocytic
Normochromic

Anisocytosis
Poikilocytosis

Howell-Jolly bodies (fragments of residual nuclear material)

Megaloblast

Large hyper-segmented nuclei

## Marrow changes

Hyperplasia – often complete cellularity in flat bones and extension down length of femur.

**Normal**                    **In PA**

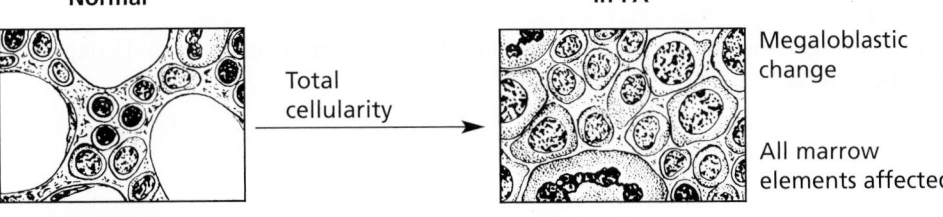

Total cellularity

Megaloblastic change

All marrow elements affected

## Associated changes
1. *Nervous system*
    (a) Subacute combined degeneration of spinal cord.
    *Note*: This serious degeneration may occur before clinical anaemia is present, and is aggravated by the administration of folic acid.
    (b) Peripheral neuropathy – both sensory and motor loss.
2. *Epithelial surfaces*
    Atrophy is common especially in the tongue and vagina – where senile atrophy is aggravated.

425

# FOLIC ACID DEFICIENCY

## FOLIC ACID (PTEROYL-GLUTAMIC ACID) DEFICIENCY

| NORMAL METABOLISM | DEFICIENCY |
|---|---|
| **Source** | **Dietary** |
| Polyglutamines in green vegetables, cereals, meat, fish and eggs (not milk) | Low intake of vegetables. Anorexia, alcoholism, poverty (elderly), infants (late weaning) |
| **Minimum Daily Requirement** | **Increased Requirements** |
| 50 μg | Pregnancy (fetal growth) |
| | Infancy and childhood (rapid growth) |
| *Body reserves* 50–100 days | Haemolysis |
| | Malignancy |
| **Absorption** | **Malabsorption** |
| As mono-glutamate in jejunum | Coeliac disease |
| | Surgical bypass |
| **Utilisation** | **Utilisation Block** |
| For DNA synthesis. Vit $B_{12}$ is necessary for synthesis of the active tetrahydrofolate form (FH4) | Drugs, e.g. methotrexate in cancer chemotherapy, also anti-convulsants, e.g. phenytoin. |

*Note:*

1. Since the marrow and blood changes in folic acid and vitamin $B_{12}$ deficiency are similar, the differential diagnosis has to be obtained by other laboratory tests – particularly the measurement of vitamin $B_{12}$ in the serum and of folic acid in RBCs. Special tests of absorption of vitamin $B_{12}$ (e.g. Schilling test) are available.
2. Since vitamin $B_{12}$ and folic acid deficiency are often associated with malabsorption, other deficiencies (e.g. iron) may co-exist.
3. All megaloblastic anaemias are macrocytic, but *not all* macrocytic anaemias are megaloblastic.
4. There is a strong association between folic acid deficiency in PREGNANCY and congenital neural tube defects.

# THE HAEMOLYTIC ANAEMIAS

## HAEMOLYTIC ANAEMIAS

In all haemolytic anaemias, there is a reduction in the life span of the red cells; due to an increased rate of red cell destruction – haemolysis.

Red cells may be destroyed:

(a) In the spleen, liver – extravascular haemolysis.
(b) In the blood stream – intravascular haemolysis, with release of haemoglobin into plasma.

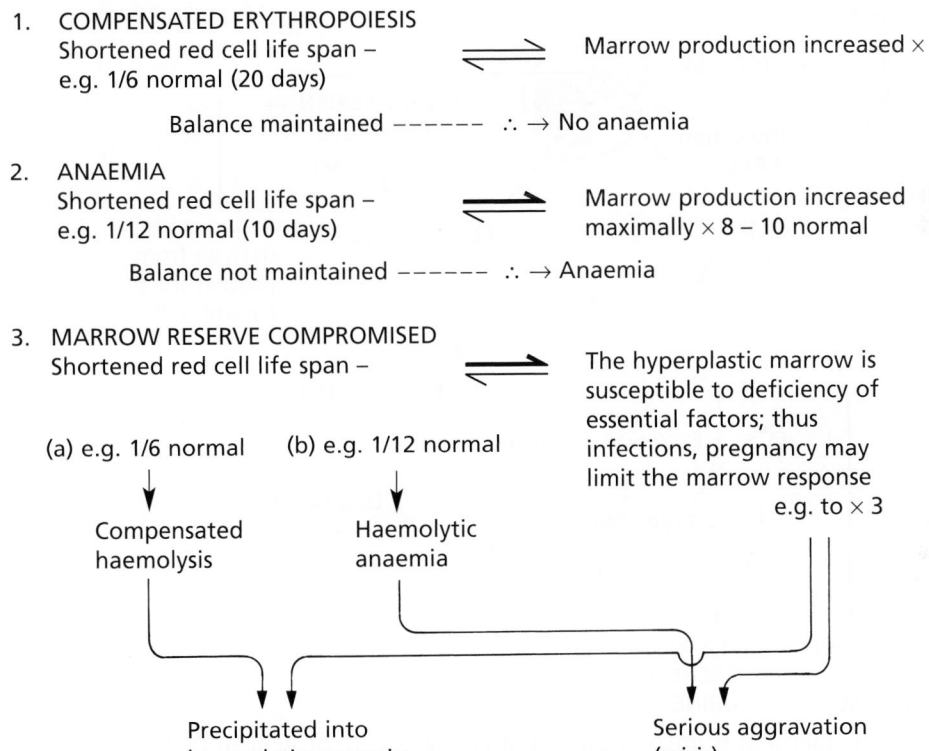

1. COMPENSATED ERYTHROPOIESIS
   Shortened red cell life span – ⇌ Marrow production increased × 6
   e.g. 1/6 normal (20 days)

   Balance maintained – – – – – – ∴ → No anaemia

2. ANAEMIA
   Shortened red cell life span – ⇌ Marrow production increased
   e.g. 1/12 normal (10 days) maximally × 8 – 10 normal

   Balance not maintained – – – – – – ∴ → Anaemia

3. MARROW RESERVE COMPROMISED
   Shortened red cell life span – ⇌ The hyperplastic marrow is susceptible to deficiency of essential factors; thus infections, pregnancy may limit the marrow response e.g. to × 3

   (a) e.g. 1/6 normal    (b) e.g. 1/12 normal

   Compensated haemolysis    Haemolytic anaemia

   Precipitated into haemolytic anaemia    Serious aggravation (crisis)

Functional reserve can compensate for a certain level of haemolysis but this fails when the degree of red cell loss is extreme or when the marrow function is compromised by other factors.

# THE HAEMOLYTIC ANAEMIAS

### Effects of the increased degradation of haemoglobin

In most haemolytic conditions, the red cells are removed and the haemoglobin degraded in the usual way, i.e. by phagocytosis by the macrophage system.

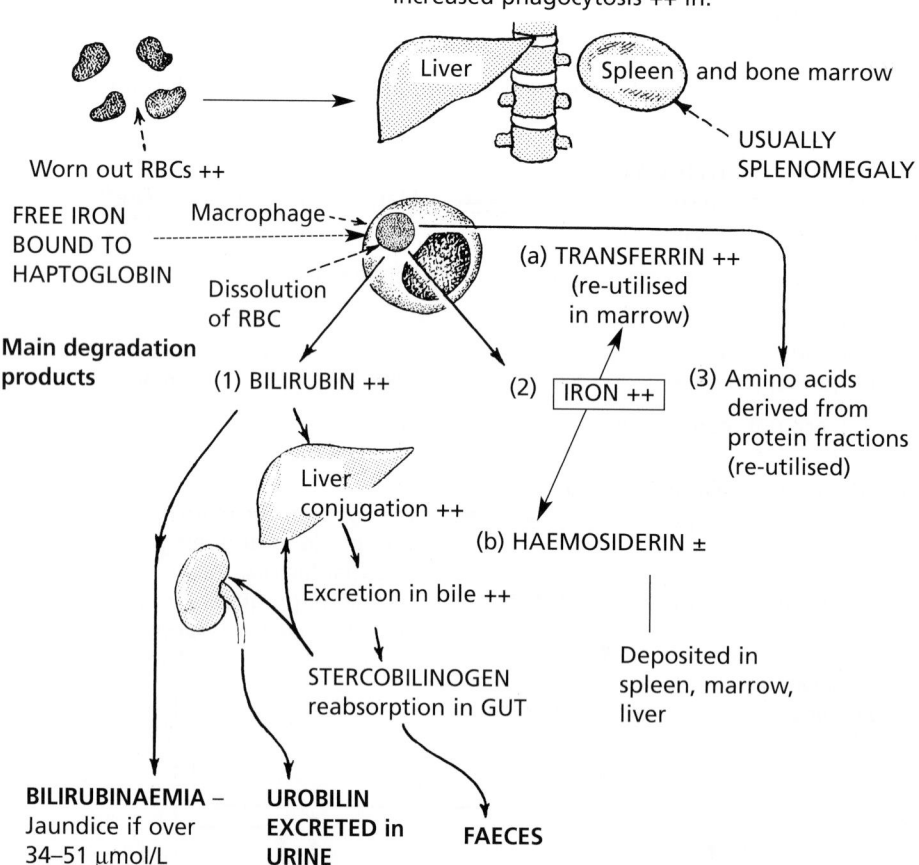

Increased phagocytosis ++ in:

Liver    Spleen  and bone marrow

USUALLY SPLENOMEGALY

Worn out RBCs ++

FREE IRON BOUND TO HAPTOGLOBIN

Macrophage

Dissolution of RBC

**Main degradation products**

(a) TRANSFERRIN ++ (re-utilised in marrow)

(1) BILIRUBIN ++    (2) IRON ++    (3) Amino acids derived from protein fractions (re-utilised)

Liver conjugation ++

(b) HAEMOSIDERIN ±

Excretion in bile ++

STERCOBILINOGEN reabsorption in GUT

Deposited in spleen, marrow, liver

**BILIRUBINAEMIA –** Jaundice if over 34–51 μmol/L

**UROBILIN EXCRETED in URINE**

**FAECES**

*Note:* 1. The bilirubin is unconjugated and is attached to protein so that renal excretion does not occur – **acholuric jaundice**.
2. Unconjugated bilirubin is toxic to the central nervous system of neonates; **kernicterus** (see p. 431) is a serious complication of haemolytic disease of the newborn.
3. If haptoglobin reserves are saturated, Hb remains free in plasma causing kidney damage and haemoglobinuria.

## REACTIVE BONE MARROW CHANGES

There is a marked hyperplasia ——— Extension of RED MARROW into long bones

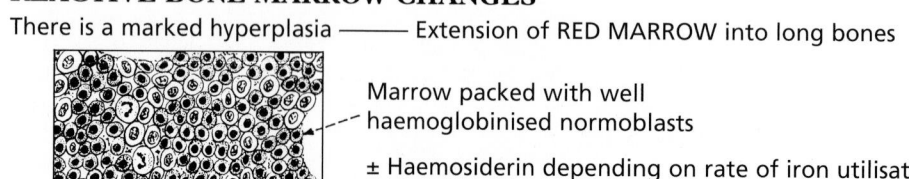

Marrow packed with well haemoglobinised normoblasts

± Haemosiderin depending on rate of iron utilisation

Many young red cells are released into the blood. The reticulocyte count may be 20–30%.

# EXTRINSIC HAEMOLYTIC ANAEMIAS

The causes of shortened red cell survival are divided into two main groups.

1. EXTRINSIC (factors outside the red cells) and 2. INTRINSIC (defects of red cells).
   Extrinsic haemolytic anaemias fall into four groups due to:
   (a) **ANTIBODIES** (either auto-immune or iso-antibodies).
   (b) **Infections.**
   (c) **Chemical damage** to the red cell.
   (d) **Physical damage** to the cell.

## 1a1 AUTO-IMMUNE HAEMOLYTIC ANAEMIA

Antibodies to cell surface antigen
Normal red cell
Intravascular lysis
Agglutination
Phagocytosis
(extravascular lysis)

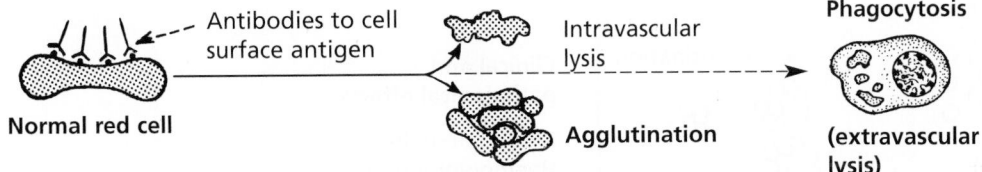

Auto-immune haemolytic anaemias are classified according to the temperature at which the reaction occurs and the presence of an underlying cause.

**WARM (37 °C – USUALLY IgG)**

**Primary** – so-called 'idiopathic haemolytic anaemia': usually in adults.

**Secondary** – associated with
(i) **lymphomas**, e.g. chronic lymphocytic leukaemia, Hodgkin lymphoma
(ii) **other cancers**
(iii) **connective tissue diseases**, e.g. systemic lupus erythematosus, rheumatoid arthritis
(iv) **drugs**, e.g. methyl-dopa

**Mechanism**:
Coating of RBC with IgG antibodies, often against Rhesus 'e' antigens.
Destruction in spleen which is often enlarged.

RBC
Spleen
Chronic haemolytic anaemia + crises

**COLD (<30 °C – USUALLY IgM)**

Idiopathic cold agglutination disease
(i) lymphomas
(ii) *Mycoplasma pneumoniae*
(iii) viral infections, e.g. measles

**Mechanism**

IgM antibody
combines with RBC
RBC
Agglutination
Blockage of peripheral vessels
Painful hands and feet
Complement activation
Intravascular lysis
Paroxysmal cold haemoglobinuria

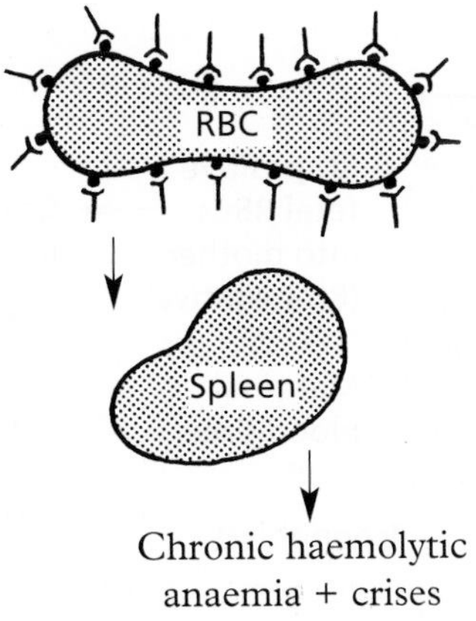

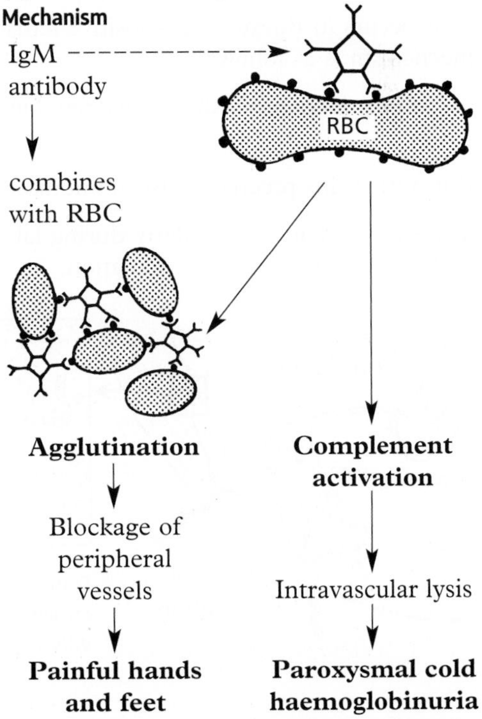

# INCOMPATIBLE BLOOD TRANSFUSION/ HAEMOLYTIC DISEASE OF THE NEWBORN

### 1a2 DESTRUCTION OF RBCS IS DUE TO ISO-ANTIBODIES

In these, the antibodies act against antigens which are derived from another individual of the same species.

*Incompatible ABO blood transfusion* is a classic example.

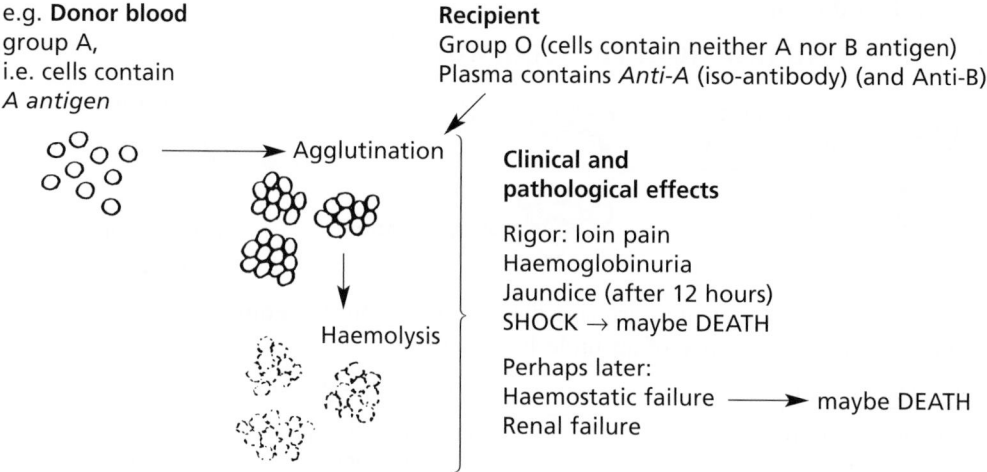

e.g. **Donor blood**
group A,
i.e. cells contain
A antigen

**Recipient**
Group O (cells contain neither A nor B antigen)
Plasma contains *Anti-A* (iso-antibody) (and Anti-B)

Agglutination

Haemolysis

**Clinical and
pathological effects**

Rigor: loin pain
Haemoglobinuria
Jaundice (after 12 hours)
SHOCK → maybe DEATH

Perhaps later:
Haemostatic failure ⟶ maybe DEATH
Renal failure

### 1a3 HAEMOLYTIC DISEASE OF THE NEWBORN (HDN)

This occurs in Rhesus (Rh)-positive fetuses conceived by Rh-negative mothers. The usual mechanism is as follows:

> *First pregnancy*: Rh-positive fetus in Rh-negative mother – no antibodies present;
> ∴ *Healthy baby*

But during this pregnancy, iso-immunisation of the mother may occur.

Towards term and particularly during labour the placental barrier is breached and fetal RBCs enter the maternal circulation.

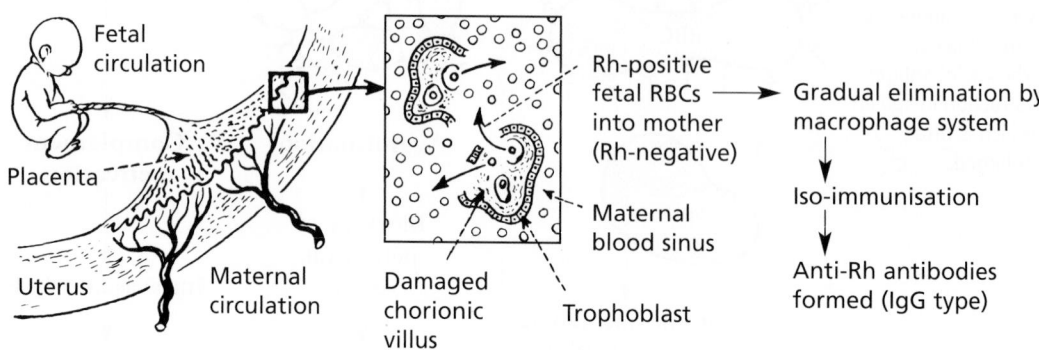

Fetal
circulation

Placenta

Uterus

Maternal
circulation

Damaged
chorionic
villus

Trophoblast

Maternal
blood sinus

Rh-positive
fetal RBCs
into mother
(Rh-negative)

⟶ Gradual elimination by
macrophage system

Iso-immunisation

Anti-Rh antibodies
formed (IgG type)

# HAEMOLYTIC DISEASE OF THE NEWBORN

The basic mechanism is influenced by three important factors:

(a) The maternal immune response tends to be proportional to the number of fetal cells entering the circulation.
(b) The maternal immune response is boosted in successive Rh-incompatible pregnancies – the highest maternal antibody titres are found in the latest of multiple pregnancies.
(c) Fetal/maternal ABO compatibility influences the Rh immune response.

| e.g. ABO COMPATIBLE | | ABO INCOMPATIBLE | |
|---|---|---|---|
| **Fetus** | **Mother** | **Fetus** | **Mother** |
| Group O Rh+ | Group O Rh− | Group A Rh+ | Group O Rh− |
| Gradual elimination of fetal cells | | Rapid destruction fetal cells | |
| ∴ Maximum immune response | | ∴ Minimum immune response | |

*Subsequent pregnancies*: all Rh-positive fetuses conceived by a mother who has acquired anti-Rh antibodies either during previous pregnancies or by blood transfusion (in this case the first fetus also) are at risk.

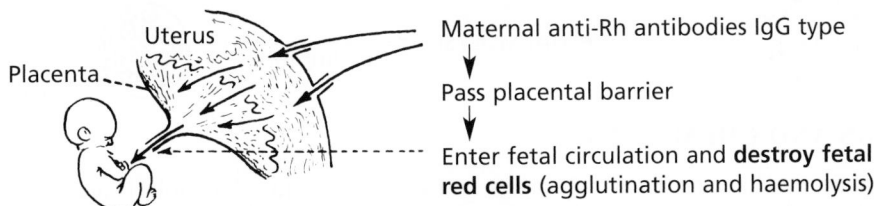

Maternal anti-Rh antibodies IgG type
↓
Pass placental barrier
↓
Enter fetal circulation and **destroy fetal red cells** (agglutination and haemolysis)

The effects are graded into three categories of severity:

(1) **Congenital haemolytic anaemia**
Usually mild anaemia and jaundice
↓
Usually self-limited

(2) **Icterus gravis neonatorum**
Rapidly developing severe **anaemia** and **jaundice**

± Brain damage due to kernicterus

Severe anoxia may cause death

(3) **Hydrops fetalis**
Stillbirth associated with severe anoxia in utero with cardiac failure and oedema
↓
**Hepatosplenomegaly** – due to extramedullary **haemopoiesis**

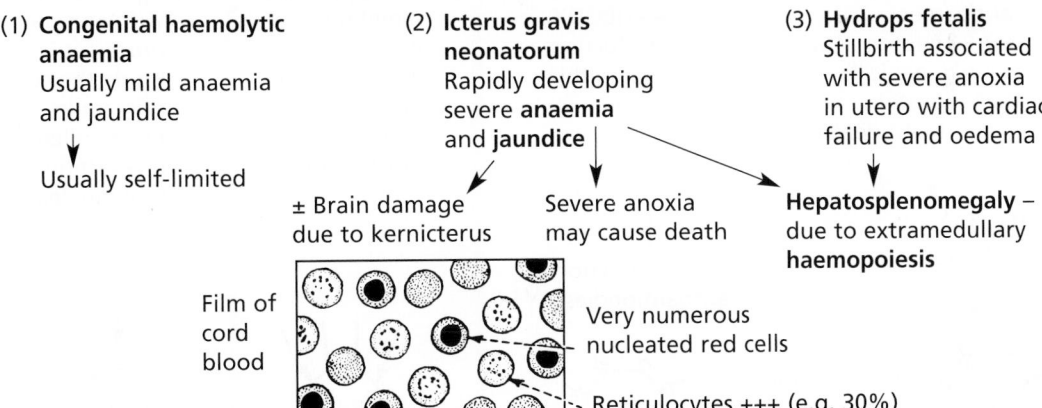

Film of cord blood

Very numerous nucleated red cells

Reticulocytes +++ (e.g. 30%)

*Modern prophylaxis*
Injection of anti-Rh antibody minimises immune response.

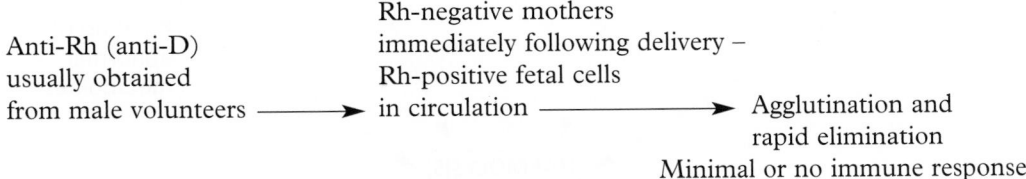

Anti-Rh (anti-D) usually obtained from male volunteers ⟶ Rh-negative mothers immediately following delivery – Rh-positive fetal cells in circulation ⟶ Agglutination and rapid elimination
Minimal or no immune response

# EXTRINSIC HAEMOLYTIC ANAEMIAS

### 1b INFECTIONS

There are three mechanisms by which infections cause haemolysis:

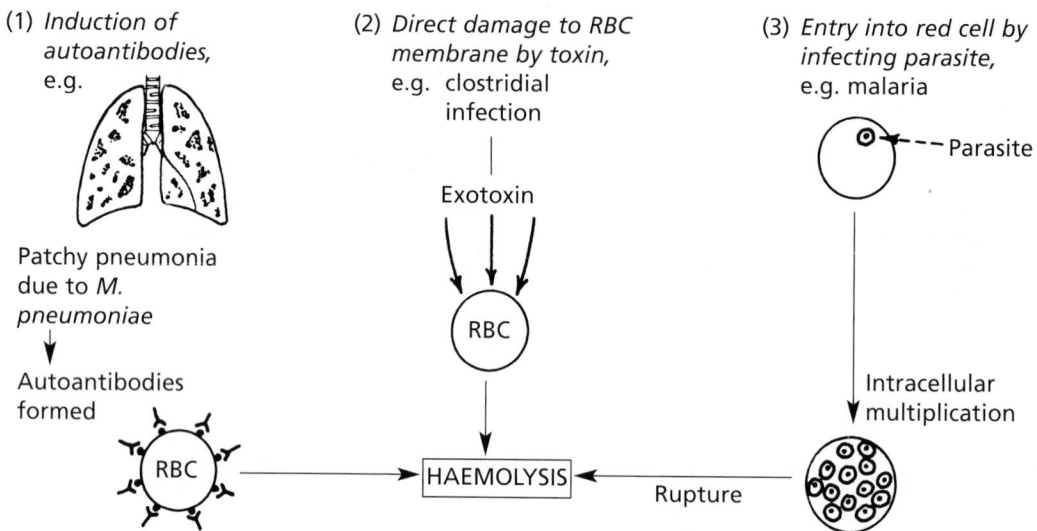

(1) *Induction of autoantibodies,* e.g.

Patchy pneumonia due to *M. pneumoniae*

↓

Autoantibodies formed

(2) *Direct damage to RBC membrane by toxin,* e.g. clostridial infection

Exotoxin

RBC

(3) *Entry into red cell by infecting parasite,* e.g. malaria

Parasite

Intracellular multiplication

Rupture

HAEMOLYSIS

### 1c DRUGS AND CHEMICALS

The three main mechanisms by which drugs and chemicals cause haemolysis are:

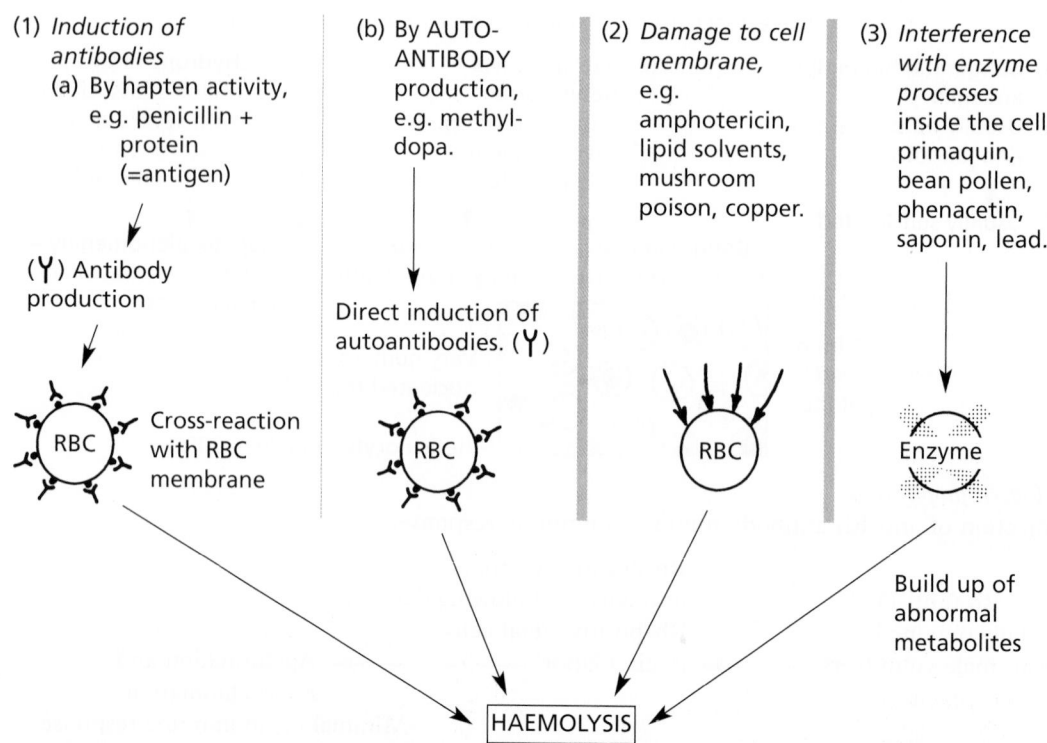

(1) *Induction of antibodies*
   (a) By hapten activity, e.g. penicillin + protein (=antigen)

(Y) Antibody production

RBC — Cross-reaction with RBC membrane

(b) By AUTO-ANTIBODY production, e.g. methyl-dopa.

Direct induction of autoantibodies. (Y)

RBC

(2) *Damage to cell membrane,* e.g. amphotericin, lipid solvents, mushroom poison, copper.

RBC

(3) *Interference with enzyme processes* inside the cell, primaquin, bean pollen, phenacetin, saponin, lead.

Enzyme

Build up of abnormal metabolites

HAEMOLYSIS

# EXTRINSIC HAEMOLYTIC ANAEMIAS

## 1d   MECHANICAL TRAUMA

The results of damage to red cells within the circulation are:

(1) Intravascular haemolysis

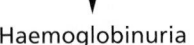

Haemoglobinuria

(2) Formation of red cell fragments (schistocytes)

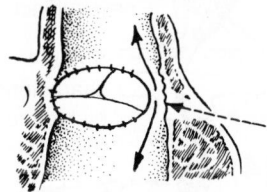

seen in blood film as 'burr', 'triangle', 'helmet' cells

The main circumstances in which red cells are damaged are:

(a) In the **heart and great vessels**

When the blood flow is subjected to undue turbulence or jet effect. An important example is prosthetic valves in the left side of the heart.

RBCs damaged by shearing stresses where valve seating is defective or through the valve itself.

(b) In the **microcirculation**

(i)   When the blood flow in arterioles is impeded by strands of fibrin.

This condition is called MICROANGIOPATHIC HAEMOLYTIC ANAEMIA and occurs in many disease states involving small blood vessels, e.g. malignant hypertension and/or intravascular coagulation.

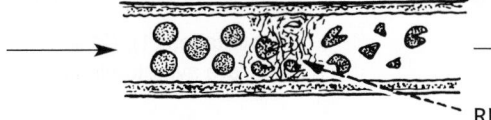

(1) Liberation of haemoglobin
(2) Emergence of fragments

RBCs being distorted and cut by fibrin sieve

(ii)   When blood vessels are subjected to direct trauma. This is seen classically in military recruits marching long distances in hard-soled boots, when the blood vessels of the soles of the feet are squeezed with every step – **march haemoglobinuria**.

The haemolysis is usually not severe enough to be of clinical significance, but haemoglobinuria may cause alarm.

**Other causes of haemolysis** include:

**Hypersplenism**

In enlargement of the spleen from any cause, the sequestration of red cells is increased so that haemolytic anaemia may result.

**Normal**

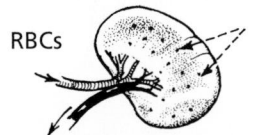

RBCs

Worn out cells (about 1% per day) removed in red pulp

RBC life span 120 days

**Hypersplenism**

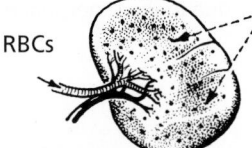

RBCs

RBCs removed in greater numbers and before they are worn out

RBC life span reduced

433

# EXTRINSIC HAEMOLYTIC ANAEMIAS – MALARIA

Malaria is an endemic disease in many parts of Africa, Asia, Central and South America. Many millions of cases occur each year and the mortality is at least 1%. The disease is particularly severe in non-immune subjects from temperate climates. In endemic areas where the 'herd' immunity is high, a low-grade chronic illness is common.

Female anopheline mosquitos act as intermediate hosts in the life cycle of the parasite, a protozoon (genus *Plasmodium*).

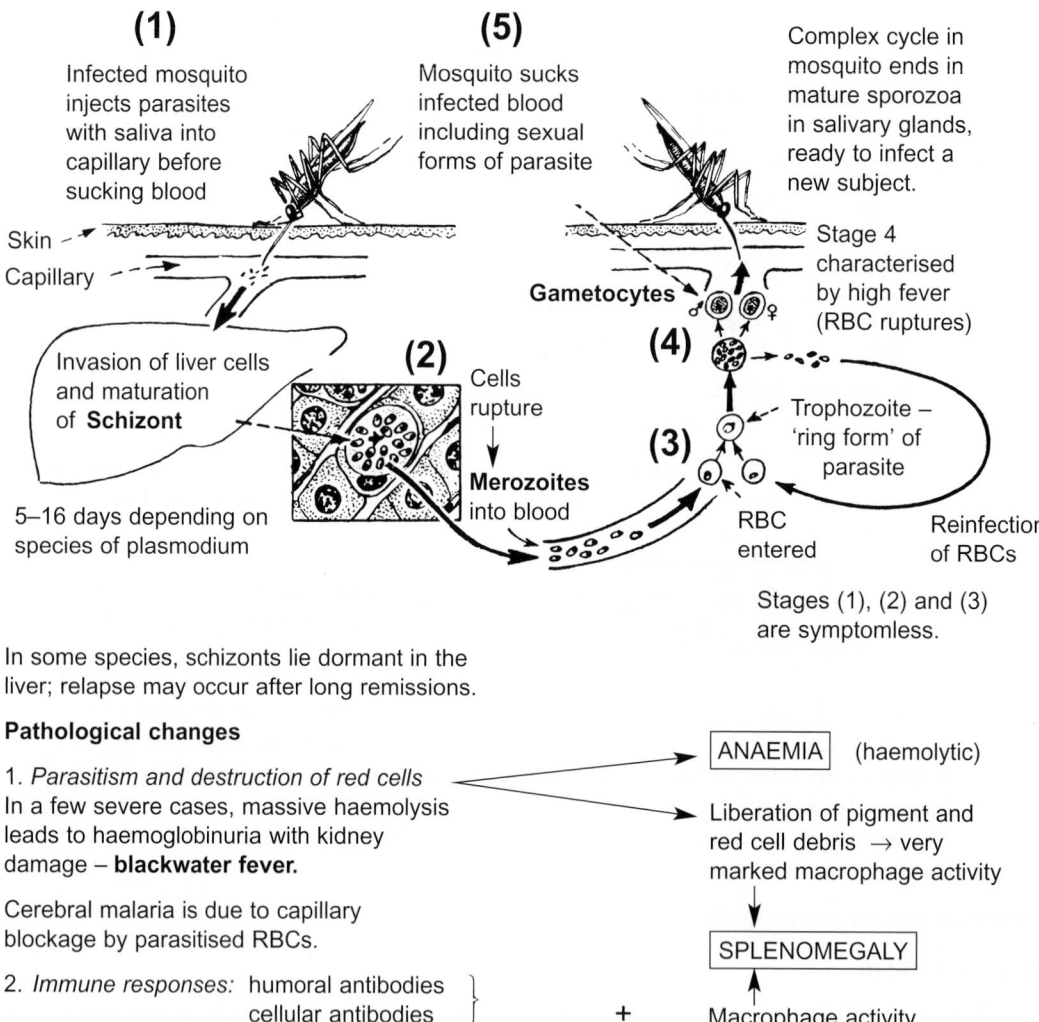

**(1)** Infected mosquito injects parasites with saliva into capillary before sucking blood

**(5)** Mosquito sucks infected blood including sexual forms of parasite

Complex cycle in mosquito ends in mature sporozoa in salivary glands, ready to infect a new subject.

Skin

Capillary

**Gametocytes** ♂ ♀

Stage 4 characterised by high fever (RBC ruptures)

Invasion of liver cells and maturation of **Schizont**

**(2)** Cells rupture

**(4)**

**(3)**

Trophozoite – 'ring form' of parasite

**Merozoites** into blood

RBC entered

Reinfection of RBCs

5–16 days depending on species of plasmodium

Stages (1), (2) and (3) are symptomless.

In some species, schizonts lie dormant in the liver; relapse may occur after long remissions.

**Pathological changes**

1. *Parasitism and destruction of red cells*
In a few severe cases, massive haemolysis leads to haemoglobinuria with kidney damage – **blackwater fever.**

Cerebral malaria is due to capillary blockage by parasitised RBCs.

2. *Immune responses:* humoral antibodies } cellular antibodies }    +

ANAEMIA    (haemolytic)

Liberation of pigment and red cell debris → very marked macrophage activity

SPLENOMEGALY

Macrophage activity

With appropriate drugs, the prognosis of most forms of malaria is good. The treatment of falciparum malaria is becoming more difficult due to the emergence of drug resistance.

# INTRINSIC HAEMOLYTIC ANAEMIAS

## 2. INTRINSIC DEFECTS – USUALLY HEREDITARY

In (a) cell membrane, (b) enzymes and (c) molecular structure of haemoglobin (haemoglobinopathies).

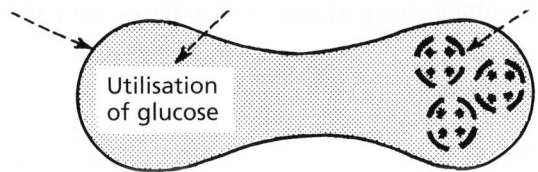

Utilisation of glucose

### a. Cell membrane defects

a1 **Hereditary spherocytosis**: the majority of cases are familial (autosomal dominant).

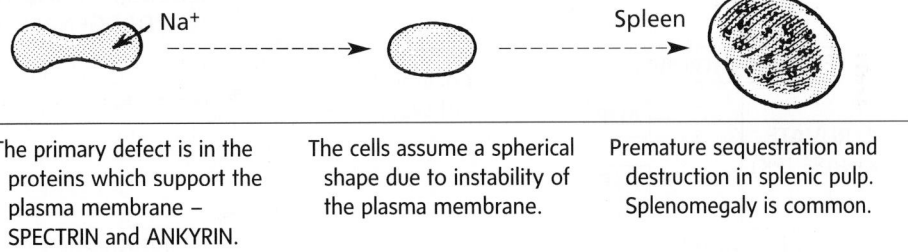

| | | |
|---|---|---|
| The primary defect is in the proteins which support the plasma membrane – SPECTRIN and ANKYRIN. | The cells assume a spherical shape due to instability of the plasma membrane. | Premature sequestration and destruction in splenic pulp. Splenomegaly is common. |

*Note*: Splenectomy is usually 'curative' but the red cell defect remains.

The severity of the haemolysis is variable; many cases are compensated and not anaemic, but crises are common, e.g. if folate deficiency supervenes. Intercurrent infections may precipitate increased red cell destruction with jaundice or temporary bone marrow hypoplasia, e.g. parvovirus infection, with severe anaemia.

The laboratory diagnosis depends on:
(1) typical blood film with spherocytes,
(2) high reticulocyte count,
(3) increased osmotic fragility of RBCs.

a2 **Hereditary elliptocytosis** is similar to spherocytosis in many respects, but it is usually not severe enough to cause anaemia or jaundice. Haemolysis is usually mild.

a3 **Hereditary abetalipoproteinaemia**: a rare disease in which the red cell membranes are abnormal and the cells become spiky (acanthocytes).

a4 **Paroxysmal nocturnal haemoglobinuria** – a rare, acquired condition in which there is a somatic mutation in myeloid stem cells. Anchorage of proteins to the red cell membrane is abnormal. The cells are particularly susceptible to the action of complement (usually activated by the alternative pathway) at low pH. Intravascular haemolysis results.

# INTRINSIC HAEMOLYTIC ANAEMIAS

b. **Enzyme defects**

Usually hereditary. Glucose is the source of energy with which the red cell metabolism is maintained. Glycolysis is effected by two classic enzyme pathways.

The following simplified diagram outlines the pathways and indicates only the main enzymes and substrates.

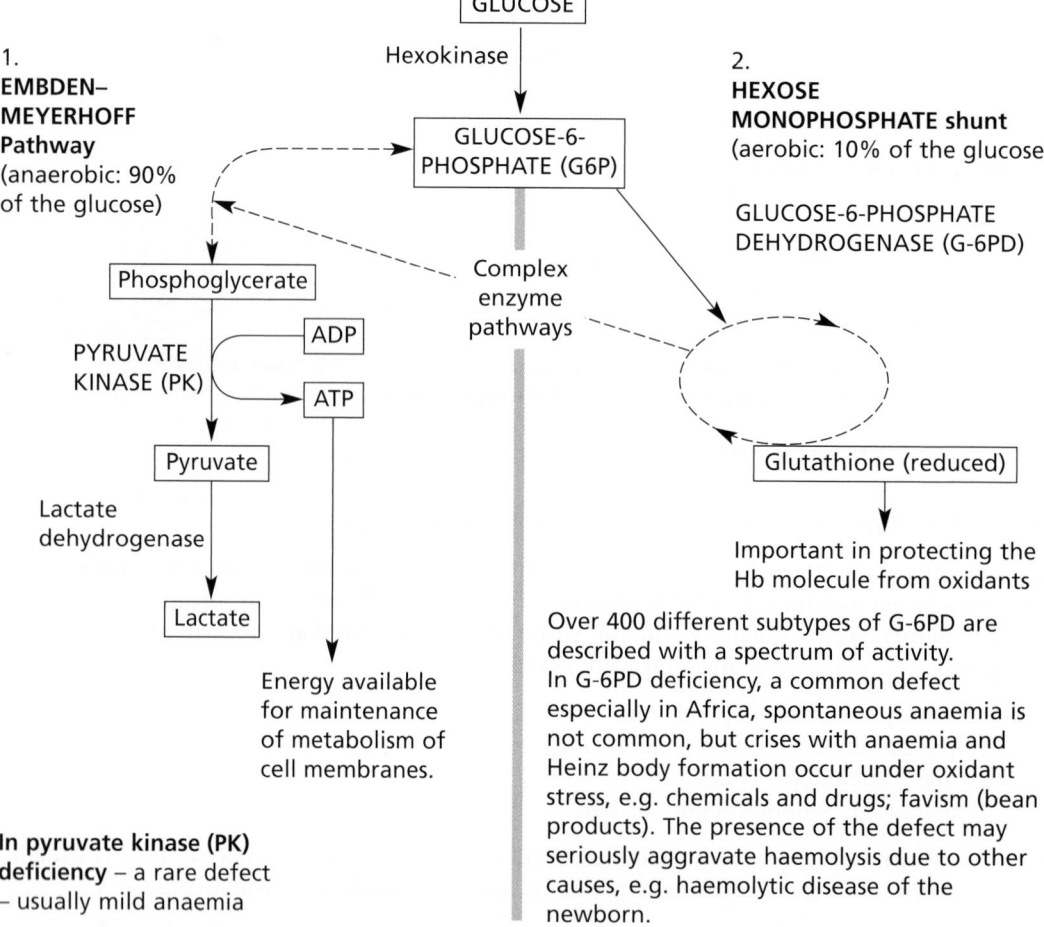

In pyruvate kinase (PK) deficiency – a rare defect – usually mild anaemia

Over 400 different subtypes of G-6PD are described with a spectrum of activity. In G-6PD deficiency, a common defect especially in Africa, spontaneous anaemia is not common, but crises with anaemia and Heinz body formation occur under oxidant stress, e.g. chemicals and drugs; favism (bean products). The presence of the defect may seriously aggravate haemolysis due to other causes, e.g. haemolytic disease of the newborn.

G-6PD deficiency shows X-linked inheritance so that in the male the defect is fully expressed, while in the female heterozygote there are two populations of red cells in the blood (1) normal cells and (2) defective cells.

In both these defects and in the rare defects of other enzymes in the pathways which have been described, the expression of the abnormal gene is very variable from case to case.

# DISORDERS OF HAEMOGLOBIN SYNTHESIS

## 2c Haemoglobinopathies

**Varieties of normal haemoglobin** are illustrated:

**Normal haemoglobin molecule**

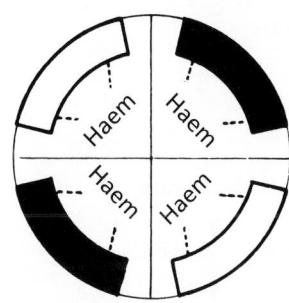

Mol. wt. = 68 000

Four subunits each consisting of a haem core with a polypeptide chain attached. The haem core is constant while the polypeptide chains occur in pairs. Four different polypeptide chains occur normally.

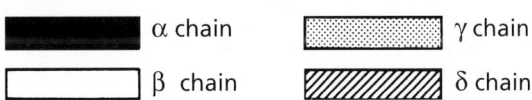

Four subunits each consisting of a haem core with a polypeptide chain attached. The haem core is constant while the polypeptide chains occur in pairs. Four different polypeptide chains occur normally.

There are three types of normal haemoglobin.

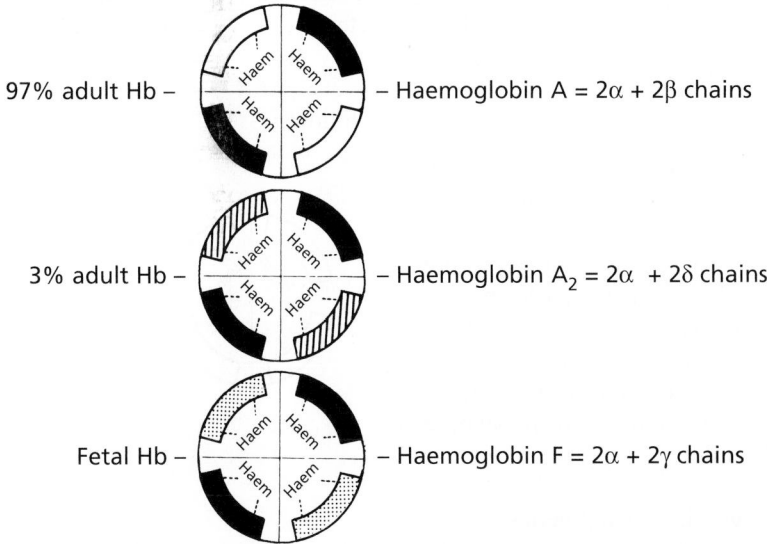

97% adult Hb – – Haemoglobin A = $2\alpha + 2\beta$ chains

3% adult Hb – – Haemoglobin $A_2$ = $2\alpha + 2\delta$ chains

Fetal Hb – – Haemoglobin F = $2\alpha + 2\gamma$ chains

Fetal haemoglobin is replaced by adult haemoglobin during the first year ('haemoglobin switching'). Note that the $\alpha$ chain occurs in all normal haemoglobins.

Two copies of the $\alpha$ chain genes ($\alpha\alpha/\alpha\alpha$) are present on chromosome 16; $\beta$, $\gamma$ and $\delta$ genes are found in a complex on chromosome 11. A number of globin-like genes are also present but are omitted for simplicity.

In the **thalassaemias** and **haemoglobinopathies** there are abnormalities in the production and structure of haemoglobin chains due to mutation of these genes.

# THE THALASSAEMIAS

These are inherited disorders in which synthesis of globin chains is diminished or absent.

They are common in the Mediterranean, Middle East and India.
α-thalassaemia – reduction of α chain synthesis.
β-thalassaemia – reduction of β chain synthesis.

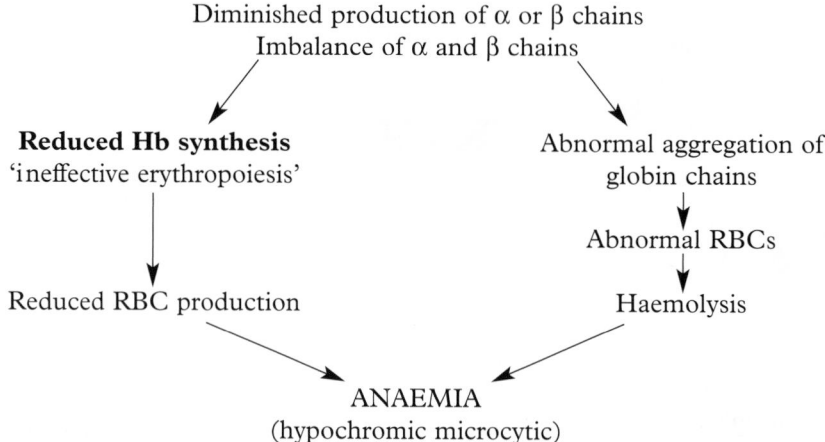

Diminished production of α or β chains
Imbalance of α and β chains

**Reduced Hb synthesis**
'ineffective erythropoiesis'

Abnormal aggregation of
globin chains

Abnormal RBCs

Reduced RBC production

Haemolysis

ANAEMIA
(hypochromic microcytic)

The severity of the disease depends on (i) the degree of globin chain abnormality and (ii) whether the patient is homozygous or heterozygous for the defect.

There are normally four α genes (αα/αα).

In the **α-thalassaemias** the genetic defects are illustrated as follows:

1. **Hb-Barts hydrops syndrome** (– –/– –): all four genes for the α chain are absent. Fetal Hb cannot be formed and the fetus dies in utero.
2. **Hb-H disease** (–α /– –): only one α gene is present. This leads to an excess of β chains which form tetramers called Hb-H. There is a moderate microcytic hypochromic anaemia with splenomegaly.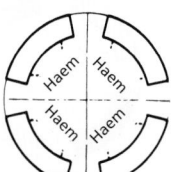
3. **α-thalassaemia** traits (–α/– α): even if two α genes are absent, the remaining two are active and the symptoms and anaemia are usually mild.

## β-Thalassaemia

**β-Thalassaemia major** – two defective β genes.
The excess of α genes leads to severe anaemia with haemolysis. The marrow becomes hyperplastic and there is atrophy of bones. The main form of haemoglobin is HbF – which persists into adult life.

**β-Thalassaemia minor** – one defective β gene.
The anaemia is mild. The red cells are microcytic and hypochromic and a mistaken diagnosis of iron deficiency anaemia can be made. These subjects act as carriers for β-thalassaemia major.

# SICKLE CELL DISEASE

This disorder is very common in Central Africa but also occurs in the Mediterranean, Middle East and India. It affects the black population of the United States and the Caribbean.

It is due to a mutation in the β chain of haemoglobin (the amino acid glutamic acid is substituted by valine) and is inherited as an autosomal recessive trait.

The effects are *mild* in heterozygotes (Hb AS) = **sickle cell trait**; they are *severe* in homozygotes (Hb SS) = **sickle cell anaemia**.

The effects are summarised as follows:

1.  **At molecular level** HbS becomes less soluble in low levels of oxygen tension.

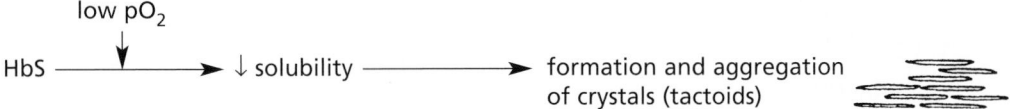

2.  **In the red cell** this causes distortion (sickling).

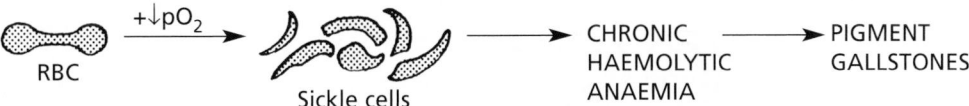

3.  **In tissues.**

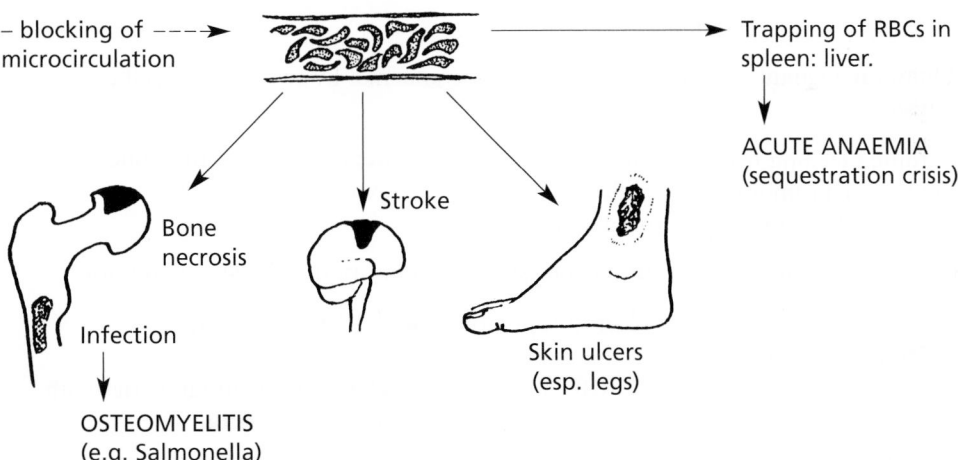

Acute sickle cell crises are often provoked by:

(1) infection, (2) cold, (3) low pO$_2$, e.g. flying in unpressurised aircraft.

In addition, infection, especially by **parvoviruses in childhood**, may provoke an **aplastic anaemia** crisis.

*Note*: HbS confers resistance to malaria: in terms of evolution this confers a survival benefit to those carrying the HbS gene.

# ANAEMIA OF CHRONIC DISORDERS

This term describes the anaemias seen commonly in patients with chronic diseases

e.g. (ia)  Chronic inflammation, e.g. rheumatoid arthritis, systemic lupus erythematosus.
    (ib)  Chronic infection, e.g. tuberculosis (TB).
    (ii)  Malignancy.

The anaemia is usually mild (Hb >9 g/dL).

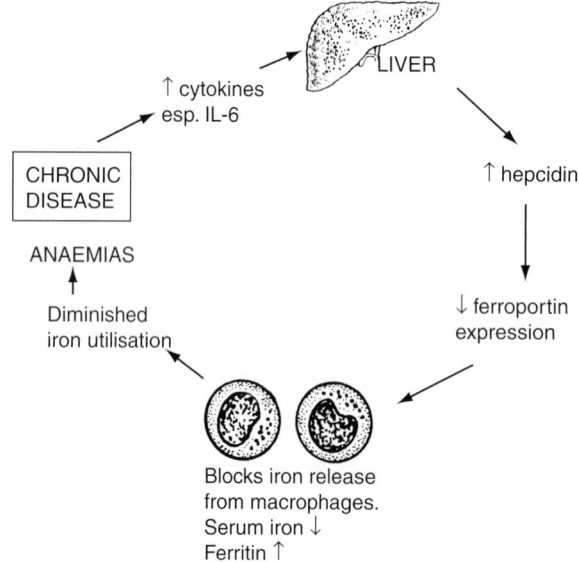

In addition, malignant tumour growth may cause anaemia by two more specific mechanisms.

(a)  Chronic bleeding from the surface of an ulcerated tumour – especially from the alimentary tract ⟶ iron deficiency.

(b)  Replacement of the bone marrow by malignant tumour.

**Normocytic normochromic anaemias** are also found in other systemic diseases.

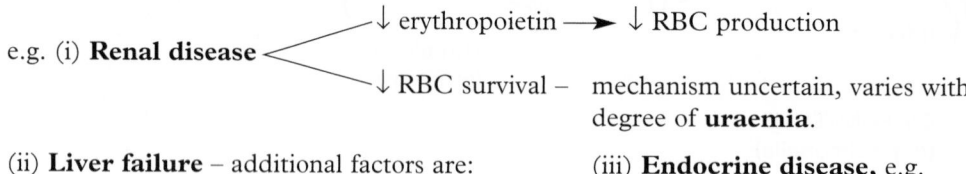

e.g. (i) **Renal disease** — ↓ erythropoietin ⟶ ↓ RBC production
↓ RBC survival – mechanism uncertain, varies with degree of **uraemia**.

(ii) **Liver failure** – additional factors are:

Liver — Bleeding varices
— Deficiency of coagulation factors
— Hypersplenism
— Alcoholic – other nutritional deficiencies

(iii) **Endocrine disease,** e.g.

hypopituitarism ⎫
hypothyroidism ⎬ — ↓ metabolism
        ⎭ — ↓ erythropoietin production

# APLASTIC ANAEMIA

In this rare disorder there is:

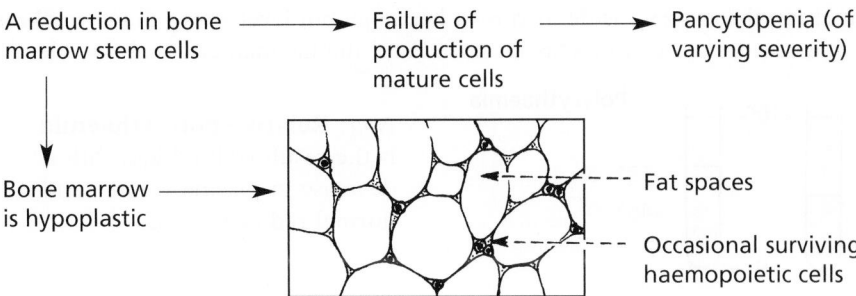

There are a number of different types

(a) **Idiopathic** – in two-thirds of cases no cause is found.
(b) **Drug induced** – this may be:
   (i) Predictable, e.g. cytotoxic chemotherapy.
   (ii) Idiosyncratic, e.g. chloramphenicol (1 in 25 000–60 000 affected), phenylbutazone.
(c) **Virus induced**, e.g. hepatitis, Epstein–Barr virus.
(d) **Auto-immune.**
(e) **Inherited**, e.g. Fanconi anaemia – autosomal recessive.

**Treatment** This consists of:
(a) Supportive therapy, e.g. blood transfusion.
(b) Attempts to restore haemopoiesis, e.g. bone marrow transplantation
                   – anabolic steroids
                   – immunosuppressive therapy
                   – withdrawal of causative drugs

**The sideroblastic anaemias**
In these rare anaemias, there is failure of synthesis of the haem component of the haemoglobin molecule. On blood film the presence of a ring of iron granules around the normoblast nucleus can be seen.

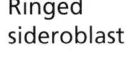
Ringed sideroblast

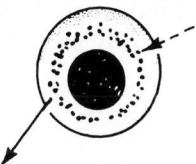

Iron granules (in mitochondria) stained by Prussian blue reaction

In a few cases, pyridoxine allows haem synthesis to proceed normally

The condition arises secondarily in many of the chronic disease states mentioned on the previous page, or as a result of drug treatment or chemical poisoning (e.g. lead). Some cases are 'primary' – representing a form of myelodysplasia.

The anaemia is usually *dimorphic*, i.e. showing hypochromic and macrocytic features combined.

# POLYCYTHAEMIA

## POLYCYTHAEMIA

Polycythaemia (erythrocytosis) is defined by a haemoglobin level above the normal range: in true polycythaemia the red cell mass is increased and the haematocrit is always elevated.

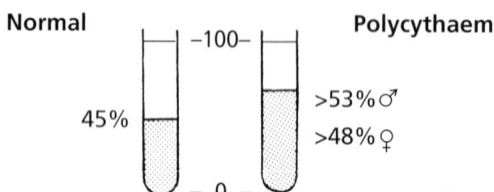

*Note*: **Relative polycythaemia** is the result of fluid loss with a decrease in plasma volume and a normal red cell mass.

### Aetiology

There are two types:

### SECONDARY POLYCYTHAEMIA

The red cell increase is the result of increased stimulation of marrow by erythropoietin. Two main groups of conditions are associated with this:

1. (Commonly) conditions causing tissue HYPOXIA
   (a) Living at high altitudes
   (b) Chronic cardiac disease especially R → L shunts
   (c) Chronic respiratory disease
   (d) Presence of abnormal haemoglobin causing defective release of $O_2$ to tissues – usually hereditary

2. (Rarely) Renal tumours and ischaemia; occasionally tumours of other organs.

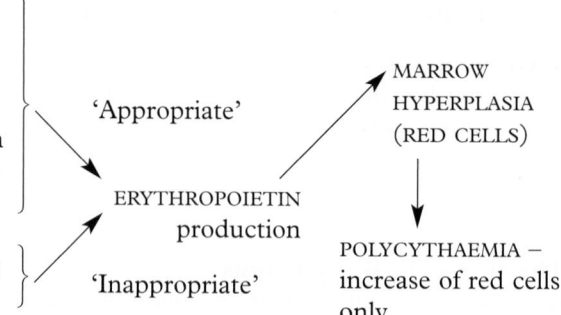

### PRIMARY POLYCYTHAEMIA (*POLYCYTHAEMIA RUBRA VERA*)

This is a myeloproliferative disorder with increased red cell production. It may be associated with an increase in other marrow elements. Splenomegaly is usually present. A minority of patients develop acute leukaemia.

### Effects of polycythaemia

(a) There is usually a distinctly florid complexion.
(b) Increased blood viscosity causes arterial and venous thrombosis.
(c) Increased marrow activity → increased uric acid metabolism → tendency to gout.

# NEUTROPHIL GRANULOCYTES

## NEUTROPHIL GRANULOCYTE (POLYMORPHONUCLEAR LEUCOCYTE)

The essential function of these cells is protection against microbial infection by phagocytosis and killing. They are produced alongside red blood cells, platelets and monocytes from a common stem cell in the marrow.

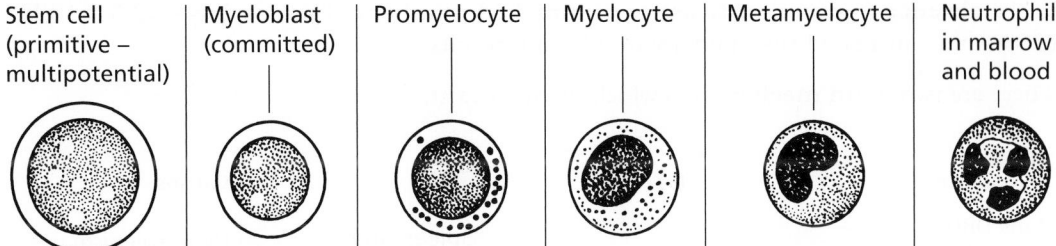

Stem cell (primitive – multipotential) | Myeloblast (committed) | Promyelocyte | Myelocyte | Metamyelocyte | Neutrophil in marrow and blood

Note the nuclear changes progressing from large open nucleus and several nucleoli to the mature condensed multi-lobed state. The cytoplasm matures with the acquisition of specific granules.

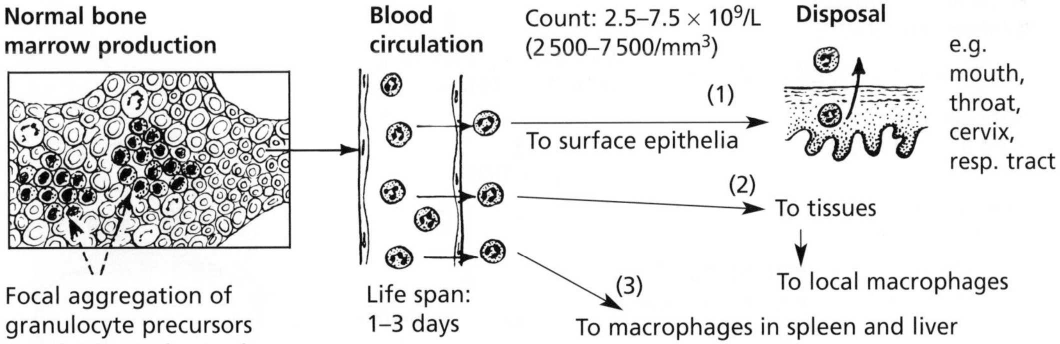

**Normal bone marrow production**

Focal aggregation of granulocyte precursors (myeloid series) mixed with other cell types. Myeloid/Erythroid ratio 3 to 8:1

**Blood circulation**

Life span: 1–3 days

Count: $2.5$–$7.5 \times 10^9$/L ($2\,500$–$7\,500$/mm$^3$)

(1) To surface epithelia

(2) To tissues → To local macrophages

(3) To macrophages in spleen and liver

**Disposal**

e.g. mouth, throat, cervix, resp. tract

An increase in the number of circulating neutrophils reflects an increased activity in the tissues at the site of an acute inflammatory reaction.

## Neutrophil activation

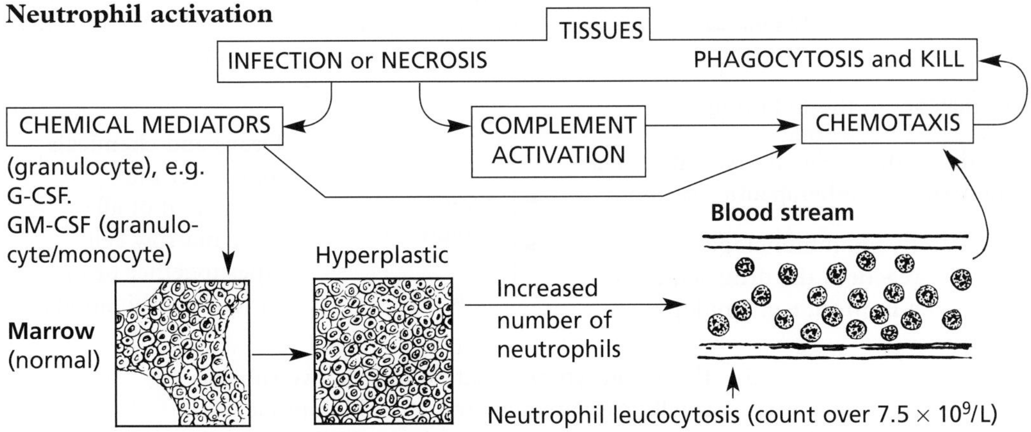

TISSUES

INFECTION or NECROSIS → PHAGOCYTOSIS and KILL

CHEMICAL MEDIATORS

COMPLEMENT ACTIVATION

CHEMOTAXIS

(granulocyte), e.g. G-CSF. GM-CSF (granulo-cyte/monocyte)

**Marrow** (normal)

Hyperplastic

Increased number of neutrophils

**Blood stream**

Neutrophil leucocytosis (count over $7.5 \times 10^9$/L)

# DISORDERS OF NEUTROPHILS – AGRANULOCYTOSIS

Neutrophil leukocytosis is a common finding in many bacterial infections. It does not however occur in: (a) some acute bacterial infections, e.g. typhoid fever, brucellosis; (b) many chronic bacterial infection, e.g. TB; (c) most virus infections unless acute bacterial infection or necrosis occurs; (d) overwhelming infections with severe toxaemia.

In the **absence (agranulocytosis)** or **diminished numbers** of neutrophils – $<2.5 \times 10/L$ $(2500/mm^3)$ increased susceptibility to infection results.

There are two **main mechanisms** which often co-exist.

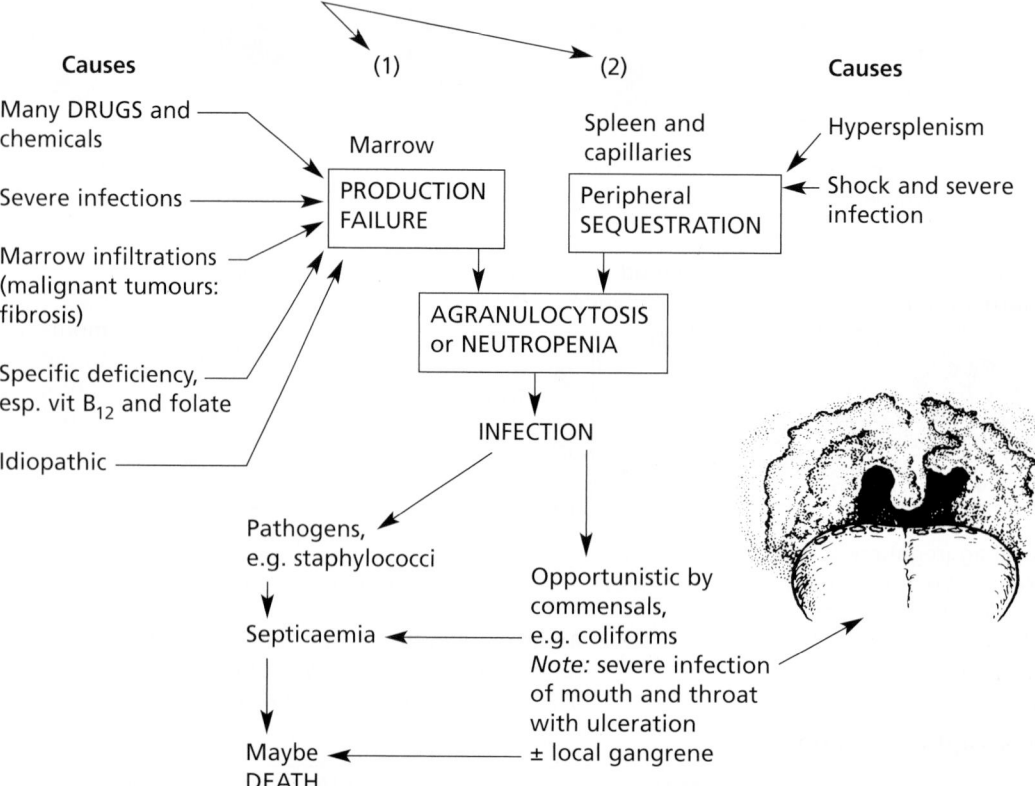

Causes      (1)      (2)      Causes

Many DRUGS and chemicals

Severe infections

Marrow infiltrations (malignant tumours: fibrosis)

Specific deficiency, esp. vit $B_{12}$ and folate

Idiopathic

Marrow
PRODUCTION FAILURE

Spleen and capillaries
Peripheral SEQUESTRATION

Hypersplenism

Shock and severe infection

AGRANULOCYTOSIS or NEUTROPENIA

INFECTION

Pathogens, e.g. staphylococci

Septicaemia

Maybe DEATH

Opportunistic by commensals, e.g. coliforms
*Note:* severe infection of mouth and throat with ulceration ± local gangrene

Drugs may act in the following ways:

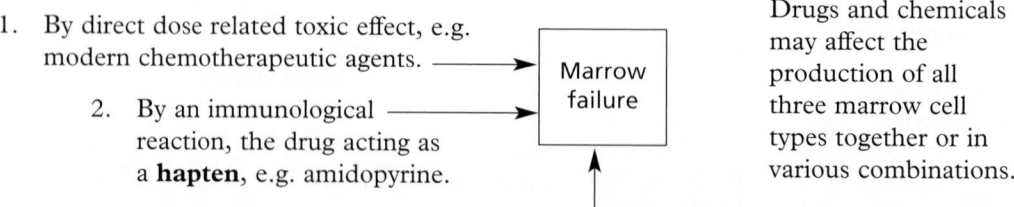

1. By direct dose related toxic effect, e.g. modern chemotherapeutic agents. ⟶

2. By an immunological reaction, the drug acting as a **hapten**, e.g. amidopyrine. ⟶

Marrow failure

Drugs and chemicals may affect the production of all three marrow cell types together or in various combinations.

3. By an idiosyncratic action in sensitive subjects small doses are effective, e.g. chloramphenicol (compare aplastic anaemia, p. 441).

# DISORDERS OF NEUTROPHILS

## Disorders of neutrophil function

Divided into three groups: (1) chemotaxis, (2) microbial phagocytosis and (3) microbial kill.

*Chemotaxis and phagocytosis* may be defective due to:

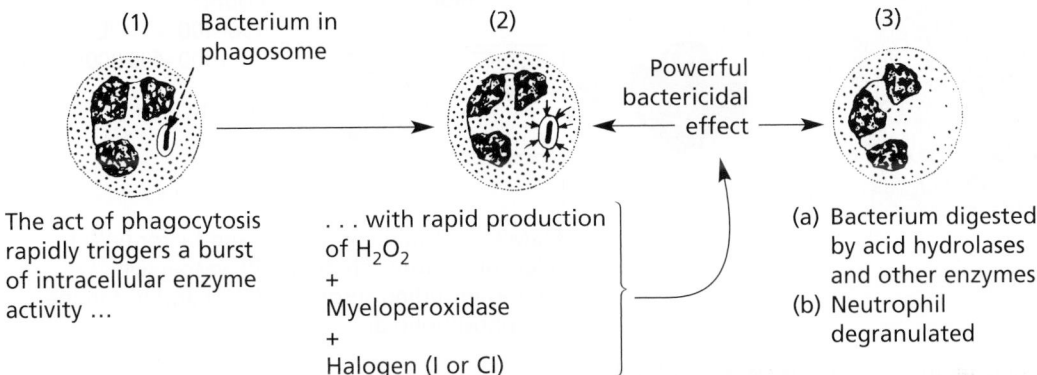

**(1)** Bacterium in phagosome
**(2)**
Powerful bactericidal effect
**(3)**

The act of phagocytosis rapidly triggers a burst of intracellular enzyme activity ...

. . . with rapid production of $H_2O_2$
+
Myeloperoxidase
+
Halogen (I or Cl)

(a) Bacterium digested by acid hydrolases and other enzymes
(b) Neutrophil degranulated

*Microbial kill* fails when there is an intracellular enzyme defect, e.g. in *chronic granulomatous disease* (CGD) and the Chediak–Higashi syndrome, where the neutrophils contain abnormal giant granules.

The normal sequence following phagocytosis is:

(a) Bacterium digested by acid hydrolases and other enzymes.
(b) Neutrophil degranulated.

## CHRONIC GRANULOMATOUS DISEASE (CGD)

It is a rare hereditary disorder in which the neutrophils have normal phagocytic function but are unable to kill certain bacteria. The disease is fully expressed only in males. It presents as multiple chronic abscesses and granulomas affecting skin, lungs, bones, spleen and liver.

The rapid production of $H_2O_2$ is defective (in the neutrophils and also in macrophages due to deficiency of NADPH-oxidase).

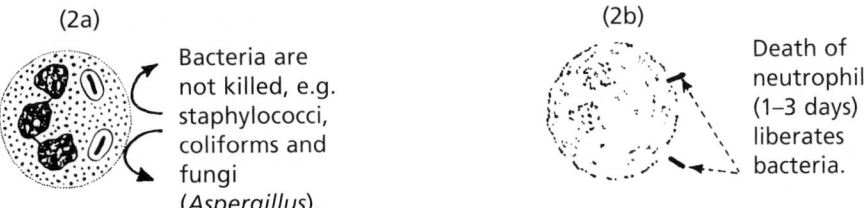

**(2a)** Bacteria are not killed, e.g. staphylococci, coliforms and fungi (*Aspergillus*).

**(2b)** Death of neutrophil (1–3 days) liberates bacteria.

About two-thirds of cases are X-linked (fully expressed in males); the remainder are recessive. The neutrophils are unable to reduce nitroblue tetrazolium (used as a diagnostic slide test).

# PLATELETS AND COAGULATION

These small, anucleate discs, derived from the cytoplasm of the bone marrow megakaryocytes, are released into the blood stream by a budding process.

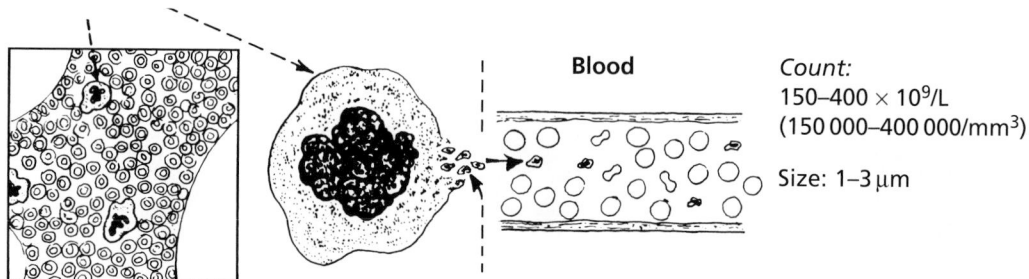

**Blood**

*Count:*
$150$–$400 \times 10^9$/L
($150\,000$–$400\,000$/mm$^3$)

Size: $1$–$3\,\mu$m

Platelets contain von Willebrand factor (vWF), adenosine diphosphate (ADP), vasoactive amines including serotonin (5HT) and histamine and phospholipid.

Their main role is in preventing blood loss after injury.

e.g. Skin wound.

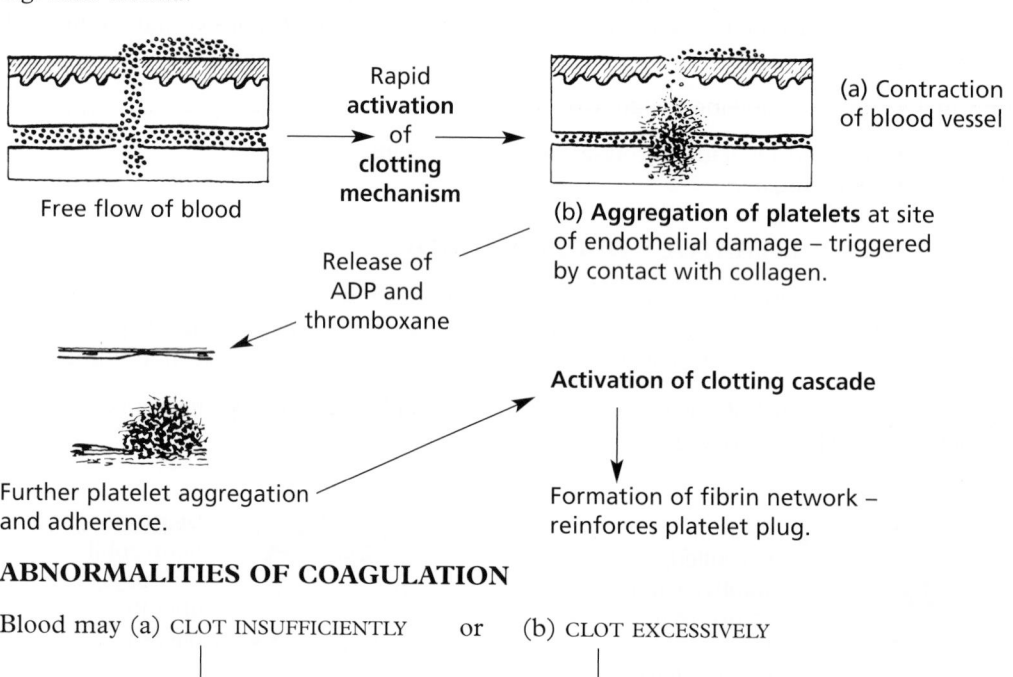

Free flow of blood

Rapid **activation** of **clotting mechanism**

(a) Contraction of blood vessel

(b) **Aggregation of platelets** at site of endothelial damage – triggered by contact with collagen.

Release of ADP and thromboxane

Further platelet aggregation and adherence.

**Activation of clotting cascade**

Formation of fibrin network – reinforces platelet plug.

## ABNORMALITIES OF COAGULATION

Blood may (a) CLOT INSUFFICIENTLY    or    (b) CLOT EXCESSIVELY

HAEMORRHAGIC TENDENCY
– too few platelets (THROMBOCYTOPENIA)
  – excess destruction.
  – decreased formation.
– abnormal platelet function.
– deficiency of clotting factors.

THROMBOSIS
– too many platelets (THROMBOCYTOSIS).
– increased viscosity –
    e.g. in polycythaemia.
– due to deficiency of inhibitors
    of clotting factors.

# DISORDERS OF PLATELETS

Disorders of the platelets include:
(a) Deficiencies of number – thrombocytopenia – lead to bleeding tendency.
(b) Defective function.

## THROMBOCYTOPENIA

Although the normal platelet count ranges from $150\text{–}400 \times 10^9/L$, a risk of dangerous spontaneous haemorrhage is unusual unless the count falls below $30 \times 10^9/L$.
The causes of thrombocytopenia fall into two main groups:

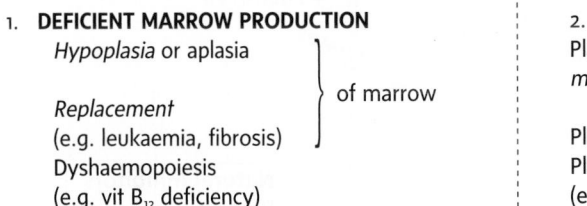

1. **DEFICIENT MARROW PRODUCTION**

   *Hypoplasia* or *aplasia* ⎤
   ⎟ of marrow
   *Replacement* ⎦
   (e.g. leukaemia, fibrosis)
   Dyshaemopoiesis
   (e.g. vit $B_{12}$ deficiency)

2. **INCREASED DESTRUCTION**

   Platelets damaged by *drugs, immune mechanisms*

   Platelets sequestered in *hypersplenism*
   Platelets utilised in *coagulation disorders*
   (e.g. DIC)

*Note:* Marrow examination throws light on the possible mechanism.

In (1) megakaryocytes are reduced in number (except in vit $B_{12}$ deficiency)

In (2) megakaryocytes are increased and immature in an attempt to make good the platelet loss

**PURPURA** is the term used for disorders involving bleeding from capillaries, with the production of small petechial spots. Mild to moderate thrombocytopenia or defective platelet formation are the usual causes. Two examples are illustrative:

1. **Idiopathic thrombocytopenic purpura** is due to **auto-immune** destruction of platelets. Antibodies are directed against platelet membrane glycoproteins.
   (a) **Acute**: mainly in children, provoked by viral infection; it is usually self-limiting in a few weeks.
   (b) **Chronic**: mainly in young women with an insidious onset and lasting many years; splenectomy is often required (the spleen is the major site of platelet destruction).
2. **Defective platelet function** has many forms – **von Willebrand disease** (vWD) is the commonest. The gene encoding vWF is located on chromosome 12. It is an autosomal dominant disorder.

vWF is a large protein which potentiates the binding of platelets to subendothelial collagen and also acts as a carrier for coagulation factor VIII.

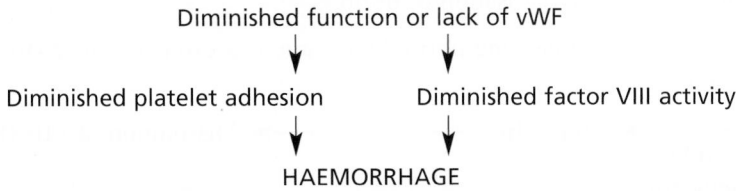

Diminished function or lack of vWF

Diminished platelet adhesion   Diminished factor VIII activity

HAEMORRHAGE

**THROMBOCYTOSIS** (increased platelet numbers) may occur in a mild form (with no clinical significance) reactive to a variety of disorders of chronic inflammation and cancer. Larger counts are seen in myeloproliferative disorders (e.g. essential thrombocytosis, chronic myeloid leukaemia) and are of serious clinical significance due to thrombosis.

# THE COAGULATION CASCADE

The coagulation of blood is the result of conversion of **FIBRINOGEN** to **FIBRIN**. The chemical pathway leading to this final phase is a complicated cascade in which inert coagulation factors are serially activated. At each step augmentation takes place.

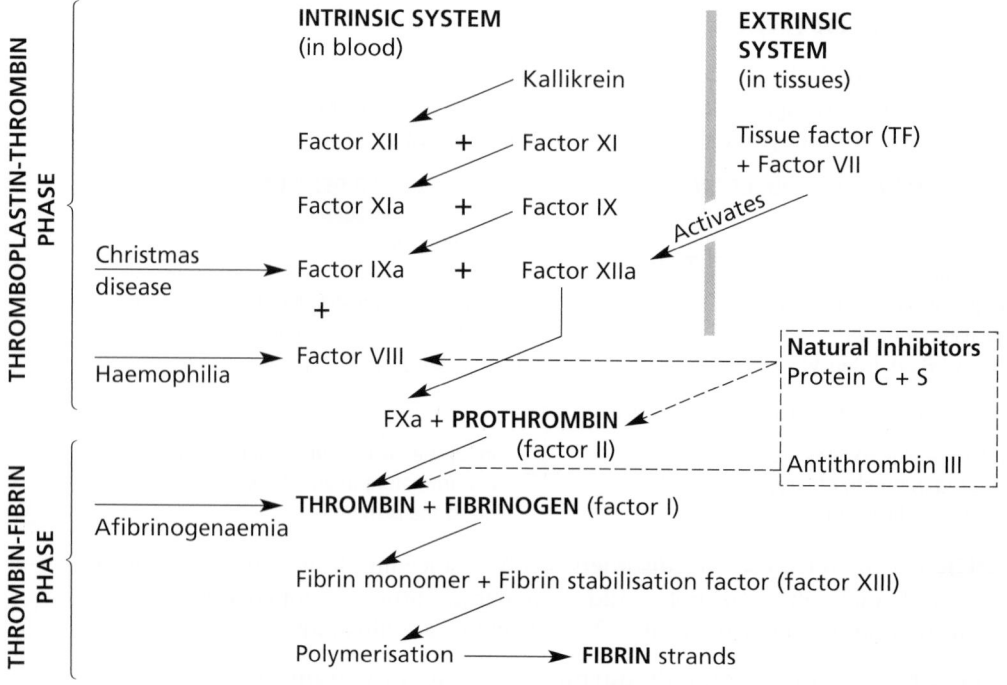

*Note*: 'a' denotes activated form.

The system contains several feed-back loops (not illustrated) which can inhibit the cascade at various levels.

Anti-thrombin III and the protein C/protein S system are powerful inhibitors preventing uncontrollable coagulation.

Vitamin K is required for the production of factors II, VII, IX and X. CALCIUM ions and phospholipids (mainly derived from platelets) are essential for many of the steps in thrombin production. Once thrombin is formed, it appears to stimulate several of the preceding reactions and also the polymerisation of fibrin.

**Fibrinolytic system** – this occurs following fibrin deposition as a protective mechanism against excess coagulation.

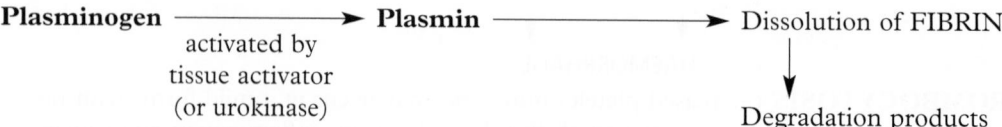

# INHERITED DEFECTS OF COAGULATION

These are less common than acquired abnormalities, but are of considerable importance.

## HAEMOPHILIA A

Haemophilia is due to deficiency of factor VIII – an essential cofactor in the activation of factor X in the intrinsic system.

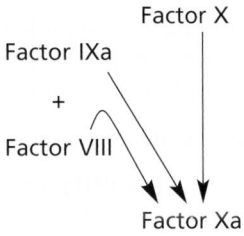

Factor VIII is encoded by a gene on the long arm of the X chromosome – haemophilia is inherited as an X-linked recessive, i.e. almost all patients are male. Their mothers are usually carriers, but about 30% of cases are due to new mutations. Around 1 in 10 000 is affected.

### Clinical features

The severity depends on the levels of factor VIII.

|  |  | LEVEL OF FACTOR VIII |
|---|---|---|
| Severe: | Frequent spontaneous bleeding | <2% of normal |
| Moderate: | Bleeding after minor trauma – rarely spontaneous | 2–10% |
| Mild: | Bleeding severe only after major trauma or surgery | 10–50% |

## Important sites of bleeding are:

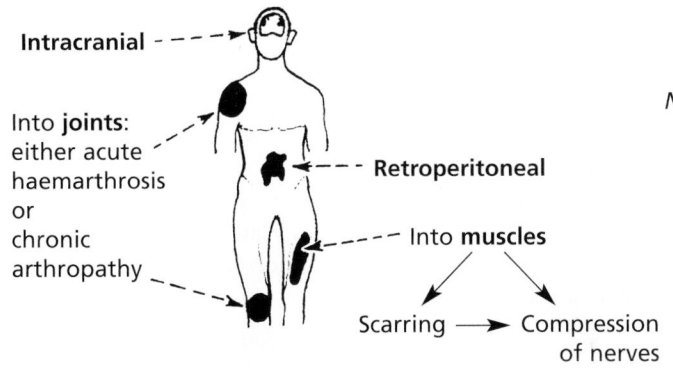

Intracranial

Into **joints**: either acute haemarthrosis or chronic arthropathy

**Retroperitoneal**

Into **muscles**

Scarring ⟶ Compression of nerves

*Note:* In the past, the use of virus infected factor VIII in treatment has caused HIV (AIDS) and hepatitis C infection. Similar concerns apply to variant CJD (p. 599).

## HAEMOPHILIA B (CHRISTMAS DISEASE)

This is due to deficiency of factor IX – also carried by a gene on the X chromosome. The clinical features are similar, but the prevalence is lower (1 in 30 000 males).

Rarely deficiencies of other coagulation factors are seen, e.g. fibrinogen, factor XI and factor V.

They are treated by infusion of the appropriate factors.

# ACQUIRED DEFECTS OF COAGULATION

This large and heterogeneous group of conditions includes:

### VITAMIN K DEFICIENCY

Vitamin K, a fat-soluble vitamin, is essential for synthesis of factors II, VII, IX and X in the liver. Deficiency leads to spontaneous bleeding, e.g. into skin and mucous membranes, and failure of blood clotting.

In **adults**, deficiency may be due to

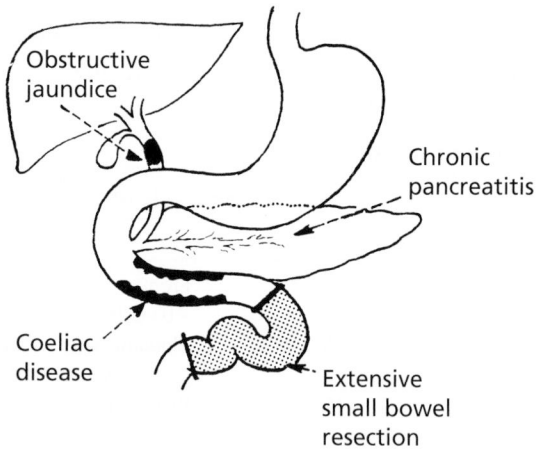

(a) MALABSORPTION (particularly of fat).
(b) DIETARY DEFICIENCY – rare
  – vitamin K is widely distributed, e.g. in green vegetables, oils.
(c) INHIBITION – by COUMARIN anticoagulants, e.g. WARFARIN.

In **neonates**, vitamin K deficiency leads to bleeding from the gastrointestinal tract and bruising. Breast milk contains little vitamin K – the disorder is uncommon in those receiving bottled milk. A severe deficiency may be seen in infants whose mothers took anticoagulants or anticonvulsants.

### LIVER DISEASE

The bleeding tendency in these patients is multifactorial.

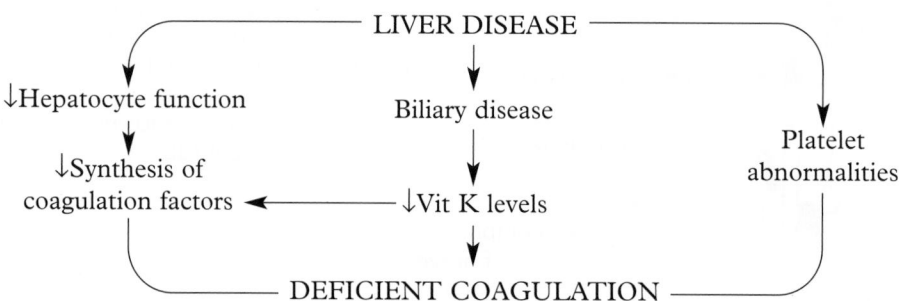

This complicates bleeding, e.g. from OESOPHAGEAL varices.

### 'ACQUIRED HAEMOPHILIA'

Rarely, antibodies develop which block the effects of serum coagulation factors, especially factor VIII. This may be idiopathic or follow auto-immune disease or drug treatment.

**Disseminated intravascular coagulation (DIC)** (see next page).

# DISSEMINATED INTRAVASCULAR COAGULATION

In this disorder the coagulation system is activated, but the consumption of platelets and clotting factors which follows leads to a paradoxical bleeding tendency.

There are numerous causes:

(a) SEPTICAEMIA – especially Gram-negative septicaemia – in meningococcal infections.
(b) SHOCK, e.g. following severe burns.
(c) OBSTETRIC DISORDERS, e.g. placental abruption, amniotic embolism, eclampsia.
(d) MALIGNANCY – especially acute promyelocytic leukaemia and mucin secreting adenocarcinomas (e.g. of stomach).
(e) IMMUNOLOGICAL DISORDERS, e.g. auto-immune diseases, incompatible blood transfusion.

**The basic mechanism** is as follows:

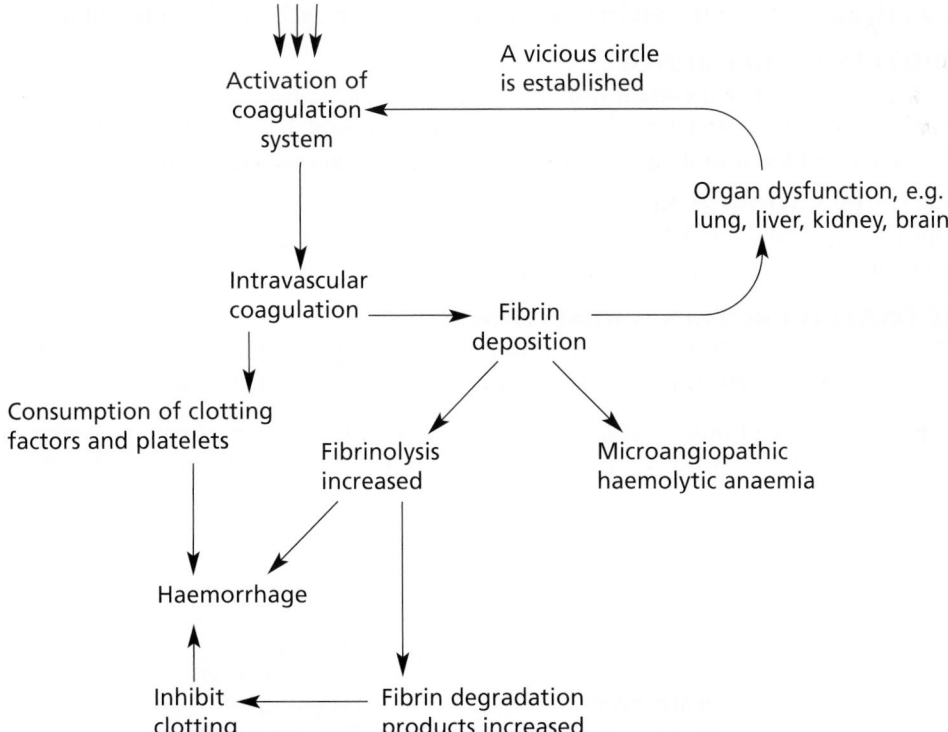

Patients frequently develop renal and hepatic failure and 'shock lung', e.g. in the haemolytic uraemic syndrome (HUS) which is often associated with toxigenic *Escherichia coli* infection – especially *E. coli* 0157 (see p. 345).

# THROMBOPHILIA – THROMBOTIC DISORDERS

The major types, causes and effects of thrombosis are discussed on pages 159–163.

Recently, a group of inherited disorders has been discovered where deficiency of NATURAL ANTICOAGULANTS leads to an increased risk of venous thrombosis. This may be deep venous thrombosis in the lower limbs or visceral, e.g. mesenteric veins. There is also an increased risk of pulmonary embolism.

The main forms are:

(a) **ANTITHROMBIN DEFICIENCY**
Antithrombin, a member of the SERPIN group of **Ser**ine protease **in**hibitors, is synthesised in the liver. It blocks the action of factors IXa, Xa and XIa and thrombin. Deficiency is due to mutation of a gene on the long arm of chromosome 1. The effects depend on the exact type of mutation. The prevalence is around 1 in 20 000.

*Note*: **Heparin**, the anticoagulant, acts by enhancing the action of antithrombin.

(b) **PROTEIN C DEFICIENCY**
This is a vitamin K-dependent protein, synthesised in the liver. Together with protein S, it blocks the action of factors Va and factor VIIIa. Around 1 in 15 000–30 000 is affected. In addition to deep thrombosis, patients also get superficial thrombophlebitis.

(c) **PROTEIN S DEFICIENCY**
This protein is secreted by the liver, platelets and endothelial cells. Its function is to bind with protein C to inhibit factors Va and VIIIa.

(d) **ACTIVATED PROTEIN C RESISTANCE**
This is an inherited disorder where a mutation affects the factor V gene. The protein is resistant to the effects of protein C – simulating protein C deficiency.

The possible role of minor deficiencies of these genetic factors in the more common forms of thrombosis is not yet established. The well-known risk factors for thrombosis are listed below.

**Acquired risk factors** for thrombosis include:

| ARTERIAL | VENOUS |
|---|---|
| Atheroma | Immobility |
| Smoking | Trauma/surgery |
| Hypertension | Malignancy |
| Myeloproliferative disorders | Oral contraceptives |
| | Obesity |

# THE LYMPHOID SYSTEM

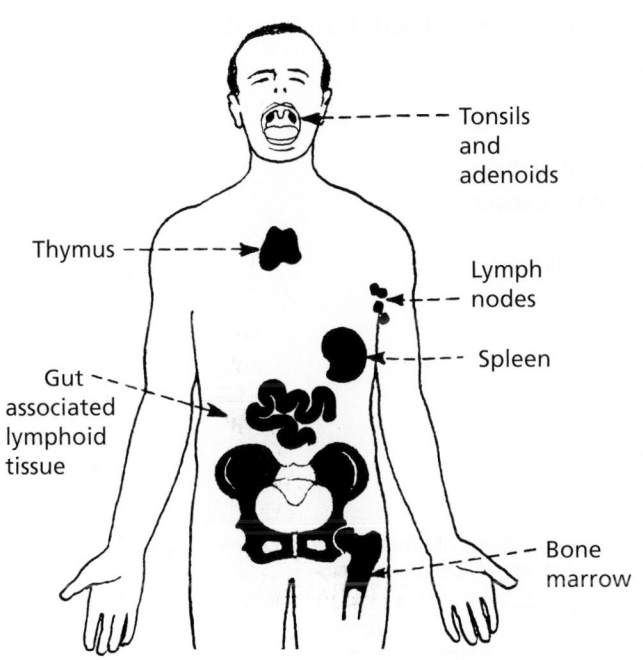

Thymus

Tonsils
and
adenoids

Lymph
nodes

Spleen

Gut
associated
lymphoid
tissue

Bone
marrow

The lymphoid organs are principally involved in:

(a) Production and maturation of lymphocytes – thymus (T cells) and bone marrow (B cells).

(b) Antigen presentation and the immune response.

(c) 'Filtration' and phagocytosis of micro-organisms and particulate material.

## LYMPH NODES

The basic structure reflects the main functions.

### CORTEX

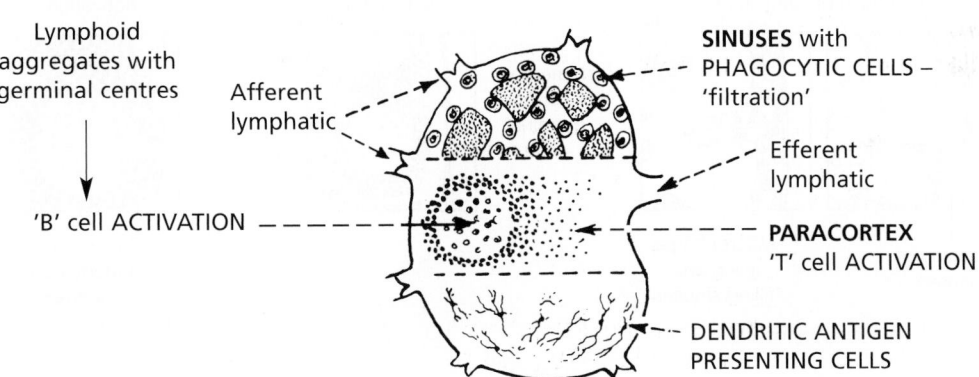

Lymphoid aggregates with germinal centres

Afferent lymphatic

'B' cell ACTIVATION

SINUSES with PHAGOCYTIC CELLS – 'filtration'

Efferent lymphatic

PARACORTEX
'T' cell ACTIVATION

DENDRITIC ANTIGEN PRESENTING CELLS

# LYMPHADENOPATHY

Lymph node enlargement may be **localised** or **generalised**. It may be due to:

(a) Reactive hyperplasia, e.g.
  – infection by bacteria or viruses.
  – particulate material.
  – immune stimulation, e.g. rheumatoid arthritis.
  – draining degradation products from a cancer.
(b) Due to neoplasia, e.g.
  – secondary deposits of carcinoma, melanoma.
  – primary lymphoid tumours.

## REACTIVE HYPERPLASIA

Several patterns are seen.

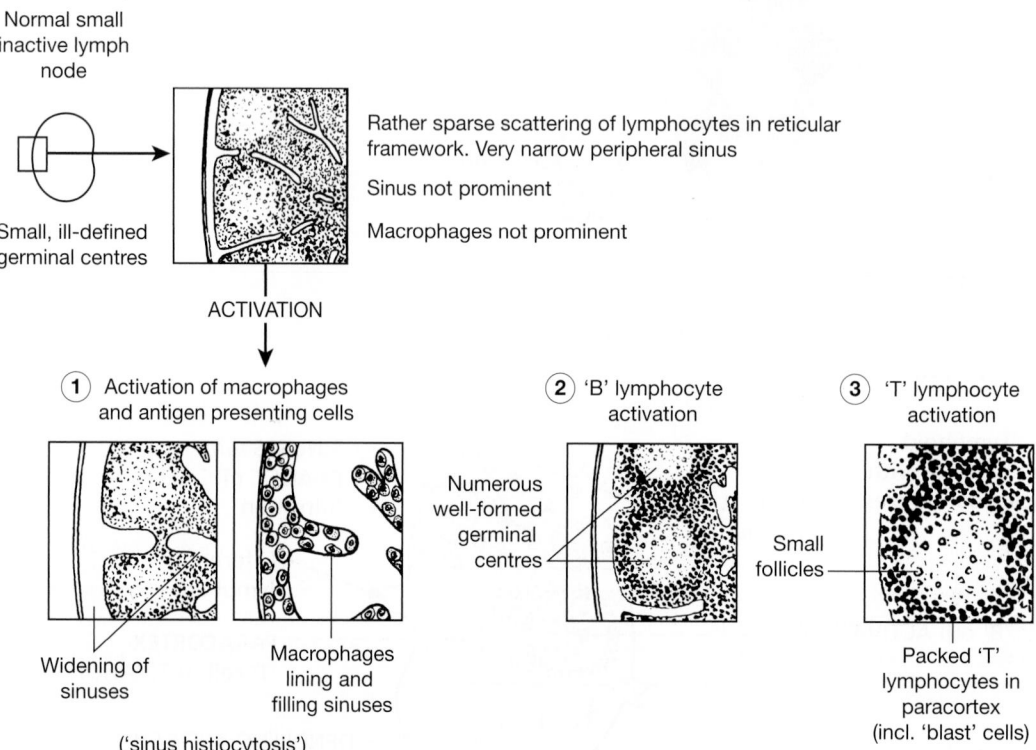

Normal small inactive lymph node

Small, ill-defined germinal centres

Rather sparse scattering of lymphocytes in reticular framework. Very narrow peripheral sinus

Sinus not prominent

Macrophages not prominent

ACTIVATION

① Activation of macrophages and antigen presenting cells

Widening of sinuses

Macrophages lining and filling sinuses

('sinus histiocytosis')

② 'B' lymphocyte activation

Numerous well-formed germinal centres

③ 'T' lymphocyte activation

Small follicles

Packed 'T' lymphocytes in paracortex (incl. 'blast' cells)

# LYMPHADENOPATHY – INFECTIONS

## ACUTE BACTERIAL LYMPHADENITIS

This is seen draining an infected area.

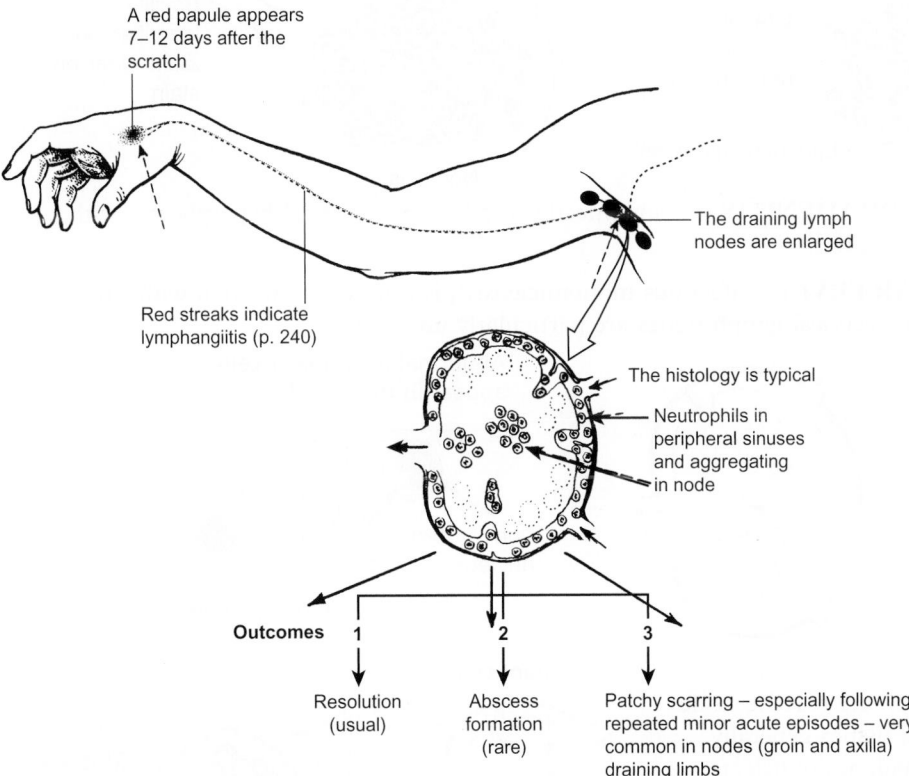

A red papule appears 7–12 days after the scratch

The draining lymph nodes are enlarged

Red streaks indicate lymphangiitis (p. 240)

The histology is typical

Neutrophils in peripheral sinuses and aggregating in node

**Outcomes** 1 2 3

Resolution (usual)

Abscess formation (rare)

Patchy scarring – especially following repeated minor acute episodes – very common in nodes (groin and axilla) draining limbs

## CAT SCRATCH DISEASE

This infection by a bacterium *Bartonella henselae* follows scratching by an infected cat. Similar histology is seen in lymphogranuloma venereum, caused by *Klebsiella granulomatis*. A small transient painless genital ulcer is followed by inguinal lymphadenopathy. The diagnosis can be confirmed by the Frei test (injection of purified chlamydial antigen stimulates a delayed hypersensitivity reaction).

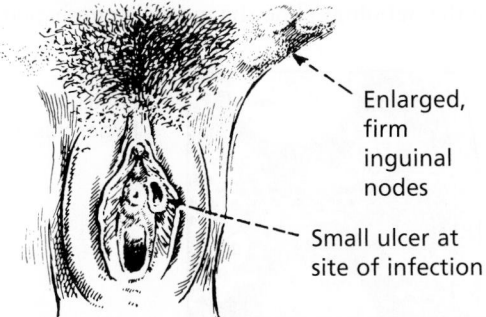

Enlarged, firm inguinal nodes

Small ulcer at site of infection

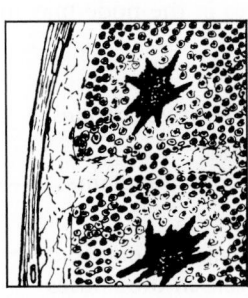

Granulomatous reaction with typical stellate abscess (neutrophils)

# LYMPHADENOPATHY

**TB** is associated with a granulomatous response (p. 55), often with necrosis. This is due to delayed-type sensitivity.

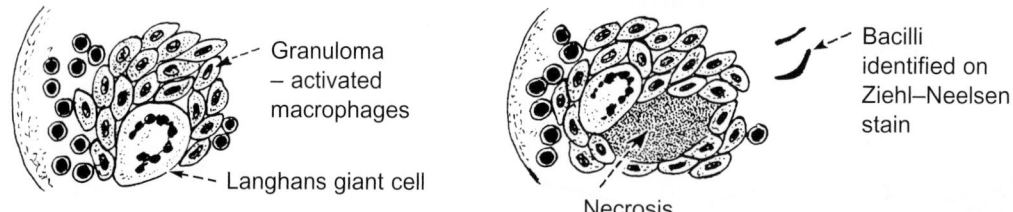

Granuloma – activated macrophages

Langhans giant cell

Necrosis

Bacilli identified on Ziehl–Neelsen stain

**VIRAL LYMPHADENITIS** – many infections induce paracortical hyperplasia – with activation of T cells.

**GLANDULAR FEVER** (infectious mononucleosis), is caused by infection with Epstein–Barr virus. The cervical lymph nodes are particularly involved.

The enlarged nodes show a striking change in the paracortex; blast cell transformation and mitoses are numerous.

Abnormal lymphoid T cells appear in the blood.

Convoluted nucleus

Blue cytoplasm

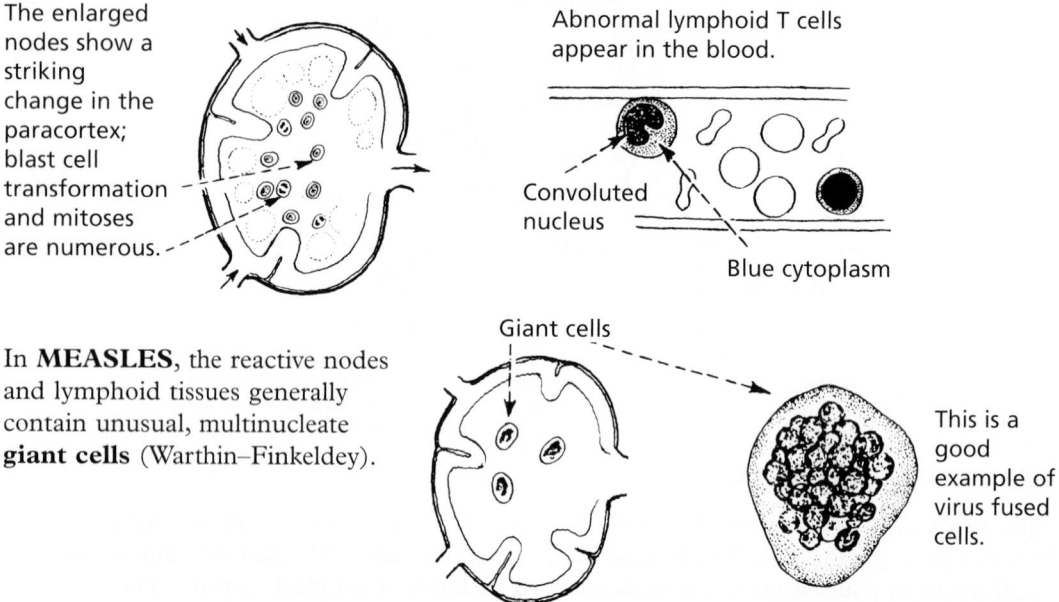

In **MEASLES**, the reactive nodes and lymphoid tissues generally contain unusual, multinucleate **giant cells** (Warthin–Finkeldey).

Giant cells

This is a good example of virus fused cells.

In **TOXOPLASMOSIS**, a protozoal disease (*Toxoplasma gondii*) which may cause serious damage to the fetus or neonate and present with lymph node enlargement in the adult, the histological appearances in the node may indicate the aetiology. The diagnosis is confirmed by serological tests.

In addition to the usual reactive changes

↓

Small epithelioid granulomas

↓

Numerous smaller monocytoid 'B' cells in the sinuses

Follicular hyperplasia

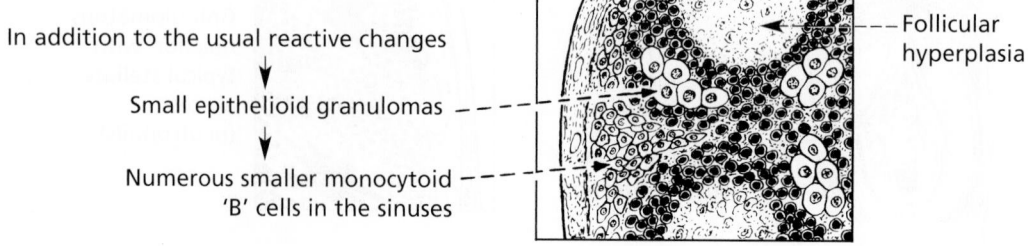

# LYMPHADENOPATHY – NON-INFECTIVE CAUSES

## FOREIGN MATERIAL

Lymph nodes to which foreign particulate material drains often show marked enlargement due to accumulation of macrophages which have ingested the foreign material.

For example:
- Carbon and silica in hilar lymph nodes.
- Silicone, e.g. in axillary lymph nodes in patients with breast implants.

**CHRONIC SKIN DISEASE** (so-called 'dermatopathic lymphadenopathy'), e.g. psoriasis, eczema and mycosis fungoides (p. 472).

The following may be seen lying free and in macrophages:
    Fat
    Melanin – from damaged skin
    Haemosiderin – from minor bleeding in skin

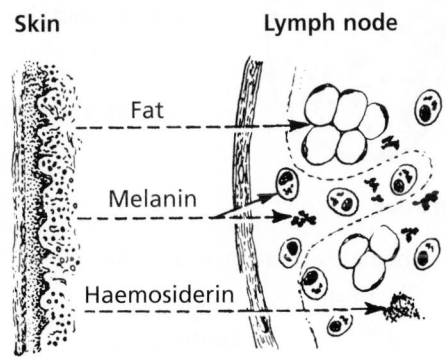

## SARCOIDOSIS

In this disease of unknown aetiology, non-necrotising granulomas are seen.

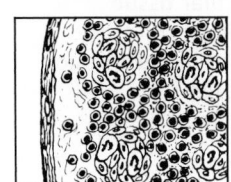

The appearances clearly resemble TB, but the granulomas remain discrete and there is no necrosis.

Sarcoid-type granulomas are also seen in the lymph nodes of patients with other granulomatous diseases, e.g. Crohn disease and in lymph nodes draining tumours.

# SPLEEN

The spleen is responsible for filtering the blood, phagocytosing debris and generating an immune response.

Normal average weight – 150 g.

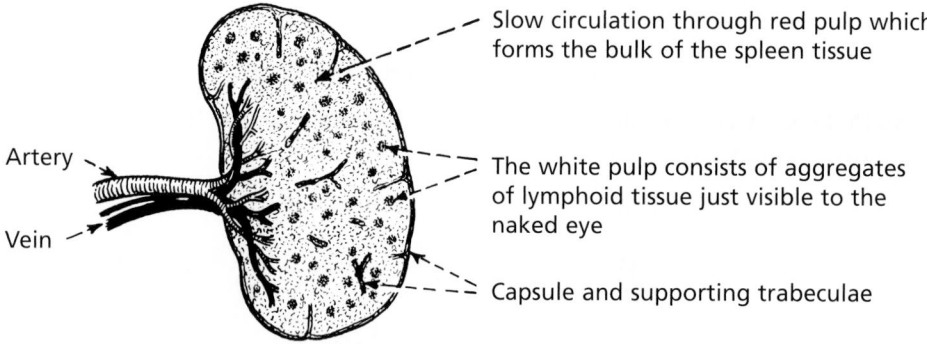

- Slow circulation through red pulp which forms the bulk of the spleen tissue

- The white pulp consists of aggregates of lymphoid tissue just visible to the naked eye

- Capsule and supporting trabeculae

Artery

Vein

## Microscopic appearance

Lymphoid aggregate – mediates IMMUNE RESPONSE.

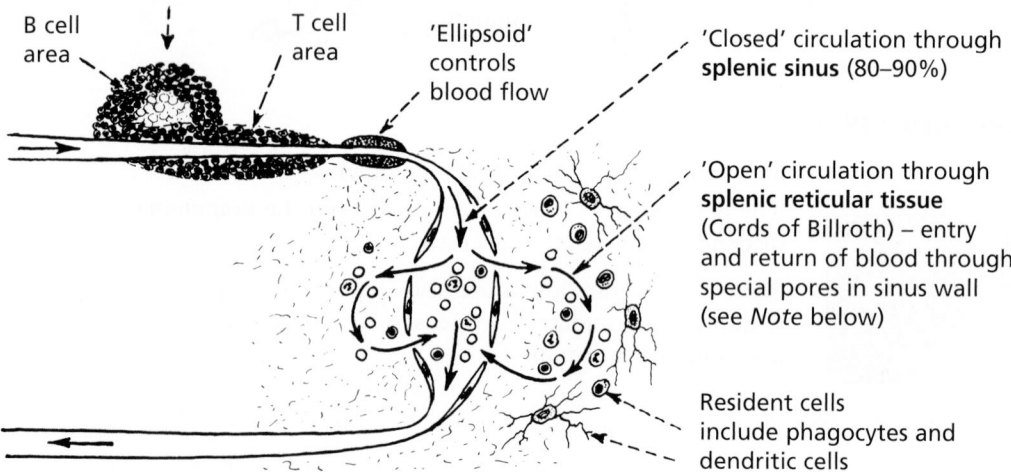

B cell area

T cell area

'Ellipsoid' controls blood flow

'Closed' circulation through **splenic sinus** (80–90%)

'Open' circulation through **splenic reticular tissue** (Cords of Billroth) – entry and return of blood through special pores in sinus wall (see *Note* below)

Resident cells include phagocytes and dendritic cells

The red pulp is the site of filtration and phagocytosis of the following:

1. Worn out cells and cell debris – especially blood cells but also cell debris derived from the body generally.
2. Microbes and their toxins.
3. Abnormal or excess material derived from metabolic processes.

*Note*: The special pores allowing re-entry of RBCs to the circulation have a 2 μm aperture: abnormal RBCs (e.g. spherocytes) cannot pass through and are trapped.

# SPLENOMEGALY

Enlargement of the spleen is an important and common clinical sign. Increase in the red pulp due to increased numbers of phagocytes and/or increased numbers of blood cells is the major component. In chronic infections, hyperplasia of the lymphoid tissue contributes.

Enlargement is associated with:
1. INFECTIONS
2. CIRCULATORY DISTURBANCES
3. DISORDERS OF THE BLOOD
4. NEOPLASIA – PRIMARY AND SECONDARY
5. STORAGE DISEASES and DEGENERATIONS

## 1. INFECTIONS

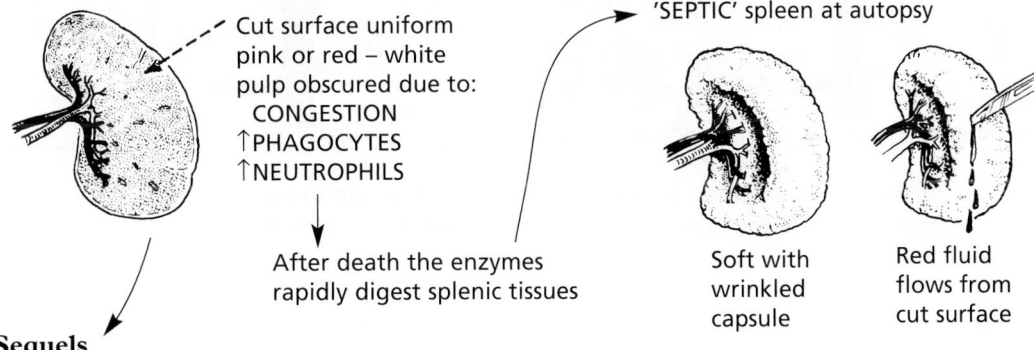

Cut surface uniform pink or red – white pulp obscured due to:
CONGESTION
↑PHAGOCYTES
↑NEUTROPHILS

After death the enzymes rapidly digest splenic tissues

'SEPTIC' spleen at autopsy

Soft with wrinkled capsule

Red fluid flows from cut surface

**Sequels**

In acute systemic bacterial infections the spleen shows slight to moderate enlargement (200–400 g).

(a) Resolution as infection resolves.
(b) Occasionally spreads through capsule to adjacent tissues, with or without abscess formation.
(c) Only extremely rarely does abscess formation occur within the spleen.

In non-pyogenic and chronic infections, there may be moderate enlargement.

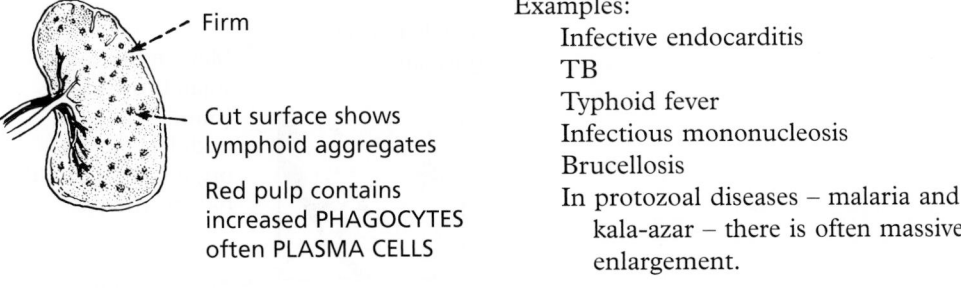

Firm

Cut surface shows lymphoid aggregates

Red pulp contains increased PHAGOCYTES often PLASMA CELLS

Examples:
Infective endocarditis
TB
Typhoid fever
Infectious mononucleosis
Brucellosis
In protozoal diseases – malaria and kala-azar – there is often massive enlargement.

# SPLENOMEGALY

### 2.  CIRCULATORY DISTURBANCES

Congestive splenomegaly occurs in two main conditions:

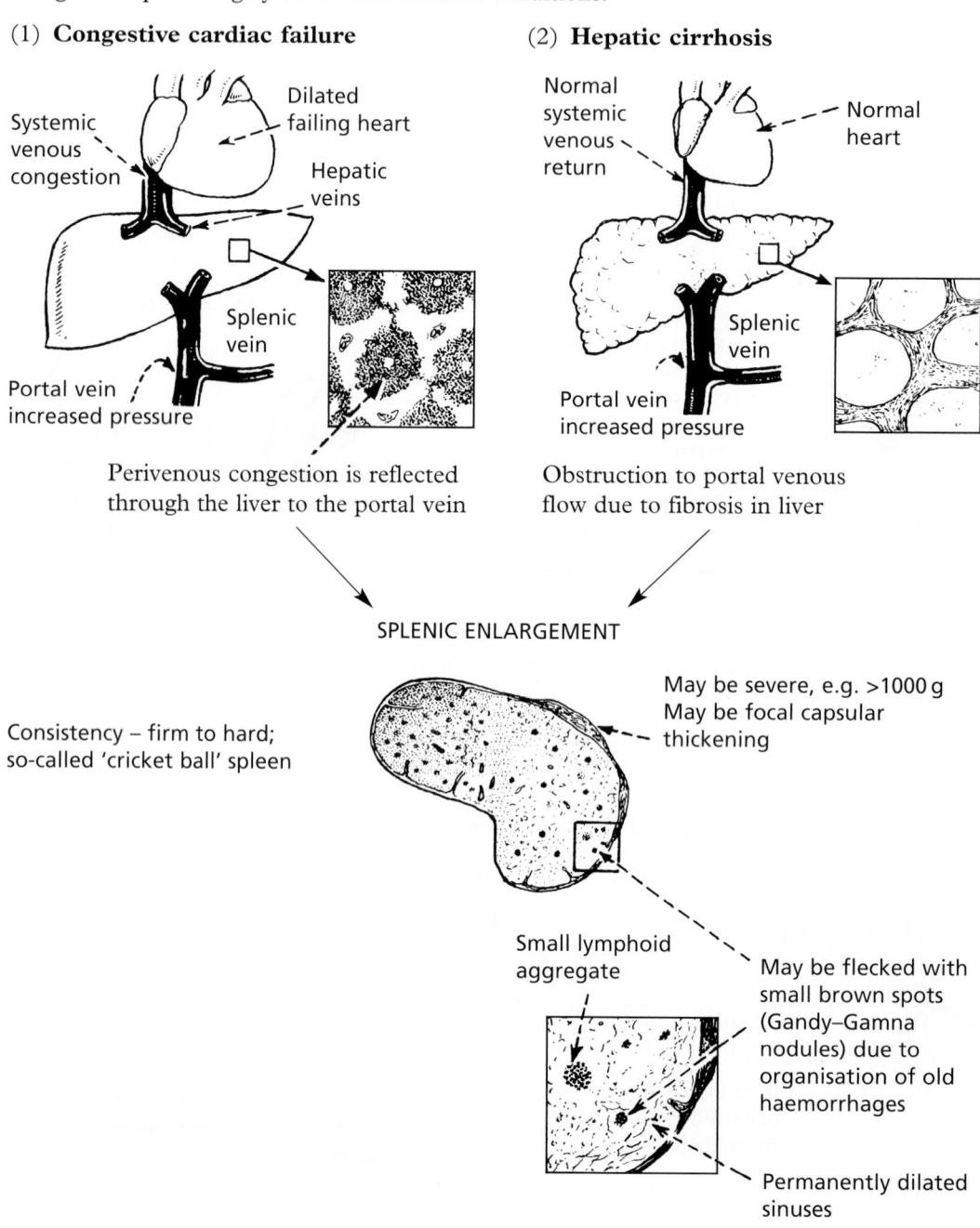

#### (1) Congestive cardiac failure

Dilated failing heart

Systemic venous congestion

Hepatic veins

Splenic vein

Portal vein increased pressure

Perivenous congestion is reflected through the liver to the portal vein

#### (2) Hepatic cirrhosis

Normal systemic venous return

Normal heart

Splenic vein

Portal vein increased pressure

Obstruction to portal venous flow due to fibrosis in liver

SPLENIC ENLARGEMENT

Consistency – firm to hard; so-called 'cricket ball' spleen

May be severe, e.g. >1000 g
May be focal capsular thickening

Small lymphoid aggregate

May be flecked with small brown spots (Gandy–Gamna nodules) due to organisation of old haemorrhages

Permanently dilated sinuses

Splenomegaly associated with portal venous hypertension may have serious haematological effects (see Hypersplenism).

# SPLENOMEGALY

## 3. DISORDERS OF THE BLOOD

Splenic enlargement is associated with blood disorders in two main circumstances:

### 1. Splenic enlargement causing blood disorders (hypersplenism).

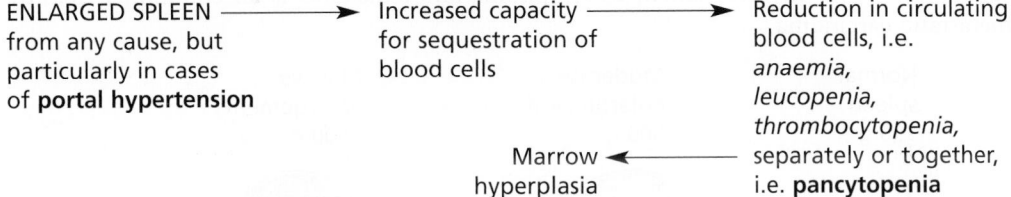

ENLARGED SPLEEN ⟶ Increased capacity ⟶ Reduction in circulating
from any cause, but           for sequestration of      blood cells, i.e.
particularly in cases         blood cells               *anaemia,*
of **portal hypertension**                              *leucopenia,*
                                                        *thrombocytopenia,*
                              Marrow ⟵ separately or together,
                              hyperplasia            i.e. **pancytopenia**

### 2. Blood disorder causing splenic enlargement.

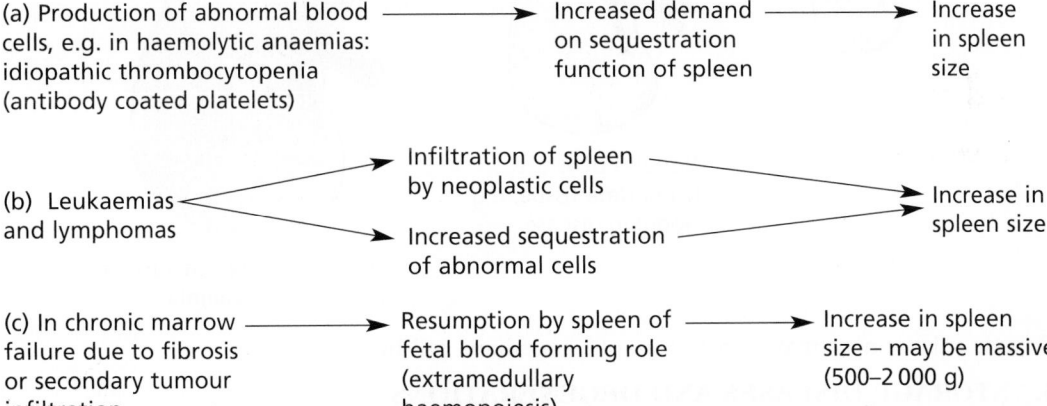

(a) Production of abnormal blood ⟶ Increased demand ⟶ Increase
cells, e.g. in haemolytic anaemias:    on sequestration      in spleen
idiopathic thrombocytopenia            function of spleen    size
(antibody coated platelets)

(b) Leukaemias ⟶ Infiltration of spleen ⟶ Increase in
and lymphomas      by neoplastic cells        spleen size
               ⟶ Increased sequestration ⟶
                  of abnormal cells

(c) In chronic marrow ⟶ Resumption by spleen of ⟶ Increase in spleen
failure due to fibrosis    fetal blood forming role   size – may be massive
or secondary tumour        (extramedullary            (500–2 000 g)
infiltration               haemopoiesis)

Sometimes these two processes combine to form a vicious circle.

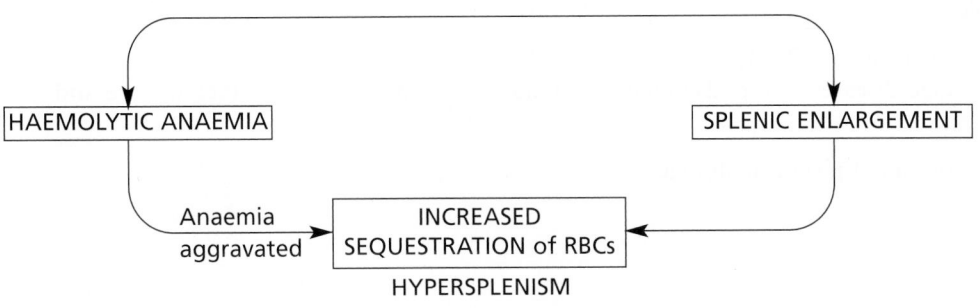

HAEMOLYTIC ANAEMIA                    SPLENIC ENLARGEMENT

Anaemia          INCREASED
aggravated   SEQUESTRATION of RBCs

HYPERSPLENISM

# SPLENOMEGALY

### 4. NEOPLASIA

(a) PRIMARY – primary tumours of the spleen are rare, the commonest being primary splenic lymphomas.

(b) SECONDARY – Splenic involvement by lymphoma and leukaemia is far commoner than by metastatic carcinoma.

Normal
spleen
150 g

Moderate
enlargement
500 g

Massive
enlargement
1500 g

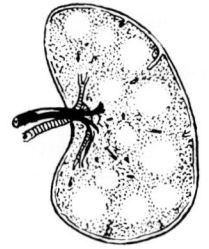

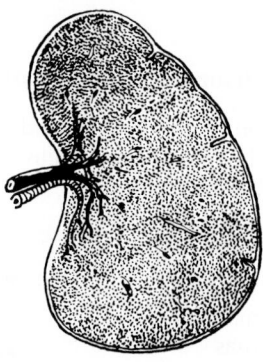

Nodules of white
lymphoma tissue, e.g
Hodgkin disease

Uniform, beefy, cut surface
in chronic leukaemia

Splenic enlargement may be a feature of Langerhans cell histiocytosis.

### 5. STORAGE DISEASES AND DEGENERATIONS

The diseases associated with this type of enlargement are rare.

Examples are:

Amyloidosis (see pp. 22–24)
Lipid storage diseases (see p. 21) including Gaucher disease, Niemann–Pick disease and Tay–Sachs disease.

Some disorders of glycogen storage.

# DISEASES OF THE SPLEEN – MISCELLANEOUS

## HYPOSPLENISM

Hyposplenism is not usually a cause of major disability. It occurs following splenectomy and in cases of splenic atrophy.

The effects are considered under two main headings:

1. **On the cells of the blood.**

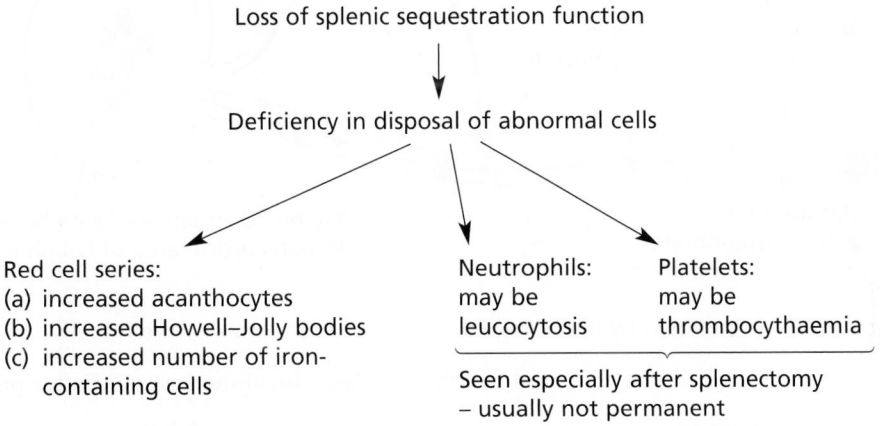

Loss of splenic sequestration function

↓

Deficiency in disposal of abnormal cells

Red cell series:
(a) increased acanthocytes
(b) increased Howell–Jolly bodies
(c) increased number of iron-containing cells

Neutrophils: may be leucocytosis

Platelets: may be thrombocythaemia

Seen especially after splenectomy – usually not permanent

2. **On resistance to infection.**

Loss of filtration of bacteria from blood ⟶ **Septicaemia** – especially caused by *Streptococcus pneumoniae* – young children are particularly susceptible and are vaccinated against this.

## INFARCTION

(i) Embolism causing infarction is not uncommon but usually clinically unimportant.

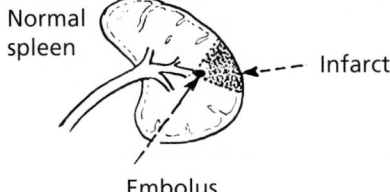

Normal spleen

Infarct

Embolus

(ii) Enlarged spleens are particularly susceptible to infarction without embolism.

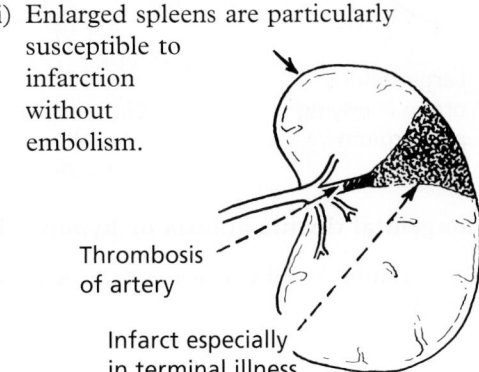

Thrombosis of artery

Infarct especially in terminal illness

# THYMUS

This 'primary' lymphoid organ is concerned with the development and maturation of T lymphocytes which are then distributed to the lymphoid tissues and to the circulating pool.

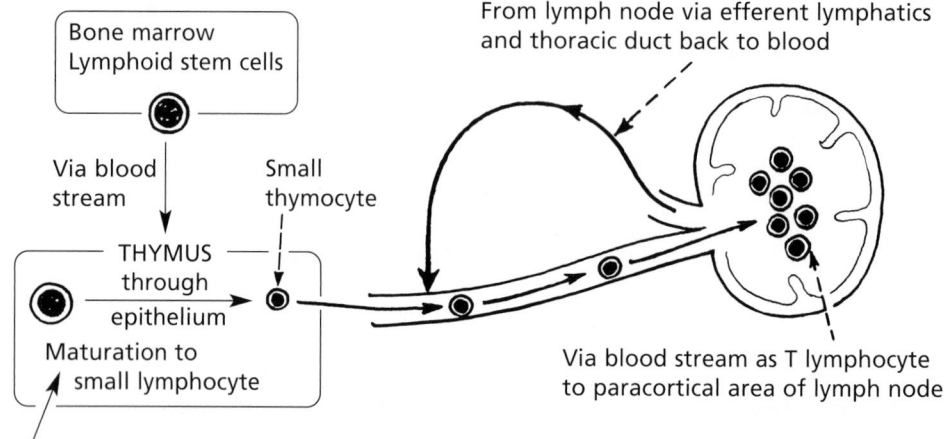

*Mechanism* – stimulation by hormones formed locally by thymic epithelial cells.

This activity is maximal in the fetal and childhood stages. Involution is rapid after puberty.

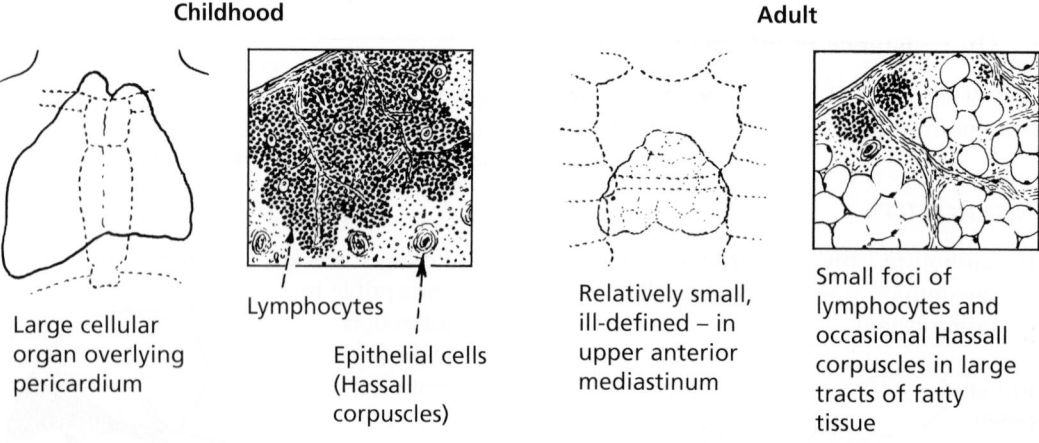

**Childhood**

Large cellular organ overlying pericardium

Lymphocytes

Epithelial cells (Hassall corpuscles)

**Adult**

Relatively small, ill-defined – in upper anterior mediastinum

Small foci of lymphocytes and occasional Hassall corpuscles in large tracts of fatty tissue

## Congenital thymic aplasia or hypoplasia

The resulting T cell deficiency is associated with disordered cell-mediated immune response.

# THYMUS

## Thymic hyperplasia

This is associated with a number of conditions:

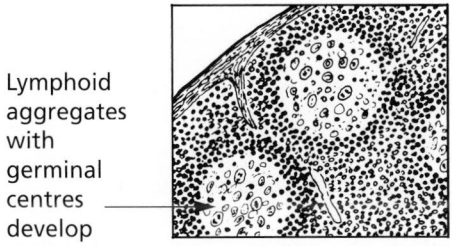

Lymphoid aggregates with germinal centres develop

Auto-immune disorders,
e.g. SLE
    Addison disease
    Thyrotoxicosis
Pancytopenia and MYASTHENIA GRAVIS

## Thymic tumours

Thymomas are rare epithelial tumours which have an admixture of lymphoid cells. They rarely metastasise. A small number are carcinomas. They may have auto-immune associations similar to thymic hyperplasia.

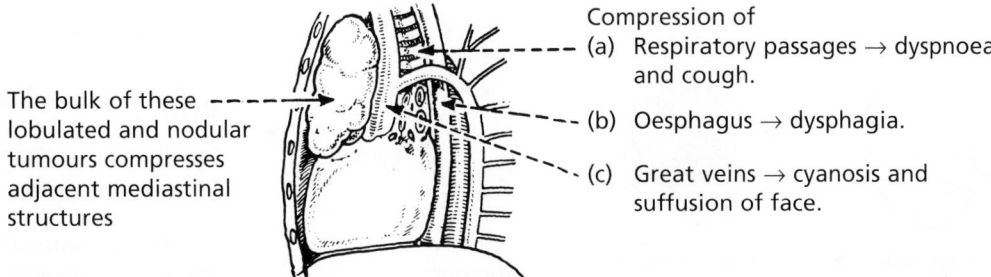

The bulk of these lobulated and nodular tumours compresses adjacent mediastinal structures

Compression of
(a) Respiratory passages → dyspnoea and cough.

(b) Oesphagus → dysphagia.

(c) Great veins → cyanosis and suffusion of face.

Other primary tumours arising in the thymus are:

(1) T cell lymphoblastic lymphomas (adolescents).
(2) Hodgkin lymphoma.
(3) Mediastinal large 'B' cell lymphoma.
(4) Germ cell tumours (e.g. teratoma).
(5) Carcinoids.

## The thymus in myasthenia gravis (MG)

MG is a disease of voluntary muscles in which weakness is the main feature. The association with the thymus is striking in that 80% of all patients with MG have either thymic hyperplasia or thymoma.

Follicular hyperplasia (80%) – seen especially in young females.
Thymoma (20%) – seen especially in middle-aged males.
The results of thymectomy in MG patients are very unpredictable.

The detailed pathological changes in MG and the mechanisms by which the thymus is linked with the disease are described on pages 152 and 663.

# NEOPLASTIC LYMPHADENOPATHY

Lymph node enlargement may be due to

(a) Invasion by SECONDARY TUMOURS – especially CARCINOMAS –
or (b) Primary lymphoid tumours – LYMPHOMAS.

## SECONDARY TUMOUR INVASION

### Carcinoma of the breast, e.g.

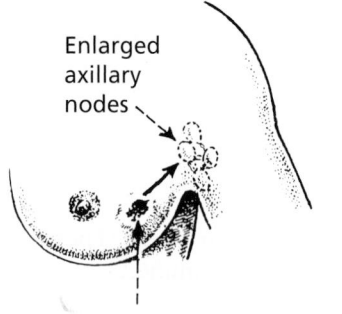

Enlarged axillary nodes

Breast carcinoma

*Note:*

(i) The nodal enlargement is not necessarily due to secondary tumour.
**Reactive hyperplasia** is also common in nodes draining tumours especially if there is ulceration. The distinction between these two causes of node enlargement can only be made with certainty by **histological examination**.

(ii) The invasion of a group of nodes occurs in a step-wise fashion: a single node (the SENTINEL node) is invaded initially and spread to adjacent nodes follows.

(a)

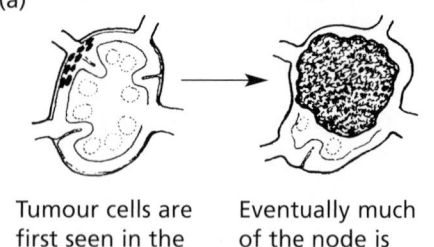

Tumour cells are first seen in the capsular sinus.

Eventually much of the node is replaced.

(b)

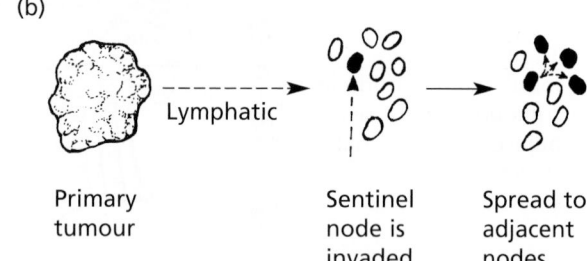

Lymphatic

Primary tumour

Sentinel node is invaded

Spread to adjacent nodes

Identification of the sentinel node may be required in the investigation of breast cancer and malignant melanoma.

## LYMPHOMAS

Lymphomas are malignant tumours derived from lymphoid cells. They may arise within lymph nodes or at other sites (extra-nodal lymphomas).

Classically, they are divided into two main groups.

(a) Hodgkin lymphoma 20–25%
   – Almost always of lymph node origin
   – Characterised by the presence of Reed–Sternberg cells
(b) Non-Hodgkin lymphoma 75–80%
   – Three-quarters arise in lymph nodes

# NON-HODGKIN LYMPHOMAS

These tumours mainly affect middle-aged to elderly patients.

They may arise

(a) Within lymph nodes     or     (b) In extra-nodal sites

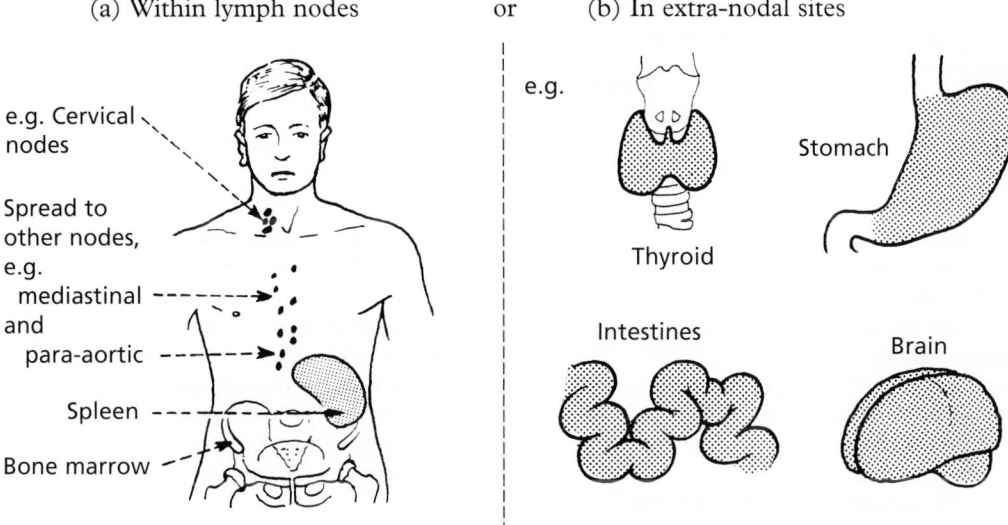

## DEGREE OF MALIGNANCY

The natural history tends to separate lymphomas into two main groups which have links with the morphological appearances.

1. *Low-grade malignancy* associated with well-differentiated relatively inactive cell types, – progress of years.
2. *High-grade malignancy* associated with primitive actively proliferating cells – progress over weeks or months.

Tend to respond well to chemotherapy.

## PATHOLOGICAL COMPLICATIONS

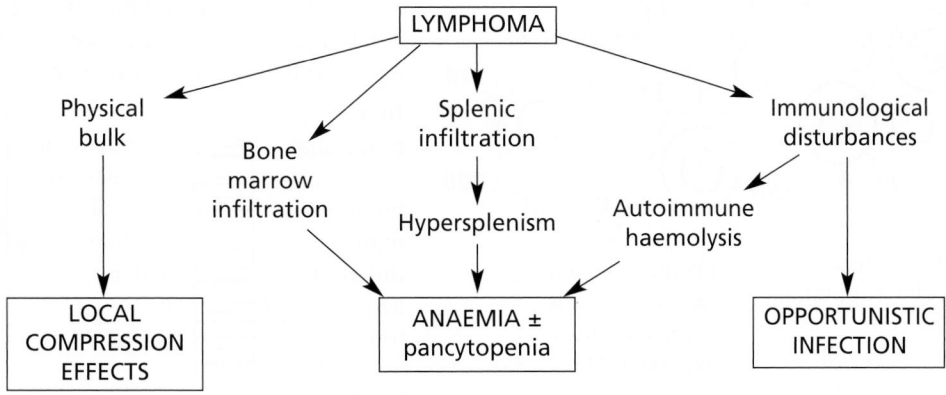

# NON-HODGKIN LYMPHOMAS

### Classification

This is a confusing area. Traditional classifications relied on morphology alone. The World Health Organisation classification, which includes immunohistochemistry and genetic data, is now generally accepted. A simplified version follows:

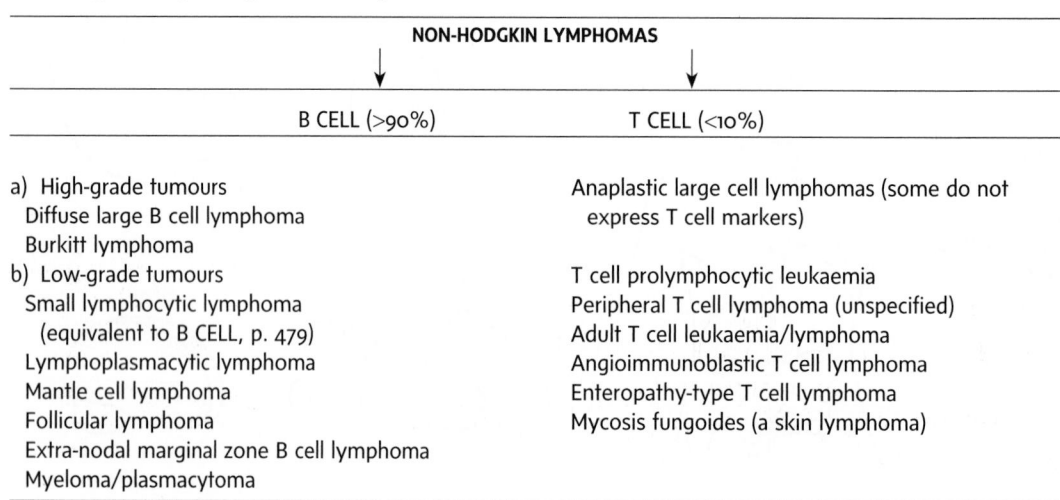

**NON-HODGKIN LYMPHOMAS**

| B CELL (>90%) | T CELL (<10%) |
|---|---|
| a) High-grade tumours<br>Diffuse large B cell lymphoma<br>Burkitt lymphoma | Anaplastic large cell lymphomas (some do not express T cell markers) |
| b) Low-grade tumours<br>Small lymphocytic lymphoma<br>(equivalent to B CELL, p. 479)<br>Lymphoplasmacytic lymphoma<br>Mantle cell lymphoma<br>Follicular lymphoma<br>Extra-nodal marginal zone B cell lymphoma<br>Myeloma/plasmacytoma | T cell prolymphocytic leukaemia<br>Peripheral T cell lymphoma (unspecified)<br>Adult T cell leukaemia/lymphoma<br>Angioimmunoblastic T cell lymphoma<br>Enteropathy-type T cell lymphoma<br>Mycosis fungoides (a skin lymphoma) |

According to this classification each type is considered separately for treatment purposes.

The classification relies on cell surface markers which distinguish the B and T cells and their subsets. B and T cell monoclonality can be detected by gene rearrangements, and some types of lymphoma have characteristic translocations.

### Subtyping of lymphoma

## IMMUNOHISTOCHEMISTRY

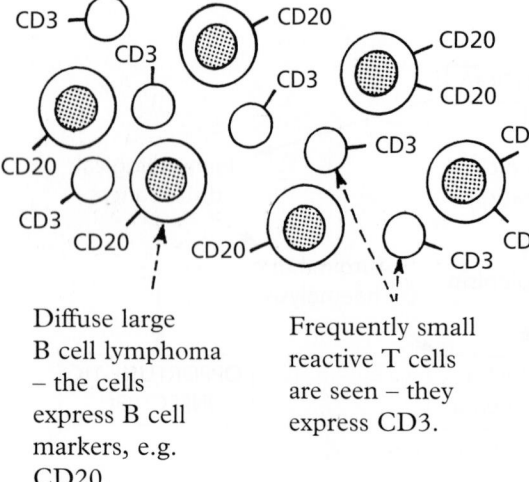

Diffuse large B cell lymphoma – the cells express B cell markers, e.g. CD20.

Frequently small reactive T cells are seen – they express CD3.

## MOLECULAR GENETIC ANALYSIS

In B cell differentiation different immunoglobulin genes are found by gene rearrangements, while in T cell differentiation a similar process occurs with T cell antigen receptors (p. 132).

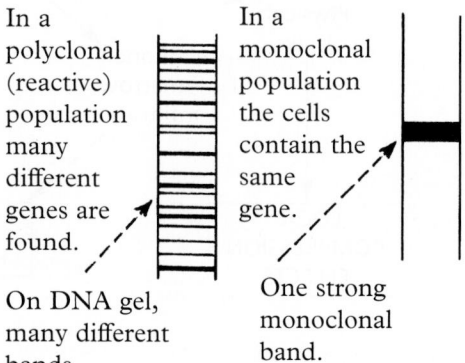

In a polyclonal (reactive) population many different genes are found.

On DNA gel, many different bands.

In a monoclonal population the cells contain the same gene.

One strong monoclonal band.

# NON-HODGKIN LYMPHOMAS

## FOLLICULAR LYMPHOMA

This is one of the commonest forms – a 'B' cell lymphoma.

The neoplastic follicles are the malignant equivalent of normal germinal centres.

The tumour cells express the anti-apoptosis gene bcl–2 which immortalises them. There is often a translocation t(14;18) which joins the bcl–2 gene (chromosome 18) to the immunoglobulin heavy chain gene (chromosome 14). This can be identified by FISH and PCR analysis.

The lymphoma is slowly progressive but often eventually fatal. Sometimes it transforms into a diffuse large 'B' cell lymphoma (DLBCL).

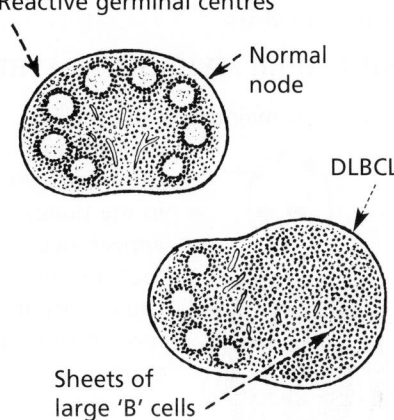

Reactive germinal centres

Normal node

DLBCL

Sheets of large 'B' cells

## BURKITT LYMPHOMA

This is a high-grade lymphoma found mainly in Equatorial Africa, New Guinea and other malaria endemic areas. Similar tumours are seen in AIDS patients. The relationship with Epstein–Barr virus has already been discussed (p. 121). The associated translocation t(8;14) activates the c-myc oncogene (p. 198). The histological appearance is typical.

Diffuse proliferation of lymphoblast-like B type cells

Cells medium-sized and uniform

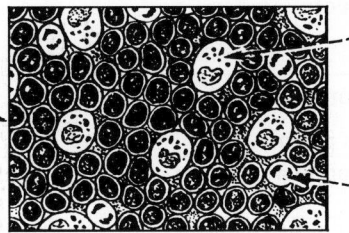

Scattering of macrophages containing debris derived from very rapid cell turnover – causing a 'starry sky' appearance

Mitoses frequent

Endemic (African type) Burkitt lymphoma typically presents with lesions in the jaw, or in the abdomen, e.g. ovary, liver, gastrointestinal tract. The less common cases in the West typically involve lymph node, marrow and gut.

The disease may respond dramatically to aggressive treatment.

## DIFFUSE LARGE B CELL LYMPHOMA (DLBCL)

This is the commonest type of lymphoma and may arise in nodes or extra-nodal sites. They rapidly disseminate. They are composed of sheets of large round cells. Treatment is with chemotherapy and anti-CD20 immunotherapy. Complete remission can be achieved in up to 80% of patients. About 50% of patients are cured.

# PLASMA CELL TUMOURS

### SOLITARY PLASMACYTOMA

A very small number of plasma cell tumours are solitary at presentation, e.g. in a long bone, the nasopharynx, a lymph node, alimentary tract. In 50% of cases, multiple myeloma occurs within 10 years.

### MULTIPLE MYELOMA (MYELOMATOSIS)

The great majority of plasma cell tumours present as widespread
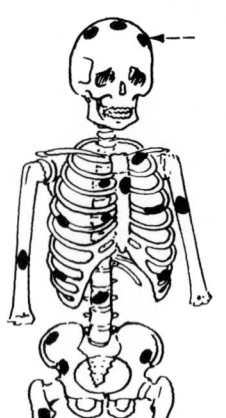
deposits in the bone marrow. Classically the lesions are seen as punched-out defects in the bones – the skull showing this appearance particularly well. These focal proliferations of plasma cells usually occur against a background of more diffuse infiltration throughout the marrow.

Binucleate cell - - -

The disease has an incidence of 10 in 100 000 per annum with an age peak in the seventh decade.

The median survival, even with treatment, is 4–6 years.

**Pathological effects** are considered under two main headings:

1.  **Tumour growth and its effects**

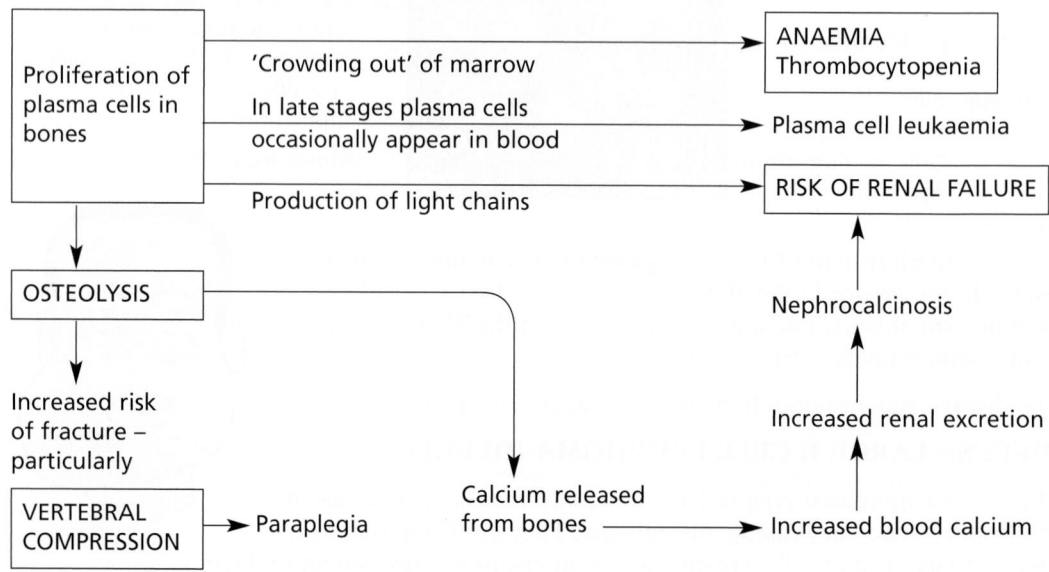

# PLASMA CELL TUMOURS

### 2.  Synthesis of immunoglobulin and its effects

Myeloma, being a monoclonal tumour, will produce a single Ig. The common heavy chains are G (60%) and A (20%). In Waldenström macroglobulinaemia the immunoglobulin is always IgM.

Light chains of κ type are encountered more frequently than λ.

The presence of a single type of Ig is reflected in the electrophoretic pattern.

The other normal immunoglobulins are always decreased.

In most cases high levels of 'M' protein cause:
1. High ESR
2. Marked rouleaux formation
3. Depending on type of Ig – increased blood viscosity.

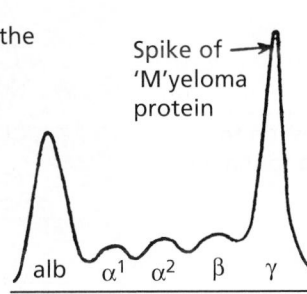

Spike of → 'M'yeloma protein

alb    α¹    α²    β    γ

### Release of light chains

In many myelomas, some of the Ig molecules are incompletely formed, and unattached light chains are released with important effects. Because of their low molecular weight the light chains:

(1) pass through the glomerular filtrate,
(a) appear in the *urine* as Bence Jones protein (precipitates during heating – redissolves between 90 °C–100 °C), and
(b) during passage through the tubules the protein precipitates as casts and also damages the epithelial cells.

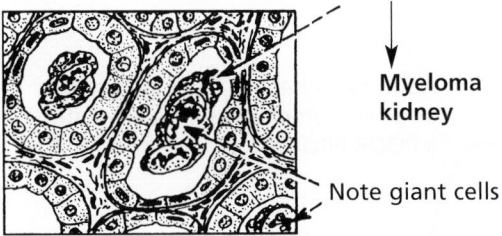

**Myeloma kidney**

Note giant cells

(2) Pass through capillaries

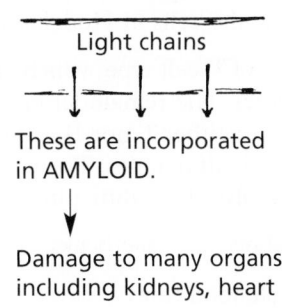

Light chains

These are incorporated in AMYLOID.

Damage to many organs, including kidneys, heart

**Infections**, often of opportunistic type and particularly pneumonias, are common because the immune response is deficient since the high levels of 'M' protein are non-functioning.

# NON-HODGKIN LYMPHOMA – T CELL

### MYCOSIS FUNGOIDES

This is a primary T cell (CD4) lymphoma of the skin occurring usually in middle age. It presents as a scaly, red macule progressing to skin plaques and then nodules.

Foci of large neoplastic cells in epidermis (Pautrier abscesses)

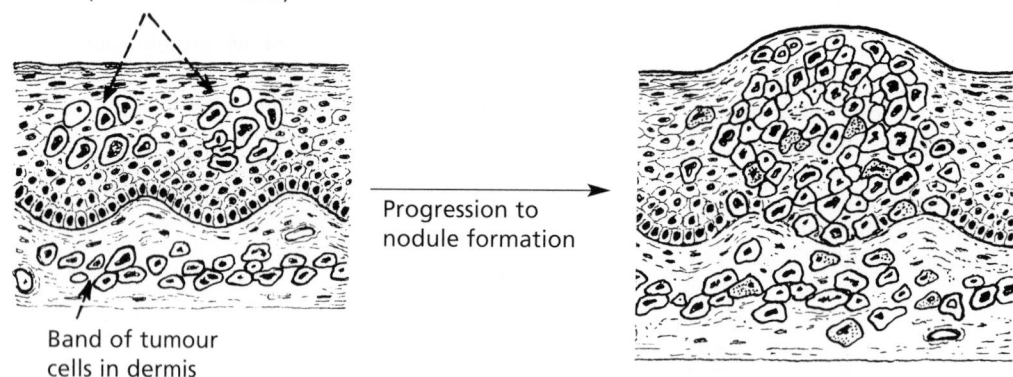

Progression to nodule formation

Band of tumour cells in dermis

After many years the lymphoma may become generalised or exfoliate into the blood (Sézary syndrome).

### ANAPLASTIC LARGE CELL LYMPHOMA

The large malignant T cells (usually expressing surface marker CD30) often spread within the sinuses of the node and may mimic the cells in Hodgkin lymphoma.

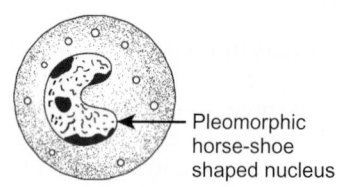

Pleomorphic horse-shoe shaped nucleus

Most cases are of T cell type, which can be proven by molecular studies. The remainder are 'null' cell type, i.e. they express neither T nor B cell markers, causing further diagnostic difficulties. The cells often express ALK-1 which helps resolve these difficulties.

The tumour shows two age peaks.

Childhood cases have a GOOD PROGNOSIS

Adult cases behave like high grade large cell lymphomas – usually with a POOR PROGNOSIS.

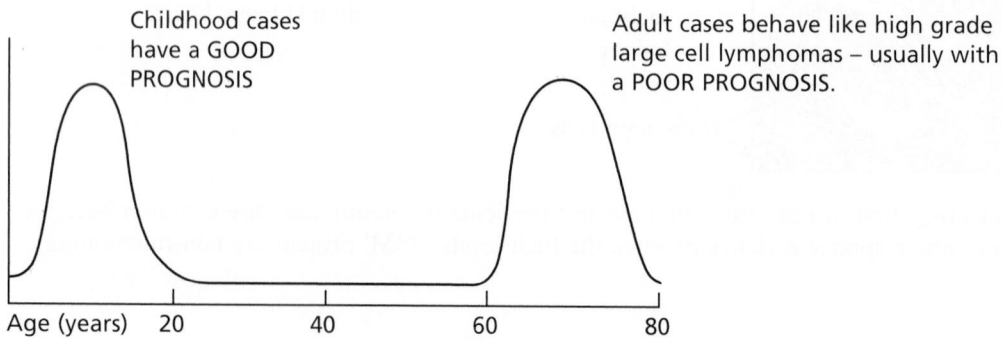

Age (years)  20  40  60  80

# HODGKIN LYMPHOMA

## Incidence

This disease accounts for 20% of lymphomas. It may occur at any age but there are two peaks of incidence.

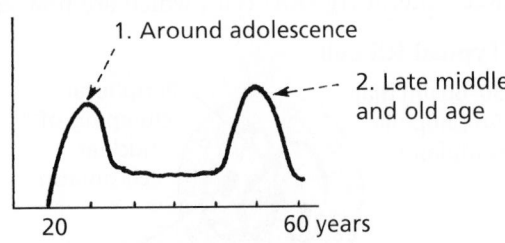

## Presentation

Most patients present with painless enlargement of one or more lymph node groups – cervical, axillary, mediastinal. One-quarter complain of systemic 'B' symptoms (see Staging) – fever, night sweats, weight loss, itch. The risk of infections is increased by immunosuppression.

## Spread and staging

The disease spreads from one group to the next directly connected by lymphatics.

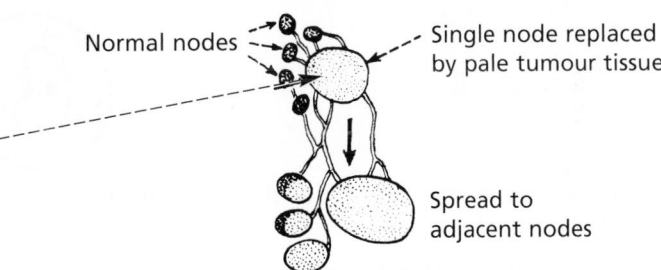

Normal nodes

Single node replaced by pale tumour tissue

Spread to adjacent nodes

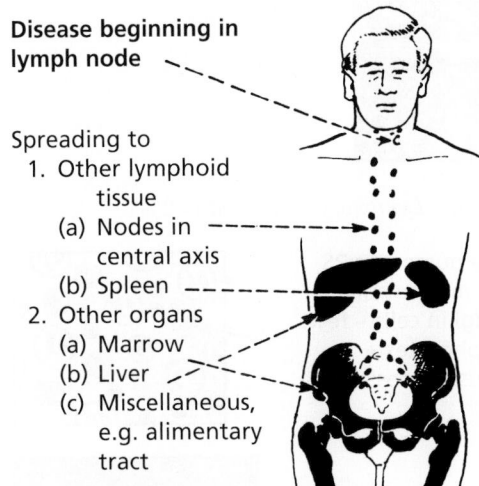

**Disease beginning in lymph node**

Spreading to
1. Other lymphoid tissue
    (a) Nodes in central axis
    (b) Spleen
2. Other organs
    (a) Marrow
    (b) Liver
    (c) Miscellaneous, e.g. alimentary tract

**Staging** (Ann Arbor system)

| | |
|---|---|
| Stage I | Disease involving single node or group of nodes |
| Stage II | Disease in more than one site – all lesions either below or above the diaphragm |
| Stage III | Disease on both sides of diaphragm |
| Stage IV | Widespread involvement of extralymphoid sites ± lymph node involvement |

The stages are further divided according to the absence (A) or presence (B) of systemic symptoms.

# HODGKIN LYMPHOMA

Hodgkin lymphoma is diagnosed on the basis of distinctive large tumour cells known as Reed–Sternberg (RS) cells, which are now known to be 'B' cells of germinal centre origin.

**Typical RS cell**

30–60 μm diam. Amphophilic cytoplasm

Peripheral clumping of nuclear chromatin

Large eosinophilic nucleoli

Mirror image nuclei

They express CD30 and CD15

**Variants of RS cell**

**1. The lacunar cell**

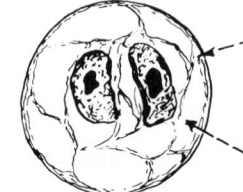

Shrinkage of cell cytoplasm towards cell wall and nucleus, leaving a clear space

**2. Mononuclear Hodgkin cell**

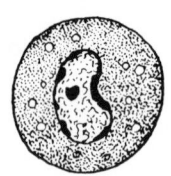

Nuclear characteristics similar to RS cell but smaller

These cells are not diagnostic of Hodgkin disease

There are two main types of Hodgkin lymphoma – classical Hodgkin lymphoma and lymphocyte-predominant:

(a) **Classical Hodgkin lymphoma**, probably caused by Epstein–Barr virus. There are four subtypes:

1. *Nodular sclerosing* (70%)

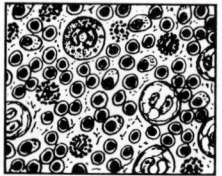

Thick bands of collagen separating Hodgkin tissue

Lacunar cells often numerous

2. *Mixed cellularity* (20%)

Plasma cells and eosinophils present in addition to RS cells and lymphocytes

3. *Lymphocyte depleted* (<2%)

Very numerous RS and mononuclear Hodgkin cells – few lymphocytes ± diffuse fibrosis

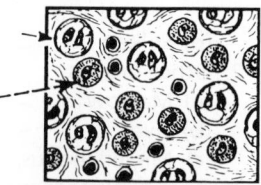

4. *Lymphocyte rich* (<2%)

(b) **Nodular lymphocyte-predominant Hodgkin lymphoma** (5%) This form affects young males and has a good prognosis. The 'popcorn cells' express 'B' cell markers and not CD30 of classic Hodgkin lymphoma – it is an unusual 'B' cell lymphoma and has an excellent prognosis.

Sheets of small lymphocytes

Scattering of unusual Hodgkin cells – 'popcorn' cells

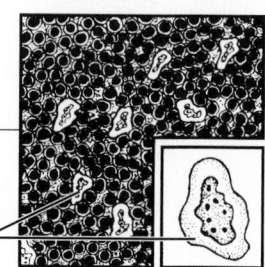

# LEUKAEMIAS

Leukaemias are primary malignant tumours of haemopoietic cells.

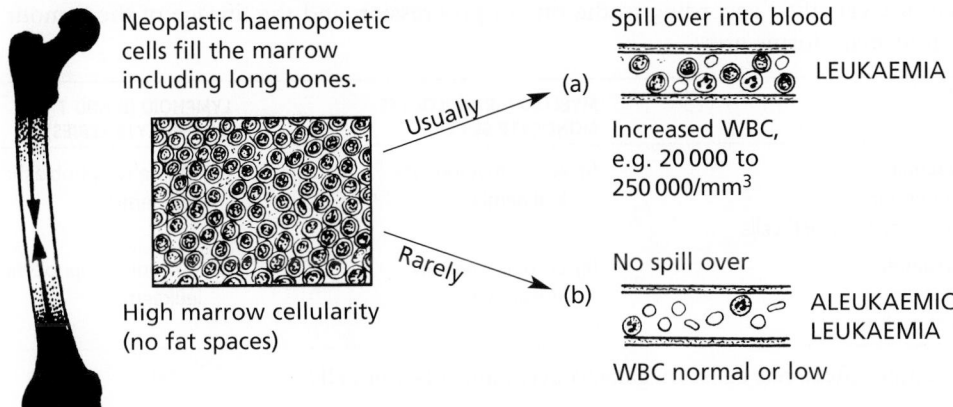

Neoplastic haemopoietic cells fill the marrow including long bones.

High marrow cellularity (no fat spaces)

*Usually* (a) Spill over into blood

**LEUKAEMIA**

Increased WBC, e.g. 20 000 to 250 000/mm$^3$

*Rarely* (b) No spill over

**ALEUKAEMIC LEUKAEMIA**

WBC normal or low

## Clinical effects

The neoplastic cells replace the normal bone marrow.

1. Deficiency of red cells ⟶ anaemia.
2. Deficiency of platelets ⟶ thrombocytopenia ⟶ bleeding.
3. Deficiency of white cells ⟶ infection.
4. Increased cell turnover ⟶ ↑DNA breakdown ⟶ ↑uric acid ⟶ gout.

## Spread of leukaemia

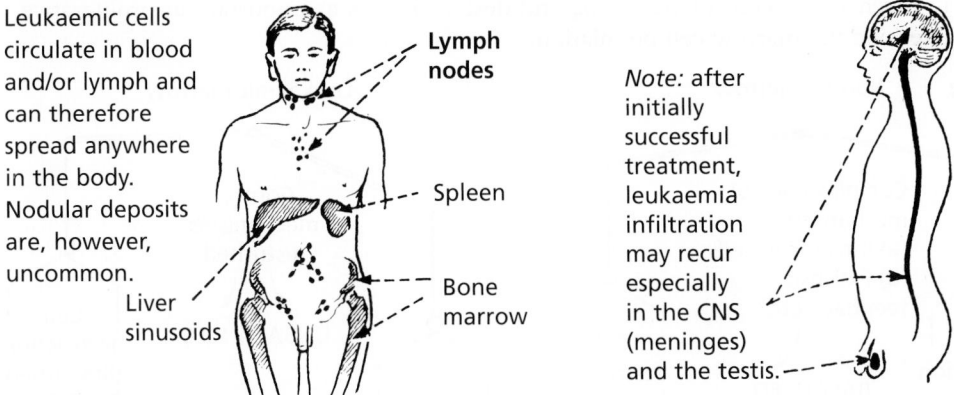

Leukaemic cells circulate in blood and/or lymph and can therefore spread anywhere in the body. Nodular deposits are, however, uncommon.

Lymph nodes

Spleen

Liver sinusoids

Bone marrow

*Note:* after initially successful treatment, leukaemia infiltration may recur especially in the CNS (meninges) and the testis.

# LEUKAEMIAS

## Classification

Leukaemias are classified according to the rate of progression and the lineage of the tumour cells. The four main forms are:

| | MYELOID (GRANULOCYTE: MONOCYTE SERIES) | LYMPHOID (B AND T LYMPHOCYTE SERIES) |
|---|---|---|
| **Acute Leukaemia**<br>– Rapid progression<br>– Numerous primitive 'blast' cells | (i) Acute myeloblastic leukaemia | (iii) Acute lymphoblastic leukaemia |
| **Chronic Leukaemia**<br>– Slow progression<br>– Cells almost mature | (ii) Chronic myeloid leukaemia | (iv) Chronic lymphocytic leukaemia |

Rare leukaemias affect red cells, megakaryocytes and plasma cells.

## Aetiology

In most cases, the cause is unknown. Risk factors include:

1. Radiation, e.g. post Hiroshima, Chernobyl, therapeutic X-rays.
2. Chemicals, e.g. chemotherapy, benzene.
3. Genetic, e.g. Down syndrome.
4. Virus, e.g. human T cell leukaemia virus-1.

## CELL KINETICS

Even in acute leukaemias, increased cell longevity beyond the normal (due to failure of response to mechanisms controlling ageing and destruction) is as important as proliferative rates in increasing the marrow cell population.

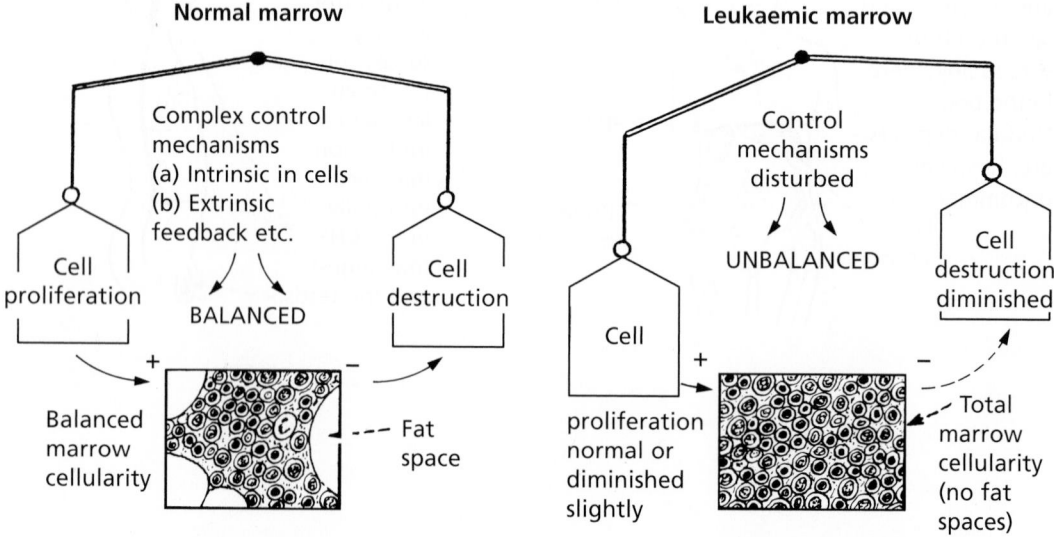

# ACUTE MYELOBLASTIC LEUKAEMIA (AML)

This is the commonest acute leukaemia of adults – 80% of patients are over 60 years old. Young adults and children may also be affected.

It may arise de novo or in association with chronic myeloid leukaemia, myeloproliferative disorders, myelodysplasia. The onset and progression to marrow failure is rapid, clinically presenting as anaemia, haemorrhage or serious infection.

**The WHO classification describes four broad categories:**

1. AML with recurrent genetic abnormalities. The differing genetic rearrangements have major implications for prognosis and treatment.
2. AML with multilineage dysplasia – usually following myelodysplastic syndrome.
3. AML, therapy-related – usually after alkylating chemotherapy.
4. AML, not otherwise classified – a wide variety showing varying degrees of differentiation, e.g. acute monocytic, acute erythroblastic, acute myelomonocytic.

## PATHOLOGY

**The marrow**

Over-run by blast cells

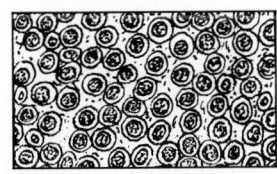

**The blood**

Decreased platelet count – **thrombocytopenia.**

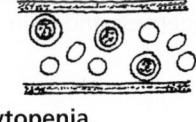

Two-thirds of cases: WBC 20 000–50 000 blast cells
One-third of cases: **aleukaemic**

Other organs may be involved: splenomegaly, hepatomegaly and lymph node enlargement. More specific pathological clinical complications are seen in two subtypes.

Promyelocytic

Primitive cell with primary myeloid granules ---

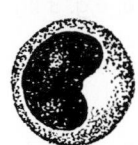

A typical chromosomal translocation t(15:17) is found.

Patients often develop disseminated intravascular coagulation.

Myelomonocytic and Monocytic

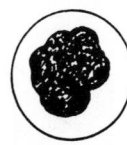

Infiltration of the gums and central nervous sytem is often seen.

# CHRONIC MYELOID LEUKAEMIA (CML)

This form of leukaemia arises from malignant transformation of a primitive stem cell – but with the production of differentiated cells – particularly neutrophils.

This is a disease of middle age. There are three phases:

1. **Chronic phase** – a period of slow evolution – 2–6 years is typical.
2. **Accelerated phase** – an increase in immature cells.
3. **Blast phase** – transformation to an acute leukaemia – myeloblastic or, very rarely, lymphoblastic.

Rarely patients develop myelofibrosis with marrow failure.

**Marrow**

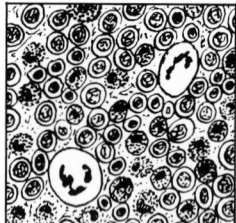

Total cellularity: cells of granulocyte series – late forms numerous (including eosinophil and basophil types). Often increase in megakaryocytes; may be increased fibrosis. Increased pressure in bones may cause tenderness and pain.

**Blood**
(a) WBC: 75 000–250 000/mm³
Differential WBC
Blasts ⎫
Promyelocytes ⎭ <5%

Majority of cells are late myelocytes and mature granulocytes

(b) ANAEMIA

(c) THROMBOCYTOPENIA
(sometimes thrombocytosis)

**Splenomegaly**

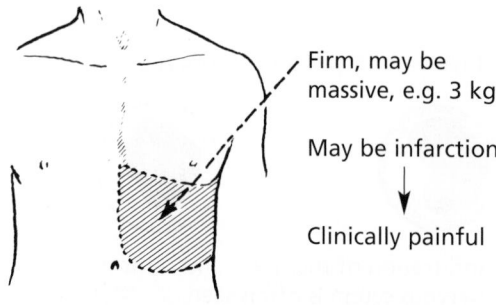

Firm, may be massive, e.g. 3 kg

May be infarction
↓
Clinically painful

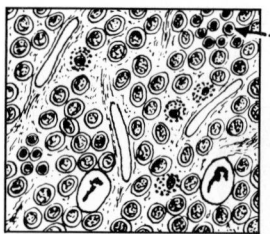

Lymphoid follicles inconspicuous

Red pulp with cells of granulocyte series
± megakaryocytes
± red cell precursors

**Philadelphia (Ph) chromosome**

In over 95% of cases of CML there is a specific cytogenetic change t(9;22)(q34;q11) with the formation of the 'Ph chromosome'.

The change involves a translocation of the c-abl gene (an oncogene) from chromosome 9 to chromosome 22 where hybridisation with the bcr gene occurs. A tyrosine kinase inhibitor (IMATINIB) which targets this pathway has been introduced and can induce complete remission.

# CHRONIC LYMPHOCYTIC LEUKAEMIA

This is a common form of leukaemia (25% of all cases) and particularly affects middle-aged and elderly patients. It is a monoclonal proliferation of small lymphocytes and is best regarded as the leukaemic form of lymphocytic lymphoma.

Most cases are of B cell type – less than 5% are of T cell lineage.

There is typically lymph node enlargement and splenomegaly.

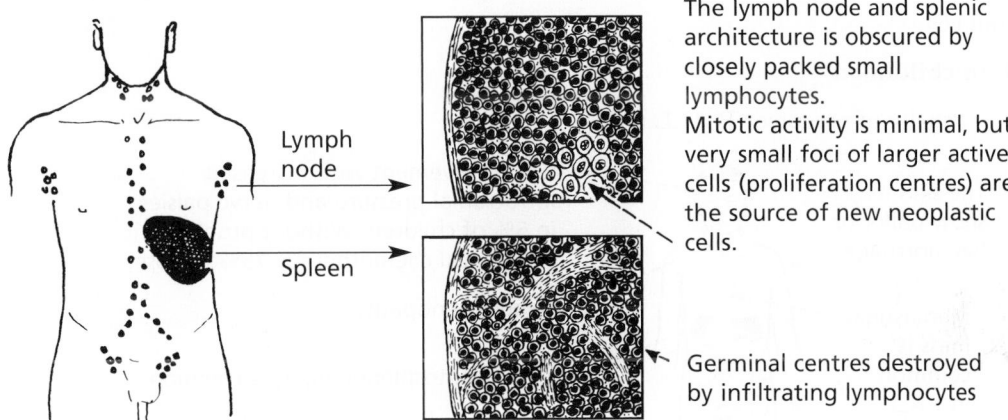

The lymph node and splenic architecture is obscured by closely packed small lymphocytes.
Mitotic activity is minimal, but very small foci of larger active cells (proliferation centres) are the source of new neoplastic cells.

Germinal centres destroyed by infiltrating lymphocytes

In some cases the lymphoid enlargement precedes the leukaemic phase.

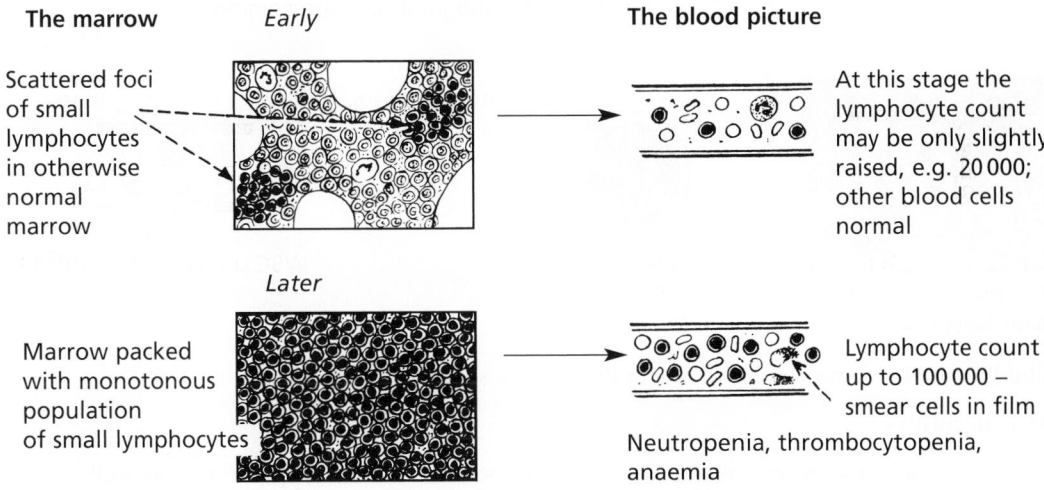

**The marrow**  *Early*  **The blood picture**

Scattered foci of small lymphocytes in otherwise normal marrow

At this stage the lymphocyte count may be only slightly raised, e.g. 20 000; other blood cells normal

*Later*

Marrow packed with monotonous population of small lymphocytes

Lymphocyte count up to 100 000 – smear cells in film

Neutropenia, thrombocytopenia, anaemia

In addition to anaemia these patients often suffer recurrent infections due to defective immunity.

In a minority of cases (approximately 5%) transformation to a high-grade 'B' cell lymphoma results (Richter syndrome).

# ACUTE LYMPHOBLASTIC LEUKAEMIA (ALL)

This term describes a group of leukaemias of lymphocytic precursors. ALL is the commonest form of childhood leukaemia but is also seen in adults.

Like AML, immunological and genotypic classification is increasingly important. Broadly, they are classified as follows:

- Precursor B cell >80%
- Precursor T cell <15%
- Null cell

### ALL in childhood

This is usually of precursor B ALL type.

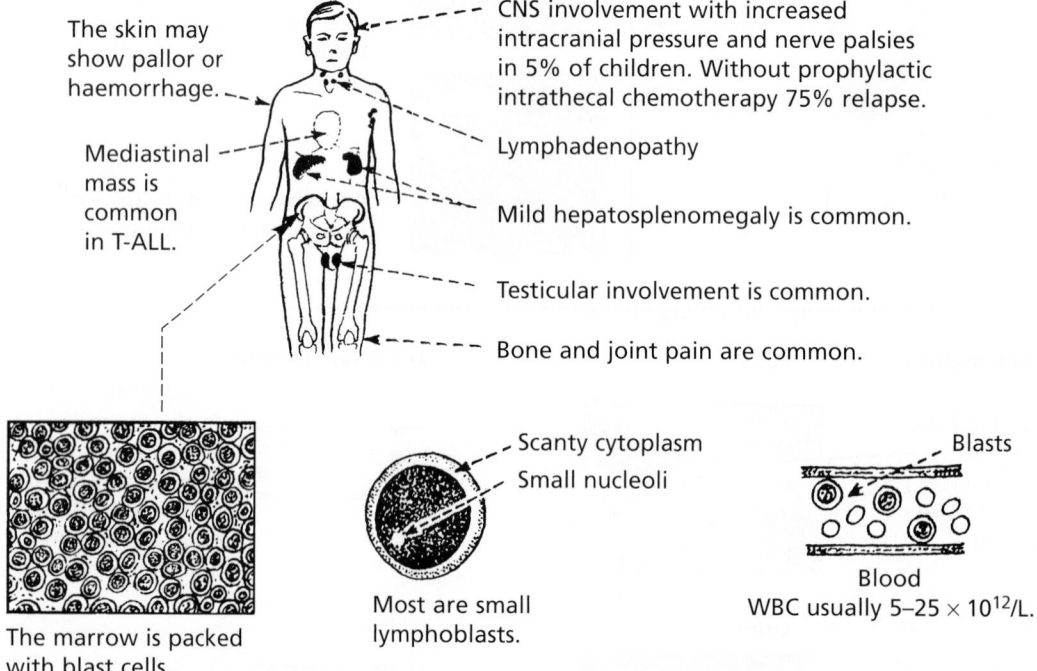

The skin may show pallor or haemorrhage.

Mediastinal mass is common in T-ALL.

CNS involvement with increased intracranial pressure and nerve palsies in 5% of children. Without prophylactic intrathecal chemotherapy 75% relapse.

Lymphadenopathy

Mild hepatosplenomegaly is common.

Testicular involvement is common.

Bone and joint pain are common.

The marrow is packed with blast cells.

Scanty cytoplasm
Small nucleoli
Most are small lymphoblasts.

Blasts
Blood
WBC usually 5–25 × 10$^{12}$/L.

Childhood ALL is now potentially curable – 70% survive 5 years.

### ALL in adults

Adults have a worse prognosis and often require bone marrow transplantation as well as chemotherapy.

# MYELOPROLIFERATIVE DISORDERS

In this group of diseases, neoplastic transformation of a haemopoietic precursor cell may lead to excess production of erythrocyte, leucocyte or platelet precursors. In many cases more than one element is affected. Transformation to acute leukaemia can occur in all forms. This can be summarised as follows:

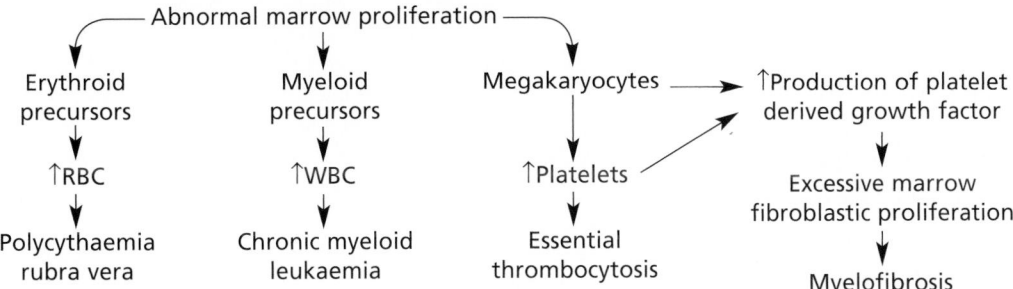

In these conditions excess marrow proliferation may be seen in liver, spleen and other organs – EXTRAMEDULLARY HAEMOPOIESIS (EHM).

## MYELOFIBROSIS

When haemopoietic cellular proliferation is overshadowed by progressive FIBROSIS of the marrow, SPLENOMEGALY (often of massive proportions) due to EXTRAMEDULLARY HAEMOPOIESIS is often found.

*Marrow:* ordinary marrow puncture usually results in a 'dry tap', therefore trephine or cutting needle biopsy is required.

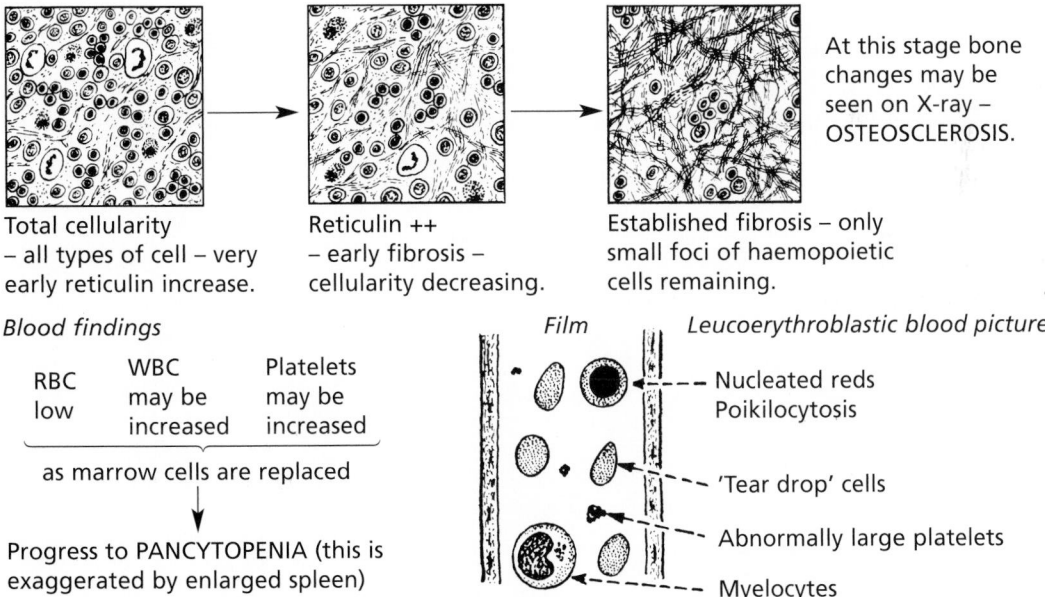

Total cellularity – all types of cell – very early reticulin increase.

Reticulin ++ – early fibrosis – cellularity decreasing.

Established fibrosis – only small foci of haemopoietic cells remaining.

At this stage bone changes may be seen on X-ray – OSTEOSCLEROSIS.

*Blood findings*

| RBC low | WBC may be increased | Platelets may be increased |
|---------|----------------------|----------------------------|

as marrow cells are replaced

Progress to PANCYTOPENIA (this is exaggerated by enlarged spleen)

*Film*     *Leucoerythroblastic blood picture*

– Nucleated reds
Poikilocytosis

– 'Tear drop' cells

– Abnormally large platelets

– Myelocytes

## MYELODYSPLASTIC SYNDROMES (MDS)

These are primary disorders of stem cells associated with several different chromosomal abnormalities. They lead to ineffective haemopoiesis of varying types, with the appearance in the peripheral blood of abnormal cells. A significant number progress to LEUKAEMIA.

# GENITOURINARY SYSTEM

## OBJECTIVES

1. To understand the aetiology and pathogenesis of the main types of glomerulonephritis.
2. To know about the pathology of the kidney in hypertension.
3. To know which infections affect the kidney and their sequelae.
4. To have a knowledge of tubulo-interstitial disorders of the kidney and their pathogenesis.
5. To know the main tumour types affecting the kidney.
6. To know about the pathology of urinary tract infection.
7. To have an understanding of the aetiology and pathogenesis of bladder tumours.
8. To know about the pathology of prostate carcinoma.
9. To have a basic knowledge of the main tumour types which arise in the testis.

# KIDNEY – STRUCTURE AND FUNCTION

The kidney has several functions:

1. Eliminating waste products.
2. Controlling electrolyte and fluid balance.
3. Contributing to acid–base balance.

By filtering plasma and modifying the filtrate to produce urine.

It produces several hormones:
   (i) *Renin*, which influences vascular tone and blood pressure.
   (ii) *Erythropoietin*, which increases red blood cell production.
   (iii) *1, 25 dihydroxy Vitamin D* – the active form is produced by $1\alpha$ hydroxylation in the kidney. It promotes calcium absorption from the gut and is required for normal bone mineralisation.

**Tests of renal function:**

1. **Blood analysis**

Many substances will show altered values in renal failure, but the following are always elevated and are commonly used in estimating the progress of the disease.
   (i) Urea – normal range 2.5–7.0 mmol/L (20–40 mg/100 mL).
   (ii) Creatinine – 50–100 mmol/L (0.6–1.2 mg/100 mL).

# KIDNEY – STRUCTURE AND FUNCTION

2. **Clearance tests** (typically creatinine clearance) give an indication of glomerular filtration rate; this is not absolute since some creatinine is secreted by renal tubules. The following formula is used to calculate the volume of blood cleared:

$$\text{Clearance} = \frac{UV}{P}$$

where:

U = urinary concentration
V = volume of urine per minute
P = plasma concentration

In practice renal function is now commonly assessed by estimated glomerular filtration rate (eGFR), which combines serum creatinine with the age and sex of patient.

Chronic Kidney Disease (CKD) can be classified as follows:

| CKD | STAGE | eGFR/mL/ min/1.73 m² |
|---|---|---|
| 1 | with an abnormality* | >90 |
| 2 | with an abnormality* | 60–89 |
| 3 | | 30–59 |
| 4 | | 15–29 |
| 5 | | <15 |

*e.g. proteinuria.

3. **Urine examination**

(a) Tests for the presence of protein, red cells, haemoglobin and neutrophils in the urine. Estimation of specific gravity and measurement of urinary output.
(b) Urinary casts. These are composed of foreign elements of various types which are moulded into cylindrical form by passage along tubules and are seen on microscopy.
(c) Culture.

The kidney is divided into:

(a) Glomeruli
(b) Tubules
(c) Interstitium
(d) Vessels

The structure and function and diseases will be discussed separately, but diseases of one may well affect others.

# GLOMERULAR STRUCTURE AND FUNCTION

The glomerulus, of which there are over 600 000 in the adult, consists of an invagination of a capillary network, derived from the afferent arteriole, into Bowman capsule – the beginning of the proximal tubule.

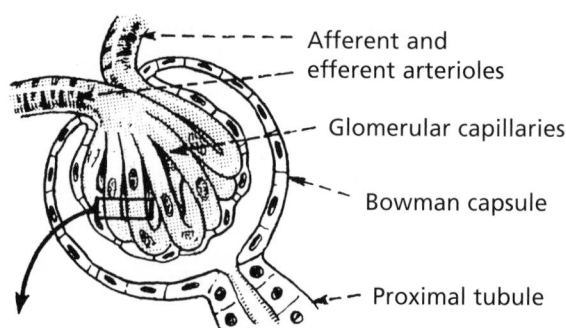

Afferent and efferent arterioles

Glomerular capillaries

Bowman capsule

Proximal tubule

The glomerulus is an efficient filter due to the large surface area of the glomerular capillaries.

### Ultrastructure

The barrier separating blood from the lumen of the matrix nephron consists of three layers:

1. Endothelium (fenestrated)
2. Basement membrane
3. Epithelium

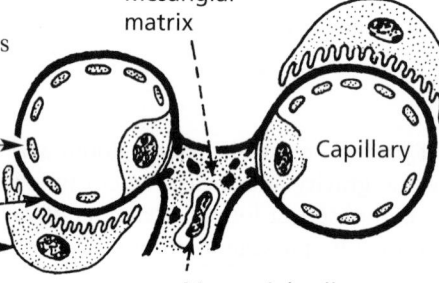

Mesangial matrix

Capillary

Mesangial cell

Mesangial cells have three functions:

1. Contract and control blood flow.
2. They are phagocytic cells and ingest proteins and immune complexes (p. 143).
3. They form matrix and secrete inflammatory mediators.

These layers form a complicated sieve controlling glomerular permeability. Wide pores (70–100 nm) in the endothelium allow all components to reach the basement membrane.

The basement membrane produced by the endothelium and epithelium has a strong anionic (negative) charge which repels major plasma proteins (also anionic). It has a central dense layer (lamina densa).

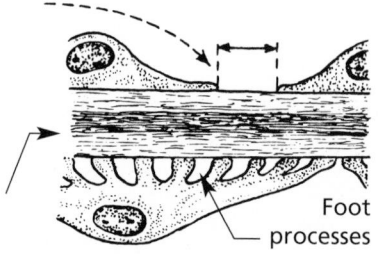

Foot processes

The epithelial cells are attached to the basement membrane by foot processes, separated by 'slit pores' 30–60 nm in diameter.

### Filtration

The glomerular filtrate is virtually protein free plasma. Its rate of production is dependent upon factors *1–4* in this diagram:

Variation in any of these factors affects the output of urine. Diminished urinary output results from a reduction in renal blood flow as in shock, from an increase in osmotic pressure as in haemoconcentration, or from obstruction to the outflow of urine.

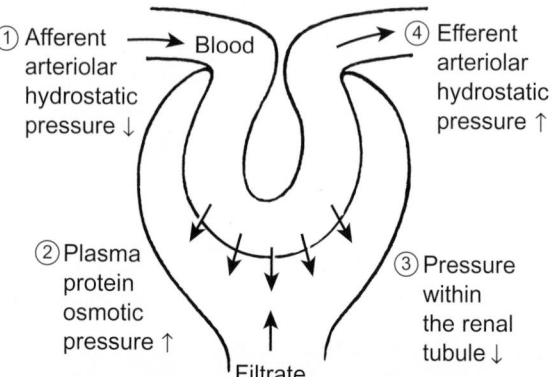

① Afferent arteriolar hydrostatic pressure ↓

Blood

④ Efferent arteriolar hydrostatic pressure ↑

② Plasma protein osmotic pressure ↑

③ Pressure within the renal tubule ↓

Filtrate

# GLOMERULAR DISEASES

**Glomerular damage results in:**

1. Reduction in urinary output
2. Proteinuria
3. Haematuria

The mechanisms underlying these changes are as follows:

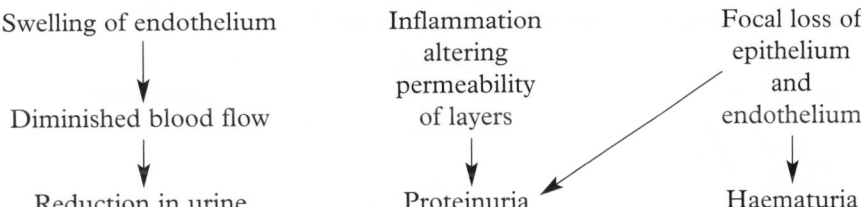

These lead to four main clinical syndromes:

1. The NEPHRITIC SYNDROME – characterised by moderate proteinuria, haematuria, oedema, oliguria and often renal impairment. Hypertension is common.
2. The NEPHROTIC SYNDROME
   Heavy proteinuria (>3.5 g/day) ⟶ Hypoalbuminaemia ⟶ Oedema
3. RENAL FAILURE – acute or chronic in type.
4. Asymptomatic haematuria or proteinuria.

The main causes are:

(a) IMMUNE DAMAGE ⟶ GLOMERULONEPHRITIS
(b) Diabetes mellitus
(c) Vascular disease, e.g. hypertension.

The cause is best determined by renal biopsy.

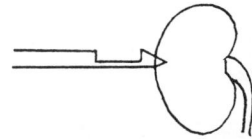 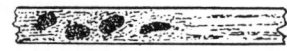

The core of tissue
obtained is examined by:

**1. Light microscopy**    **2. Immunofluorescence**    **3. Electron microscopy**

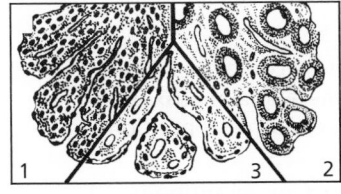     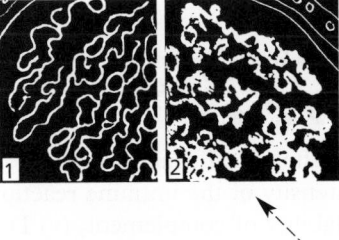     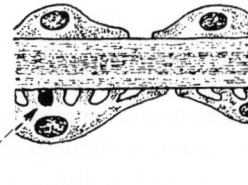

Shows 1. increase in cells,
      2. details of basement
          membrane and
      3. mesangial matrix.

Immune complexes
can be detected.
    1. Linear
    2. Granular

Detailed cellular and
membrane damage
can be seen.

The main forms of glomerular disease are described in the following pages.

# GLOMERULONEPHRITIS – DISEASE MECHANISMS

The mechanism in most forms of GN is:

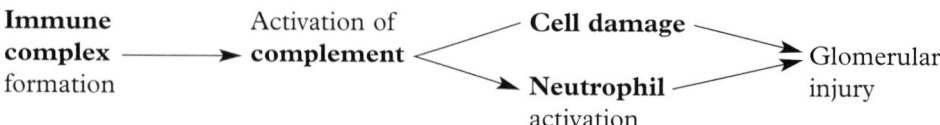

The glomerulus is central to immune complex deposition and formation due to its **fenestrated endothelium** and **high intraluminal pressure**.

Immune complexes can occur in glomeruli as follows:

1. Deposition of circulating complex.   2. In situ formation of complexes.
(a) Deposited antigens   (b) Glomerular antigens

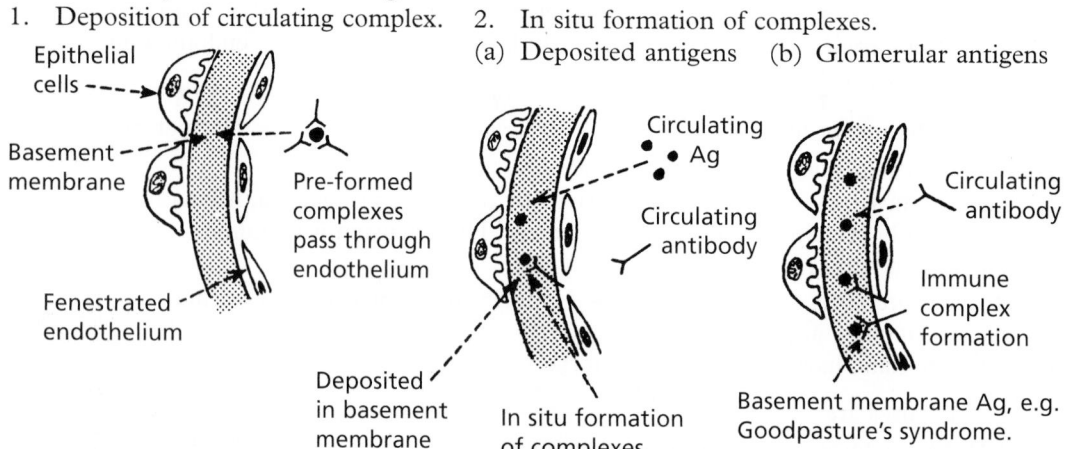

**Localisation of complexes**

This depends on the size of the complexes, their shape and electrical charge, and their ability to penetrate the basement membrane.

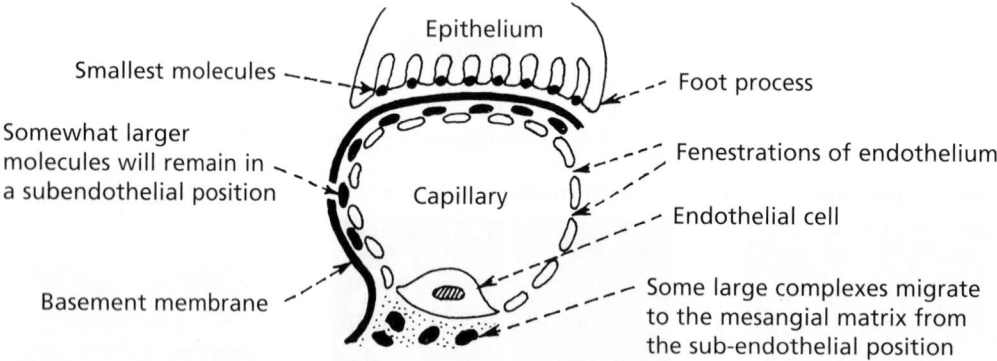

Other factors modifying the pathological changes are:

(i) amount of antigen, (ii) intensity of the immune reaction, (iii) type of antibody (especially IgA), (iv) availability of complement, (v) Degradation of complexes by macrophages and mesangial cells, (vi) secondary tubular damage has important effects on renal function.

*Note:* In addition to its damaging consequences, complement activation does **solubilise complexes,** allowing their disposal. Thus complement deficiency may predispose to immune complex disease, e.g. in systemic lupus erythematosus (SLE).

# ACUTE DIFFUSE PROLIFERATIVE (POST-INFECTIOUS) GLOMERULONEPHRITIS

This disease classically follows 2–3 weeks after an infection – usually pharyngitis due to Group A haemolytic streptococci. It is commonest in children and young adults who develop the NEPHRITIC SYNDROME: oliguria, proteinuria, haematuria (urine is smoky and dark), moderate hypertension and facial (periorbital) oedema. This disease is now uncommon in fully developed countries.

The lesion is essentially acute inflammation of all glomeruli.

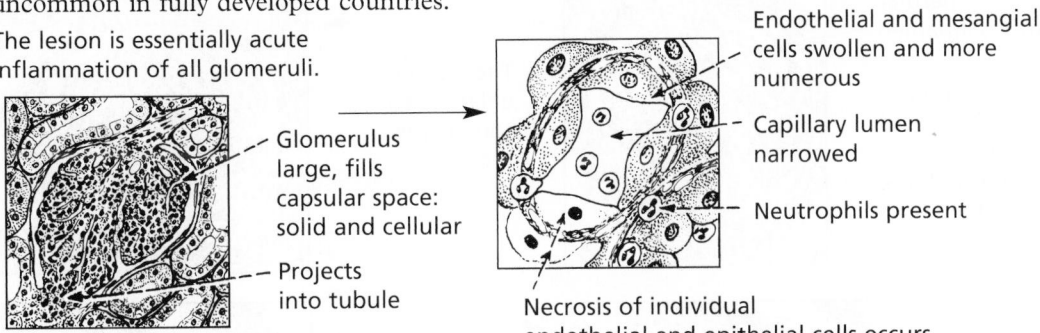

Glomerulus large, fills capsular space: solid and cellular

Projects into tubule

Endothelial and mesangial cells swollen and more numerous

Capillary lumen narrowed

Neutrophils present

Necrosis of individual endothelial and epithelial cells occurs

Immune complexes are identified by:

### 1. **Electron microscopy**

Hump-shaped electron-dense granular deposits seen in subepithelial position.

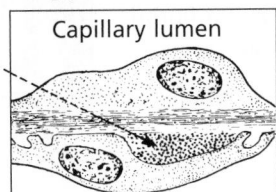

Capillary lumen

### 2. **Immunofluorescence**

This demonstrates granular deposition of IgG and C3 (complement component 3).

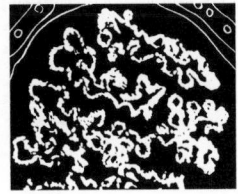

The clinical findings can be correlated with pathology as follows:

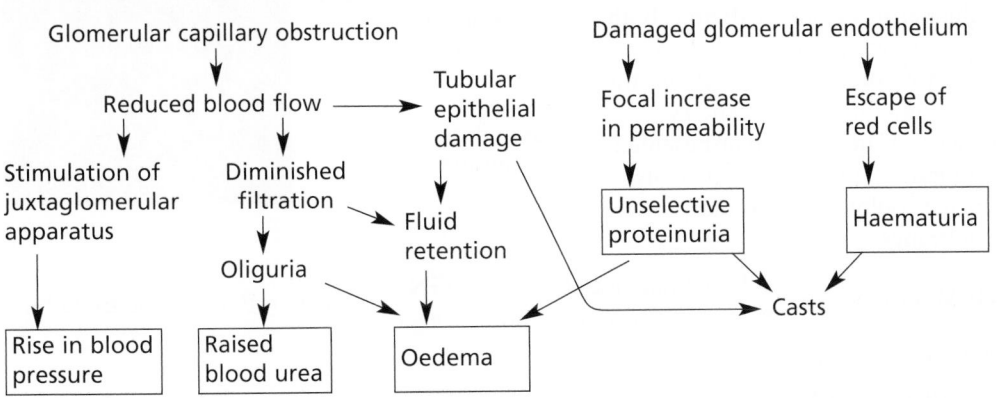

Glomerular capillary obstruction
↓
Reduced blood flow → Tubular epithelial damage
↓
Stimulation of juxtaglomerular apparatus
↓
Diminished filtration
→ Fluid retention
↓
Oliguria
↓
Rise in blood pressure

Raised blood urea

Oedema

Damaged glomerular endothelium
↓
Focal increase in permeability
↓
Unselective proteinuria

Escape of red cells
↓
Haematuria

→ Casts

**Prognosis** – the disease usually resolves in 1–2 weeks, particularly in children, but in adults complications are more common.

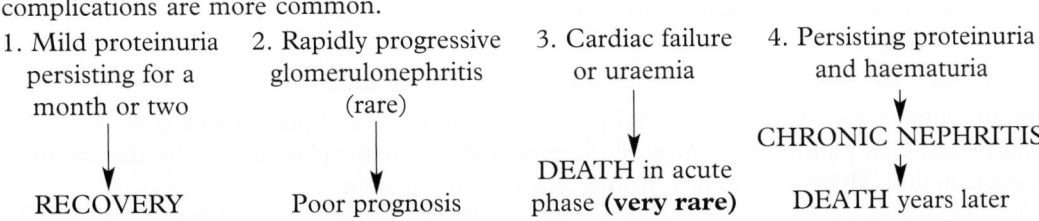

1. Mild proteinuria persisting for a month or two
↓
RECOVERY

2. Rapidly progressive glomerulonephritis (rare)
↓
Poor prognosis

3. Cardiac failure or uraemia
↓
DEATH in acute phase (**very rare**)

4. Persisting proteinuria and haematuria
↓
CHRONIC NEPHRITIS
↓
DEATH years later

489

# CRESCENTIC (RAPIDLY PROGRESSIVE) GLOMERULONEPHRITIS

This is a clinical syndrome and not a specific aetiological form of glomerulonephritis. The histological hallmark is **crescent formation** in >50% of glomeruli. Without treatment, this disease progresses to end-stage renal failure in weeks or months.

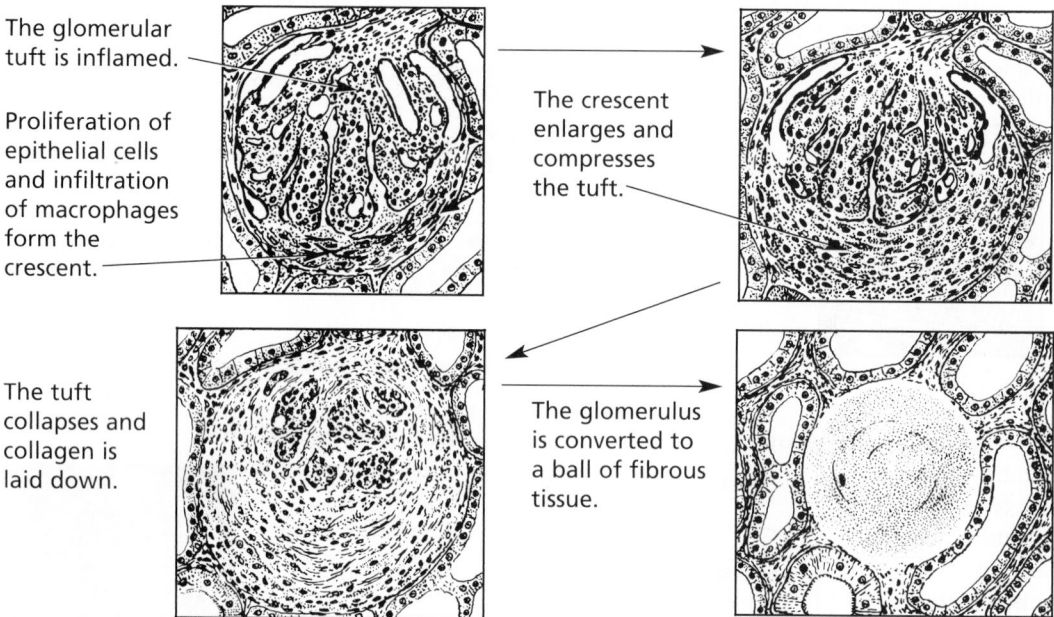

The glomerular tuft is inflamed.

Proliferation of epithelial cells and infiltration of macrophages form the crescent.

The crescent enlarges and compresses the tuft.

The tuft collapses and collagen is laid down.

The glomerulus is converted to a ball of fibrous tissue.

Many types of glomerulonephritis can progress to crescentic GN. Examples include:

1. **Goodpasture syndrome**
   In this serious disorder there is both renal and often pulmonary damage. Immunofluorescence (IF) shows the cause – an antibody to Type IV collagen in the glomerular basement membrane (anti-GBM) which also damages pulmonary alveolar membranes.

   IF Immunofluorescence shows linear deposits of IgG and C3 in the capillary basement membranes

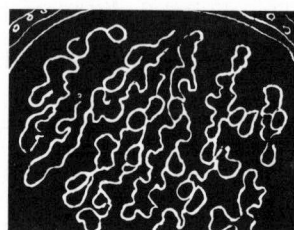

Anti-GBM antibody
→ Renal damage (crescentic GN)
→ Lung damage (haemorrhage)
} Renal and/or pulmonary failure

RPGN may complicate:

2. **Vasculitis** – e.g. Wegener granulomatosis, microscopic polyarteritis nodosa.
3. **SLE.**
4. **Acute diffuse proliferative glomerulonephritis**, especially in adults.
5. **IgA nephropathy.**

**Prognosis** – without treatment, most patients die within 6 months.

Immunosuppressive drugs (e.g. steroids, cyclophosphamide) and plasma exchange (to remove anti-GBM antibodies) improve the prognosis but many patients require dialysis or transplantation. Hypertension is a further serious complication.

# MEMBRANOUS GLOMERULONEPHRITIS

This accounts for around 30% of cases of the nephrotic syndrome in adults; some patients present with asymptomatic proteinuria.

**Aetiology**

In around 85% of cases THERE ARE autoantibodies to antigens expressed by podocytes. The remainder are secondary to

1. Drugs, e.g. penicillamine, – in treatment of rheumatoid arthritis.
2. Tumours, e.g. carcinoma of lung, colon, melanoma.
3. Infections, e.g. malaria, HIV, hepatitis B, syphilis.
4. Collagen disorders, e.g. SLE.

**Pathology** – There is generalised thickening of capillary basement membrane.

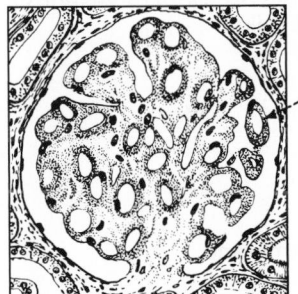

Tuft enlarges

Diffuse hyaline thickening of capillary

Glomeruli not hypercellular

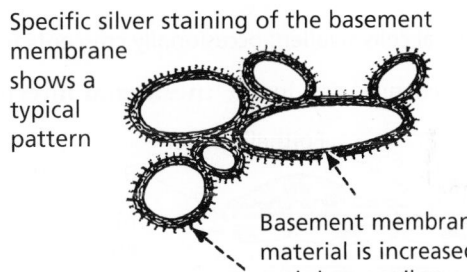

Specific silver staining of the basement membrane shows a typical pattern

Basement membrane material is increased and shows spikes

Immunofluorescence reveals deposition of IgG in the capillary walls.

Electron microscope findings explain this appearance.

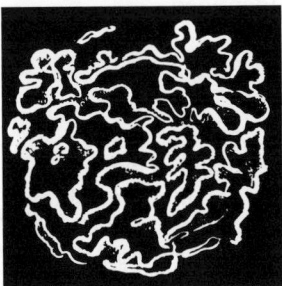

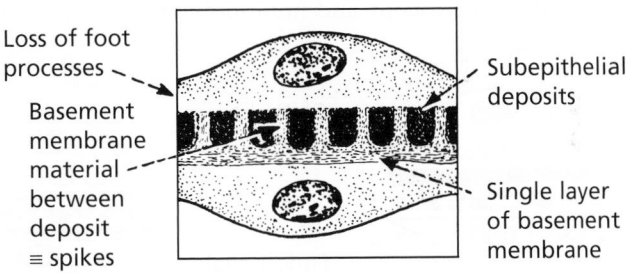

Loss of foot processes

Basement membrane material between deposit ≡ spikes

Subepithelial deposits

Single layer of basement membrane

In the later stages there is a massive increase in basement membrane material. Silver staining shows

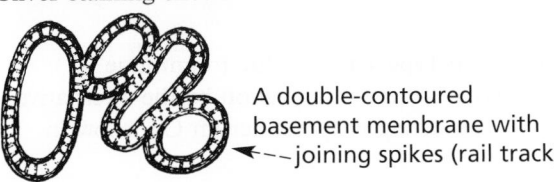

A double-contoured basement membrane with joining spikes (rail track)

Electron microscope shows

Two layers of basement membrane

Deposits

Capillary lumen

Tubular changes – in the early stages, protein droplets and lipid globules appear in the tubular epithelium. If the disease progresses there is atrophy of the tubules and interstitial fibrosis.

**Prognosis** – in about 25% of patients the disease remits spontaneously, the remainder continue to have proteinuria and in 40% chronic renal failure eventually supervenes.

# MESANGIOCAPILLARY (MEMBRANOPROLIFERATIVE) GLOMERULONEPHRITIS

In this form of glomerulonephritis there is an increase both in **cells** and **mesangial matrix** within glomeruli.

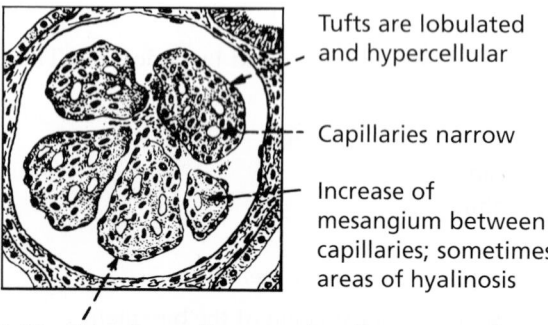

Tufts are lobulated and hypercellular

Capillaries narrow

Increase of mesangium between capillaries; sometimes areas of hyalinosis

Epithelial cells swollen; occasionally crescents form

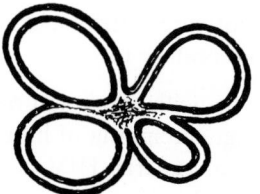

Silver staining of basement membrane

Duplication of basement membrane as in membranous glomerulonephritis, but without spikes

These changes are due to **'mesangial interposition'**

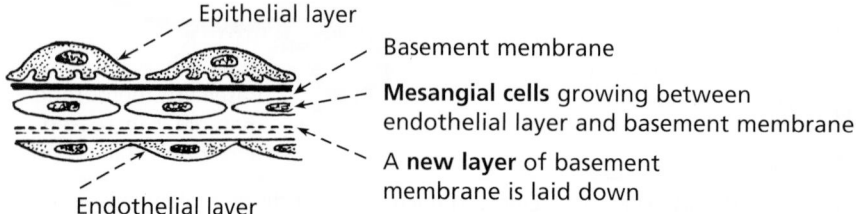

Epithelial layer

Basement membrane

**Mesangial cells** growing between endothelial layer and basement membrane

A **new layer** of basement membrane is laid down

Endothelial layer

Using electron microscopy and immunofluorescence, two types are identified.

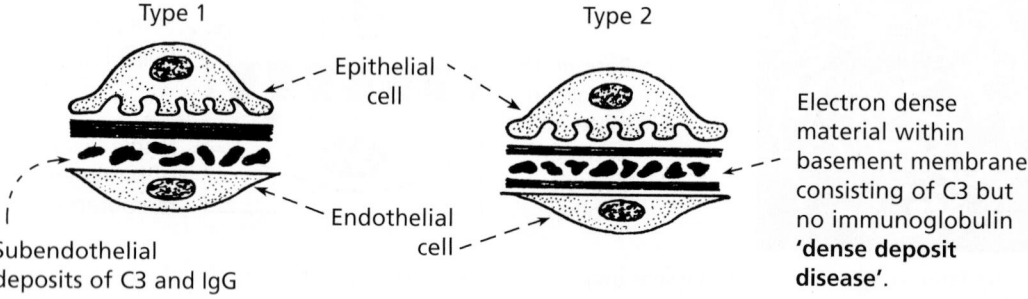

Type 1

Type 2

Epithelial cell

Endothelial cell

Subendothelial deposits of C3 and IgG

Electron dense material within basement membrane consisting of C3 but no immunoglobulin **'dense deposit disease'**.

## Aetiology

Complement activation is a feature of both forms. In Type 1 this is due to immune complexes by the classical pathway (p. 139). In Type 2 there is activation by the alternative pathway by an autoantibody which stabilises C3 converting enzyme. Serum C3 is low in both forms.

## Clinical features

Children and young adults are usually affected. They present with the **nephrotic syndrome** (50%), the nephritic syndrome or asymptomatic haematuria or proteinuria.

In half of patients there is progression to renal failure (with hypertension) within a decade. The disease often recurs in the subsequently transplanted kidney.

# FOCAL GLOMERULONEPHRITIS

In contrast to the glomerular diseases discussed already, focal glomerulonephritis affects only a proportion of glomeruli (focal) and only part of those glomeruli (segmental).

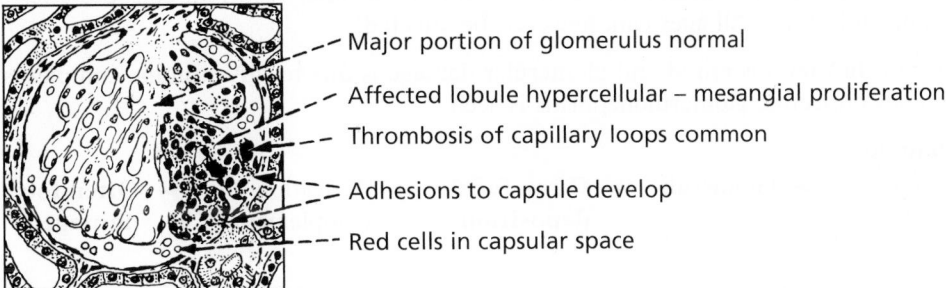

– Major portion of glomerulus normal

– Affected lobule hypercellular – mesangial proliferation

– Thrombosis of capillary loops common

– Adhesions to capsule develop

– Red cells in capsular space

In some cases, part of the tuft becomes necrotic and there is related inflammation (focal segmental necrotising glomerulonephritis). Crescents are sometimes seen. This pattern is seen in:

- Systemic vasculitis, e.g. polyarteritis nodosa.
- IgA nephropathy and Henoch–Schönlein purpura.
- SLE.
- Some cases of Goodpasture syndrome.
- Infective endocarditis.

The pattern is associated with haematuria or nephrotic syndrome. Segmental lesions heal by fibrosis.

## FOCAL SEGMENTAL GLOMERULOSCLEROSIS (FSGS)

In this pattern of disease, a segment of glomerulus undergoes sclerosis without inflammation, but with an increase in mesangial matrix.

Primary FSGS presents as nephrotic syndrome with progression to chronic renal failure. It may recur within a transplanted kidney.

Secondary FSGS may complicate a variety of pre-existing conditions including HIV and IgA nephropathy.

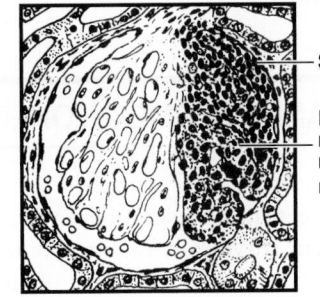

– Sclerosis

Increase in mesangial matrix, but not cells

# IGA NEPHROPATHY

This is the commonest form of glomerulonephritis worldwide. It can present with microscopic or macroscopic haematuria or the nephrotic syndrome and may lead to chronic renal failure. It typically affects young males, who often suffer recurrent episodes after upper respiratory infections. All ages can, however, be affected.

The serum IgA level is raised and glomerular damage is due to IgA immune complexes. Sometimes crescentic glomerulonephritis is seen.

**Mechanism**

IgA immune complexes in blood → Glomeruli → **Often focal deposition** → Activation of complement (C3) → **Often focal damage**

Shows deposits of IgA and C3 within the mesangium: the capillary loops are not usually affected.

Immunofluorescence

*Note:* The focal deposition is dependent on the molecular size of the complex and failure of mesangial clearance.

Henoch–Schönlein purpura has similar renal changes but also skin rash and gastrointestinal symptoms.

# MINIMAL CHANGE GLOMERULONEPHRITIS

This is the major cause of nephrotic syndrome in children. It typically remits spontaneously and responds to a short course of steroids. Recurrences are quite common.

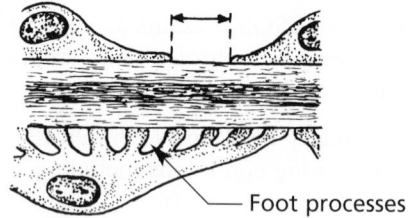

**Normal**

Foot processes

The glomeruli are histologically normal, but electron microscopy reveals fusion of podocyte foot processes. This is a finding in many causes of proteinuria. No immune complexes are found on immunofluorescence or electron microscopy.

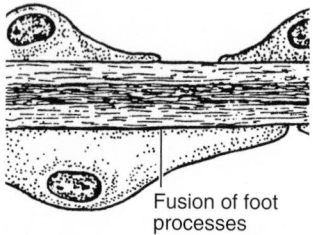

**Minimal change**

Fusion of foot processes

# CHRONIC GLOMERULONEPHRITIS (GN)

This is the end stage of many forms of glomerulonephritis, but most patients present at this stage without a history of previous renal disease.

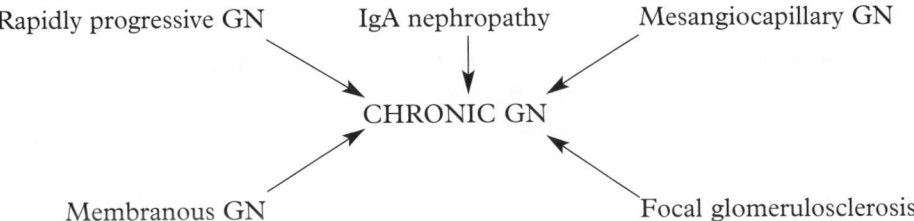

Rapidly progressive GN    IgA nephropathy    Mesangiocapillary GN

CHRONIC GN

Membranous GN    Focal glomerulosclerosis

**Pathology –** the kidneys are both small – granular contracted kidney.

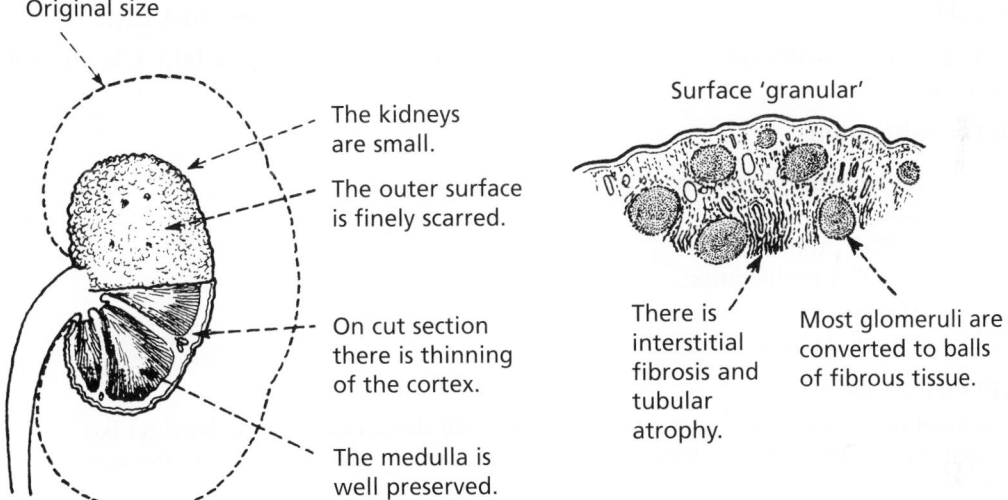

Original size

The kidneys are small.

The outer surface is finely scarred.

On cut section there is thinning of the cortex.

The medulla is well preserved.

Surface 'granular'

There is interstitial fibrosis and tubular atrophy.

Most glomeruli are converted to balls of fibrous tissue.

In chronic glomerulonephritis a vicious cycle is set up.

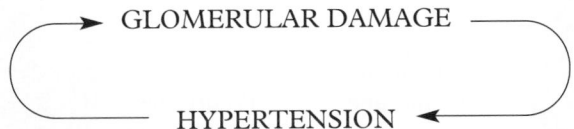

GLOMERULAR DAMAGE

HYPERTENSION

Patients may first present with chronic renal failure, or this may develop after years of glomerulonephritis.

# GLOMERULAR DISEASE IN SYSTEMIC DISORDERS

### SYSTEMIC LUPUS ERYTHEMATOSUS (SLE)

At least 50% of patients with SLE have clinical evidence of renal involvement, and almost all will have abnormalities on renal biopsy.

The main consequences are: (1) Proteinuria ⟶ nephrotic syndrome.
                                  (2) Microscopic haematuria.
                                  (3) Hypertension.
                                  (4) Progression to renal failure.

The renal changes form a spectrum.

Minimal abnormalities                                        Diffuse proliferative glomerulonephritis

                           Focal glomerulonephritis

**MILD** ⟶ **SEVERE**

On immunofluorescence, IgG and C3 are almost always present and IgA, IgM, Clq and C4 are often also seen.

### WHO classification

(i)  No lesion by light microscopy.
(ii)  Mesangial proliferation.
(iii) Focal (<50%) proliferation.
(iv) Diffuse (>50%) proliferation.
(v)  Membranous.
(vi) Chronic renal damage.

### AMYLOIDOSIS

The general features of amyloidosis have already been described (p. 22). Amyloid is deposited around the capillary basement membranes of the glomeruli and in the renal vessels and interstitium.

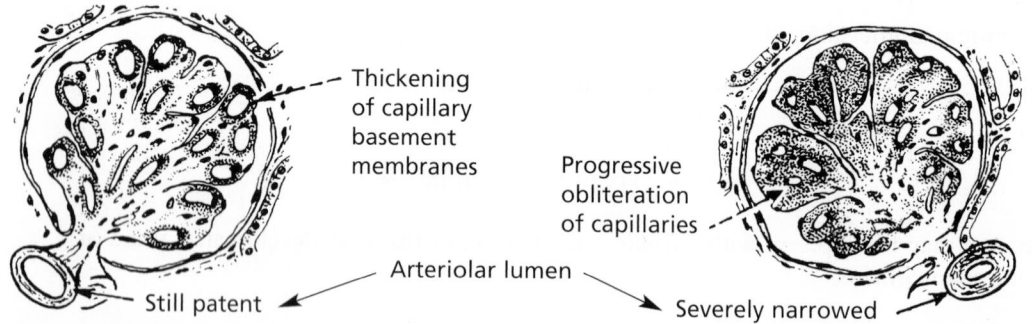

— Thickening of capillary basement membranes

Progressive obliteration of capillaries —

— Arteriolar lumen —

Still patent ⟵        ⟶ Severely narrowed

Gross proteinuria leading to nephrotic syndrome is common. Interstitial fibrosis results from tubular degeneration. There is ischaemia due to glomerular and arteriolar lesions. Chronic renal failure results.

### Parasitic glomerulopathies

The kidney and particularly the glomeruli are damaged in many parasitic infections in the tropics. **Malaria** and **schistosomiasis** are especially important.

# THE KIDNEY AND HYPERTENSION

There are two aspects to the relationship of the kidney and high blood pressure.

(a) Many renal diseases lead to hypertension (p. 220).

(b) Hypertension leads to renal damage.

A vicious circle can be set up:

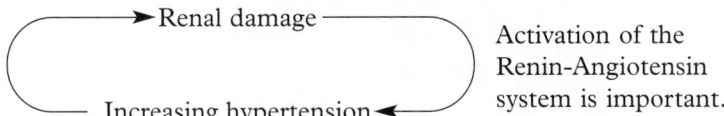

Activation of the Renin-Angiotensin system is important.

The renal consequences of benign and malignant hypertension differ, but in each, vascular changes are important.

## BENIGN HYPERTENSION

**Afferent arterioles**

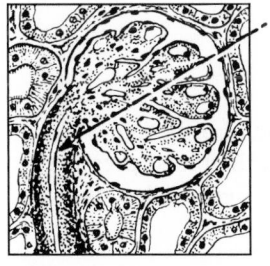

Thickening and hyalinisation of the vessel wall due to deposition of fibrin and basement membrane matrix.

These arteriolar changes lead to glomerular ischaemia.

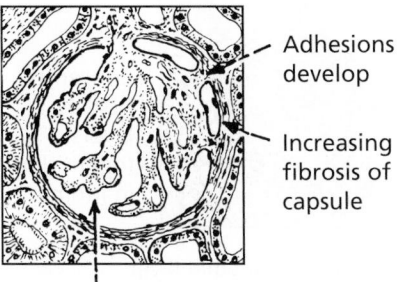

Adhesions develop

Increasing fibrosis of capsule

Capillaries collapse and disappear

**Interlobular arteries**

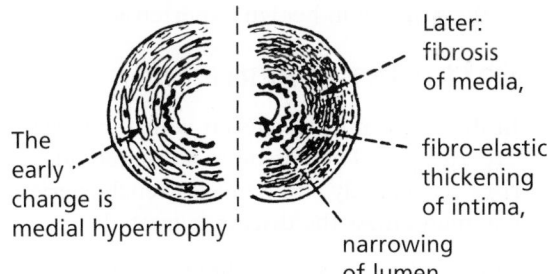

The early change is medial hypertrophy

Later: fibrosis of media,

fibro-elastic thickening of intima,

narrowing of lumen.

*Late*

*Late*

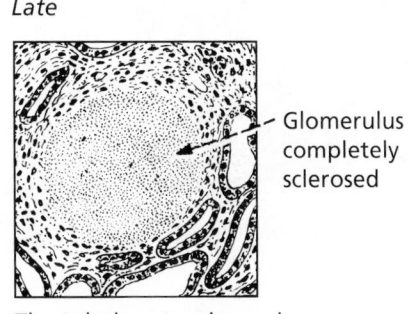

Glomerulus completely sclerosed

The tubules atrophy and there is interstitial fibrosis.

These changes are patchy in distribution so that renal failure rarely occurs.

# THE KIDNEY AND HYPERTENSION

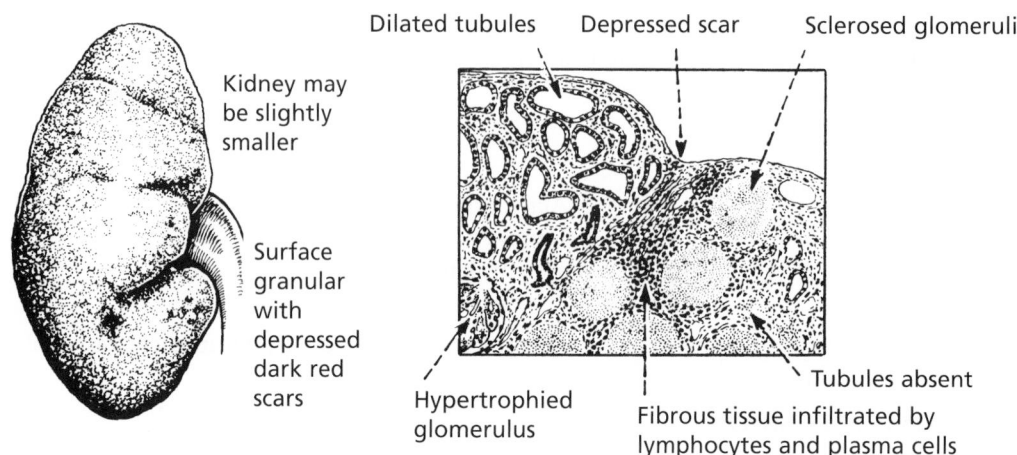

It is now thought that small emboli from atheroma of the aorta are responsible for much of the scarring in benign hypertension.

## MALIGNANT HYPERTENSION

In this form of hypertension which may arise *de novo* or on a background of benign hypertension. There is often an underlying cause for the hypertension; the blood pressure rises very rapidly and damages renal arteries, arterioles and glomeruli. Renal failure is common unless the disease is treated.

Afferent arterioles: the hallmark is **fibrinoid necrosis**.
Fibrinoid necrosis heals with the production of an 'onion-skin' lesion.

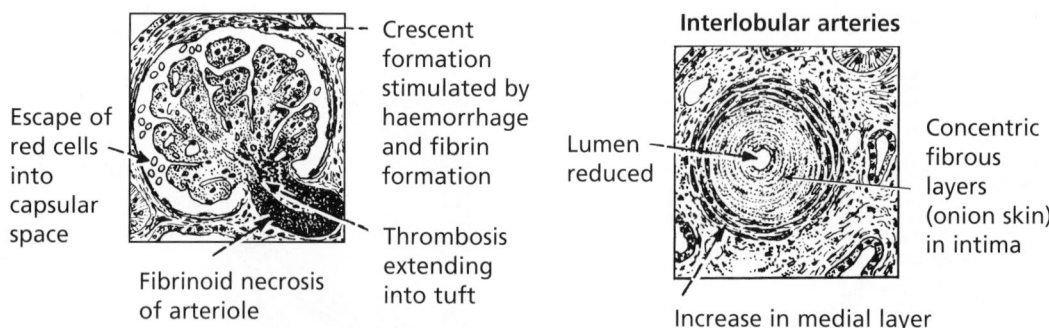

These changes account for the gross appearance.

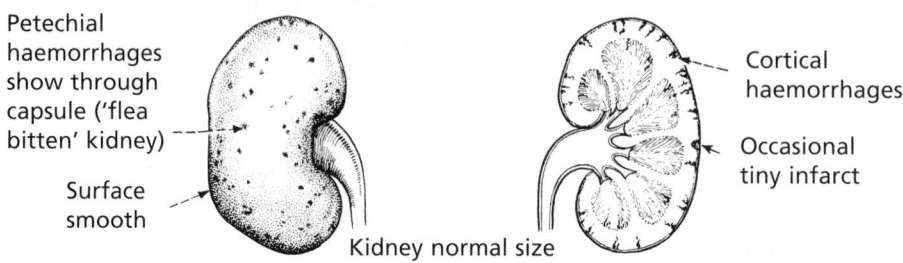

# CHRONIC RENAL FAILURE

Progressive renal damage in many kidney diseases eventually leads to chronic renal failure. The major causes include:

(a) Chronic glomerulonephritis.

(b) Chronic pyelonephritis and interstitial nephritis.

(c) Diabetic nephropathy.

(d) Obstructive uropathy.

(e) Polycystic kidneys.

In many cases the underlying cause cannot be determined.

The severity of renal failure is monitored by the serum urea, creatinine and by the glomerular filtration rate (GFR).

Chronic kidney disease

Stage 1 Slight kidney damage

2 Mild decrease in kidney function

3 Moderate decrease in kidney function

4 Severe decrease in kidney function

5 Renal failure requires dialysis or transplantation

The rate of decline depends on the underlying cause

**Compensatory mechanisms:**

As nephrons are lost, the surviving nephrons show (1) COMPENSATORY HYPERTROPHY and are (2) CONTINUALLY ACTIVE with no 'down time'. (In the normal kidney, the nephrons do not all function simultaneously.)

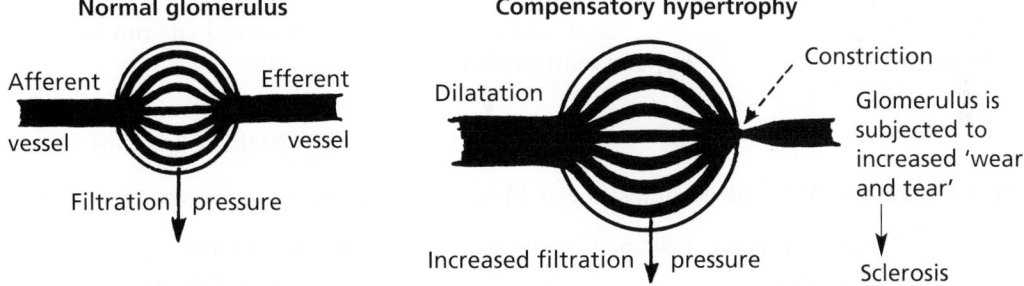

**Normal glomerulus**

Afferent vessel

Efferent vessel

Filtration pressure

**Compensatory hypertrophy**

Dilatation

Constriction

Glomerulus is subjected to increased 'wear and tear'

Increased filtration pressure

Sclerosis

**Effects of chronic renal failure:**

1. **WATER and ELECTROLYTE BALANCE**

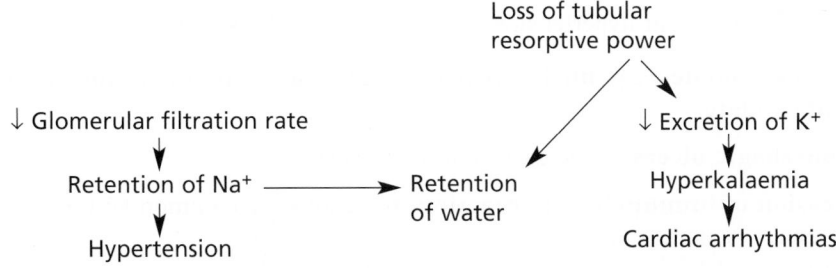

Loss of tubular resorptive power

↓ Glomerular filtration rate

Retention of Na⁺ ⟶ Retention of water

Hypertension

↓ Excretion of K⁺

Hyperkalaemia

Cardiac arrhythmias

Urine concentration is lost.

# CHRONIC RENAL FAILURE

### 2.  DISTURBANCE OF ACID–BASE BALANCE

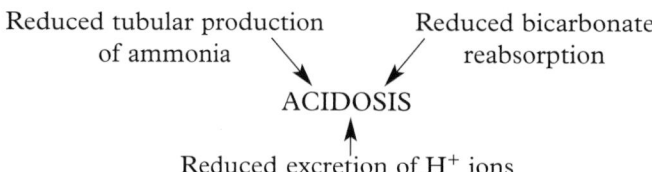

Reduced tubular production of ammonia

Reduced bicarbonate reabsorption

ACIDOSIS

Reduced excretion of $H^+$ ions

### 3.  URAEMIA

The kidney also fails to excrete nitrogenous waste products, which accumulate. Although urea concentrations rise and are used to monitor renal function, retention of urea is not in itself harmful.

In uraemia, patients are lethargic. Anorexia, nausea and vomiting are common, with confusion, convulsions and death.

### 4.  HORMONAL ABNORMALITIES

Three main hormones are involved: erythropoietin, parathyroid hormone and vitamin D.

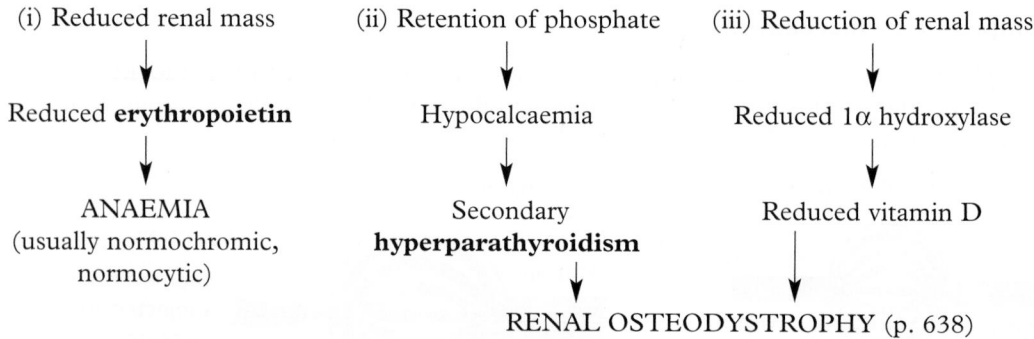

(i) Reduced renal mass

Reduced **erythropoietin**

ANAEMIA
(usually normochromic, normocytic)

(ii) Retention of phosphate

Hypocalcaemia

Secondary **hyperparathyroidism**

(iii) Reduction of renal mass

Reduced 1α hydroxylase

Reduced vitamin D

RENAL OSTEODYSTROPHY (p. 638)

### 5.  HYPERTENSION – this is almost inevitable and several consequences are possible.

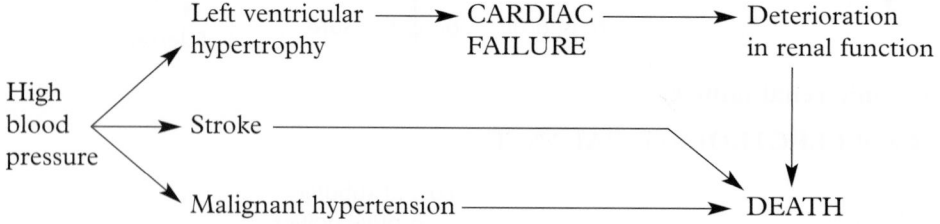

High blood pressure

Left ventricular hypertrophy → CARDIAC FAILURE → Deterioration in renal function

Stroke

Malignant hypertension → DEATH

6. **Fibrinous exudates,** e.g. **fibrinous pericarditis,** 'uraemic pneumonitis' with pleural exudate.

7. **Haemorrhagic ulcers** of the gastrointestinal tract.

8. **Depression of immunological reaction.** Infections are common and will in turn affect renal function.

# INFECTIONS OF THE KIDNEY AND URINARY TRACT

The kidney can become infected through two main routes.

(1) **Ascending infection** usually associated with **lower urinary tract infection** (obstruction and/or vesico-ureteric reflux are often present). This is by far the commoner route and gives rise to PYELONEPHRITIS.
(2) Blood borne (haematogenous) infection by pyogenic organisms (e.g. from septicaemia) or in tuberculosis (the latter now uncommon).

# ACUTE PYELONEPHRITIS

This is an acute ascending pyogenic infection and the patient exhibits the usual general features of pyrexia, nausea, vomiting, headaches, rigors, etc., plus localising signs, e.g. frequency, dysuria, loin pain and sometimes haematuria.

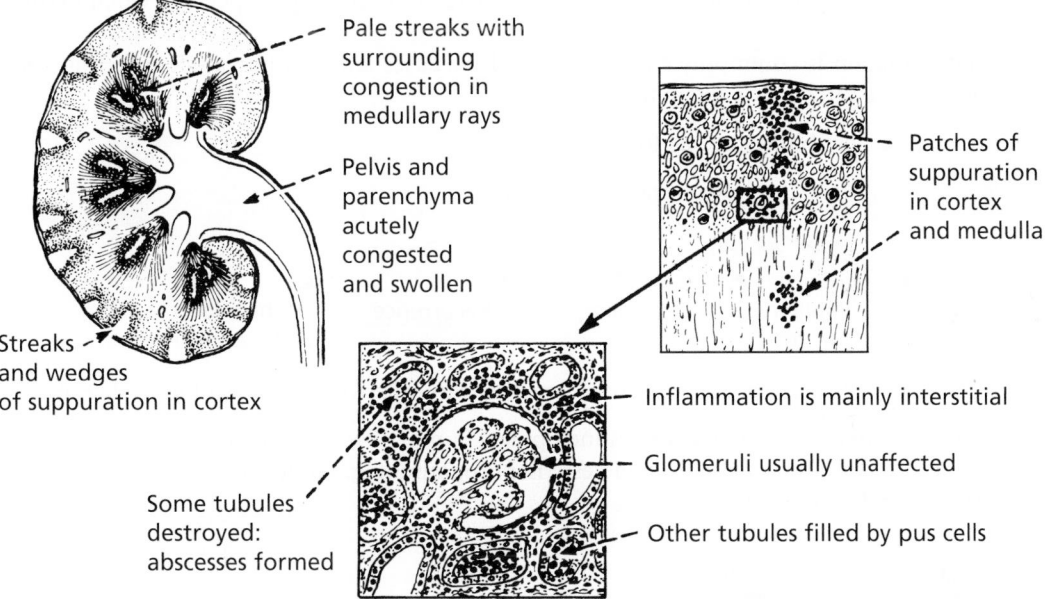

Pale streaks with surrounding congestion in medullary rays

Pelvis and parenchyma acutely congested and swollen

Streaks and wedges of suppuration in cortex

Some tubules destroyed: abscesses formed

Patches of suppuration in cortex and medulla

Inflammation is mainly interstitial

Glomeruli usually unaffected

Other tubules filled by pus cells

### Bacteriology

Large numbers of bacteria are found in the urine, several hundred thousand per mL in the acute phase.

The commonest infecting organism is *Escherichia coli*, but other faecal bacteria may also be found, e.g. proteus, *Streptococcus faecalis*.

# ACUTE PYELONEPHRITIS

### Causes

**In women**, cystitis is common, particularly in the sexually active. Ascending infection is often provoked by vesico-ureteric reflux during micturition. Pyelonephritis may occur in pregnancy.

**In men**, urinary tract obstruction is usually found, typically due to prostatic enlargement.

A number of causes of obstruction are seen in both sexes, e.g. calculi or tumours in the renal pelvis, tumours pressing on the ureter, calculi in ureters and tumours of the bladder.

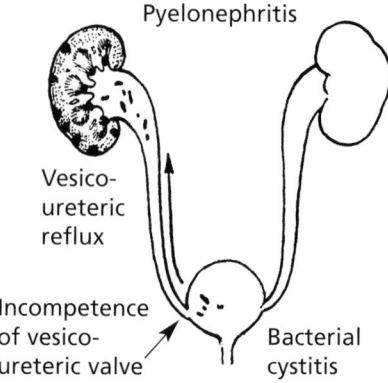

### Influence of urinary tract obstruction

Obstruction of the urinary tract acts in three ways to promote infection:
1. The urine tends to stagnate and encourages growth of bacteria.
2. A tendency to vesico-ureteric reflux during micturition develops especially when cystitis occurs.
3. Catheterisation is commonly carried out in these cases and can introduce infection. In this case the infection is likely to be mixed.

**Progress:** The possibilities are as follows:

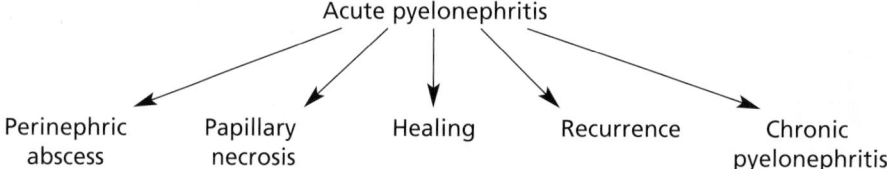

Perinephric abscess and papillary necrosis are now rare due to specific antibiotic therapy.

**Papillary necrosis** (maximal at the kidney poles) is most likely to occur in cases associated with urinary obstruction, diabetes, analgesic nephropathy (e.g. paracetamol, aspirin), sickle cell anaemia and severe hypotension.

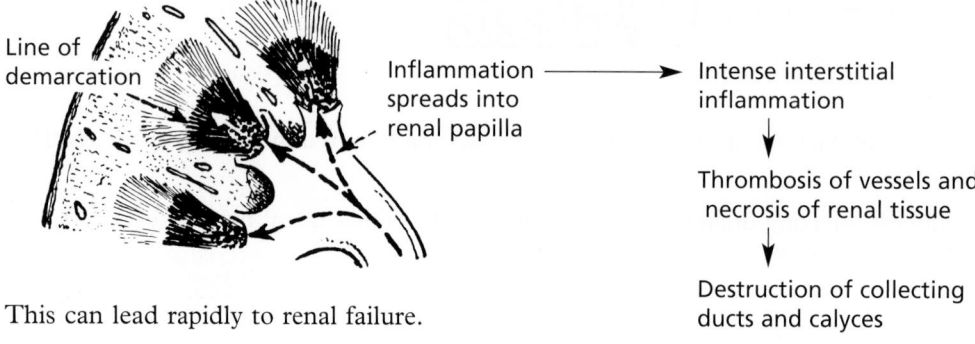

This can lead rapidly to renal failure.

# CHRONIC PYELONEPHRITIS

Chronic pyelonephritis is essentially the result of repeated attacks of inflammation and healing. Vesico-ureteric reflux in early life, often associated with congenital anomalies of the urinary tract, is now regarded as important. The process can be visualised as follows:

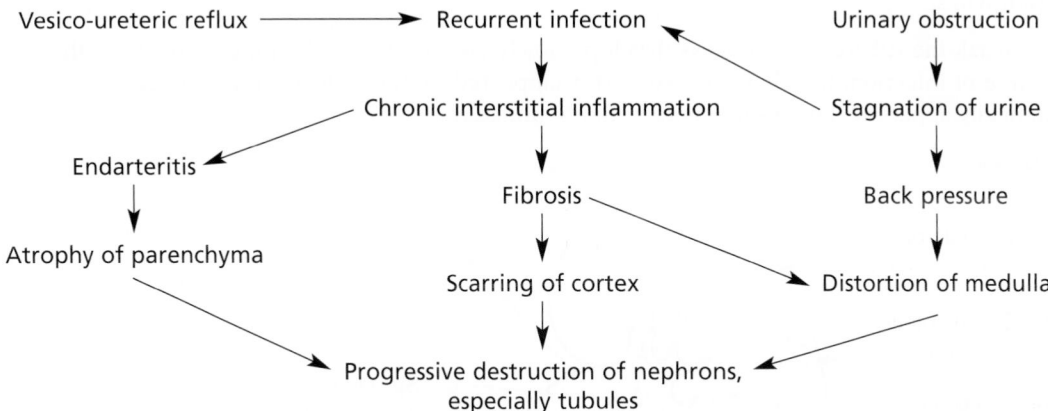

Kidney function may be further diminished by the onset of hypertension. In cases with urinary obstruction, the external size of the kidney may remain normal or even be increased. Those with no underlying abnormality, commoner in the female, show progressive contraction of the kidney which becomes greyish white.

Microscopically, there is interstitial fibrosis, inflammation and loss of parenchyma.

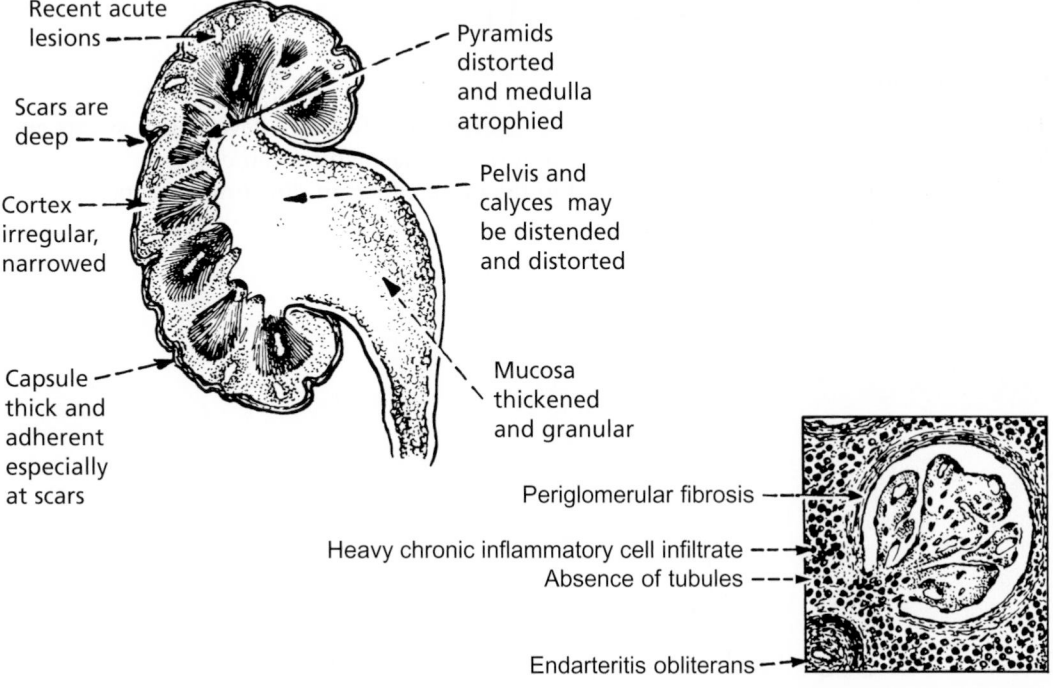

Depending on the cause, only one or both kidneys may be affected to variable degrees (c.f. chronic glomerulonephritis).

503

# TUBERCULOSIS OF THE KIDNEY

Tuberculosis of the kidney is uncommon in many Western countries. It is due to **blood spread of the infection** from another site, e.g. the lungs. Even less commonly, there may be an ascending infection from some other part of the genitourinary system, e.g. the epididymis.

As usual, the tuberculous process develops slowly and lesions in the lungs, which are the source of infection, may have healed and disappeared by the time kidney damage is clinically apparent. The disease is commonly unilateral.

### Stages

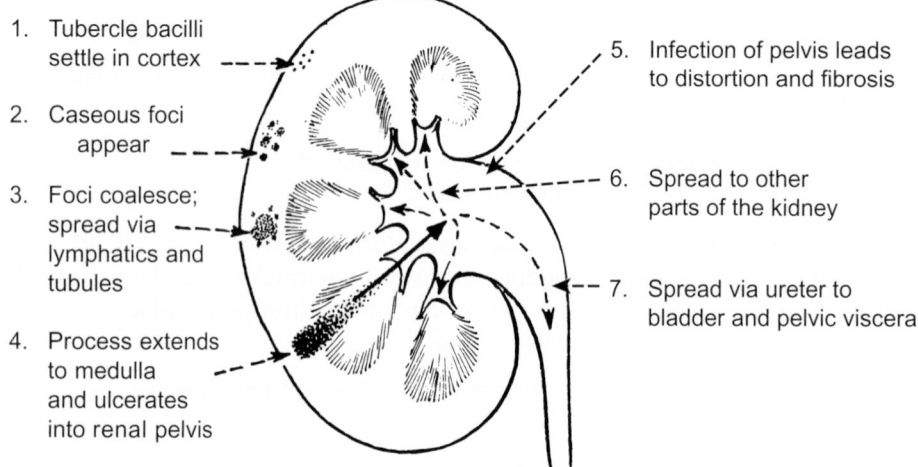

1. Tubercle bacilli settle in cortex

2. Caseous foci appear

3. Foci coalesce; spread via lymphatics and tubules

4. Process extends to medulla and ulcerates into renal pelvis

5. Infection of pelvis leads to distortion and fibrosis

6. Spread to other parts of the kidney

7. Spread via ureter to bladder and pelvic viscera

### Clinical features

The patient may show the general features of tuberculous infection – fever, night sweats and loss of weight. Lumbar discomfort or pain, dysuria and haematuria can develop. Mycobacteria can usually be demonstrated in the urine either on direct microscopic examination or by culture.

# INTERCURRENT RENAL CONDITIONS

## DIABETES

Renal complications are common in diabetes. Up to 30% of diabetic patients develop proteinuria, usually after many years, and may go on to chronic renal failure.

The renal lesion is a special form of the 'small vessel disease' seen systemically in insulin-dependent diabetes, e.g. diabetic retinopathy. Rarely, similar changes can be seen in non-diabetics.

**Diabetic glomerulosclerosis**. This takes one of two forms:

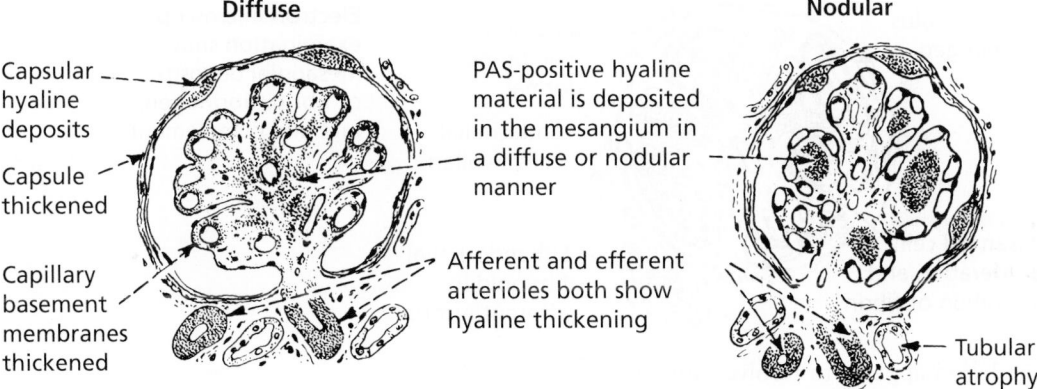

**Diffuse**

Capsular hyaline deposits

Capsule thickened

Capillary basement membranes thickened

PAS-positive hyaline material is deposited in the mesangium in a diffuse or nodular manner

Afferent and efferent arterioles both show hyaline thickening

**Nodular**

Tubular atrophy

The basement membrane thickening is due to deposition of abnormally glycosylated proteins. The nodular form is often termed the Kimmelstiel–Wilson lesion. Progressive closure of capillaries can occur together with fibrous obliteration of the capsular space and the whole glomerulus. Haemodynamic changes, especially hyperfiltration, lead to sclerosis. Secondary tubular atrophy follows.

## Clinical effects

Screening for microalbuminuria is important to detect early disease. Proteinuria may result in the nephrotic syndrome. Hypertension leads to further renal damage: control of blood pressure, and of diabetes itself, is important to delay the onset of renal failure. Inhibitors of angiotensin activity are particularly effective.

## Pyelonephritis

This is common in diabetes and may be complicated by papillary necrosis.

## Atheroma

This disease is common in the renal arteries and their branches in diabetes. It increases the renal ischaemia.

# RENAL FUNCTION AND PREGNANCY

Four conditions affecting renal function may arise in pregnancy.

1. **Acute pyelonephritis** is relatively common, possibly due to (a) the effects of uterine pressure on the ureters and (b) relaxation of smooth muscle, allowing ureteric dilatation and reflux.
2. **Pre-eclampsia and eclampsia**. This is a syndrome characterised by hypertension, increasing unselective proteinuria and oedema. Placental ischaemia with stimulation of vasoconstriction leads to disseminated intravascular coagulation (DIC). The main kidney lesion is glomerular; tubular changes are secondary.

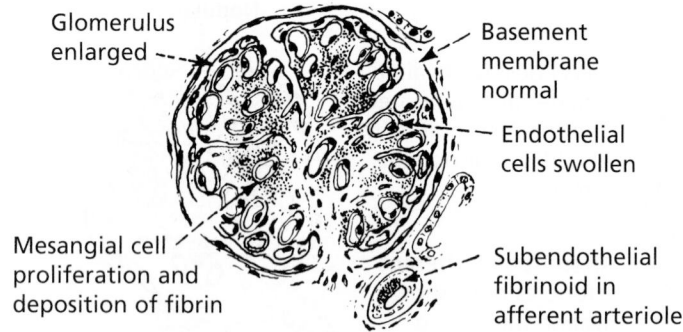

Glomerulus enlarged

Basement membrane normal

Endothelial cells swollen

Mesangial cell proliferation and deposition of fibrin

Subendothelial fibrinoid in afferent arteriole

Electron microscopy examination shows mesangial deposits of fibrin, fibrinogen, IgM and complement.

The lesion appears to resolve rapidly after birth.

**Acute tubular necrosis** is associated with complications of pregnancy causing SHOCK, e.g. septic abortion, retroplacental haemorrhage and postpartum haemorrhage.

In more severe cases **bilateral cortical necrosis** may occur especially if DIC is superadded.

Severe liver and cerebral damage may also occur.

# RENAL TUBULE – STRUCTURE AND FUNCTION

The renal tubules modify the glomerular filtrate. Initially isotonic and neutral, it becomes hypertonic and quite strongly acid. Within 24 hours, 180 L of filtrate are reduced to 1.5 L of urine. The main functions of this process are:

(a)  To get rid of waste products, particularly those of protein metabolism.
(b)  To aid in maintaining the normal acid–base balance.
(c)  To conserve fluid, electrolytes and other essential substances.

Three mechanisms are involved:

1.  Active absorption of substances from the filtrate by the tubular epithelium.
2.  Passive interchange between the filtrate and the interstitial tissues to maintain osmotic equilibrium.
3.  Secretion by the tubular epithelium.

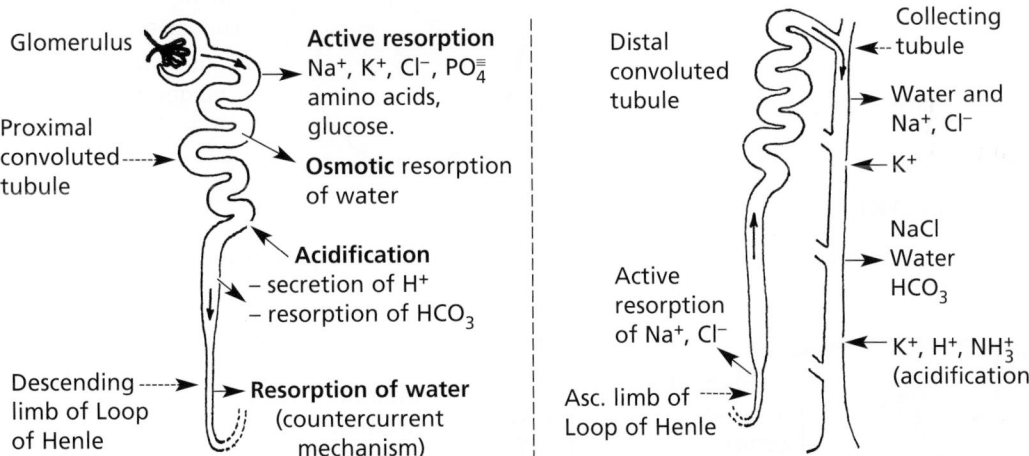

*Note:* Active reabsorption requires energy, and there is a limit to the capacity of the process – maximal tubular capacity (Tm). When this is exceeded, the particular substance involved will appear in the urine. Glucose is an example. In diabetes, the amount of glucose in the filtrate far exceeds the absorptive capacity, and glycosuria results.

**Effects of tubular damage**

Damage to the tubules results in gross biochemical changes.

1.  Loss of mechanisms controlling balance of electrolytes, water and urea.
2.  Upset in acid–base balance.
3.  Loss of substances in urine normally completely or almost completely reabsorbed – glucose, potassium, amino acids.

Glomerular lesions and pathological changes in the renal pelvis also upset tubular function by interfering with blood supply.

# ACUTE KIDNEY INJURY (AKI) (ACUTE TUBULAR NECROSIS)

This arises in two circumstances:

1. Due to ischaemia during a state of shock, e.g. due to haemorrhage, burns, trauma, acute intestinal obstruction, incompatible transfusion and acute pancreatitis.
2. Nephrotoxic: due to directly toxic substances, e.g. carbon tetrachloride, cis-platinum, lithium, mercury and various drugs, e.g. antibiotics, radiocontrast drugs.

The gross appearance of the kidneys is the same in both groups.

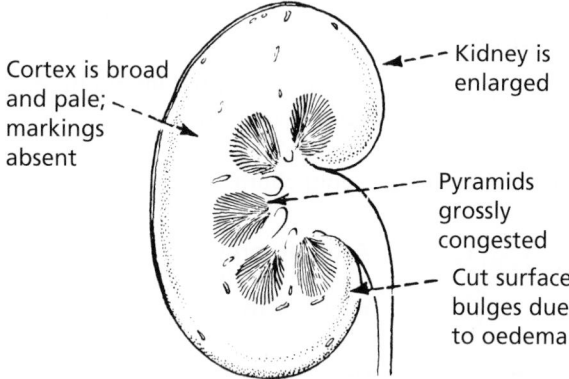

Cortex is broad and pale; markings absent

Kidney is enlarged

Pyramids grossly congested

Cut surface bulges due to oedema

### Ischaemic AKI

The lesions are the result of ischaemia, and this determines the part of the kidney affected and the portion of the tubule damaged.

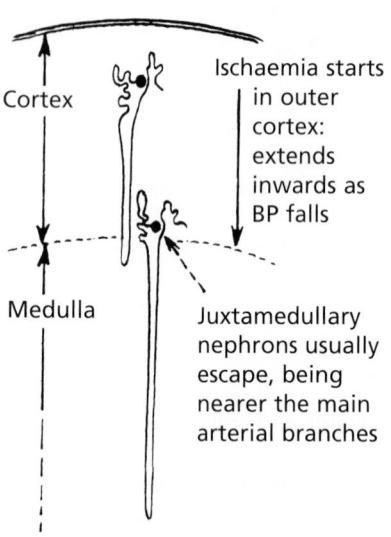

Cortex

Ischaemia starts in outer cortex: extends inwards as BP falls

Medulla

Juxtamedullary nephrons usually escape, being nearer the main arterial branches

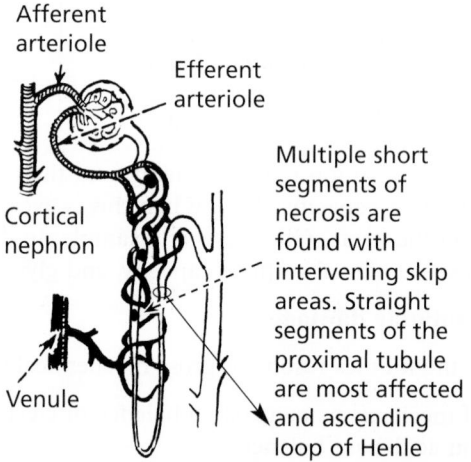

Afferent arteriole

Efferent arteriole

Cortical nephron

Venule

Multiple short segments of necrosis are found with intervening skip areas. Straight segments of the proximal tubule are most affected and ascending loop of Henle

Casts are found in the distal tubules, consisting largely of Tam–Horsfall protein and plasma proteins.

# ACUTE KIDNEY INJURY (ACUTE TUBULAR NECROSIS)

## Toxic AKI

The lesions are evenly distributed, affecting all nephrons. They are maximal in the proximal tubules and are the direct result of the toxin, the action of which is intensified by the concentrating activity of the tubule.

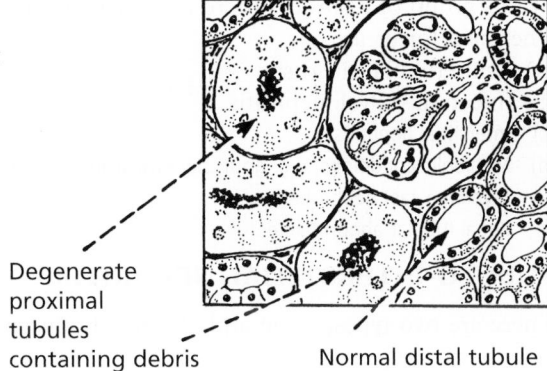

Degenerate proximal tubules containing debris

Normal distal tubule

## Clinical effects

There are two clinical phases:

### 1. *Oliguria*

The glomerular filtration rate is greatly reduced due to reduced renal blood flow.
Unselective reabsorption of the filtrate occurs through the damaged tubule. The effects are:

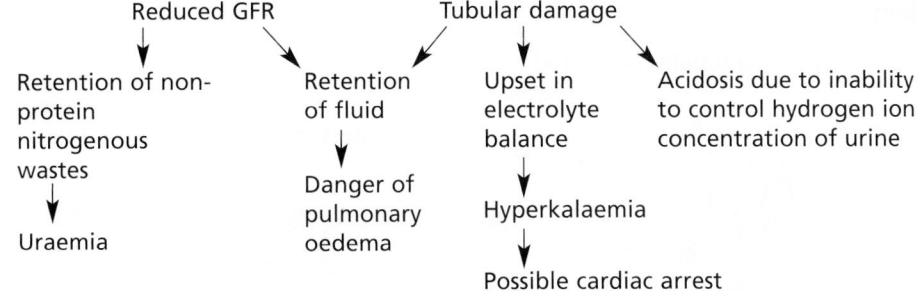

Reduced GFR → Tubular damage

- Retention of non-protein nitrogenous wastes → Uraemia
- Retention of fluid → Danger of pulmonary oedema
- Upset in electrolyte balance → Hyperkalaemia → Possible cardiac arrest
- Acidosis due to inability to control hydrogen ion concentration of urine

### 2. *Diuresis*

This occurs following healing of the lesions. The damaged tubular epithelium is replaced by a simple type which has not yet developed selective activities. Large volumes of dilute urine are passed.

The clinical results are:

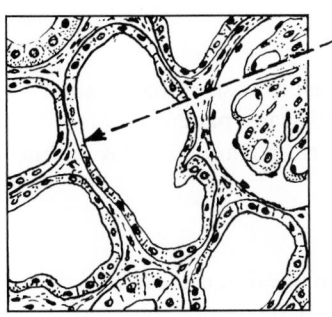

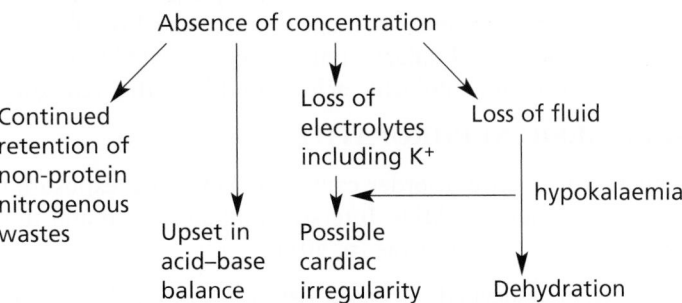

Absence of concentration

- Continued retention of non-protein nitrogenous wastes
- Upset in acid–base balance
- Loss of electrolytes including $K^+$ → Possible cardiac irregularity
- Loss of fluid → Dehydration
- hypokalaemia

The tubular epithelium has a great capacity for regeneration and ultimately regains its selective powers and the prognosis is good.

# TUBULO-INTERSTITIAL DISEASES

In this group of disorders there is damage to the renal tubules and to the interstitial tissues. The main forms are:

(a) Acute tubular necrosis  } Page 501
(b) Infection – Pyelonephritis

(c)  Interstitial nephritis

(d)  Metabolic conditions, e.g. gout, nephrocalcinosis, hypokalaemia

(e)  Myeloma cast nephropathy

(f)  Renal tubular abnormalities

## TUBULO-INTERSTITIAL NEPHRITIS

There are two types, acute and chronic, both typically associated with an immunological reaction to drugs.

*ACUTE:* symptoms develop 10–14 days after exposure to drugs, e.g. methicillin, and NSAIDs, e.g. mefenamic acid. Patients are febrile; there is haematuria, proteinuria. Arthralgia is common. Renal impairment varies in severity – may cause ACUTE RENAL FAILURE.

### Pathology

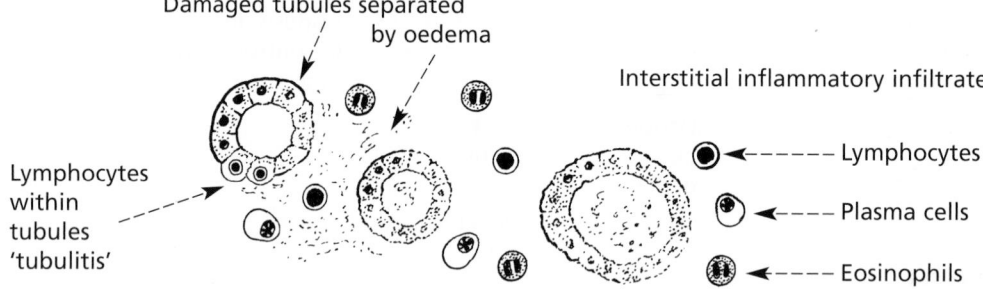

Prognosis (i)  Complete remission may follow withdrawal of drug and/or treatment with steroids.
      (ii)  Continuing exposure → chronic renal impairment.

*CHRONIC:* long-standing interstitial nephritis leads to interstitial fibrosis, inflammation and continuing tubular damage with tubular loss and atrophy. Many patients present with chronic renal failure. 'Balkan nephropathy' found in the river Danube valley is due to ingestion of aristolochic acid, found in herbal remedies.

## ANALGESIC NEPHROPATHY

This is a distinctive disorder caused by long-term exposure to analgesics, e.g. phenacetin (historically) and NSAIDs. Interstitial inflammation and tubular damage may proceed rapidly to papillary necrosis (p. 501).

There is an associated increased risk of transitional cell carcinoma of the kidney and ureter (p. 522).

Both minimal change and membranous glomerulonephritis may complicate NSAID therapy.

# METABOLIC TUBULAR LESIONS

These are due to metabolic defects.

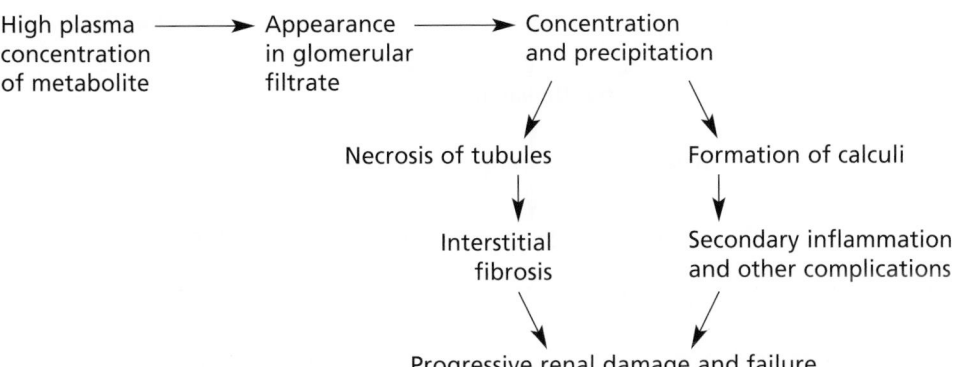

High plasma ⟶ Appearance ⟶ Concentration
concentration      in glomerular        and precipitation
of metabolite       filtrate

Necrosis of tubules          Formation of calculi

Interstitial          Secondary inflammation
fibrosis              and other complications

Progressive renal damage and failure

The following are some examples:

(a) **Hypercalcaemic nephritis**
Calcium is deposited in tubular epithelial cells with subsequent fibrosis and calcification
– **nephrocalcinosis**.

The usual causes of hypercalcaemia are malignant tumours, primary
hyperparathyroidism, hypervitaminosis D and sarcoidosis.

(b) **Urate nephropathy** occurs in patients with long standing hyperuricemia and **gout**.
Increased primary secretion of uric acid leads to uric acid crystal formation in the acid
environment of the distal tubule. Renal uric acid stones can occur.

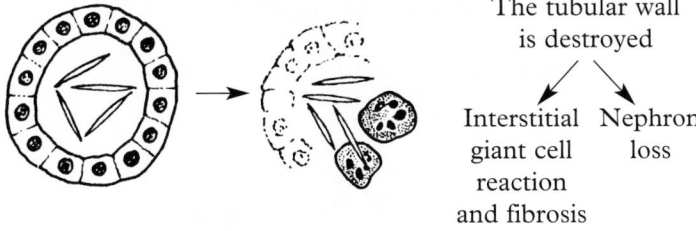

The tubular wall
is destroyed

Interstitial   Nephron
giant cell      loss
reaction
and fibrosis

(c) **Myeloma cast nephropathy**
This is dealt with on pages 470 and 471.

## RENAL TUBULAR ACIDOSIS

The tubules, either due to an inherited defect or to damage secondary to other renal
diseases, are unable to produce an acid urine.

There are two main forms:
1. In Type I the defect is in the distal tubule.
2. In Type II the function of the proximal tubule is abnormal and there are usually other
   abnormalities in addition to acidosis, e.g. in the Fanconi syndrome there is
   aminoaciduria, glycosuria and hypophosphatemia.

# THROMBOTIC MICROANGIOPATHIES (HAEMOLYTIC URAEMIC SYNDROME)

This is a rare complication of many conditions.

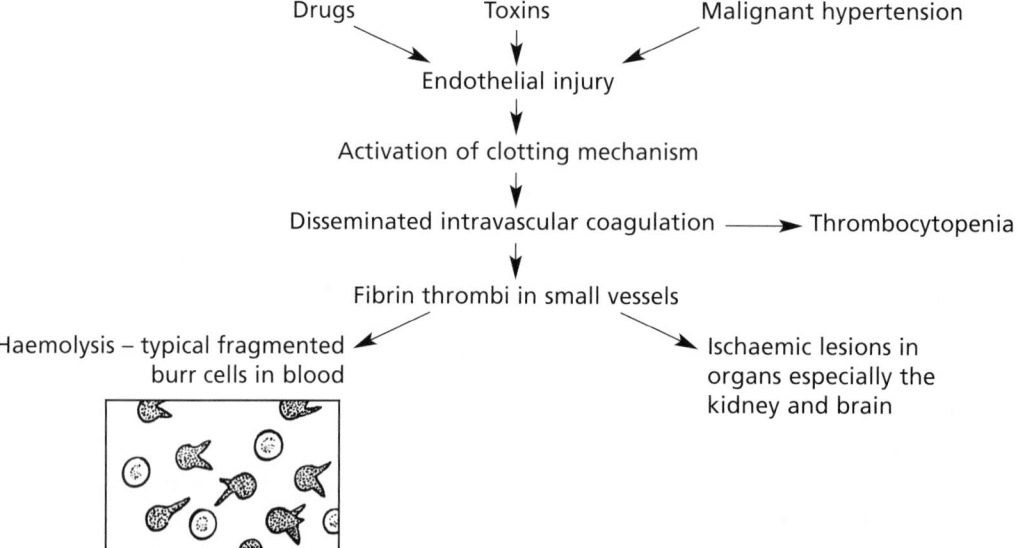

Drugs           Toxins           Malignant hypertension

Endothelial injury

Activation of clotting mechanism

Disseminated intravascular coagulation   ⟶   Thrombocytopenia

Fibrin thrombi in small vessels

Haemolysis – typical fragmented burr cells in blood

Ischaemic lesions in organs especially the kidney and brain

The renal lesions are similar to those seen in malignant hypertension. There is fibrinoid necrosis of the afferent arterioles and capillaries of the glomeruli, resulting in tubular necrosis. In the most extreme cases, bilateral cortical necrosis of the kidneys may occur. Clinical manifestations include renal failure, haemolytic anaemia, hypertension and sometimes purpura with thrombocytopenia.

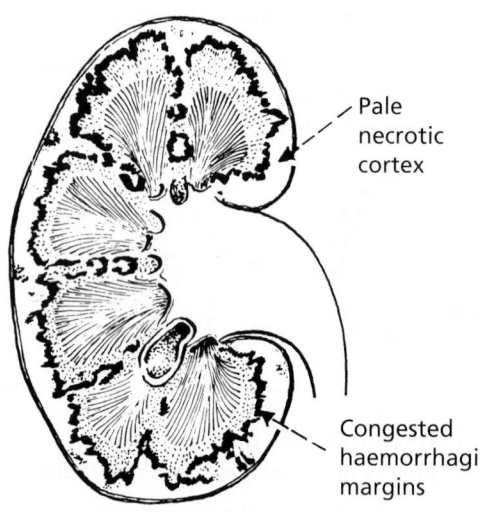

Pale necrotic cortex

Congested haemorrhagic margins

**Aetiology**

Activation of the clotting system can occur in many widespread circumstances:

1. In children there is a close association with gastrointestinal infections: particularly by *E. coli* 0157 which produces a verocytotoxin.
2. Shock, e.g. following abruptio placentae in pregnancy, endotoxic shock.
3. Malignant hypertension.
4. Drugs, e.g. immunosuppressives.

# PATHOLOGICAL COMPLICATIONS OF RENAL REPLACEMENT THERAPIES

The prognosis of end-stage renal failure has been greatly improved by (1) dialysis and (2) renal transplantation. The following possible pathological complications are important:

1. **Dialysis**

(a) *Haemodialysis*
   (i) **Local** – infection and thrombosis at site of vessel access.
   (ii) **Systemic** – aluminium toxicity: historically, severe dementia or severe osteomalacia was caused by using water containing excess aluminium. Aluminium and other impurities are now removed.

   Amyloidosis largely affecting osteoarticular tissues (e.g. carpal tunnel syndrome: joint stiffness, bone cysts) due to raised circulating $\beta_2$ microglobulin. Visceral involvement is rare and late.

(b) **Continuous Ambulatory Peritoneal Dialysis** – infective peritonitis: especially due to staphylococci, Gram-negative organisms and fungi.
   Sclerosing peritonitis is a non-infective complication with fibrous thickening of the peritoneum; this may result in small bowel obstruction or necrosis.

2. **Renal transplantation**
   Rejection is the main complication, depending on the extent of HLA matching between donor and recipient. The Banff classification is used to type rejection, of which there are four forms:

(a) *Hyperacute rejection* – within minutes or hours

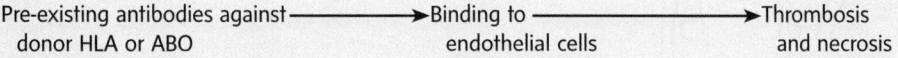

Pre-existing antibodies against ⟶ Binding to ⟶ Thrombosis
   donor HLA or ABO        endothelial cells        and necrosis

(b) *Acute cellular rejection* – within days to months

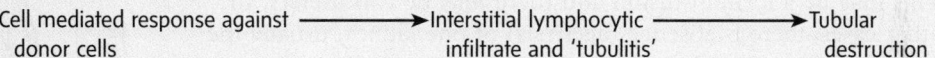

Cell mediated response against ⟶ Interstitial lymphocytic ⟶ Tubular
   donor cells        infiltrate and 'tubulitis'        destruction

(c) *Acute humoral rejection* – days to months

Cell mediated immune ⟶ Infiltration of vessel wall by ⟶ Thrombosis
   response to epithelial cells        lymphocytes 'endotheliitis'        and necrosis

(d) *Chronic rejection* – months to years

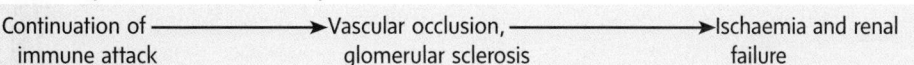

Continuation of ⟶ Vascular occlusion, ⟶ Ischaemia and renal
   immune attack        glomerular sclerosis        failure

### Other complications

1. Cyclosporin and tacrolimus toxicity
2. Opportunistic infections
3. Increased incidence of tumours, particularly LYMPHOMAS

Associated with therapeutic immuno-suppression.
*Note:* Many lymphoproliferative disorders are due to Epstein–Barr virus infection and some respond to reduction in immuno-suppressive therapy.

4. Recurrence of original renal disease, e.g. IgA nephropathy in transplanted kidney.

# CONGENITAL DISORDERS

There are many forms of malpositions and malformations of the kidney:

1.  **Ectopic kidney (pelvic kidney)**

    One or both kidneys fail to reach the normal adult position. The condition causes difficulty:
    (a) During childbirth.
    (b) In differential diagnosis of pelvic neoplasms and infections.
    (c) When the renal artery originates at the normal level and the long vessel creates problems in arterial supply.

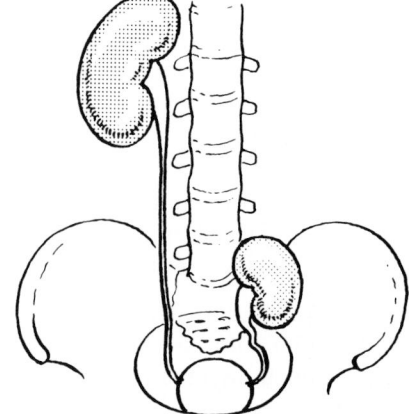

2.  **Fusion of kidneys**

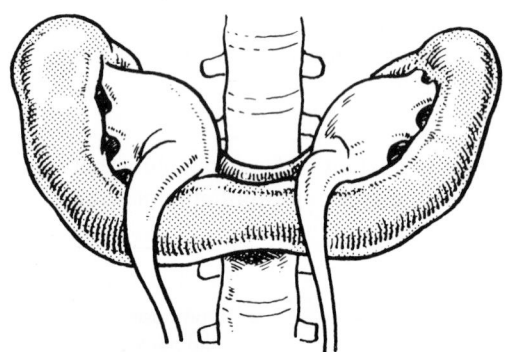

This is usually partial, producing the so-called 'horse-shoe' kidney. The ureters may be partially obstructed leading to hydronephrosis, infection and stones.

3.  **Single kidney**

    This may be a form of fusion and there may be two ureters. In other cases, there is absence (agenesis) of one kidney, usually the left. There is no interference with renal function unless, of course, the single kidney becomes diseased.

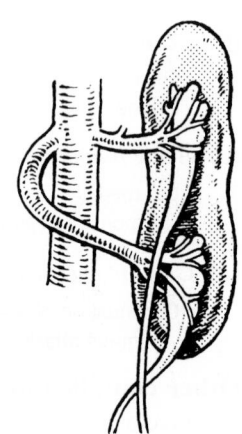

4.  **Bilateral agenesis (Potter syndrome)**

    This is incompatible with life. The affected infants have a distinctive appearance, with low set ears, receding chin, parrot beak nose and wide set eyes.

# POLYCYSTIC KIDNEY DISEASE

This occurs in two main forms:

1. **Autosomal Dominant Polycystic Kidney Disease (ADPKD)**

   This is relatively common, and accounts for 5–10% of cases of chronic renal failure. The kidneys are converted into a mass of cysts with loss of renal parenchyma.

   It is an inherited autosomal dominant trait due to two genes, *PKD-1* (85% of cases) which encodes a protein polycystin-1, and *PKD-2* (15%) which encodes polycystin 2 and is associated with milder disease.

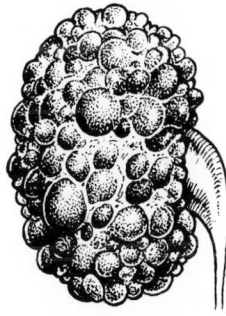

Kidney greatly enlarged: (often exceeds 1 kg)

Cysts vary in size (largest 3–4 cm)

Many are brownish (fluid serous or mucoid)

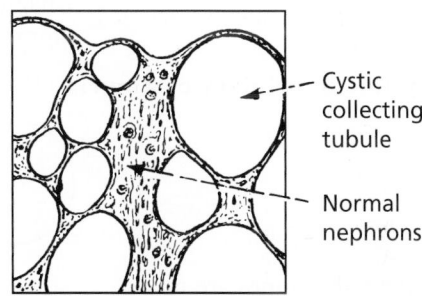

Cystic collecting tubule

Normal nephrons

The precise defect is unclear but defects of the cilia of tubular epithelial cells appear responsible. There is cyst formation in some of the collecting tubules, causing a mixture of normal and abnormal nephrons. Cystic change develops after birth and is progressive, resulting in atrophy of normal nephrons by pressure.

Cysts also occur in the liver. Death from cerebral haemorrhage is more frequent than expected, partly due to the hypertension secondary to the kidney disorder and in some cases due to 'berry aneurysms' of cerebral arteries at the circle of Willis.

It is usually discovered during the third and fourth decades.

2. **Autosomal Recessive (Childhood) Polycystic Kidney Disease**

This is a rare condition, which may present in the perinatal period or later in childhood.

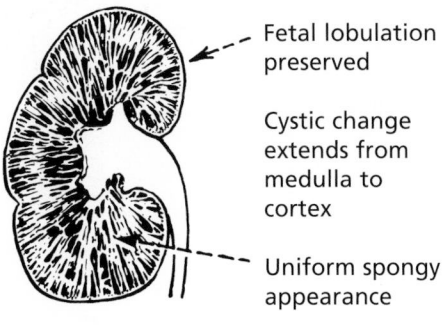

Fetal lobulation preserved

Cystic change extends from medulla to cortex

Uniform spongy appearance

The nephrons are said to be normal in number and formation. Cystic dilatation is situated in the terminal branches of the collecting tubules. The disease, if severe, is incompatible with life, and death occurs shortly after birth. It is an autosomal recessive trait due to mutations of the *PKHD-1* gene which encodes a protein, fibrocystin. Congenital hepatic fibrosis often dominates in children who survive infancy.

# URINARY CALCULI

Stones may form in the renal pelvis, ureter or bladder.

Four basic types of renal calculi are recognised.

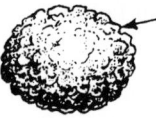 Surface is rough; colour brown, probably due to old blood pigment

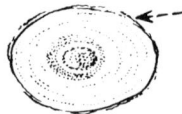 Flaking surface, greyish white

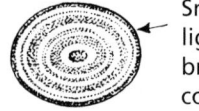 Smooth light brown colour

(1) **Calcium oxalate** (~80%).

(2) **Triple phosphates** (magnesium phosphate ammonium) (15%).

(3) **Uric acid and urates** (5%).

(4) **Cystine in primary cystinuria** (1%).

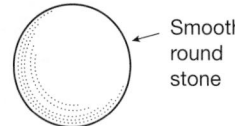 Smooth round stone

Commonly the stones are mixed.

**Mode of formation.** There are two steps – *nucleation* followed by *aggregation*:

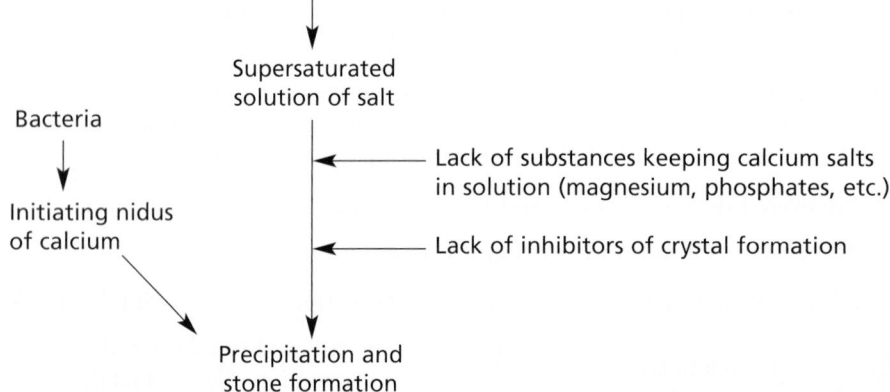

Excess excretion of stone substance (e.g. oxalate) + Calcium

Supersaturated solution of salt

Bacteria

Initiating nidus of calcium

Lack of substances keeping calcium salts in solution (magnesium, phosphates, etc.)

Lack of inhibitors of crystal formation

Precipitation and stone formation

# URINARY CALCULI

## Predisposing factors

1. **Urinary pH**. Urate and oxalate stones form in an acid urine; phosphate stones in alkaline urine.
2. **Dehydration** – causing increased urinary concentration.
3. **Stasis**. Obstruction to urine flow encourages salt precipitation.
4. **Infection** is one of the most important factors.
5. **Metabolic factors**. These can operate by altering the pH of the urine and especially by increasing the output of substances, e.g.

   (a) Hypercalciuria and hyperphosphaturia. These may be caused by: hyperparathyroidism, primary or secondary to renal failure, Vitamin D overdose, diet, e.g. excessive milk and alkalis over years in peptic ulcer cases, immobilisation leading to loss of calcium from bones.
   (b) Oxaluria. Due to:
   Congenital metabolic defect (primary oxaluria), Intestinal over absorption in enteric diseases and vegetarians.
   (c) Urate excess.
   (d) Rare stones, e.g. cystine, xanthine, are related to inborn metabolic defects.

## Effects

This can lead to:

- Renal colic.
- Hydronephrosis.
- Infection, e.g. pyelonephritis.

With the development of stasis and infection, further stone formation is encouraged:

### Staghorn calculus

This large single stone is associated with suppuration and ulceration of the pelvis and calyces. It is composed mainly of phosphates.

Stones and infection in the pelvis can lead to squamous metaplasia of the epithelium. In a few instances this may develop into squamous carcinoma.

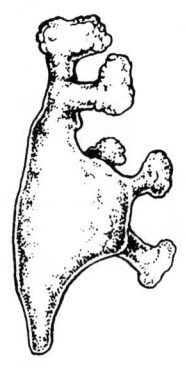
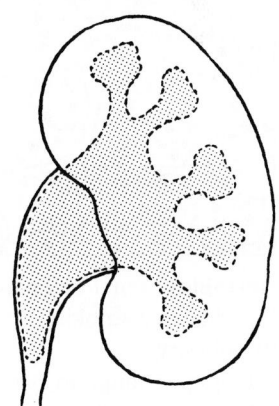

## BLADDER CALCULI

These may have passed down the ureter. In the bladder they can increase greatly in size, due to the deposition of phosphates. Cystitis is common. Stones may actually form in the bladder when there is urethral obstruction and chronic cystitis.

# TUMOURS OF THE KIDNEY

### MALIGNANT TUMOURS

Many types of benign and malignant tumours occur in the kidney. The three most common malignant tumours are: renal cell carcinoma, transitional cell carcinoma and nephroblastoma (Wilms tumour).

### 1. Renal cell carcinoma

This is the commonest (90%) primary malignant renal tumour and arises from tubular epithelium. It has a typical appearance.

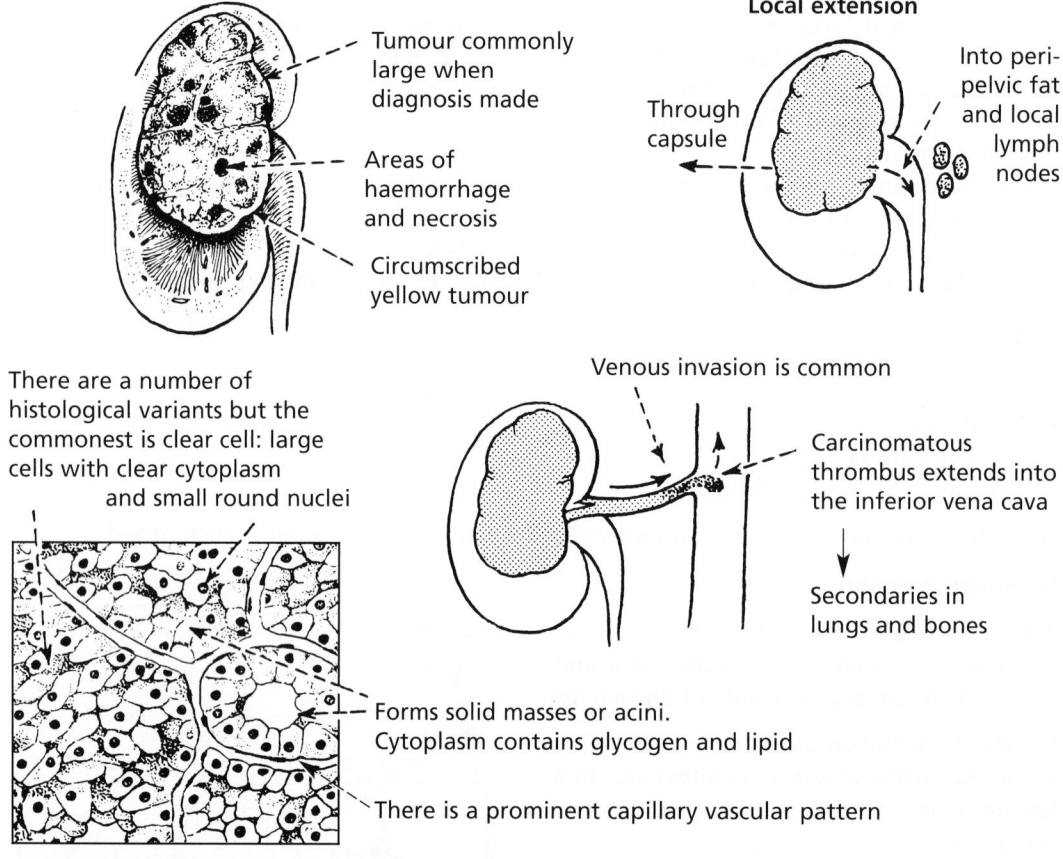

Tumour commonly large when diagnosis made

Areas of haemorrhage and necrosis

Circumscribed yellow tumour

**Local extension**

Through capsule

Into peri-pelvic fat and local lymph nodes

There are a number of histological variants but the commonest is clear cell: large cells with clear cytoplasm and small round nuclei

Venous invasion is common

Carcinomatous thrombus extends into the inferior vena cava

Secondaries in lungs and bones

Forms solid masses or acini. Cytoplasm contains glycogen and lipid

There is a prominent capillary vascular pattern

**Aetiology**: renal cell carcinoma is associated with:
(a) cigarette smoking
(b) obesity
(c) cystic change in patients on haemodialysis
(d) genetic predisposition, e.g. the von Hippel–Lindau syndrome (renal cysts, cerebellar haemangioblastoma) – associated with a gene on chromosome 3

# TUMOURS OF THE KIDNEY

**Systemic effects**

Patients with renal carcinoma may have:

(i) Hypercalcaemia – parathyroid-related hormone peptide production (PTHrP).
(ii) Hypertension – increased renin production by tumour or in adjacent kidney.
(iii) Polycythaemia – increased erythropoietin.

## 2. Transitional cell carcinoma

This tumour arises from the epithelium of the renal pelvis and is similar to the commoner transitional cell carcinoma of the bladder, with which it shares aetiological factors.

Patients usually present with haematuria.

## 3. Nephroblastoma (Wilms' tumour)

This is one of the commonest malignant tumours of childhood usually presenting between 2 and 5 years. About 10% are bilateral. It is an embryonic type of tumour derived from 'nephrogenic rests', and forms a large well-circumscribed growth which rapidly invades blood vessels, giving rise to pulmonary secondaries. With modern therapy 90% long-term survival rates are achieved.

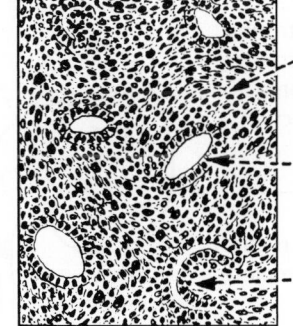

Much of the tumour consists of spindle cells resembling sarcoma

This merges with tubules and acini

Occasionally there are primitive glomerular structures

There may be skeletal muscle differentiation.

Mutation of the Wilms tumour gene (*WT-1*) on chromosome 11 and a variety of other genes appear to be responsible for the development of this tumour.

## BENIGN TUMOURS

1. **Oncocytoma**. This benign epithelial tumour accounts for 5% of surgically removed tumours. It arises from cells of the collecting ducts. The cells are large with eosinophilic nuclei due to many mitochondria.
2. **Papillary adenoma**. This is a small (<5 mm) nodular proliferation of tubular-type epithelium.
3. **Angiomyolipoma**. This mass of fat, blood vessels and smooth muscle may occur sporadically or in tuberous sclerosis.

# DISEASES OF THE URINARY TRACT

The urinary tract is a collecting and discharge system. There are four main pathological processes affecting its function: (1) obstruction, (2) infection, (3) calculus formation and (4) neoplastic disease.

## OBSTRUCTION

Acute obstruction, if complete, causes rapid cessation of urine production. If both kidneys are involved, renal failure quickly follows. Chronic obstruction is more common and leads to anatomical changes.

## HYDRONEPHROSIS

This is a dilatation of the renal pelvis and calyces, due to chronic incomplete or intermittent obstruction.

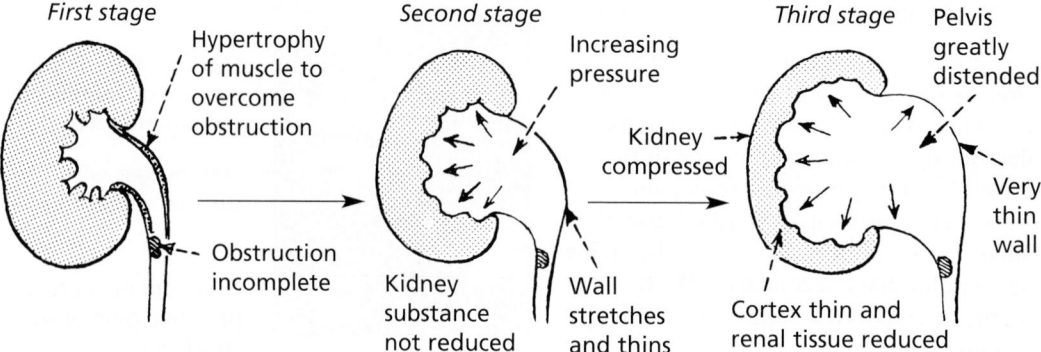

First stage — Hypertrophy of muscle to overcome obstruction — Obstruction incomplete

Second stage — Increasing pressure — Kidney substance not reduced — Wall stretches and thins

Third stage — Kidney compressed — Pelvis greatly distended — Very thin wall — Cortex thin and renal tissue reduced

Microscopically, there is tubular atrophy and glomerular scarring. Superimposed infection is common and aggravates the renal damage.

### Aetiology

The condition may affect one or both kidneys. This is related to the site of obstruction.

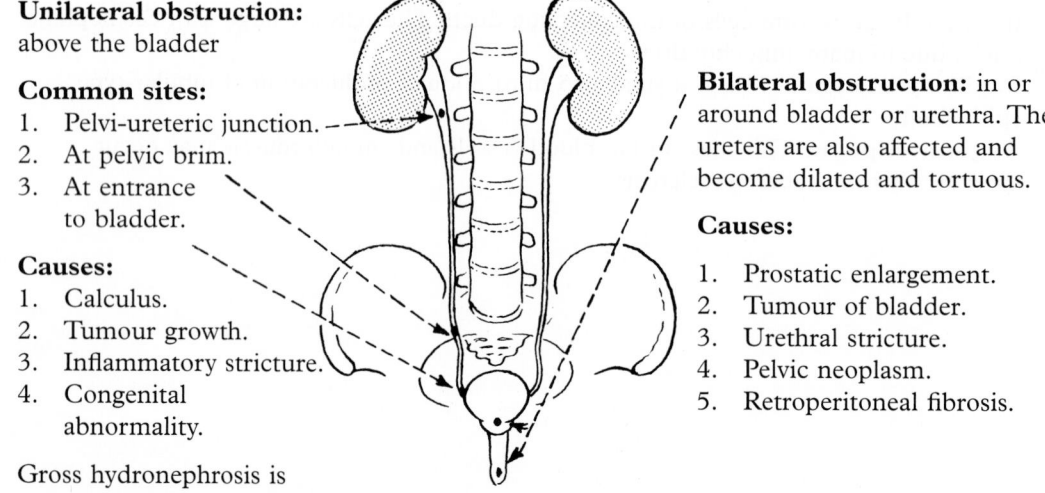

**Unilateral obstruction:** above the bladder

**Common sites:**
1. Pelvi-ureteric junction.
2. At pelvic brim.
3. At entrance to bladder.

**Causes:**
1. Calculus.
2. Tumour growth.
3. Inflammatory stricture.
4. Congenital abnormality.

Gross hydronephrosis is more commonly unilateral.

**Bilateral obstruction:** in or around bladder or urethra. The ureters are also affected and become dilated and tortuous.

**Causes:**
1. Prostatic enlargement.
2. Tumour of bladder.
3. Urethral stricture.
4. Pelvic neoplasm.
5. Retroperitoneal fibrosis.

# URINARY TRACT INFECTION

### Acute cystitis
The bladder shows the usual signs of inflammation. Small haemorrhages are common in the oedematous mucosa. The causes have already been discussed.

### Chronic cystitis
This is the result of repeated attacks of acute cystitis. It is usually associated with obstruction of the urethra causing stasis of urine.

Mixed infection including *Bacillus proteus* is common and, together with urea-splitting organisms forming ammonia, result in an alkaline urine. Phosphates precipitate and can form crumbling whitish calculi.

### Interstitial cystitis
This disorder usually affects women who complain of intermittent pain, frequency and dysuria without bacterial infection.

Mast cells are commonly seen in the mucosa which may show typical ulcers (Hunner ulcers). The cause is unknown.

### Tuberculous cystitis
This is always secondary to a tuberculous infection elsewhere, usually in the kidney. Less commonly, the epididymis is the source of infection. Small tubercles form in the submucous layer, usually at the bladder base. These ulcerate and secondary infection is common.

### Urethritis
Acute inflammation of the urethra is commonly due to gonococcus. Another form is however now more common in Western countries: non-gonococcal urethritis. It is caused in the main by *Chlamydia trachomatis*, a Gram-negative bacterium. It is associated with prostatitis, epididymitis, pharyngitis, conjunctivitis and perihepatitis. Diagnosis is by molecular testing of voided urine.

It is also associated with reactive arthritis, see p. 655.

### Schistosomiasis
Infection of the bladder with *Schistosoma haematobium* results in chronic granulomatous inflammation with urinary obstruction and haematuria. There is a strong association with the development of squamous cell carcinoma of the bladder.

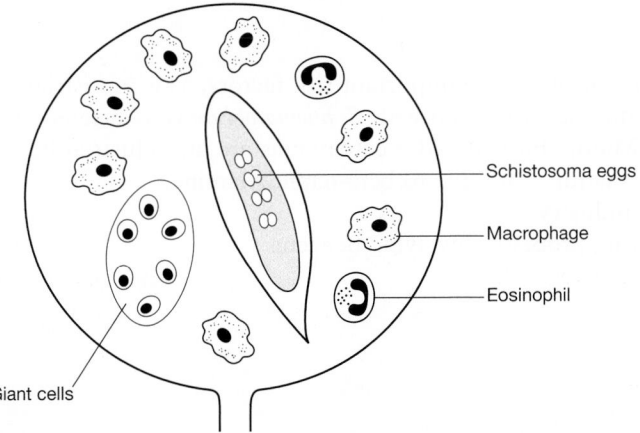

Schistosoma eggs

Macrophage

Eosinophil

Giant cells

# TUMOURS OF THE UROTHELIUM

### TRANSITIONAL CELL CARCINOMA

**Transitional cell** carcinomas occur in the bladder, ureters and renal pelvis. They arise from the stratified transitional epithelium lining the tract and are all considered to be CARCINOMAS but show a wide spectrum of malignant potential. They are graded I to III according to the World Health Organisation (WHO) classification. They can be papillary or solid in growth pattern.

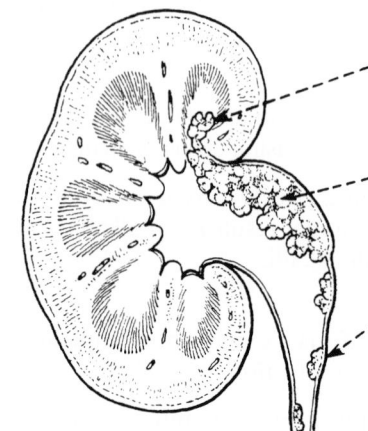

Invasion into renal parenchyma is often seen.

Papillary tumour arising in renal pelvis.

Multiple tumours may be seen in the ureter – representing a field change. At surgery the entire ureter is usually resected.

**GRADE I** – these are usually **papillary tumours** with uniform, well-differentiated epithelial covering showing no mitotic activity, a slender stalk and delicate branching fronds. Haemorrhage is common.

**GRADE II** – these also are mainly **papillary**. The epithelial cells show mitoses and nuclear pleomorphism.

**GRADE III** – are often solid sessile tumours. They show marked nuclear pleomorphism, mitotic activity and aggressive growth. Ulceration and necrosis are common: invasion into the bladder muscle and lymphatic invasion are usual.

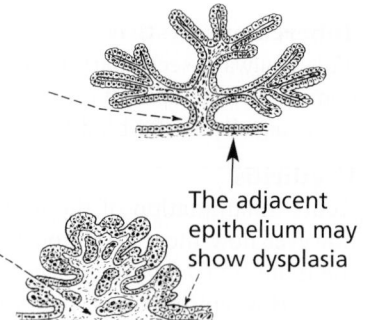

The adjacent epithelium may show dysplasia

Squamous carcinoma and adenocarcinoma are rare tumours. Rhabdomyosarcoma may occur in the bladder in children.

(i) Urothelial tumours are often multiple and recurrence is common: long-term surveillance is important.

(ii) Progression from a low grade to higher grades is frequent.

### Aetiology

Smoking and analgesic abuse are important risk factors, as is industrial exposure, e.g. rubber and dye industries. Infection with *S. haematobium* is associated with squamous carcinoma in the Middle East. Bladder carcinomas are an industrial hazard:

(a) In aniline dye manufacture due to beta-naphthylamine.

(b) In the rubber industry.

(c) In manufacturing processes involving benzene.

# THE PROSTATE

The prostate surrounds the bladder neck and urethra. Although traditionally divided into five lobes, it is now regarded as having four major zones, which tend to be affected by different disorders.

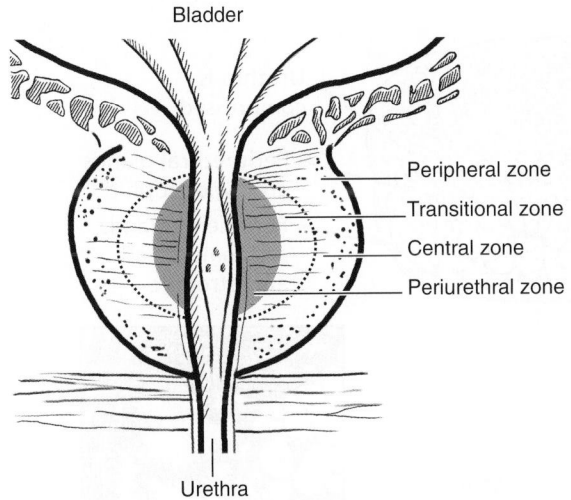

Bladder

Peripheral zone

Transitional zone

Central zone

Periurethral zone

Urethra

Its internal structure is a series of branching glands in a fibromuscular stroma.

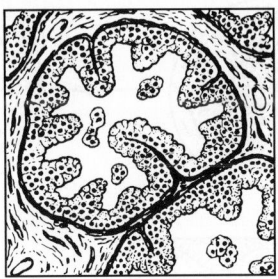

There are three main disorders of the prostate:

1. Prostatitis
2. Benign prostatic hyperplasia
3. Prostatic carcinoma

## Prostatitis

There are three forms:

1. *Acute bacterial prostatitis* – associated with urinary tract infections – usually by Gram-negative bacilli such as *E. coli*. Instrumentation, e.g. catheterisation, may provoke the episode.
2. *Chronic bacterial prostatitis* – due to repeated urinary tract infections, usually by the same group of organisms.
3. *Chronic abacterial prostatitis* – the cause of this is unknown. The patient complains of urinary symptoms such as dysuria and frequency, low back pain and perineal discomfort.
4. *Granulomatous prostatitis* – can be seen in a variety of situations, e.g. TB and following BCG therapy for bladder cancer. Ruptured ducts and acini may stimulate a granulomatous reaction which can mimic cancer.

# DISEASES OF THE PROSTATE

### BENIGN PROSTATIC HYPERPLASIA

This is an extremely common finding in over 70% of men over 60 years. The prostate is enlarged, often over 100 g (normal prostate 20 g). The transitional and periurethral zones are most affected.

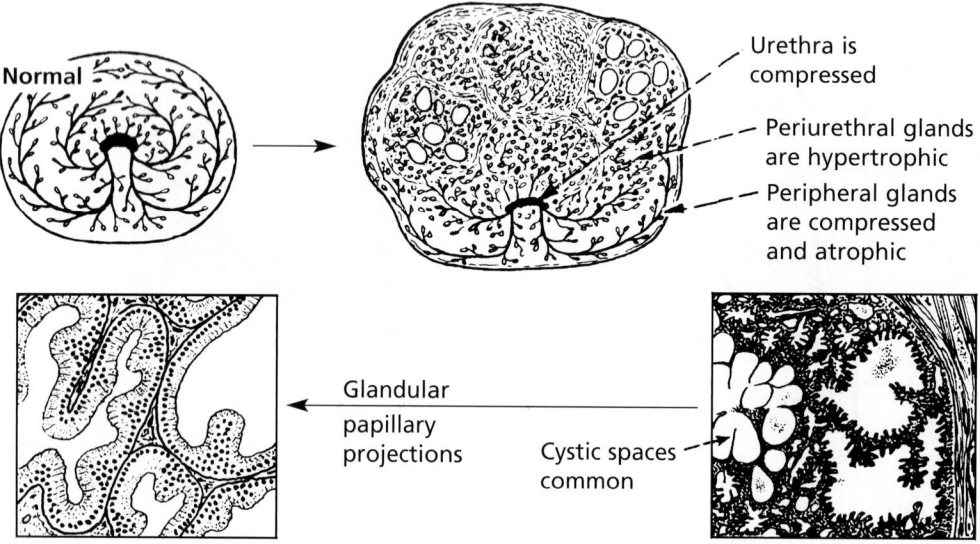

**Normal**

Urethra is compressed

Periurethral glands are hypertrophic

Peripheral glands are compressed and atrophic

Glandular papillary projections

Cystic spaces common

### Aetiology

Androgens are responsible for prostatic proliferation with conversion of testosterone to dihydrotestosterone by the enzyme $5\alpha$-reductase, found mainly in prostatic stromal cells.

Use of $5\alpha$-reductase inhibitors is effective treatment in many cases; often combined with $\alpha$ adrenergic blockers.

### Complications

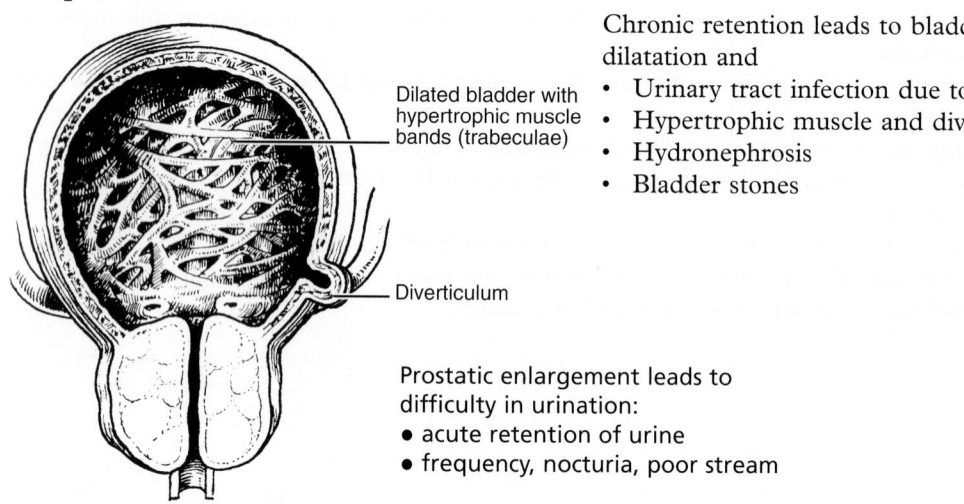

Dilated bladder with hypertrophic muscle bands (trabeculae)

Diverticulum

Chronic retention leads to bladder dilatation and
- Urinary tract infection due to stasis
- Hypertrophic muscle and diverticula
- Hydronephrosis
- Bladder stones

Prostatic enlargement leads to difficulty in urination:
• acute retention of urine
• frequency, nocturia, poor stream

Nodularity of lateral lobes with compression of urethra

# ADENOCARCINOMA OF THE PROSTATE

This is now the commonest cancer in men in the United Kingdom and a significant cause of cancer death. It is rare below the age of 40 and rises to very high prevalence in men over 80.

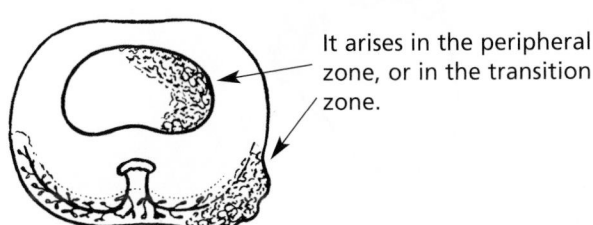 It arises in the peripheral zone, or in the transition zone.

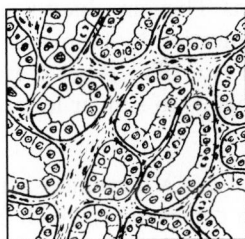 Closely set small irregular acini lined by a single layer of epithelium.

### Histological grading

The GLEASON system (grades 2 through 10) indicates the degree of differentiation from (2) very well differentiated to (10) aggressive anaplastic tumours. Grading correlates well with prognosis.

### Spread

1. Direct spread occurs throughout the prostate and outwards to the pelviprostatic tissue.
2. Lymphatic spread is the main mode of extension. There is a rich lymphatic plexus and the perineural lymphatics are particularly affected. The pelvic nodes are invaded and subsequently the abdominal chain.
3. Bone metastases tend to be common, especially in the vertebrae. This is due to retrograde spread from the prostatic venous plexus to the vertebral veins. These secondaries are often characterised by the formation of new dense bone around them (osteosclerosis).

### Biochemical tests

1. Prostatic specific antigen (PSA) measured in the blood is a useful diagnostic marker.
2. When bone metastases occur, blood alkaline phosphatase may also rise due to osteoblastic activity.

Prostatic intraepithelial neoplasia (PIN), analogous to CIN (p. 537), has been recognised as a pre-invasive stage of the disease. High-grade PIN is strongly associated with development of invasive cancer.

# DISEASES OF THE PENIS

### TUMOURS OF THE PENIS

Papillomatous proliferations (condylomata acuminata), usually arise in the coronal sulcus or glans. They are due to sexually transmitted infection by Human Papilloma Virus (HPV) Types 6 and 11, and are analogous to similar lesions in the female genitalia.

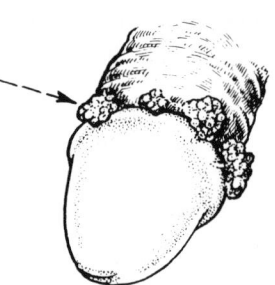

Peyronie disease is a fibromatosis related to Dupuytren contracture, which causes bending of the penis.

### Precancerous lesions

Epithelial dysplasia and carcinoma-in-situ can affect the penis (Bowen disease). This is related to HPV infection (Type 16).

### Carcinoma of the penis

Accounts for less than 1% of all male malignancy and affects middle-aged and elderly men. The site of growth is usually in the preputial area, often in the coronal sulcus, but it extends to involve the glans penis. Two forms of growth occur:

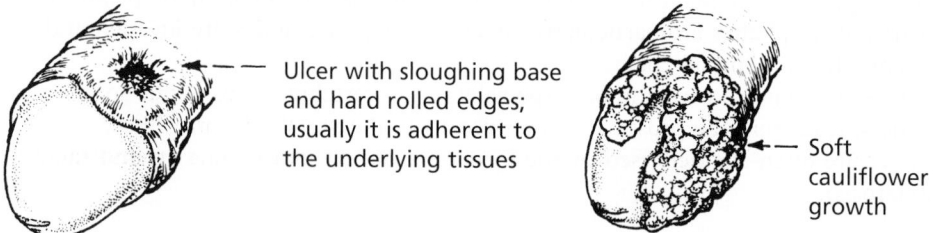

Ulcer with sloughing base and hard rolled edges; usually it is adherent to the underlying tissues

Soft cauliflower growth

The growth spreads by the lymphatics to the regional (inguinal) nodes. Distant metastases occur late. The prognosis is reasonably good, 5-year survival rate being greater than 50%.

### Aetiology

1. Males circumcised in childhood virtually never develop carcinoma; the risk is greatly increased in the presence of poor penile hygiene.
2. HPV Types 16 and 18 are the initiating carcinogens.

### Inflammation

A wide variety of infections affect the penis, and are usually sexually transmitted. They include bacteria, e.g. syphilis and gonorrhoea, and viruses, e.g. genital herpes.

### CANCER OF THE SCROTUM

This is a lesion which is rarely seen nowadays. Previously it was an occupational disease due to exposure to carcinogenic agents, e.g. soot, industrial oils, arsenic, etc.

# DISEASES OF THE TESTIS

## EPIDIDYMITIS AND ORCHITIS

Acute inflammation due to bacteria is uncommon in these organs. Spread of urinary infection via the vas deferens does occasionally occur and may result in suppuration. Gonorrhoea and chlamydia are seen in young men.

In 20% of adult cases of mumps, the epididymis and testis become acutely inflamed. The condition is usually unilateral, but if bilateral there is a distinct danger of subsequent infertility.

**Acute inflammation** of the testis may be confused with **torsion**. Torsion generally occurs within the tunica vaginalis and leads to obstruction of the testicular vessels. Infarction results, with destruction of the tissue. Recurrent minor degrees of torsion can cause atrophy. Since the torsion may be bilateral, prophylactic surgery may reduce the risk of a second event.

### Chronic granulomatous orchitis

This is a condition of unknown origin. The testis is infiltrated by macrophages, plasma cells and lymphocytes. Atrophy of the germinal epithelium occurs and the testis becomes fibrotic.

### Tuberculosis

The epididymis is affected first; spread may have come from the prostate or vas deferens.

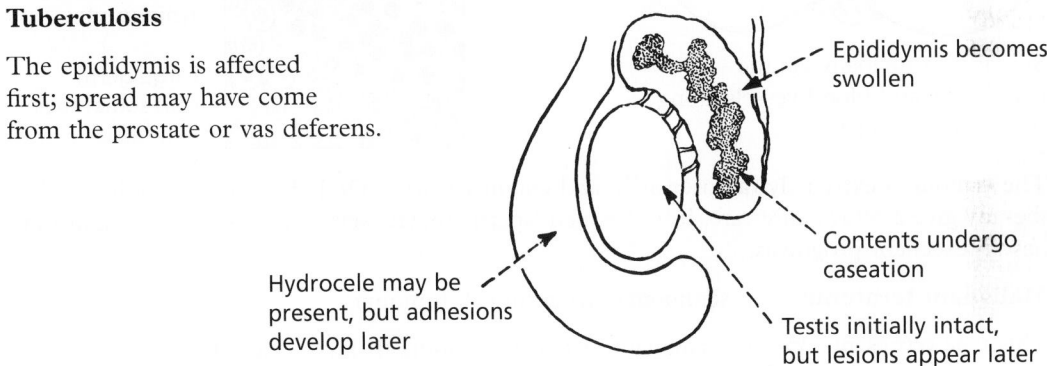

Epididymis becomes swollen

Contents undergo caseation

Testis initially intact, but lesions appear later

Hydrocele may be present, but adhesions develop later

### Syphilis

Apart from the primary sore on the penis, the only other genital site involved is the testis. These are common in the tertiary stage. Two types of lesion are seen.

1. **Gumma**

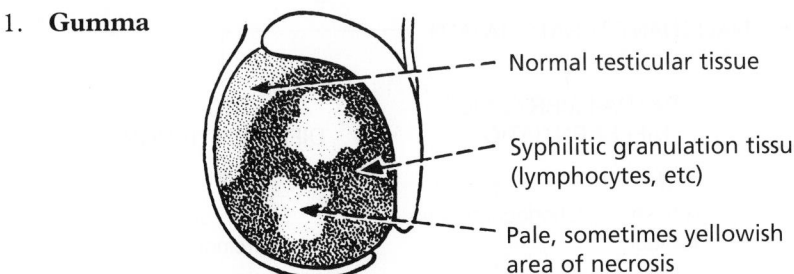

Normal testicular tissue

Syphilitic granulation tissue (lymphocytes, etc)

Pale, sometimes yellowish area of necrosis

2. **Granulomatous lesion** leading to scar formation with destruction of seminiferous tubules.

# TUMOURS OF THE TESTIS

### GERM CELL TUMOURS OF THE TESTIS

These tumours make up 2% of cancers in men and the incidence is rising steeply in Western countries. They are the commonest form of malignancy in young men. Tumours are more common in undescended testes.

The two main tumour types are SEMINOMA and TERATOMA.

**Seminoma** This corresponds to the dysgerminoma in the female. It is rare before puberty and has its peak incidence in adults in their 30s. It accounts for 50% of all testicular tumours.

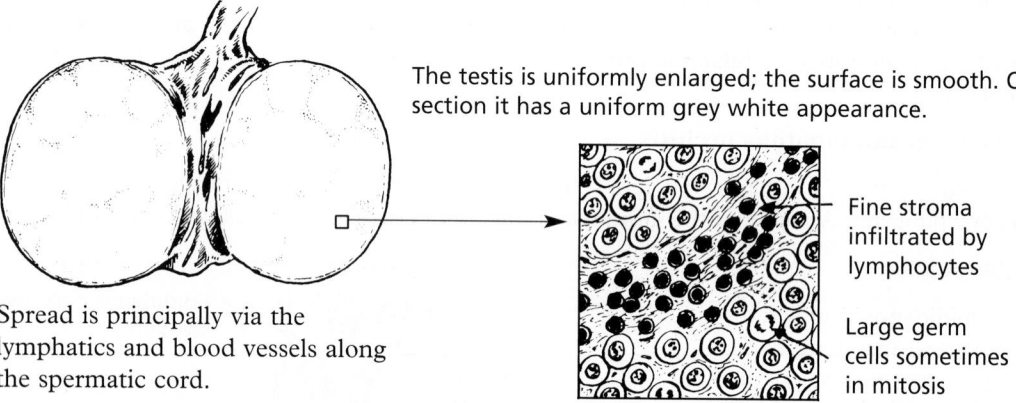

The testis is uniformly enlarged; the surface is smooth. On section it has a uniform grey white appearance.

Spread is principally via the lymphatics and blood vessels along the spermatic cord.

Fine stroma infiltrated by lymphocytes

Large germ cells sometimes in mitosis

The tumour is extremely radiosensitive and chemosensitive. Orchidectomy and adjuvant therapy give a >95% cure rate. In older men 'spermatocytic seminoma' is a rare variant but has an excellent prognosis.

**Malignant teratoma** (non-seminomatous germ cell tumour)

This type represents 35% of malignant testicular tumours. It takes origin from totipotent germ cells capable of differentiating into derivatives of ectoderm, endoderm and mesoderm. It is customary to classify them according to the degree and type of differentiation exhibited.

The tumours form a spectrum of well differentiated to anaplastic highly malignant growths. The 2004 WHO classification is used most commonly.

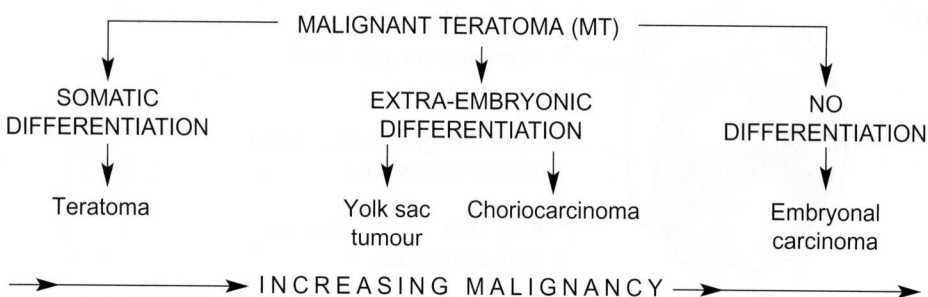

# TUMOURS OF THE TESTIS

These tumours, unlike seminoma, are usually irregular in shape and show focal haemorrhage and necrosis; in the better differentiated tumours small cysts are common.

1. Embryonal carcinoma – this is an undifferentiated tumour composed of pleomorphic tumour cells.
2. Teratoma – in these tumours the cells differentiate along somatic cell lines e.g. formation of intestinal glands, squamous epithelium, cartilage etc.
3. Yolk sac tumour – these are the commonest tumour to occur in children under 3 years. They produce AFP which is used to monitor disease progression.
4. Choriocarcinoma – these are tumours which differentiate along trophoblastic lines. They produce HCG.

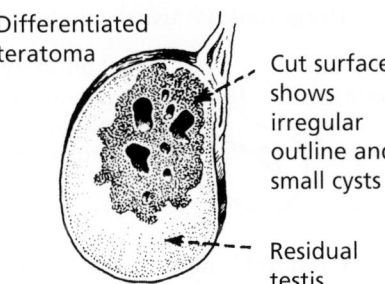

Differentiated teratoma

Cut surface shows irregular outline and small cysts

Residual testis

Many germ cell tumours are mixed tumours, i.e. they contain more than one element, most commonly embryonal carcinoma and teratoma.

## Spread

The usual mode of spread is by lymphatics to para-aortic lymph nodes. Vascular invasion with lung metastases also occurs.

## Prognosis

Modern therapy has greatly improved the overall prognosis.

## Intratubular germ cell neoplasia

There is an 'in situ' form of germ cell tumour, often found in association with the malignant tumours described above and represents a precursor form.

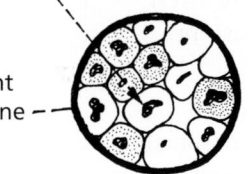

Large cells resembling those of seminoma

Tubular basement membrane intact

## MISCELLANEOUS TUMOURS

The following tumours are rare: Sertoli tumours
Leydig cell tumours
Lymphoma

It should be remembered that leukaemia often involves the testes (p. 475).

Rarely paratesticular sarcomas occur, e.g. rhabdomyosarcoma in children and liposarcoma in adults.

# INFERTILITY

There are numerous causes which affect females or males. The causes are classified as follows:

1. **Pregonadal** – usually endocrine disorders of pituitary or adrenal origin.

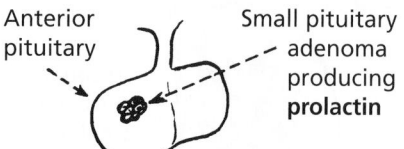

Anterior pituitary

Small pituitary adenoma producing **prolactin**

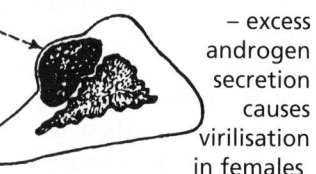

Adrenal cortical adenoma or genetic abnormality –

– excess androgen secretion causes virilisation in females

2. **Gonadal** – failure of production of gametes.

| Male | Female |
|---|---|
| **Klinefelter syndrome** | **Turner syndrome** |
| XXY | XO |

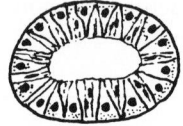

Gonadal dysgenesis – ovaries represented by small slender functionless tissue – '**streak gonads**'

Tubules lined only by Sertoli cells:
– spermatocyte arrest,
– often maldescent.

Polycystic ovary syndrome (Stein–Leventhal syndrome) Ovarian tissue replaced by multiple cysts.

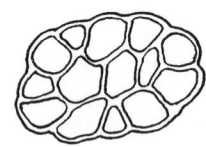

(i) Chromosomal defects
(ii) Germ cell aplasia
(iii) *Iatrogenic causes*: **irradiation**, **chemotherapy**, hormones, e.g. the 'pill' and oestrogens in treatment of prostatic carcinoma

3. **Postgonadal** – obstruction of passage of gametes.

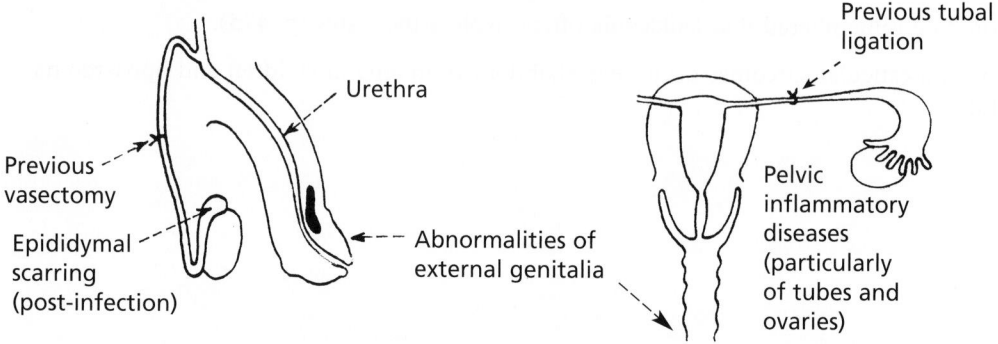

Previous tubal ligation

Urethra

Previous vasectomy

Epididymal scarring (post-infection)

Abnormalities of external genitalia

Pelvic inflammatory diseases (particularly of tubes and ovaries)

*Note:* In some cases of infertility no cause can be detected.

# FEMALE GENITAL SYSTEM AND BREAST

## OBJECTIVES

1. To know the main inflammatory and neoplastic disorders which affect the vulva and vagina.
2. To have knowledge of common pathologies of the uterus and in particular the main tumours affecting the cervix and endometrium.
3. To understand the main pathologies affecting the ovaries especially tumours and the commoner histological subtypes.
4. To have a basic understanding of gestational trophoblast disease.
5. To have knowledge of the main benign conditions which affect the breast.
6. To know the main histological types of breast carcinoma, its pattern of spread and prognostic factors.

# FEMALE GENITAL TRACT – ANATOMY AND PHYSIOLOGY

The following diagrams summarise normal anatomy and physiology:

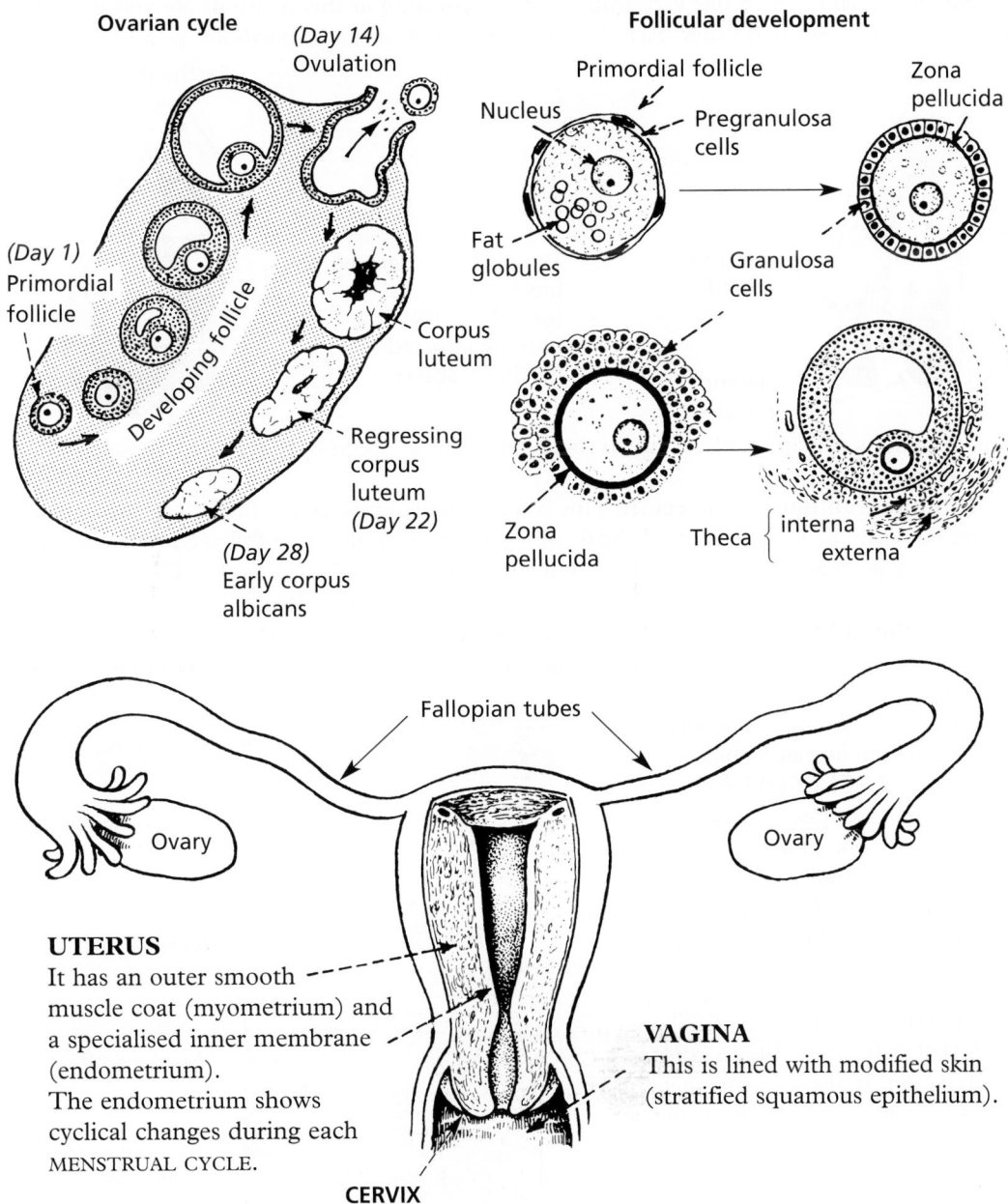

**Ovarian cycle**

*(Day 14)* Ovulation

*(Day 1)* Primordial follicle

Developing follicle

Corpus luteum

Regressing corpus luteum *(Day 22)*

*(Day 28)* Early corpus albicans

**Follicular development**

Primordial follicle

Nucleus

Pregranulosa cells

Zona pellucida

Fat globules

Granulosa cells

Zona pellucida

Theca { interna / externa

Fallopian tubes

Ovary

Ovary

**UTERUS**
It has an outer smooth muscle coat (myometrium) and a specialised inner membrane (endometrium).
The endometrium shows cyclical changes during each MENSTRUAL CYCLE.

**VAGINA**
This is lined with modified skin (stratified squamous epithelium).

**CERVIX**

# DISEASES OF VAGINA AND VULVA

**VULVAL INFLAMMATION** is common in post-menopausal women. It is related to atrophy of the skin, which has very thin epithelial covering at this phase of life and is easily abraded. Inflammation at other periods of life frequently involves Bartholin gland.

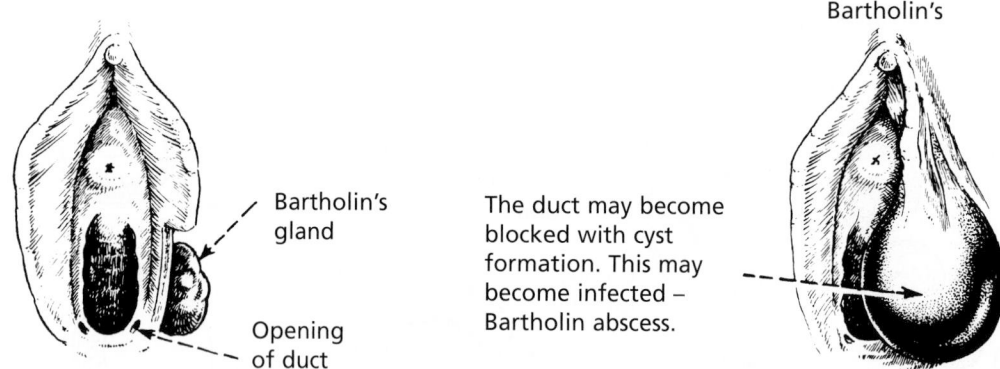

Bartholin's gland

Opening of duct

The duct may become blocked with cyst formation. This may become infected – Bartholin abscess.

Bartholin's

Two conditions which mainly occur in the tropics and are seen only very occasionally in temperate countries are:

1. **Lymphogranuloma venereum**. This is a chlamydial infection which starts as an ulcer on the vulva or in the vagina. It heals in a short time, only to be followed by a chronic suppurative reaction in the inguinal and sometimes pelvic lymph nodes. This leads to extensive scarring and sometimes fistulous openings in the pelvic viscera.

2. **Granuloma inguinale**. This begins as a papule on the vulva, perineum or vagina. It ulcerates and can spread widely, causing extensive destruction of tissue. Histologically, it is a granuloma and the infecting organism (*Klebsiella granulomatis*) can be seen in macrophages.

LICHEN SCLEROSUS presents as white plaques (leukoplakia). It is most common in post-menopausal women and may have an auto-immune basis. There is inflammation and thinning of the epidermis.

LICHEN SIMPLEX CHRONICUS is due to chronic irritation. It also presents as an area of leukoplakia. There is epithelial thickening and excess keratin.

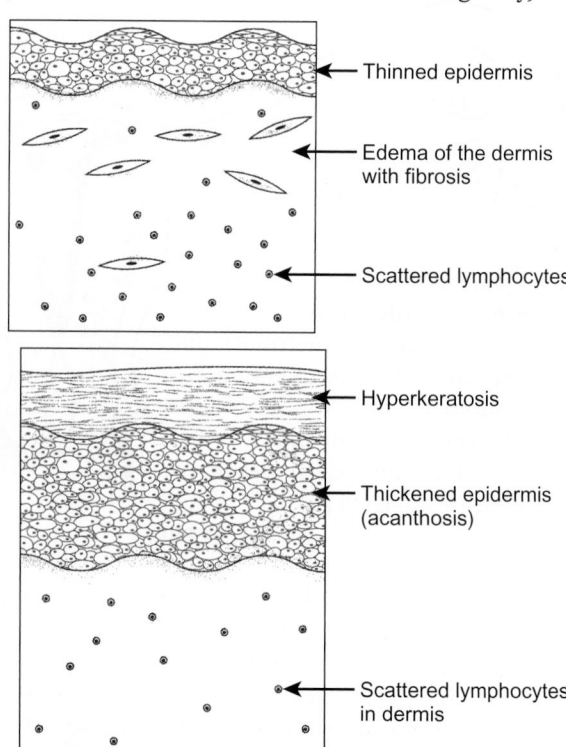

Thinned epidermis

Edema of the dermis with fibrosis

Scattered lymphocytes

Hyperkeratosis

Thickened epidermis (acanthosis)

Scattered lymphocytes in dermis

# DISEASES OF VAGINA AND VULVA

**VULVAL INTRAEPITHELIAL NEOPLASIA (VIN)** also presents as white patches but shows varying degrees of dysplasia. It is pre-malignant.

The degree of dysplasia varies, eventually amounting to carcinoma in situ in some cases. These changes are now numerically graded VIN I, II and III (analogous to cervical intraepithelial neoplasia (CIN)).

## TUMOURS OF THE VULVA

Benign tumours are common. CONDYLOMATA ACUMINATA are papillomas due to infection by human papilloma virus (HPV) Types 6 or 11. Koilocytosis (see p. 537) in the superficial keratinocytes is characteristic.
Sweat gland tumours (hidradenomas) may also occur.

### Carcinoma of the vulva

This is a rare condition found usually in women in the sixth and seventh decades of life.

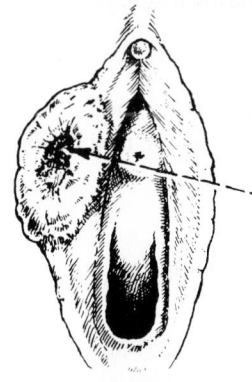

Starting as an indurated plaque it becomes ulcerated

The inguinal glands on both sides are invaded at an early stage. The tumour is usually a squamous carcinoma.

Atrophic post-menopausal vulva.

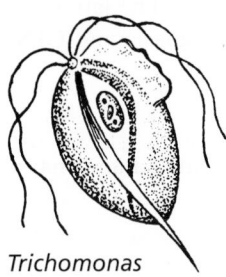

*Trichomonas vaginalis*

Vaginal discharge is a common complaint, especially in parous women. In many cases it is related to chronic cervicitis. There are however a number of inflammatory conditions which arise primarily in the vagina.

Gonococcal infection may produce an acute inflammation with purulent discharge but it is often asymptomatic.

Purulent discharge is also associated with infection by a protozoon, *Trichomonas vaginalis*. The discharge tends to be frothy. It is commonly transmitted during sexual intercourse. The male can also be infected.

***Candida albicans*** infection is common in pregnancy, in diabetes and in patients undergoing antibiotic or immunosuppressive therapy.

**PRIMARY TUMOURS of the VAGINA** are rare. Squamous carcinoma occurs in the upper vagina and may lead to fistula formation between the vagina and the bladder or rectum. Vaginal intraepithelial neoplasia may be associated with CIN and VIN. Historically, clear cell adenocarcinoma was sometimes found in adolescent girls, due to the effect on the foetus of administration of diethylstilbestrol to the patient's mother during early pregnancy. It arose in a background of vaginal adenosis – a proliferation of glands within the vaginal wall.

# DISEASES OF THE CERVIX

The cervix constitutes the lower one-third of the uterine body.

It is in two parts: endocervical and ectocervical, with different lining epithelium.

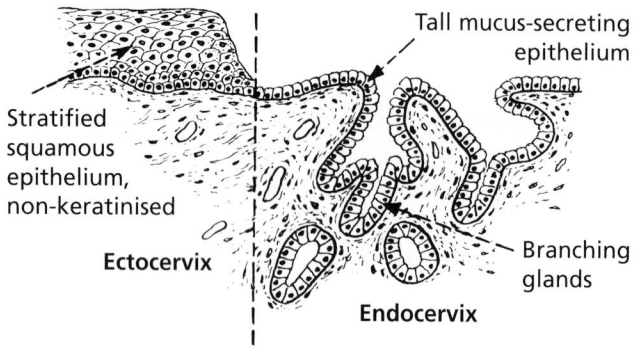

Stratified squamous epithelium, non-keratinised

**Ectocervix**

Tall mucus-secreting epithelium

Branching glands

**Endocervix**

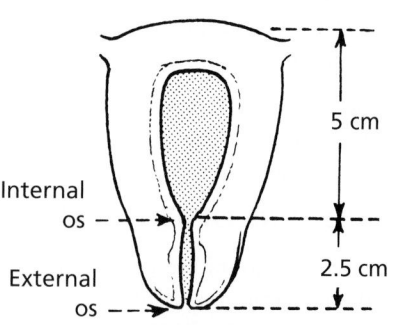

Internal os

External os

5 cm

2.5 cm

The remainder of the cervical wall consists of circular smooth muscle lying in abundant fibroelastic tissue.

At the internal os, the structure gradually merges with that of the uterus proper, the branching glands giving place to the simple tubules of the endometrium, and the proportion of muscle increases greatly.

## CERVICITIS

Inflammation of the cervix may be acute or chronic. Acute cervicitis may be due to gonorrhoea or follow cervical laceration at childbirth.

Chronic cervicitis is commoner and may be due to *Candida*, *Trichomonas* (p. 535) and *Chlamydia*. The last is associated with reactive lymphoid follicles (follicular cervicitis).

Viral infections of the cervix include herpes simplex virus (Type II) and HPV. The latter can cause simple viral warts or be associated with cervical intraepithelial dysplasia and CIN and invasive carcinoma (p. 538).

## CERVICAL POLYP

This is a local proliferation of endocervical mucosa which becomes pedunculated and may protrude through the cervix.

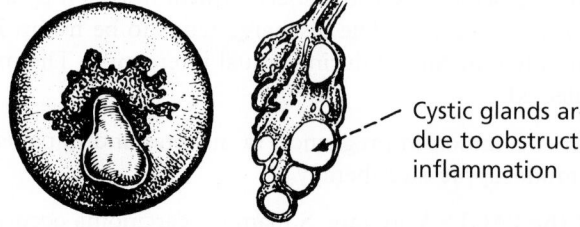

Cystic glands are common due to obstruction by chronic inflammation

# CERVICAL INTRAEPITHELIAL NEOPLASIA (CIN)

**The transformation zone**

From puberty onwards and particularly in pregnancy the squamo-columnar junction presents on the vaginal surface of the external os. This is the area where **squamous metaplasia** occurs. It is important because cervical squamous carcinoma and its precursor, CIN, begin there. Within this metaplastic epithelium, **dysplastic** changes may develop. They are graded as CIN I, II and III. Later, in some cases, invasive squamous carcinoma develops.

**CIN I = mild dysplasia**

Upper two-thirds: Stratified.

Basal one-third: High nucleo-cytoplasmic ratio; pleomorphic nuclei

**CIN II = moderate dysplasia**

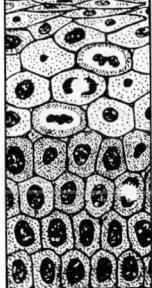

Superficial stratification

Cellular abnormalities extending up into middle one-third

**CIN III = severe dysplasia and carcinoma in situ**

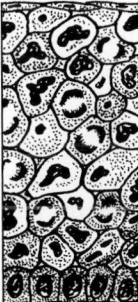

May be one or two layers of stratified epithelium on surface.

Remainder: immature; large nuclei; mitoses.

Koilocytes (cells with a wrinkled pyknotic nucleus and perinuclear cytoplasmic clearing) are often seen in the suprabasal layers and indicate HPV infection.

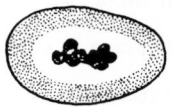

## CYTOLOGY AND CIN

The cervical screening programme aims to detect CIN and thus prevent the development of invasive carcinoma. Cellular preparations from the squamo-columnar junction obtained by a cervical brush are stained by the Papanicolaou method (liquid-based cytology). The cells can be examined for dysplasia – so-called 'dyskaryosis'. Inflammatory changes, e.g. due to *Candida* infection, may be seen.

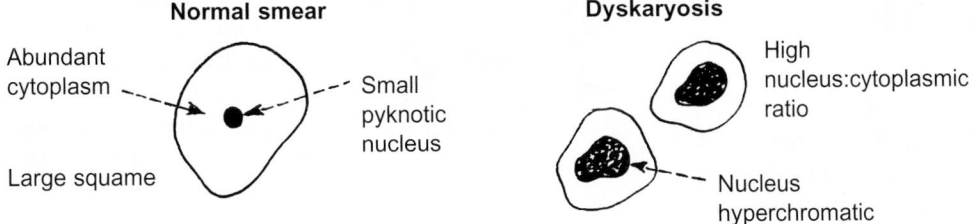

**Normal smear**

Abundant cytoplasm

Small pyknotic nucleus

Large squame

**Dyskaryosis**

High nucleus:cytoplasmic ratio

Nucleus hyperchromatic

The cytology is a SCREENING TEST. Patients with abnormalities are referred for colposcopy where abnormal epithelium turns white on exposure to acetic acid (acetowhite). Punch biopsy is then undertaken to identify CIN. If present, this is then followed by laser loop excision of the transformation zone.

# CARCINOMA OF CERVIX

### CARCINOMA

The tumour is a squamous carcinoma in 90% of cases, and an adenocarcinoma in 10%. Most squamous carcinomas arise at the squamo-columnar junction: most adenocarcinomas arise within the endocervical canal.

### Aetiology

Cervical cancer is caused by infection with strains of HPV, a sexually transmitted disease. For this reason vaccination against HPV is now offered to girls of secondary school age.

The cervix becomes indurated with necrosis and ulceration

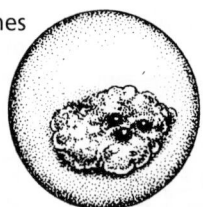

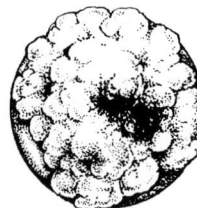

Later, a large fungating mass is produced

**Microinvasive carcinoma** is the earliest stage of invasive cancer – where spread is less than 5 mm in depth. This is associated with an excellent prognosis.

### Spread

Until a very late stage, the disease is confined to the pelvic cavity. The patient commonly dies before distant metastases appear.

Local spread takes place in several directions:

1. **Downward extension.**

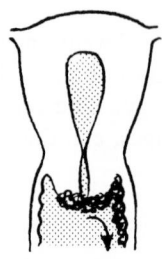

The ureters come very close to the cervix in their travel to the bladder, and are often involved in extension of the tumour to the parametrium. The ureters may be obstructed by pressure or invasion. Renal infection and failure follow.

2. **Lateral extension.** The anatomy of this region is important.

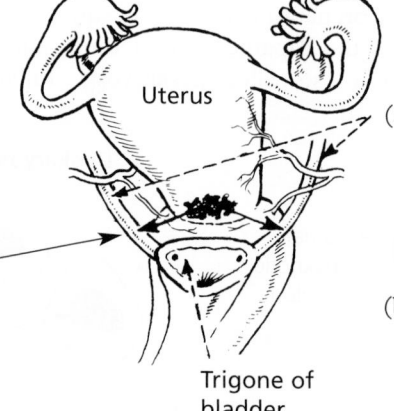

Uterus

Trigone of bladder

(a) The growth encircles the external os. In some cases it causes obstruction of the cervical canal and pyometra may develop.

(b) Direct extension to the vagina follows.

# CARCINOMA OF CERVIX

3. **Anterior and posterior extension.**

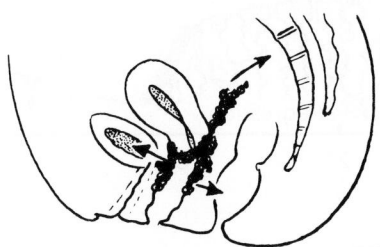

Direct invasion of the bladder or rectum results in fistulous communications. Spread along the uterosacral ligaments involves the sacral nerves, causing intractable pain.

4. **Lymphatic spread.**
This occurs early and involves the chains of lymph nodes in the pelvis.

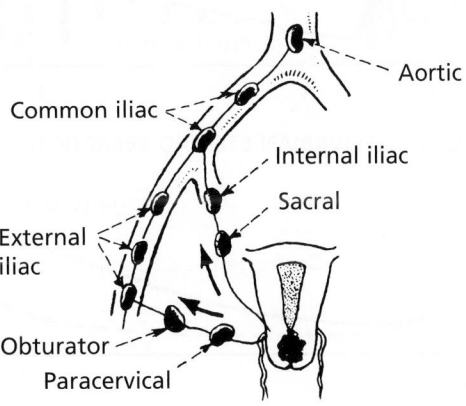

## Prognosis

With modern treatment there is an 80% 5-year cure rate when the disease is diagnosed early, i.e. confined to the cervix; cure rate falls significantly if spread to the pelvis has occurred.

Previously death was commonly due to a combination of renal failure and sepsis. Fatal haemorrhage from eroded vessels also occurred. With better local control death is usually due to metastases.

# CYCLICAL ENDOMETRIAL CHANGES

**Menstruation**

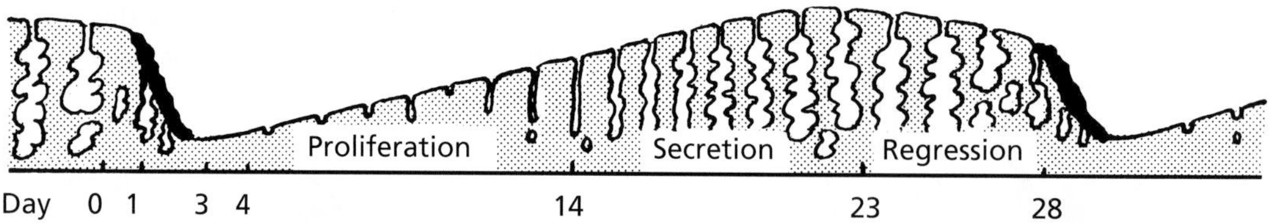

Proliferation    Secretion    Regression

Day    0  1    3  4                    14                    23                    28

## ASSOCIATED OVARIAN STEROID SECRETION

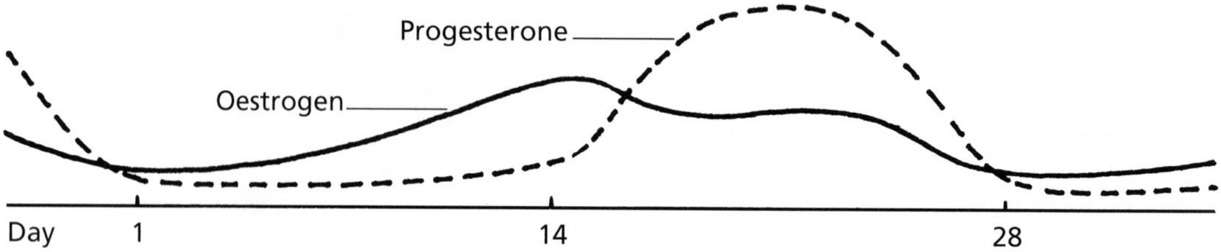

Progesterone

Oestrogen

Day    1                    14                    28

### Proliferative phase

This is induced by oestrogen produced by developing ovarian follicles, stimulated by FSH from the pituitary.

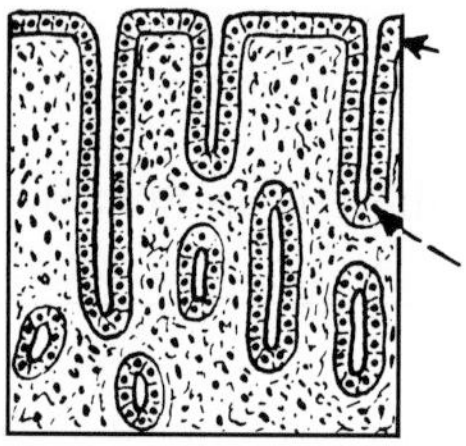

Stromal cells, narrow spindles to begin with, become plump.

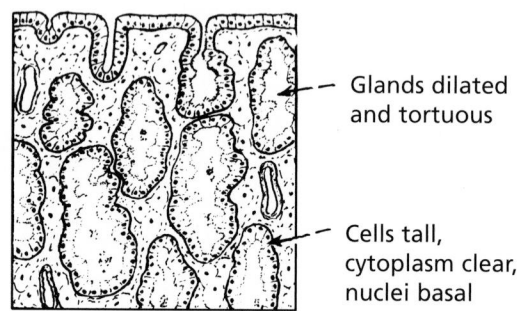

Epithelium is cuboidal, growing taller as ovulation is approached

Glands are simple, narrow tubes dilating prior to ovulation. (Triggered by a surge of FSH and LH)

### Secretory phase

Progesterone produced by the corpus luteum stimulates secretion by the glands. Oestrogen is also produced. The stromal cells enlarge (pseudo-decidual change), oedema is present and vascularity greatly increased.

Glands dilated and tortuous

Cells tall, cytoplasm clear, nuclei basal

### Premenstrual phase

Endometrial growth ceases 5–6 days before menstruation. Prior to menstruation, it shrinks due to decreased blood flow and discharge of secretion. This increases the tortuosity of glands and blood vessels. Finally, apoptosis occurs and the endometrium is shed.

# DISEASES OF THE ENDOMETRIUM

**Endometritis** may be acute or chronic. In its acute form there is an infiltrate of neutrophils and in chronic endometritis there is a lymphoplasmacytic infiltrate. Causes include:

1. Pelvic inflammatory disease (*Neisseria gonorrhoeae, Chlamydia trachomatis*).
2. Retained products of conception.
3. Intrauterine device–related.

### Tuberculous endometritis

This is now uncommon in the United Kingdom. Histologically there are epithelioid granulomas within the endometrium. Diagnostic biopsy should be done as late in the cycle as possible to allow the granulomas to develop.

## ENDOMETRIOSIS

This consists of deposits of endometrium outside the uterine cavity.

In most cases, the disease is confined to the pelvis and the genital tract.

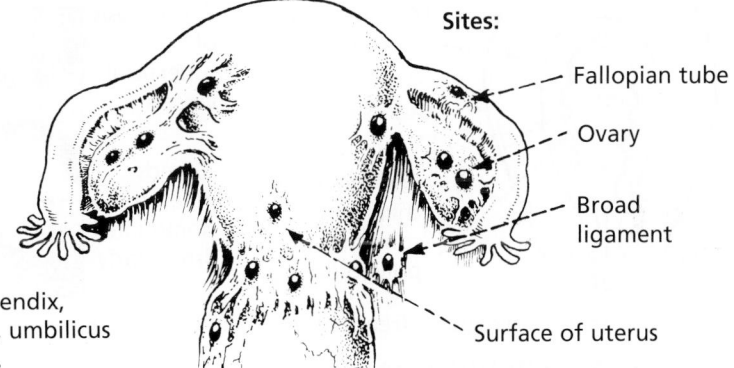

**Sites:**
— Fallopian tube
— Ovary
— Broad ligament
— Surface of uterus

**Other sites:** caecum and appendix, bladder, rectum, umbilicus laparotomy scar.

These deposits show cyclical changes. The result is haemorrhage into the local tissues at the time of menstruation. Adhesions develop, often leading to infertility. Malignant change to endometrioid adenocarcinoma occurs rarely.

### Aetiology

Three theories have been proposed:
1. Retrograde spill of menstrual debris – perhaps the most favoured.
2. Metaplasia of tissues into Müllerian duct elements.
3. Lymphatic and blood-borne emboli of endometrial tissue.

## ADENOMYOSIS

Deep down growths of endometrium occur within the myometrium. There is an accompanying overgrowth of muscle and connective tissue. Two macroscopic forms occur:

1. **Diffuse**
   Deposits are confined to inner part of myometrium. Foci of endometrium often brownish in colour.

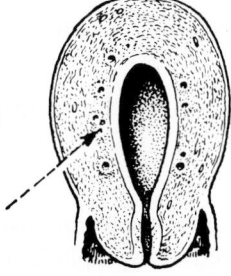

2. **Localised**
   Resembling fibroid but with brownish foci.

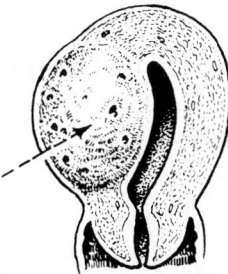

The endometrial deposits communicate with the uterine cavity, but despite this they often contain altered blood in the glands which become cystic. The diffuse type is commoner. Adenomyosis is not related to endometriosis.

# ENDOMETRIAL HYPERPLASIA

**Endometrial hyperplasia** occurs in three forms: simple hyperplasia, complex hyperplasia and atypical hyperplasia. Of these, atypical hyperplasia is most important as it is associated with an increased risk of malignancy. Progressive molecular genetic alterations occur on the pathway to cancer.

### SIMPLE HYPERPLASIA
This tends to occur in the peri-menopausal period. It is due to excess oestrogen stimulation – particularly associated with **anovulatory** cycles, but rarely with oestrogen therapy or oestrogen-secreting tumours.

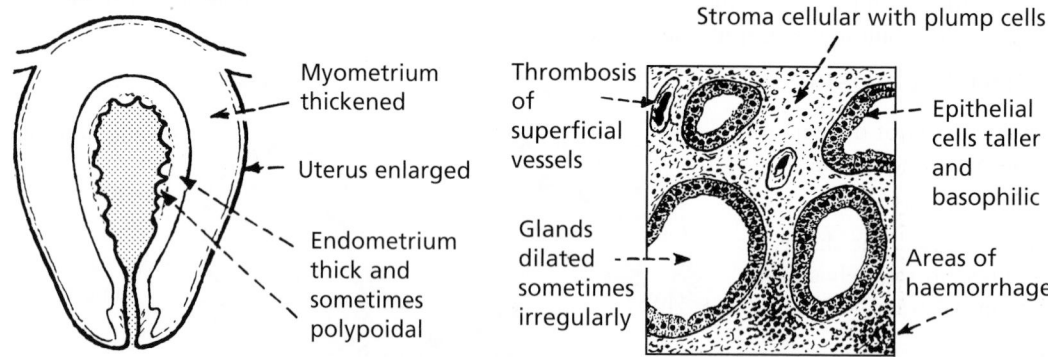

Clinically, there is irregular, frequent and heavy bleeding.

### COMPLEX HYPERPLASIA
In this form hyperplasia is often focal, and glands, but not stroma, are affected. Thus the glands appear crowded, but show no atypia. There is no increased risk of malignancy.

### ATYPICAL HYPERPLASIA
In this condition the hyperplasia is focal and cytological atypia with mitotic figures is common. Intervening endometrium may show simple hyperplasia. The importance of atypical hyperplasia is its relationship to the development of adenocarcinoma, i.e. it is considered to be pre-cancerous.

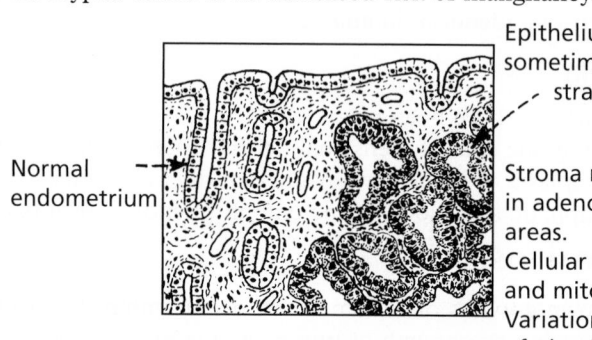

Up to 40% have co-existing carcinoma in hysterectomy specimens.

### ENDOMETRIAL POLYP
This is a localised proliferation of endometrial glands which becomes pedunculated.

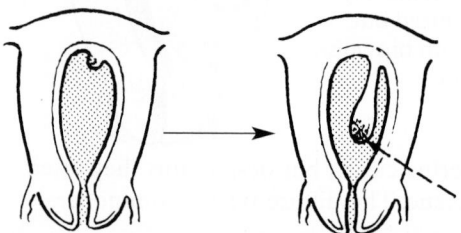

Sometimes polyps are associated with general endometrial hyperplasia. Progressive elongation of the pedicle may lead to venous congestion and bleeding.

# ENDOMETRIAL CARCINOMA

This common gynaecological cancer particularly affects post-menopausal patients, who typically present with vaginal bleeding.

**CARCINOMA**

This growth may form a *localised* plaque or polyp.

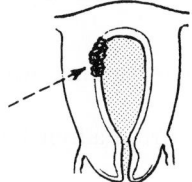

In some cases it appears as a *diffuse* change involving much of the endometrium. It grows initially within the endometrial layer, bulging into the uterine cavity.

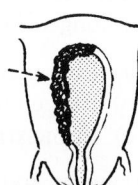

Most growths are well-differentiated adenocarcinomas (endometrioid). These are graded from I–III

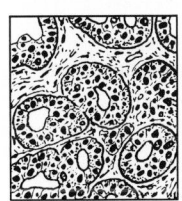

GRADE I

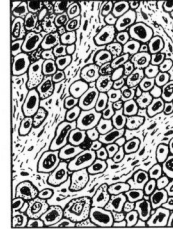

GRADE III

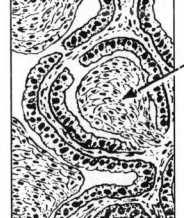

Areas of squamous metaplasia are relatively common; they have no prognostic implication

In some cases with a particularly poor prognosis malignant squamous epithelium is admixed with the adenocarcinoma – so-called 'ADENOSQUAMOUS' carcinoma.

The endometrium possesses no lymphatics and invasion of the myometrium takes place slowly.

**Local extension**: this may take place in several directions.

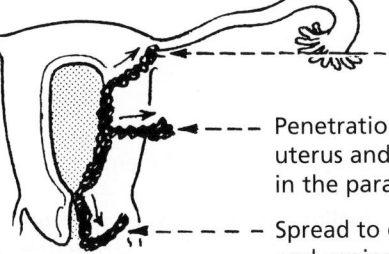

Spread towards tube

Penetration of uterus and growth in the parametrium

Spread to cervix and vagina

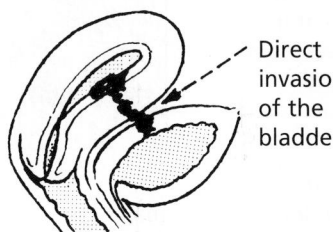

Direct invasion of the bladder

**Metastases**

1. **Via lymphatics.**

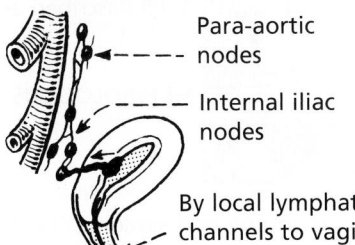

Para-aortic nodes

Internal iliac nodes

By local lymphatic channels to vagina

2. **Via blood vessels.** Secondary deposits in the vagina and ovaries may be due to this mode of spread.

3. **Via fallopian tube.**

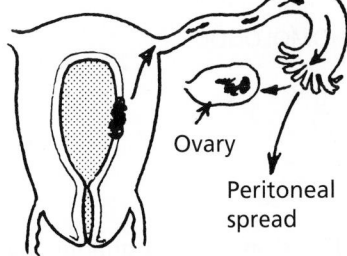

Ovary

Peritoneal spread

4. **Distant metastases.** At a late date, secondaries may appear in the liver, lungs and bones. These may be the result of lymphatic or blood spread.

The most important prognostic factor is the stage of the tumour, usually expressed in the FIGO (International Federation of Gynaecology and Obstetrics system).

# ENDOMETRIAL CARCINOMA

### Aetiology

Endometrial carcinoma is uncommon before the fifth decade. The most important factor is prolonged OESTROGENIC stimulation due to:

(a) Endogenous overproduction, e.g. in cases of oestrogen-secreting ovarian tumours.
(b) Exogenous oestrogen therapy.
(c) In OBESITY: increased conversion of androstenedione (from adrenals) to oestrone.

ATYPICAL HYPERPLASIA is an important precancerous stage.

Other endometrial malignancies:

## ENDOMETRIAL STROMAL SARCOMAS

These rare tumours may be of low grade or high grade.

**Low-grade tumours** – infiltrate extensively through the lymphatics of the myometrium. The cells are cytologically bland and mitoses are few. About one-fifth of patients eventually die from the disease.

**High-grade stromal sarcomas** – are highly malignant spindle-celled tumours, with poor prognosis. It may be difficult to separate these from uterine leiomyosarcomas.

## CARCINO-SARCOMA (MALIGNANT MIXED MÜLLERIAN TUMOURS)

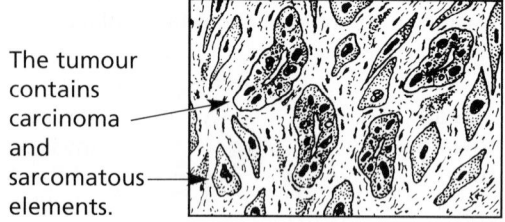

The tumour contains carcinoma and sarcomatous elements.

If these resemble endometrial stroma, the tumour is described as

HOMOLOGOUS

Sometimes stromal elements include malignant cartilage; sometimes striated muscle.

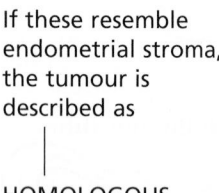

The tumour is then described as

HETEROLOGOUS

These uncommon tumours have features both of endometrial carcinoma and sarcoma. They often present as soft fleshy masses protruding through the cervix into the vagina.

# DISEASES OF THE MYOMETRIUM

Tumours of the myometrium are extremely common.

## LEIOMYOMA (FIBROID)

This is a circumscribed growth derived from uterine muscle.

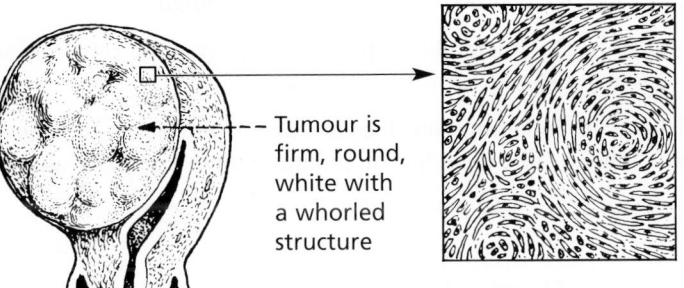

Tumour is firm, round, white with a whorled structure

The cells are typical long spindle muscle cells, arranged in interlacing bundles

They vary in size from tiny (mm) growths to several cm in diameter and are frequently multiple.
Fibroids may be found in any part of the uterus.

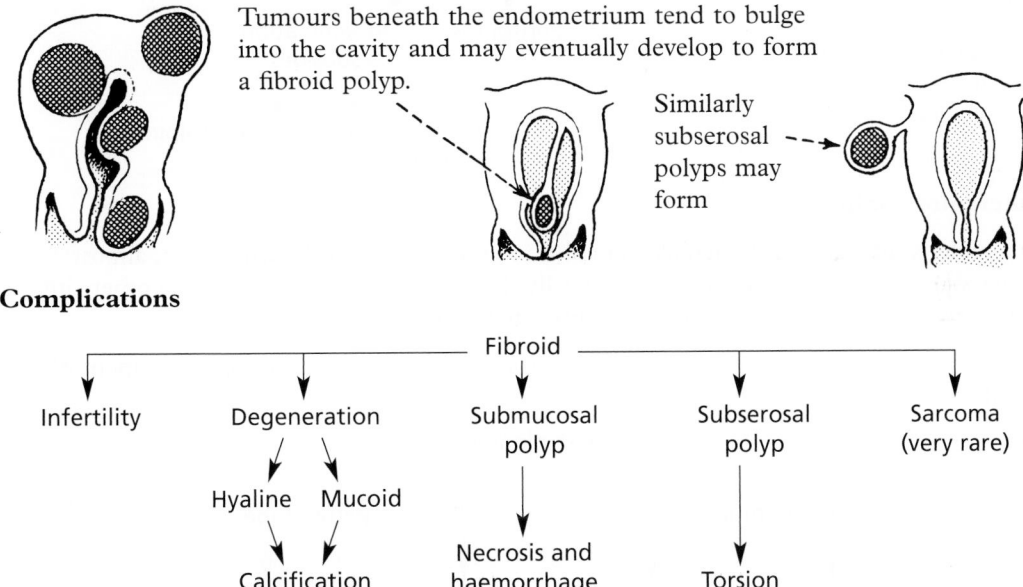

Tumours beneath the endometrium tend to bulge into the cavity and may eventually develop to form a fibroid polyp.

Similarly subserosal polyps may form

### Complications

Fibroid
- Infertility
- Degeneration
  - Hyaline
    - Calcification
  - Mucoid
    - Calcification
- Submucosal polyp
  - Necrosis and haemorrhage
- Subserosal polyp
  - Torsion
- Sarcoma (very rare)

Leiomyoma is one of the commonest tumours, occurring in 15–20% of women over the age of 35. Growth ceases at the menopause.

## LEIOMYOSARCOMA

This is a rare tumour which may arise from a preceding leiomyoma, but usually does not. Some tumours are highly malignant but in others with few mitotic figures it is difficult to predict the outcome – these are known as Smooth Muscle Tumours of Uncertain Malignant Potential (STUMP).

# DISEASES OF THE FALLOPIAN TUBE

### Acute salpingitis

This is the result of ascending infection from the endometrium: some cases follow abortion and puerperal infection. *Chlamydia* may cause acute salpingitis.

The inflammation is usually bilateral and primarily involves the tubal plicae which are congested and oedematous; with a purulent exudate.

If resolution of the acute inflammation does not occur (antibiotic therapy is important), chronic salpingitis follows. The term 'pelvic inflammatory disease' is used.

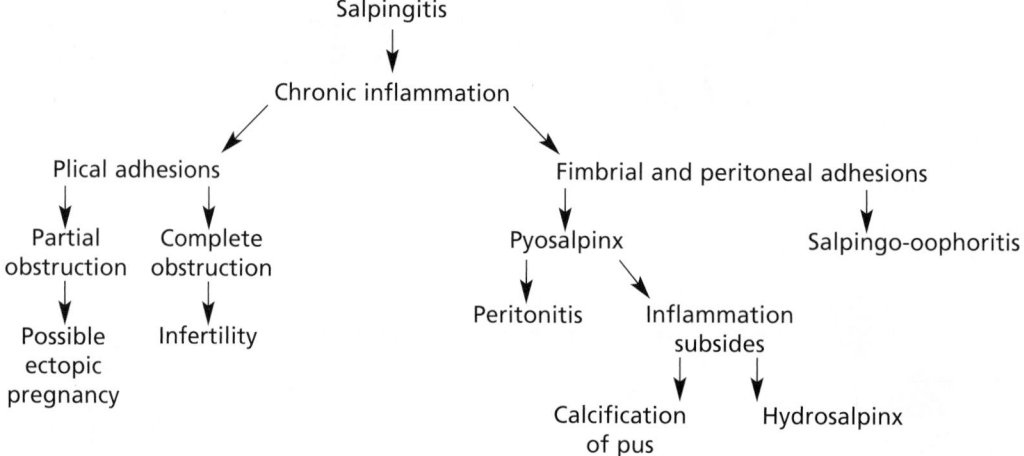

### Tuberculous salpingitis

Tuberculous infection of the female genital tract, for some unexplained reason, almost always starts in the fallopian tube. It is usually due to blood spread from some other site; only very occasionally it is secondary to tuberculous peritonitis.

The complications are those expected of a chronic salpingitis with the added element of caseation.

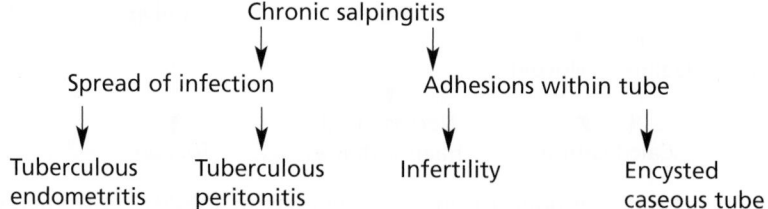

### Tumours of the fallopian tube

Benign tumours such as fibroma and leiomyoma occasionally occur. Small cysts of congenital origin are common around the fimbrial ends of the tubes.

Carcinoma, usually a papillary adenocarcinoma, is extremely rare. There may be a profuse watery secretion which appears as a vaginal discharge. There is an association with *BRCA* mutations.

# DISEASES OF THE OVARIES

## OOPHORITIS

Inflammation of the ovaries is always secondary to disease of the fallopian tubes or peritoneum. The inflamed fimbrial end of the tube becomes adherent to the ovary and direct spread of infection occurs. Tubo-ovarian inflammation is also associated with the presence of an intra-uterine contraceptive device (p. 541). Important local complications may follow.

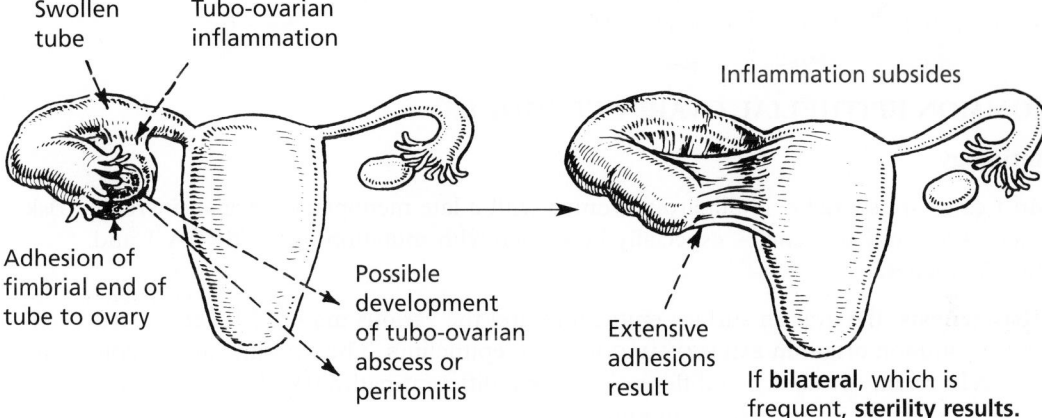

Swollen tube

Tubo-ovarian inflammation

Inflammation subsides

Adhesion of fimbrial end of tube to ovary

Possible development of tubo-ovarian abscess or peritonitis

Extensive adhesions result

If **bilateral**, which is frequent, **sterility results**.

The ovary may be similarly involved in tuberculous salpingitis, and caseating lesions can occur.

## FOLLICULAR CYSTS

These may be single or multiple. The maximum diameter of a normal Graafian follicle is 1.5–2 cm. Single follicular cysts may be several centimetres in diameter.

Bilateral, multiple small cysts of this nature occur in polycystic ovarian disease and are associated with obesity, hirsutism and oligomenorrhoea (Stein-Leventhal syndrome, polycystic ovary syndrome).

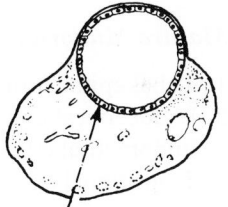

Granulosa cells lining cyst

## THECA LUTEIN CYSTS

These are cysts from which the granulosa cells have disappeared, leaving cysts surrounded by luteinised thecal tissue.

# DISEASES OF THE OVARIES

Many types of ovarian tumours exist. Various classifications have been suggested; none is completely satisfactory. The following is a simple working classification:

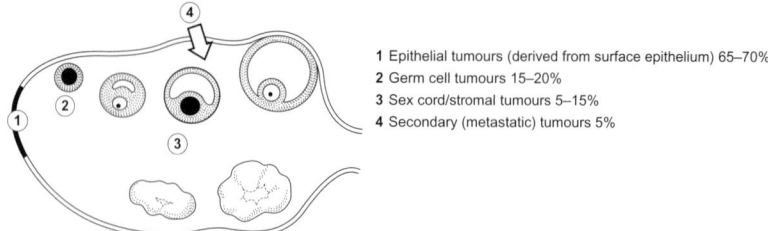

1 Epithelial tumours (derived from surface epithelium) 65–70%
2 Germ cell tumours 15–20%
3 Sex cord/stromal tumours 5–15%
4 Secondary (metastatic) tumours 5%

## COMMON EPITHELIAL OVARIAN TUMOURS

### Aetiology

Most cases are sporadic. Nulliparous women with a late menopause have an increased risk. There is a family tendency – especially in women with mutation of the BRCA-1 and BRCA-2 genes.

**Histogenesis**: the ovarian surface epithelium and the various mature Müllerian structures have a common origin in EMBRYONAL COELOMIC epithelium. The ovarian surface epithelial stem cells retain the ability to differentiate along different pathways: this explains the histological appearance of these tumours.

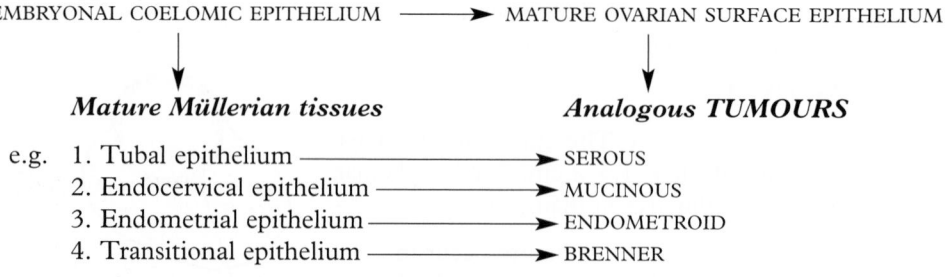

EMBRYONAL COELOMIC EPITHELIUM ⟶ MATURE OVARIAN SURFACE EPITHELIUM

*Mature Müllerian tissues*          *Analogous TUMOURS*

e.g.  1. Tubal epithelium ⟶ SEROUS
2. Endocervical epithelium ⟶ MUCINOUS
3. Endometrial epithelium ⟶ ENDOMETROID
4. Transitional epithelium ⟶ BRENNER

The histological features relate to a spectrum of behaviour:

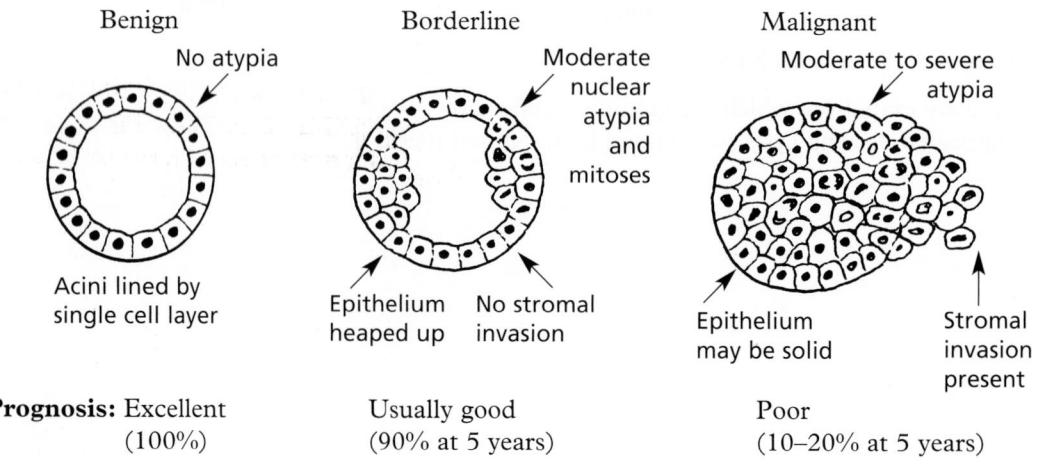

| Benign | Borderline | Malignant |
|---|---|---|
| No atypia | Moderate nuclear atypia and mitoses | Moderate to severe atypia |
| Acini lined by single cell layer | Epithelium heaped up — No stromal invasion | Epithelium may be solid — Stromal invasion present |
| **Prognosis:** Excellent (100%) | Usually good (90% at 5 years) | Poor (10–20% at 5 years) |

# COMMON EPITHELIAL OVARIAN TUMOURS

## 1. SEROUS TUMOURS

### (a) Serous cystadenoma

Twenty-five percent of all ovarian tumours are of this variety. In a third of cases they are bilateral, but they almost never reach the large size of the mucinous tumours.

Smooth surface

(unilocular or multilocular)

Some tumours have small loculi with papillary formations, making them appear solid.

Intracystic papilla. May be few and sessile or pedunculated with fronds often complex in structure

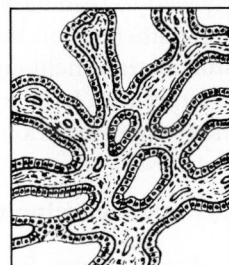

Epithelium cuboidal with central nuclei. Fluid is watery.

Psammoma bodies with concentric layers of calcification are commonly seen.

### Complications

1. Torsion may occur.
2. Malignant transformation is common and 30% of malignant tumours are bilateral.

### (b) Serous cystadenocarcinoma

This is the commonest malignant tumour of the ovary. Usually it takes the form of exuberant papillomatous growths extending over the surface and obliterating the ovarian structure. It is often bilateral. They are classified as low grade or high grade. Low-grade tumours are associated with *KRAS* and *BRAF* mutations and high-grade tumours with *p53* mutations.

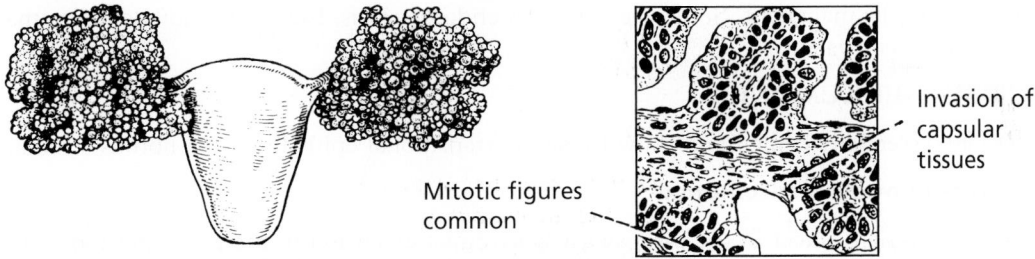

Mitotic figures common

Invasion of capsular tissues

## 2. MUCINOUS TUMOURS

### (a) Mucinous cystadenoma

This accounts for 20% of all ovarian tumours. It can reach a very large size and is typically multilocular. Twenty-five percent are bilateral.

Slightly nodular due to loculi

The cut surface shows the multilocular mosaic pattern

Mucin secretion

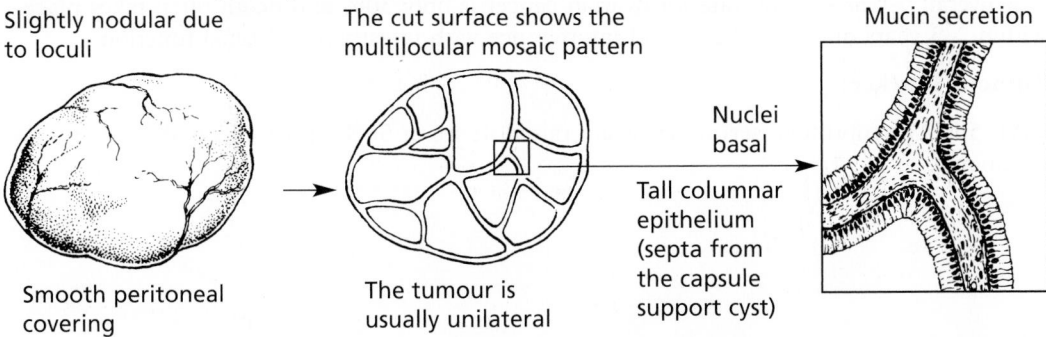

Nuclei basal

Tall columnar epithelium (septa from the capsule support cyst)

Smooth peritoneal covering

The tumour is usually unilateral

# CARCINOMA OF THE OVARY

### Complications

(i) **Torsion of the pedicle**. This is not uncommon with a large ovarian tumour of any type.

(ii) **Rupture**. This may lead to seeding of the mucin-secreting epithelium on the peritoneum.

(iii) **Malignant transformation** including borderline tumours. Cells are large, with large irregular nuclei. Mitoses are common; slight secretion present.

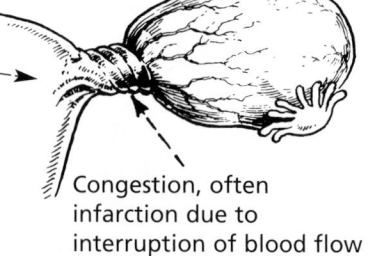

Congestion, often infarction due to interruption of blood flow

### (b) Mucinous cystadenocarcinoma

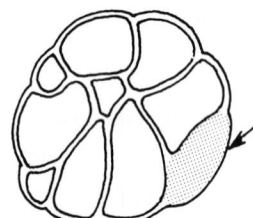

This accounts for 20% of all cases of primary carcinoma of the ovary. It almost always arises as a malignant transformation of a benign cystadenoma.

Areas of solid growth appear in the cyst wall.

### 3. ENDOMETRIOID TUMOUR

These are solid or cystic tumours and are histologically similar to those of the endometrium. They are usually malignant. Some cases arise in endometriosis. Endometrioid adenofibroma is the benign equivalent.

### 4. BRENNER TUMOURS

These are essentially benign and show islands of transitional epithelium in a fibrous stroma.

### Progress in ovarian carcinoma

Spread of ovarian cancer in the early stages is by direct extension to the pelvic peritoneum. The serous carcinoma seeds widely in the peritoneal cavity and only later are lymphatics invaded and metastases appear.

The mucinous variety rarely spreads by lymphatics.

The overall 5-year survival rate for ovarian cancer is only 30% and death often takes place within 2–3 years due to cachexia and interference with intestinal and renal function.

### Tumour marker

CA125 is a glycoprotein: serum levels are raised in about 50% of patients with ovarian carcinoma.

# TUMOURS OF THE OVARY – SEX CORD STROMAL

These may be divided into two broad groups:

1.  Those tending to produce excess oestrogen: granulosa cell tumours and thecomas.
2.  Those producing androgens and virilisation: Sertoli-Leydig cell tumours, hilus cell tumours and lipid cell tumours.

### Granulosa cell tumour

This is composed of cells resembling the granulosa cells lining Graafian follicles. They vary in size from a few mm to large cystic structures. Commonly, the smaller varieties are found deep in the ovarian substance. This tumour may be found at any age: 5% occur in children; 50% in the child-bearing years; 40% are post-menopausal.

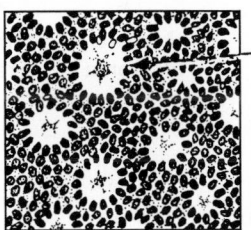

Rosettes of cells with nuclei radially arranged are common (Call-Exner bodies).

All granulosa cell tumours are potentially malignant. They may recur, sometimes many years after removal.

Measurement of serum **inhibin** (a glycoprotein produced by granulosa cells) is useful in following progress.

### Thecoma

This is a spindle-celled tumour, found mainly during the third, fourth and fifth decades of life. It is benign and rarely recurs.

Function of these tumours varies widely. Oestrogenic effects consist of:

1.  Precocious puberty in children.
2.  Hyperplasia of endometrium. This may be atypical and carcinoma develops occasionally.

**Fibromas** are histologically similar but do not produce hormones. They may be associated with pleural effusion (Meigs syndrome).

### Sertoli-Leydig cell tumours (androblastoma)

Tubules lined by SERTOLI cells, sometimes pyramidal with clear cytoplasm.

LEYDIG cells occasionally with Reinke crystalloids in their cytoplasm

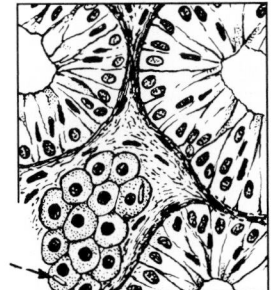

This typifies the virilising tumour group. It is a rare tumour. The degree of virilisation varies. Usually a small yellow tumour within the ovary, it is characteristic on microscopy. Some of these tumours are malignant and consist of poorly differentiated spindle cells with occasional tubule formations.

The androgens, if secreted, result in:

1.  Atrophy of breasts and external genitalia.
2.  Deepening of voice, temporal recession of hair.
3.  Growth of facial and body hair.
4.  Enlargement of clitoris.

# TUMOURS OF THE OVARY – GERM CELL

### GERM CELL TUMOURS

These arise from primitive germ cells capable of differentiating in many ways. The following diagram indicates the main varieties of tumour produced.

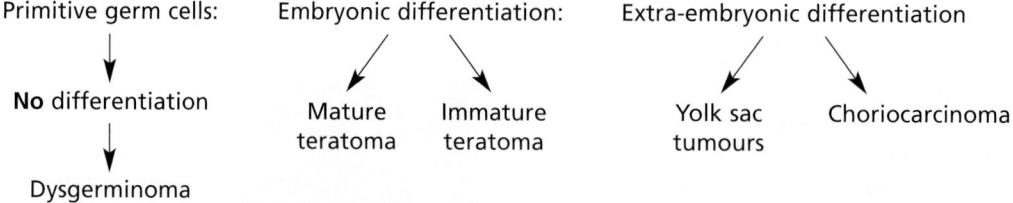

Primitive germ cells:       Embryonic differentiation:        Extra-embryonic differentiation

**No** differentiation        Mature        Immature        Yolk sac        Choriocarcinoma
                             teratoma      teratoma        tumours

Dysgerminoma

### Dysgerminoma

This is a solid tumour, usually ovoid with a smooth capsule, greyish colour and rubbery consistency. Like all germ cell tumours it is commoner in younger age groups. It is sometimes bilateral. Some cases are found in association with gonadal dysgenesis.

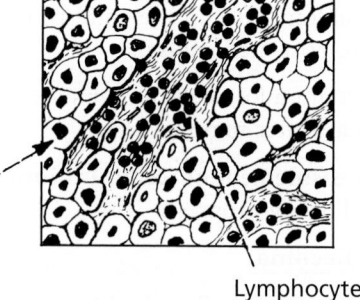

Lymphocytes

Microscopically, it consists of large clear round cells with large nuclei resembling germ cells. These are arranged in alveoli separated by fine connective tissue infiltrated by lymphocytes. These histological appearances are identical to those of seminoma of the testis.

Dysgerminomas are malignant tumours which spread to para-aortic lymph nodes. They are radio-sensitive and also respond to chemotherapy.

# TUMOURS OF THE OVARY – GERM CELL

## Teratomas

These are of two main varieties: (1) mature and (2) immature.

### Mature cystic teratoma (dermoid cyst)

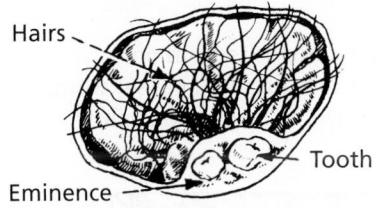

This is one of the commonest ovarian tumours and it occurs at all ages.

It is unilocular with an eminence on one aspect from which hairs grow. Teeth may be present. The cyst is lined by stratified squamous epithelium. Sebaceous glands, nervous tissue, respiratory, intestinal epithelium and thyroid tissue may also be present.

Very occasionally the squamous epithelium may undergo malignant change.

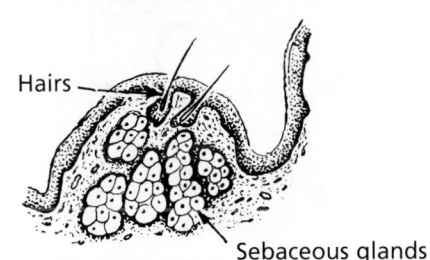

### Immature teratoma

The tumours are predominantly solid and are malignant. They contain immature tissues, typically of primitive nerve tissue and mesenchymal tissue. They may metastasise to the peritoneum where the nerve tissue may differentiate (gliomatosis peritonei).

Chemotherapy has greatly improved the prognosis in these cases.

Solid tumours are occasionally seen consisting only of thyroid tissue (struma ovarii) or carcinoid tumour cells.

### Extra-embryonic tumours (yolk sac tumours, choriocarcinoma)

These are very rare and highly malignant, but modern chemotherapy has greatly improved the prognosis.

# TUMOURS OF THE OVARY – GERM CELL AND SECONDARIES

### SECONDARY TUMOURS

The ovaries are often the site of metastases from the breast, lung, intestinal system, etc. They are commonest during the child-bearing years.

### Krukenberg tumour

This is a very characteristic secondary tumour due to metastatic deposits from an undiscovered carcinoma, usually from the gastrointestinal tract in a premenopausal woman. Both ovaries are involved. They are firm and fibrous, of equal size, smooth and slightly lobulated. No adhesions are present.

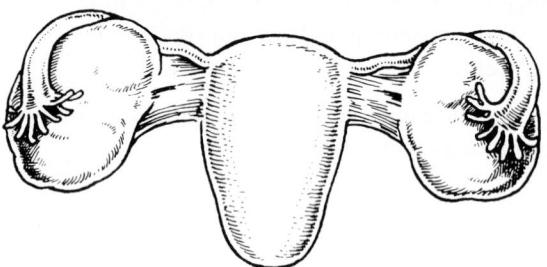
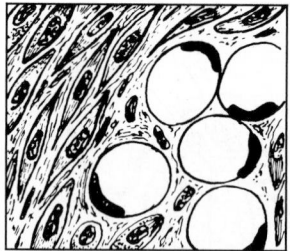

Histologically there are large tumour cells, eccentric nuclei and clear cytoplasm containing mucin (signet ring cells) lying in a spindle-celled stroma.

# ECTOPIC PREGNANCY

This means implantation of the fertilised ovum outside the uterine cavity, usually in the fallopian tube.

**Aetiology**

Most commonly the tube has been previously damaged by salpingitis, leading to partial blockage of the tube. There has been an increased incidence of ectopic pregnancy in women fitted with intrauterine contraceptive devices.

**Sites of implantation**

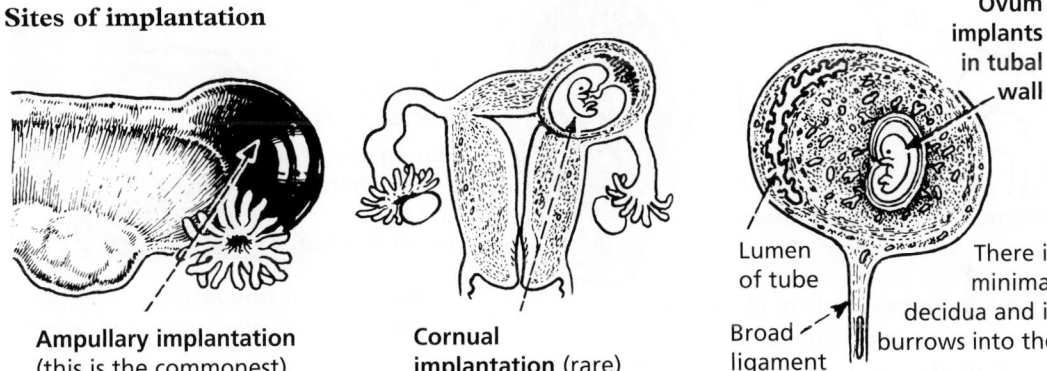

**Ampullary implantation**
(this is the commonest)

**Cornual implantation** (rare)

Ovum implants in tubal wall

Lumen of tube

Broad ligament

There is minimal decidua and it burrows into the

**Uterine changes**

Decidua develops

Uterus enlarges

Erosion of the tubal tissues by the ovum results in **rupture**.

This is the commonest finding.
The direction of rupture varies:

(1) Rupture into the lumen of the tube and leakage into peritoneal cavity.

(2) Rupture directly into the peritoneal cavity. If the implantation is cornual, there may be a further complication: damage to the uterine arteries with **arterial bleeding**.

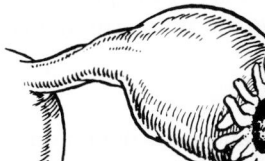

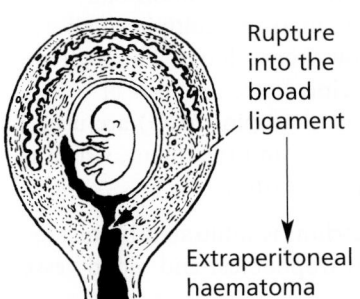

Rupture into the broad ligament

Extraperitoneal haematoma

(3) Exceedingly rarely the whole pregnancy – ovum and placental tissue – aborts into the peritoneal cavity where it reimplants. Usually development is limited and the foetus dies, but continuation of the pregnancy almost to term has been reported.

# GESTATIONAL TROPHOBLAST DISEASE

This term describes proliferative conditions of placental tissue.

## HYDATIDIFORM MOLE

This occurs in two forms:

1. **Complete**. This occurs when an ovum lacking its nucleus is fertilised by one or two sperm. The pregnancy lacks a foetus. The uterus is filled by cysts of varying size.

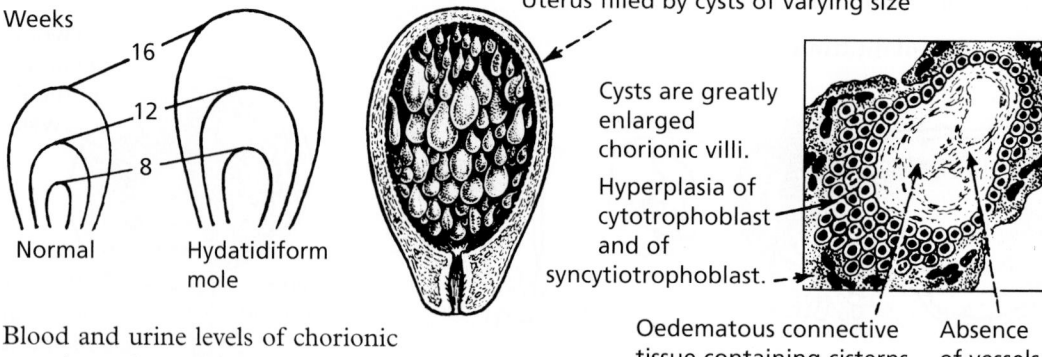

Weeks

Normal    Hydatidiform mole

Uterus filled by cysts of varying size

Cysts are greatly enlarged chorionic villi.

Hyperplasia of cytotrophoblast and of syncytiotrophoblast.

Oedematous connective tissue containing cisterns    Absence of vessels

Blood and urine levels of chorionic gonadotropin are high.

> *Prevalence*: uncommon in the West (1 in 1 500 pregnancies) but common in the East (1 in 120 pregnancies).
> *Genetics*: both sets of chromosomes are paternal, usually 46XX.
> *Progress*: abortion is the usual outcome; there is a 2–3% risk of CHORIOCARCINOMA developing.
> An **invasive mole** is a complete mole in which the villi may penetrate the myometrium and invade blood vessels with pulmonary 'metastases'. There is usually complete regression after hysterectomy.

2. **Partial mole**. This occurs when an ovum is fertilised by two sperm resulting in a triploid karyotype 69XXY or 69XXX. Part of the placenta shows cystic change and a foetus, usually malformed, may be present. While trophoblast may persist there is no risk of choriocarcinoma.

## CHORIOCARCINOMA

This is a malignant tumour of trophoblast and is by definition of foetal origin. It usually follows hydatidiform mole. Pleomorphic cytotrophoblast and syncytiotrophoblast, showing numerous mitoses, invade blood vessels causing haemorrhage and early lung metastases

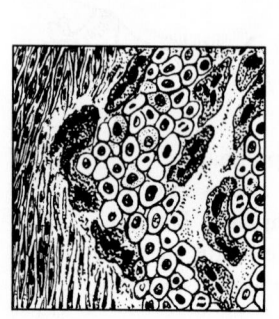

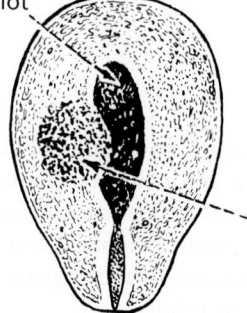

Clot

either as a single large 'cannon-ball' haemorrhagic mass or multiple small emboli ('snow-storm' lung). The high blood and urine concentrations of chorionic gonadotropin (hCG) are used to monitor progress and treatment, which is now usually successful.

The myometrium is infiltrated by masses of malignant trophoblast and blood vessels are eroded.

# BREAST STRUCTURE AND FUNCTION

The breast is a greatly modified sweat gland which has evolved to produce and secrete milk during lactation.

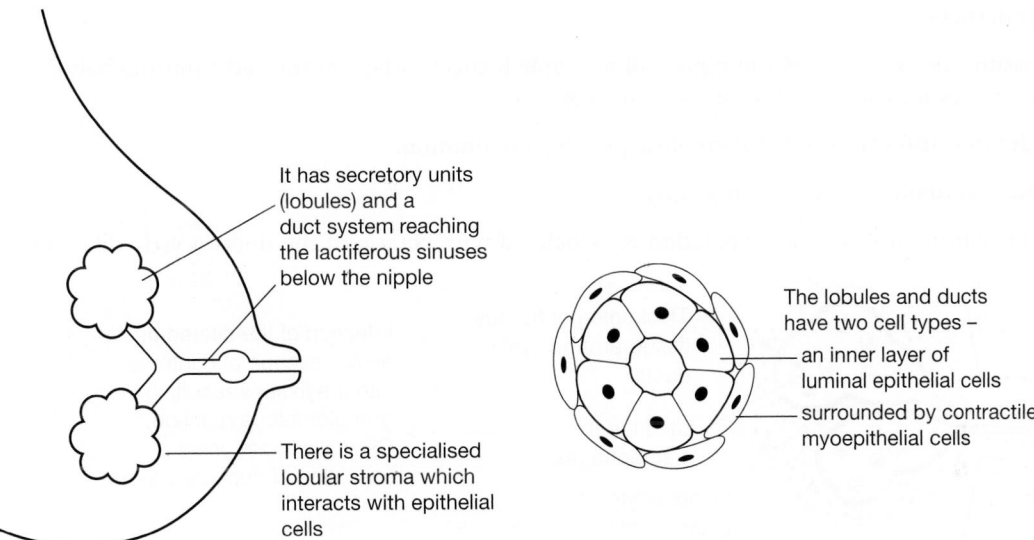

It has secretory units (lobules) and a duct system reaching the lactiferous sinuses below the nipple

There is a specialised lobular stroma which interacts with epithelial cells

The lobules and ducts have two cell types –

an inner layer of luminal epithelial cells

surrounded by contractile myoepithelial cells

The breast responds to oestrogen and progesterone both during the menstrual cycle and, especially, during pregnancy in preparation for lactation.

# BENIGN DISEASES OF THE BREAST

### Inflammatory disorders

**Acute infection** is an occasional complication of **lactation**. It presents with pain and tenderness.

Fissures or abrasions of the nipple allow staphylococci to be transmitted from the baby. Abscesses may form in the breast with scarring.

**Chronic infection,** e.g. tuberculosis, is very uncommon.

### Duct ectasia (plasma cell mastitis)

This chronic inflammatory reaction is associated with ectasia of the ducts (cystic dilatation).

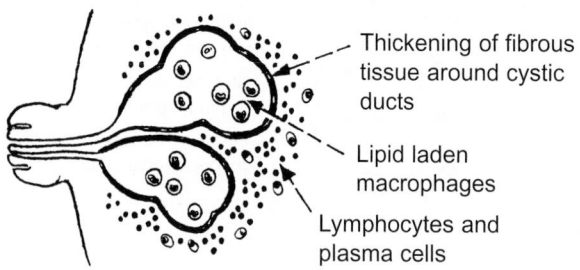

Thickening of fibrous tissue around cystic ducts

Lipid laden macrophages

Lymphocytes and plasma cells

Infection of the dilated ducts allows escape of contents into the tissues resulting in granulomatous reaction. Clinically it may raise suspicion of duct carcinoma.

**Traumatic fat necrosis** may present as a mass mimicking carcinoma. There is necrotic fat with lipid-rich macrophages, giant cells and later, fibrosis.

In some cases of **silicone implant**, there is leakage of silicone with fibrosis and granulomatous inflammation in the surrounding 'capsule'.

### Fibrocystic change

This change presents as a lump or lumpiness of the breast in pre-menopausal women.

1. **Fibrosis**. There is progressive hyalinisation of the stroma.
2. **Cyst formation**. Obstruction of ducts leads to dilatation of the ducts and acini. The lining epithelium may show apocrine metaplasia.
3. (a) **Adenosis**. This is an increase in the number of lobules and in the size of existing lobules.
   (b) **Sclerosing adenosis**
   This is a localised condition which may simulate carcinoma. There is proliferation of acini and stroma, with fibrosis.

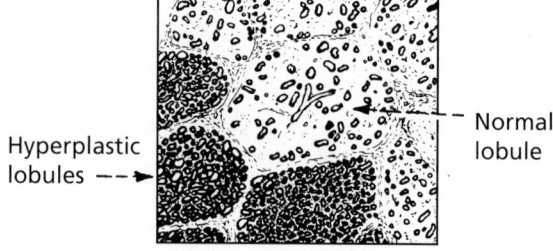

Hyperplastic lobules - - ➤

Normal lobule

# BENIGN DISEASES OF THE BREAST

4.  **Epithelial hyperplasia** means proliferation of the epithelial component of the breast and is important because some forms are associated with an increased risk of breast cancer.

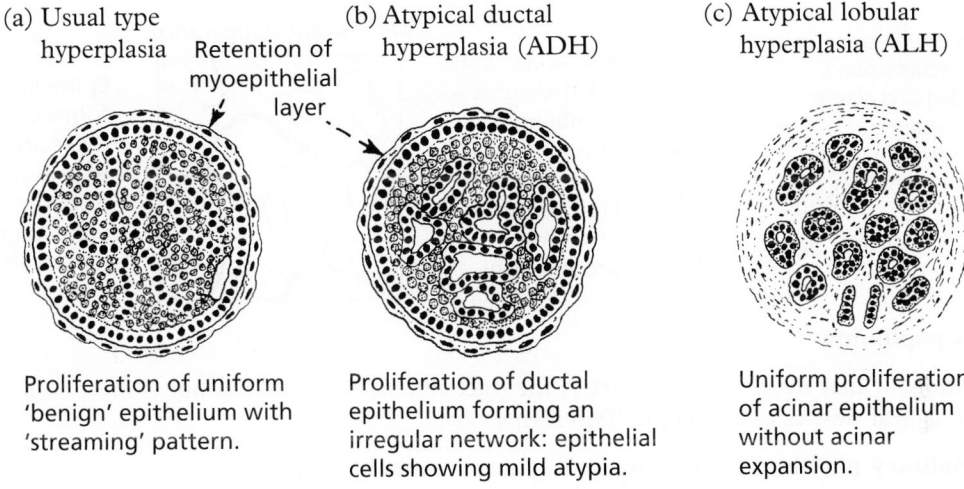

(a) Usual type hyperplasia

Retention of myoepithelial layer

(b) Atypical ductal hyperplasia (ADH)

(c) Atypical lobular hyperplasia (ALH)

Proliferation of uniform 'benign' epithelium with 'streaming' pattern.

Proliferation of ductal epithelium forming an irregular network: epithelial cells showing mild atypia.

Uniform proliferation of acinar epithelium without acinar expansion.

Fibrocystic change is very common, and the various changes are due to abnormal and exaggerated responses of the breast tissues to the cyclical physiological menstrual hormonal stimuli.

**Radial scar**

This small (up to 1 cm diameter), firm lesion shows a central dense fibrous core with radiating fingers of fibrosis entrapping and distorting glandular elements. It is benign but can be confused with carcinoma even on histological examination.

Similar but larger lesions, also detected by mammography, are known as **complex sclerosing lesions**.

# BENIGN BREAST TUMOURS AND IN SITU CARCINOMA

### Fibroadenoma

This is the commonest benign tumour of the breast. It is usually single, occurring in young women. It presents clinically as a small, firm, mobile lump.

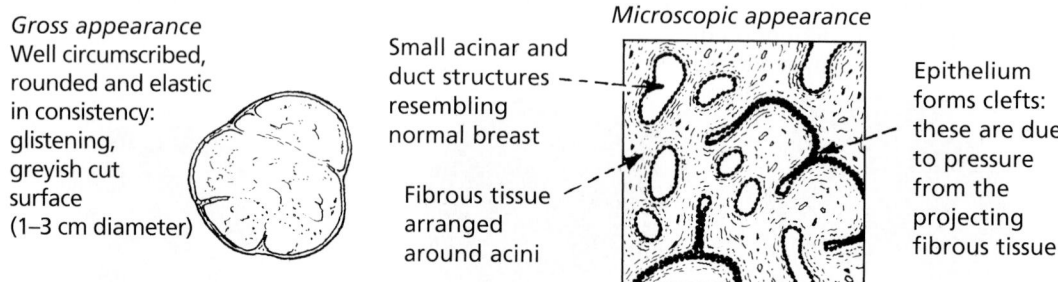

*Gross appearance*
Well circumscribed, rounded and elastic in consistency: glistening, greyish cut surface
(1–3 cm diameter)

Small acinar and duct structures resembling normal breast

Fibrous tissue arranged around acini

*Microscopic appearance*

Epithelium forms clefts: these are due to pressure from the projecting fibrous tissue

### Duct papilloma

This tumour may develop in any part of the duct system of the breast, but is most common in the lacteal sinuses at the nipple. Two forms exist:

1.  **Solitary papilloma**. These are almost always near the nipple.

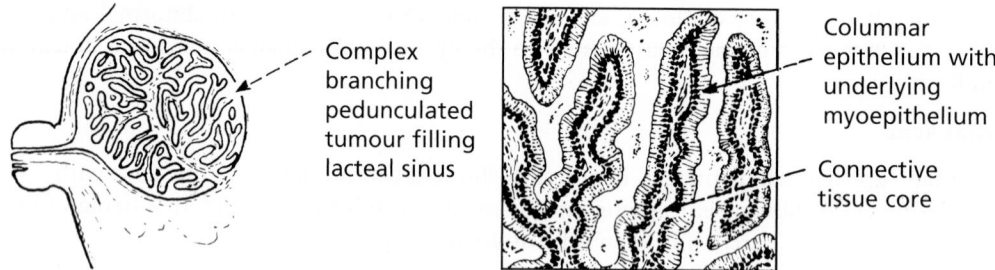

Complex branching pedunculated tumour filling lacteal sinus

Columnar epithelium with underlying myoepithelium

Connective tissue core

Prominent myoepithelium gives a double layer of cells covering the fronds.

2.  **Multiple papillomas**
    These may be distributed throughout the duct system. There is a small increased risk of cancer developing.

    In both forms, there may be discharge from the nipple which may be blood stained. Cytological examination of the discharge will reveal benign epithelial cells.

# BENIGN BREAST TUMOURS AND IN SITU CARCINOMA

### Ductal carcinoma in situ (DCIS)

The cells lining the ducts show cytological features of malignancy but have not yet invaded the stroma. Focal calcification allows it to be detected by mammographic screening or it may present as a palpable mass.

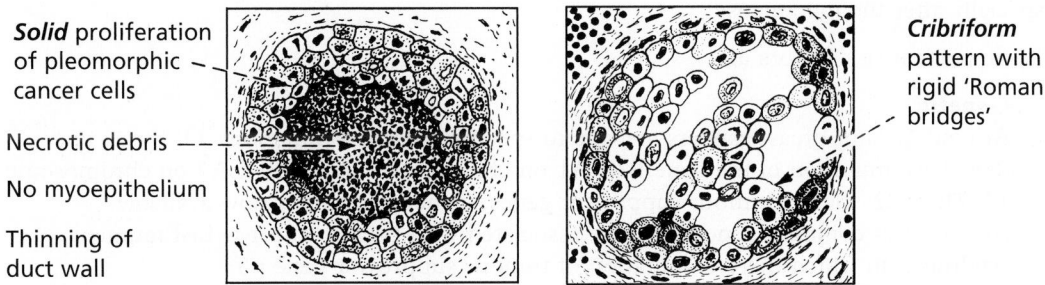

*Solid* proliferation of pleomorphic cancer cells

Necrotic debris

No myoepithelium

Thinning of duct wall

*Cribriform* pattern with rigid 'Roman bridges'

DCIS is graded 1, 2 or 3 depending on how abnormal the cells are. The higher the grade, the higher the risk of invasive malignancy. Intraepithelial spread of DCIS into the nipple skin gives rise to Paget's disease.

**Lobular carcinoma in situ.** This lesion is usually multifocal and bilateral. The breast acini of affected lobules are distended by fairly uniform cells which grow into the duct system or break through basement membrane to become infiltrative carcinoma, either of lobular or ductal type.

# CARCINOMA OF THE BREAST

This is the commonest form of malignancy in women and rarely occurs in men. It may be found in any part of the breast but most frequently it is found in the upper outer quadrant.

### Aetiology

Breast cancer is uncommon below the age of 30 years. The risk steadily increases with age, especially after the menopause.

The important risk factors are:

1. **Genetic**
   Around 10% of breast cancers are due to specific inherited mutations. Of these, one-third have mutation of the gene BRCA1 on chromosome 17 or BRCA2 on chromosome 13. These are classic tumour suppressor genes. Genetic testing is now available. Another less common genetic disease associated with breast cancer is Li-Fraumeni syndrome, in which there is mutation of tumour suppressor gene p53.
2. **Sex hormone associations**
   (a) Commoner in nulliparous women.
   (b) Early menarche and late menopause increase risk – prolonged cyclical exposure to sex hormones.
   (c) Breast feeding reduces risk.

### INFILTRATING DUCTAL CARCINOMA

This is the commonest form and presents as a firm to hard lump. The following illustrations show a large carcinoma with significant local spread. Modern screening methods aim to detect the disease at a much earlier stage.

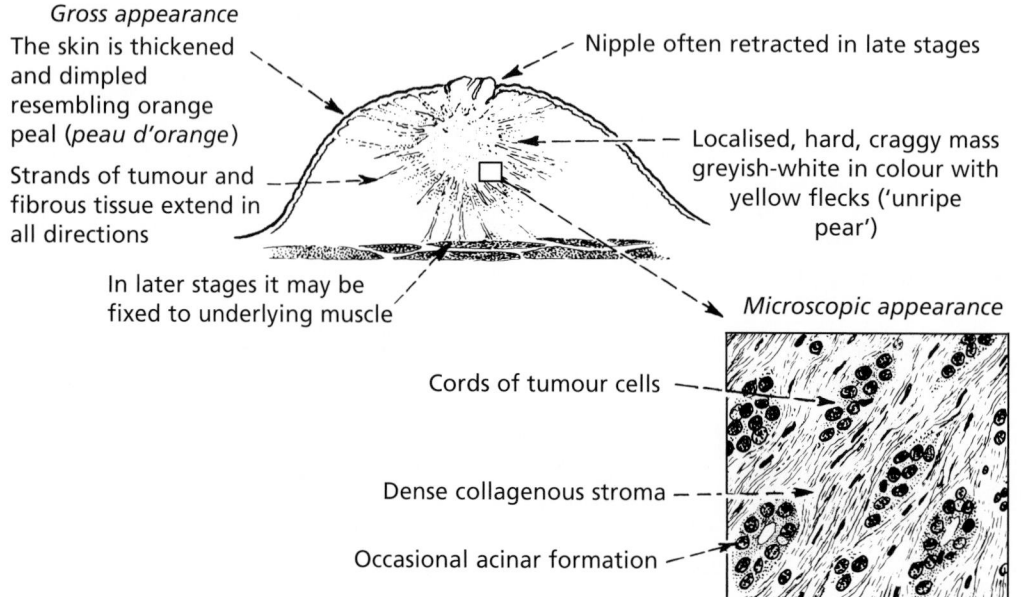

*Gross appearance*

The skin is thickened and dimpled resembling orange peal (*peau d'orange*)

Strands of tumour and fibrous tissue extend in all directions

In later stages it may be fixed to underlying muscle

Nipple often retracted in late stages

Localised, hard, craggy mass greyish-white in colour with yellow flecks ('unripe pear')

*Microscopic appearance*

Cords of tumour cells

Dense collagenous stroma

Occasional acinar formation

# CARCINOMA OF THE BREAST

## INFILTRATING LOBULAR CARCINOMA

Ten percent of breast cancers are of this type. There is a 10% chance of a similar tumour arising in the contralateral breast. They may be multifocal. Microscopically the tumour infiltrates the tissues as single files of malignant cells.

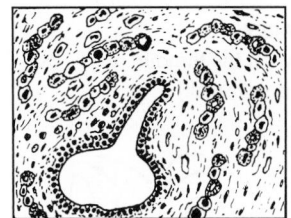

Infiltrating lobular carcinoma

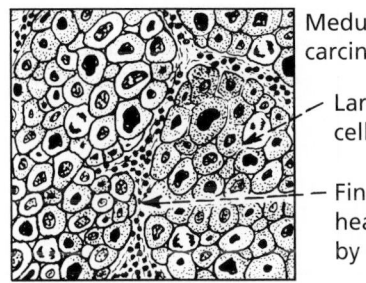

Medullary carcinoma

Large tumour cells

Fine stroma often heavily infiltrated by lymphocytes

**More rare forms** of breast cancer are TUBULAR CARCINOMA – showing well-differentiated tubular structures. MEDULLARY CARCINOMA – a highly cellular tumour with a florid lymphocytic infiltrate and a 'pushing margin', and MUCINOUS CARCINOMA where the malignant cells lie in pools of mucin.

**Local spread**: in late stages there may be infiltration of the skin with ulceration. Intra-epithelial spread of tumour may also occur. The classical example is PAGET'S DISEASE OF THE NIPPLE. Tumour cells spread along the duct system and out onto the skin surface.

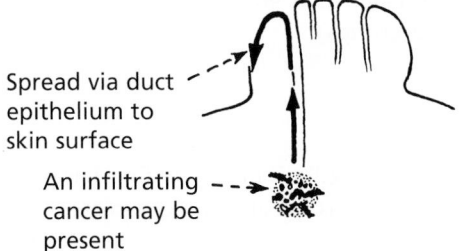

Spread via duct epithelium to skin surface

An infiltrating cancer may be present

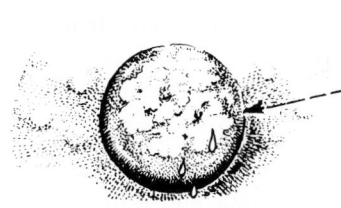

Nipple is red, swollen and inflamed

*Microscopic examination* reveals:

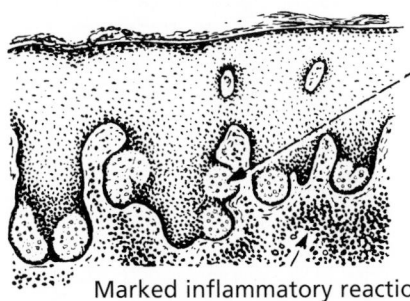

Packets of pale cells in the epithelium

Marked inflammatory reaction in dermis with plasma cells.

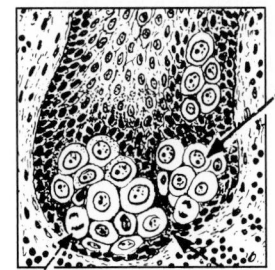

Paget cells (nuclei large with prominent nucleoli; cytoplasm clear)

Occasional mitosis

# CARCINOMA OF THE BREAST

**Metastatic spread**: this is by lymphatics and blood vessels.

| EARLY (when the tumour is still small) | via **LYMPHATICS** | via **BLOOD STREAM** |
|---|---|---|
| | 1. to axillary nodes from all sites of breast; <br> 2. through internal mammary lymphatics to thorax (esp. in cancers sited medially). | to bone marrow where cells can lie dormant for long periods. |
| **LATE** | Local spread via skin lymphatics causing: <br> (a) Widespread lesion – skin becomes stiff and board-like: 'cancer-en-cuirasse'. <br> (b) Blockage of dermal lymphatics: oedema of skin except at anchorage points, 'peau d'orange'. | Secondaries appear in many viscera, particularly liver, lung and bone (spine, long bones). |

## Prognosis

The prognosis is influenced by the following factors, the first three of which are components of the TNM (tumour-node-metastasis) staging system.

1. Size – lesions under 2 cm have a 5-year survival of greater than 90%.
2. Number of lymph nodes involved (divided into three groups):
   (a) no nodes involved
   (b) 1–3 nodes
   (c) ≥4 nodes

Sentinel node biopsy is currently the mainstay for staging the axilla. This is the first lymph node draining the breast tissue and if this contains tumour, i.e. is 'positive', a complete axillary clearance is performed.

3. Distant metastases – patients with haematogenous spread are rarely curable.
4. Histological grade (graded 1, 2, 3) on the basis of:
   (a) extent of tubule formation
   (b) nuclear pleomorphism
   (c) mitotic activity

# CARCINOMA OF THE BREAST

5.   Hormone receptor status – oestrogen receptor positive tumours respond better to tamoxifen and other antioestrogen drugs. Progesterone receptors are also detected. Demonstration of overexpression HER2/NEU allows treatment by monoclonal antibodies (herceptin) directed against the protein.

These factors are summarised in prognostic indices such as the Nottingham Prognostic Index, based on size, lymph node status and grade.

### Screening for breast cancer

The aim of screening is to detect either pre-malignant conditions or cancer at an early stage and is very important where there is a family history of cancer. Mammography is capable of detecting intra-duct carcinoma and pre-cancerous lesions. Focal calcification is an important indicator but is not diagnostic of malignancy because it also occurs in benign lesions. Whatever method of screening is used, the diagnosis must be established on morphological evidence using fine needle aspiration or more commonly needle biopsy.

**Other rare tumours of** the breast include PHYLLODES TUMOUR – large and usually benign, affecting elderly women; occasionally sarcoma of the stroma is present. Soft tissue sarcomas and primary lymphoma are rare.

### THE MALE BREAST

Breast disease is uncommon in men. Abnormal enlargement – gynaecomastia – may occur in a temporary form at puberty or as a permanent feature in Klinefelter syndrome (XXY). Oestrogen metabolic imbalance (e.g. in liver disease) or excess intake (e.g. treatment of prostatic cancer) are other causes. All tumours are rare but breast cancer does occur.

# NERVOUS SYSTEM

## OBJECTIVES

1. To understand the functional anatomy and physiology of the nervous system and how these apply to common pathological presentations.
2. To understand the pathology of cerebral infarction and haemorrhage.
3. To describe traumatic injuries to the CNS and their effects.
4. To recall the main causes of dementia and have a basic understanding of the pathological changes.
5. To recall the distribution and effects of common infections of the CNS.
6. To have a basic understanding of demyelinating and degenerative disease of the CNS.
7. To briefly describe the effect of metabolic disorders and toxins on the CNS.
8. To describe the mechanisms of hydrocephalus and the common causes.
9. To recall neoplasms that affect the central and peripheral nervous system.

# NERVOUS SYSTEM – ANATOMY AND PHYSIOLOGY

Considerations of anatomy and physiology have important applications to diseases of the CNS, particularly their effects and spread.

The anatomy of the various coverings is important.

**The skull and vertebrae** form a rigid compartment protecting the delicate CNS tissues.

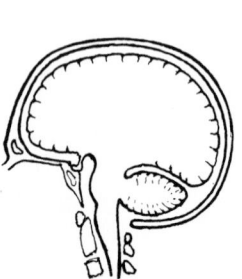

This rigidity has serious disadvantages when pressure inside the skull increases, e.g. an expanding lesion soon takes up the small reserves of space available and the delicate brain tissues are progressively compressed, with very serious results.

**Meninges and cerebrospinal fluid (CSF)**

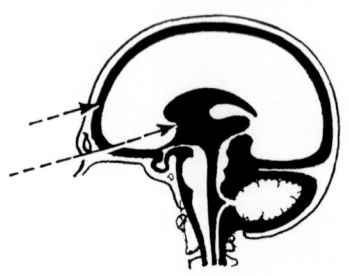

Diseases (particularly infections) at this site are usually *widespread* over the whole brain and cord surfaces, e.g. meningitis. Impediment to the flow of CSF causes serious effects – hydrocephalus.

# NERVOUS SYSTEM – ANATOMY AND PHYSIOLOGY

The detailed arrangement of the meninges is important.
The thick **dura**, closely applied to the skull, acts as the periosteum – its rigid reflections (falx cerebri and tentorium cerebelli) complicate the effects of increased intracranial pressure.

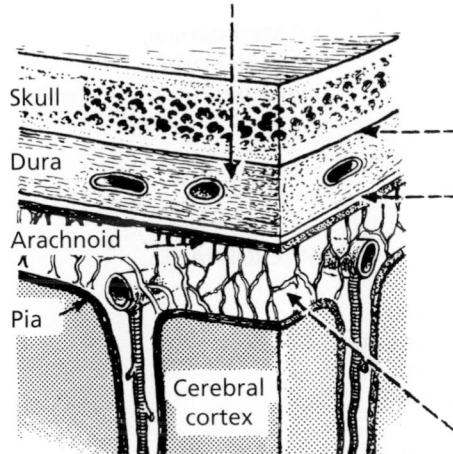

Skull

Dura

Arachnoid

Pia

Cerebral cortex

**Extradural** lesions tend to be localised; they have to strip the dura from the bone.

**Subdural** lesions remain local but can spread more widely since the arachnoid and dura are loosely attached.

The **arachnoid**, a delicate membrane, is loosely attached to the dura and sends trabeculae across the subarachnoid space which contains the cerebral blood vessels and the CSF.

Disease in the **subarachnoid** space can spread widely over the whole surface of the brain and spinal cord but is prevented from penetrating into the brain tissue by the **pia**.

The **pia** is invaginated into the brain substance along with the small penetrating vessels.

The dura, arachnoid and pia act as barriers which selectively separate the CSF and the blood from the CNS tissues.

It is important to understand that, although the CSF is very similar in composition to the extracellular fluid of the brain, changes in the CSF only very indirectly reflect changes in the CNS in disease.

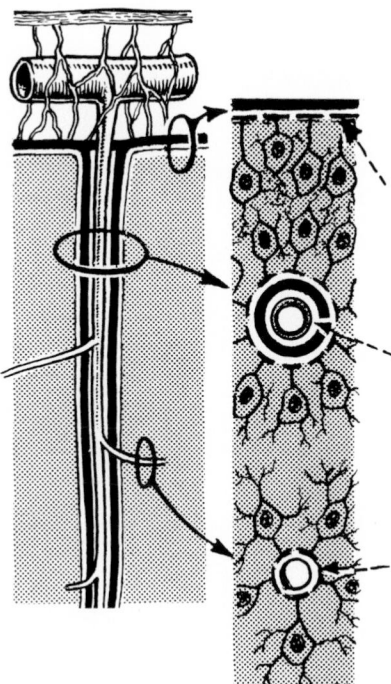

The pia's barrier function is reinforced by the membrane formed by the foot processes of astrocytes:

1. on the brain surface.
2. around the penetrating vessels. The potential space between the vessel wall and the pia is called the Virchow–Robin space.

3. at capillary level the pia is not present, but the foot processes along with the capillary endothelium and basement membrane form a specialised and selective 'blood-brain barrier'.

569

# NERVOUS SYSTEM – ANATOMY AND PHYSIOLOGY

Thus the pia and the membrane formed by the foot processes of the astrocytes separate types of tissue derived from two embryological layers.

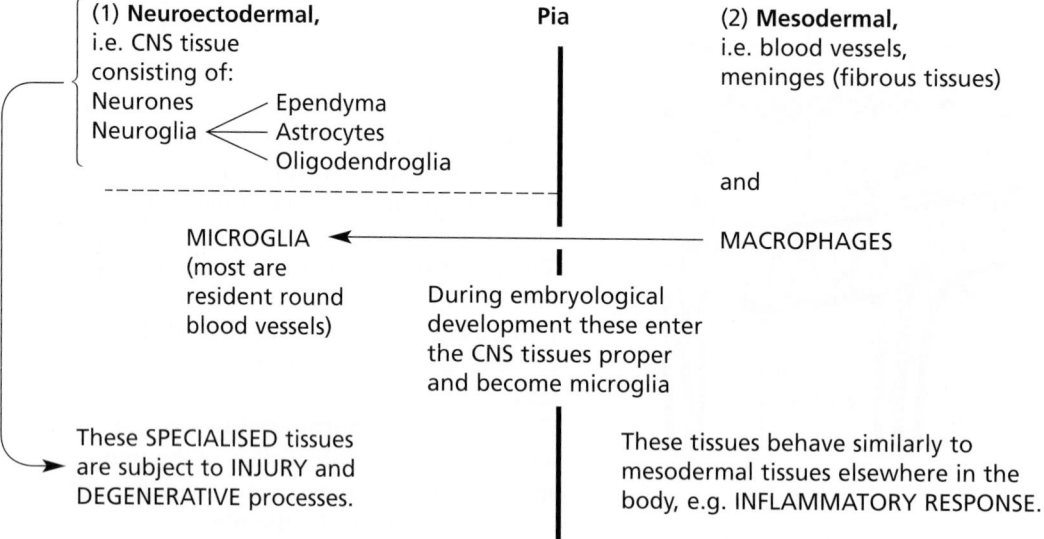

# NEURONAL DAMAGE

**NEURONES** are sensitive to damage by a wide variety of agents including anoxia, hypoglycaemia, virus infections and intracellular metabolic disturbances (e.g. associated with vitamin B deficiencies).

There are two main types, depending on the rapidity of the changes.

1. *Rapid NECROSIS* – associated with acute failure of function.

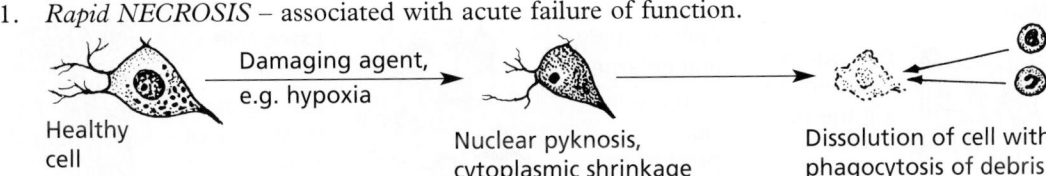

Healthy cell

Nuclear pyknosis, cytoplasmic shrinkage

Dissolution of cell with phagocytosis of debris

2. *Slow ATROPHIC CHANGES* – associated with gradual loss of function.

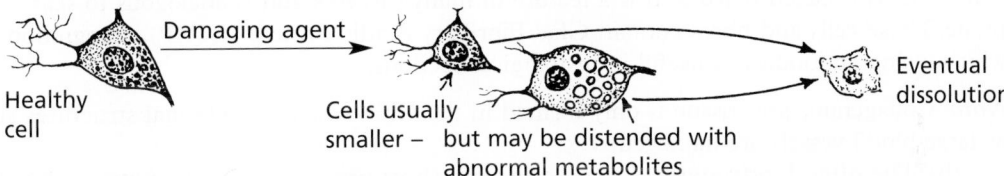

Healthy cell

Cells usually smaller – but may be distended with abnormal metabolites

Eventual dissolution

The process of ageing involves cumulative atrophy and disappearance of neurones; in some individuals the process is speeded up resulting in *presenile dementia*.

*Note*: There is no regeneration of destroyed neurones.

A large group of disorders of cerebral function seen in psychiatric practice have (as yet) no morphological evidence of nerve cell damage. They are caused by disturbances of poorly understood biochemical control mechanisms within the brain.

In addition to the PRIMARY degenerations described above, neurones are subject to SECONDARY degeneration in certain circumstances.

1. ***Retrograde degeneration*** – when the main axon is damaged there is degeneration of the neurone as well as the classical distal degeneration of the axon.

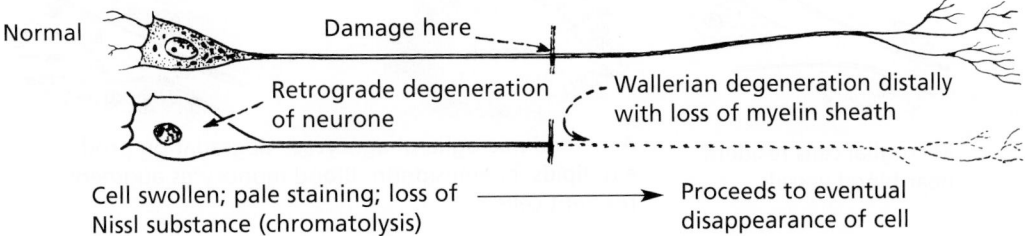

Normal

Damage here

Retrograde degeneration of neurone

Wallerian degeneration distally with loss of myelin sheath

Cell swollen; pale staining; loss of Nissl substance (chromatolysis) ⟶ Proceeds to eventual disappearance of cell

2. ***Trans-synaptic degeneration*** – in closely integrated neurone systems, neurone loss may be followed by degeneration of associated neurones across synapses.

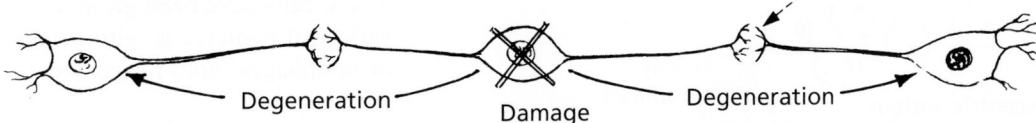

Degeneration — Damage — Degeneration

# GLIAL REACTIONS

The glial cells react vigorously in many diseases of the CNS.

1. The **NEUROGLIAL** cells have supportive and nutritive functions.
   (a) The **astrocytes** with their numerous fibrillary processes give structural support. They are less susceptible to damage than neurones.

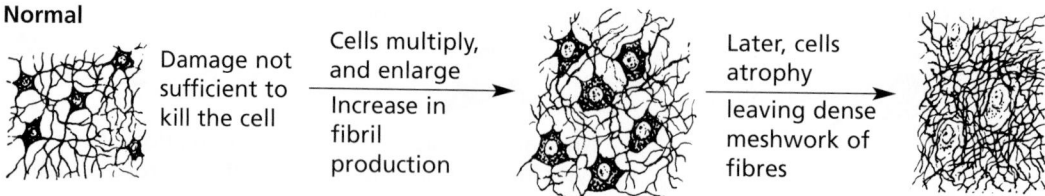

This process is called GLIOSIS. It is a feature of many diseases and is analogous to scar tissue. These cells and fibres contain Glial Fibrillary Acidic Protein (GFAP), recognition of which, using antibodies, is useful in histological sections.

*Note*: Collagenous scar tissue is only formed in the CNS when mesodermal structures such as large blood vessels are damaged.

   (b) The **oligodendrocytes** – small cells with short processes – have a nutritive function in respect of neurones and especially myelin. This reaction is best seen when neurones are damaged.

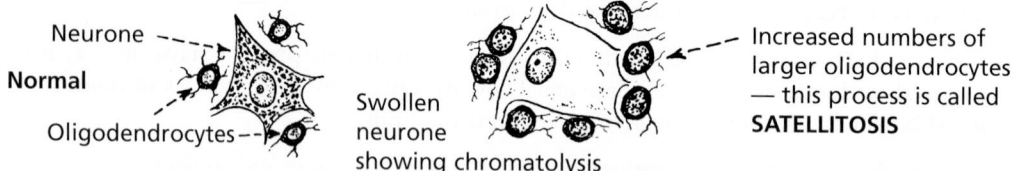

2. The **MICROGLIAL** cells are members of the mononuclear-phagocytic system. Reaction is best seen when there is necrosis of tissues.

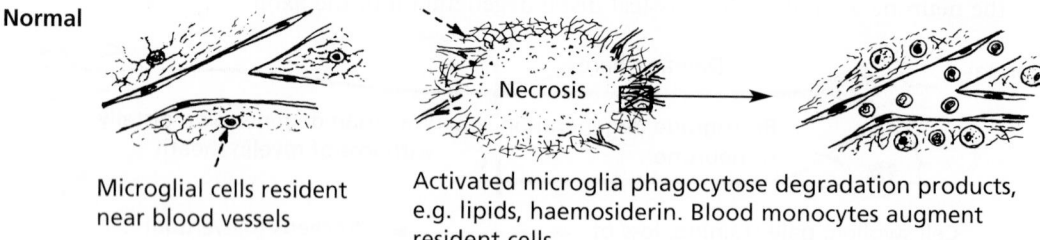

Microglial cells are well seen in and around infarcts; the activated cells which have ingested lipids are strikingly different from the small inactive microglia.

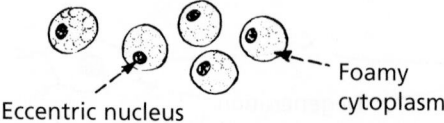

These cells have been given a variety of names, e.g. 'gitter' cells, or lipophages (lipid phagocytes).

# INCREASED INTRACRANIAL PRESSURE

**INCREASED INTRACRANIAL PRESSURE** (ICP) occurs in two main circumstances:

1. Due to the presence of an EXPANDING LESION.
2. Due to obstruction of the free flow of the CSF – this causes hydrocephalus and is dealt with on page 615.

## INTRACRANIAL EXPANDING LESIONS

These lesions may occur within the brain substance or in the meninges. Important examples are:

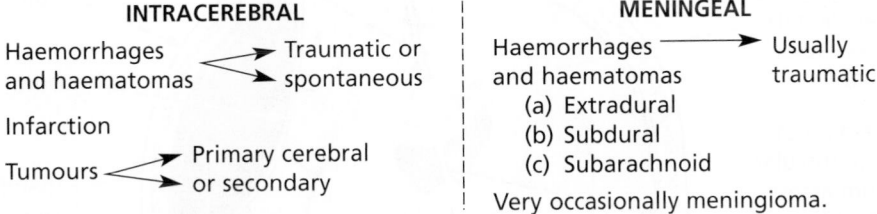

The situation is often aggravated by cerebral OEDEMA.

The severity of the effects are modified by two important factors:

(1) the size of the lesion and (2) the rapidity of expansion.

There are three stages in the progress of increased ICP.

(1) The stage of **Compensation**

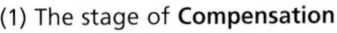

(2) The stage of **Decompensation**

At this stage there are herniations and distortions of the brain with their associated complications including:
- Reduction in level of consciousness;
- Dilatation of pupil ipsilateral to mass lesion and papilloedema;
- Bradycardia with raised blood pressure ('Cushing' effect);
- Cheyne-Stokes respiration.

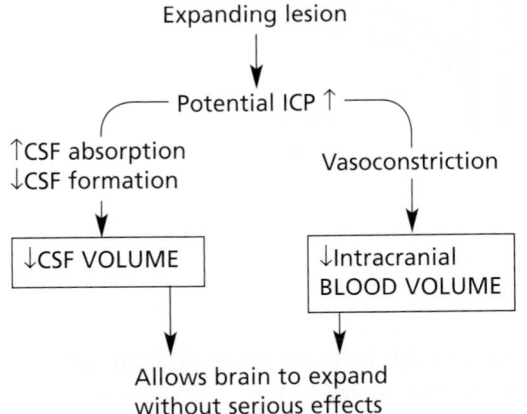

(3) A vicious circle is established leading to the stage of vasomotor paralysis.

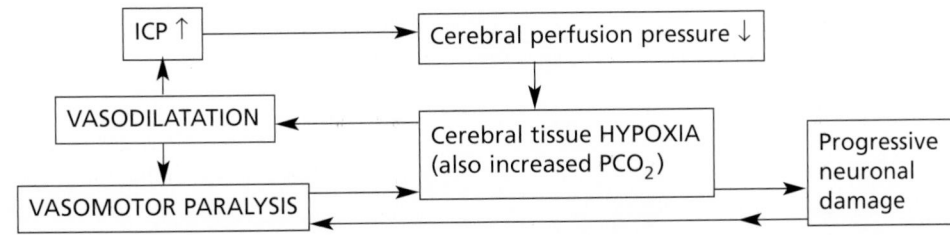

# INCREASED INTRACRANIAL PRESSURE

### EFFECTS

### Distortions and dislocations of the brain substance

These are to some extent dependent on the site of the initiating lesion; the effects of a unilateral expanding lesion are illustrated.

(1) Flattened cerebral convolutions (diminished subarachnoid space)

(2) Herniation of cingulate gyrus under the falx (supracallosal hernia)

(3) Movement of interventricular septum across the mid-line with distortion of ventricles

(4) Herniation of parahippocampal gyrus past the free edge of the tentorium cerebelli (tentorial hernia)

(5) Midbrain pushed against tentorium of opposite side (Kernohan notch); may give rise to paradoxical signs

(6) Cerebellar tonsils and medulla pushed down into foramen magnum

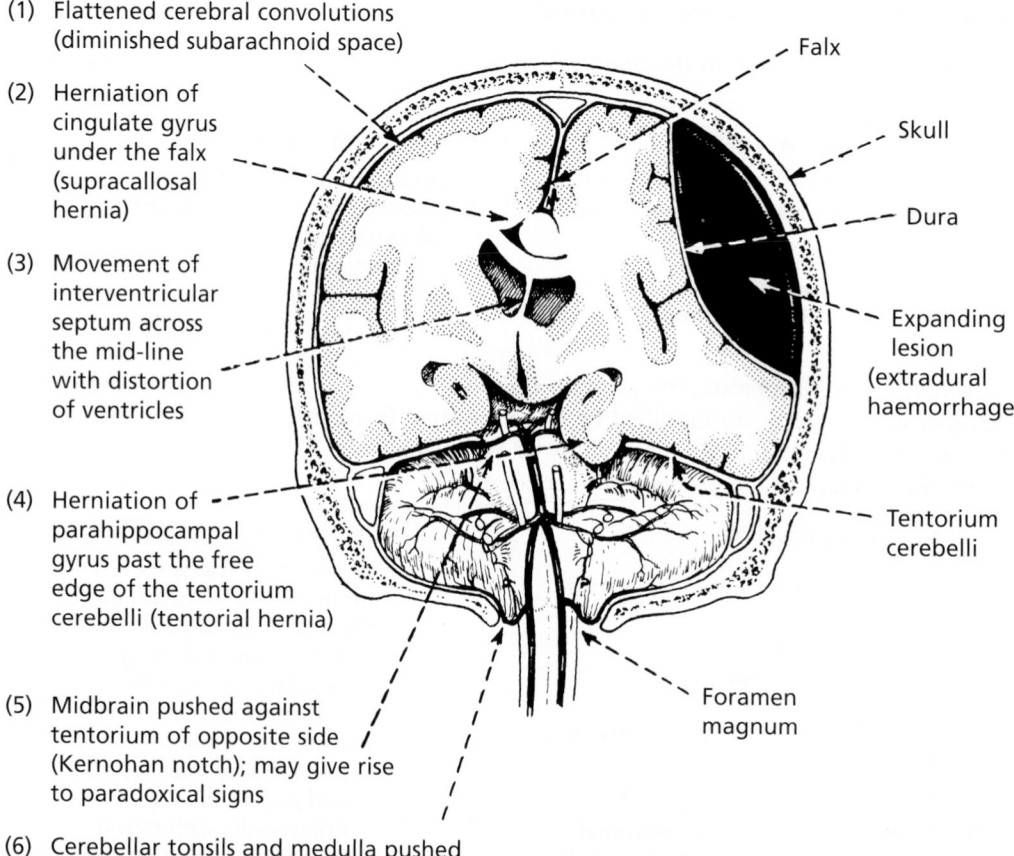

Falx

Skull

Dura

Expanding lesion (extradural haemorrhage)

Tentorium cerebelli

Foramen magnum

*Note:* The sudden removal of even small amounts of CSF by **LUMBAR PUNCTURE** may precipitate medullary 'coning' with fatal results due to damage to the 'vital centres'.

# CEREBRAL OEDEMA

Swelling of the brain, of which oedema is the major component, is an important complication of many brain diseases because the enlargement either initiates or aggravates increased intracranial pressure.

The process may be localised or generalised depending on the type of initiating disorder.

| LOCALISED CONDITIONS | GENERALISED CONDITIONS |
|---|---|
| Examples:<br>Infarcts and local ischaemia<br>Haematomas (due to vessel rupture and injury)<br><br>Tumours | Examples: intoxications<br>Metabolic disturbances, e.g. hypoglycaemia<br>Generalised hypoxia<br>Severe head trauma<br>Malignant hypertension |

The pathological mechanism is as follows:

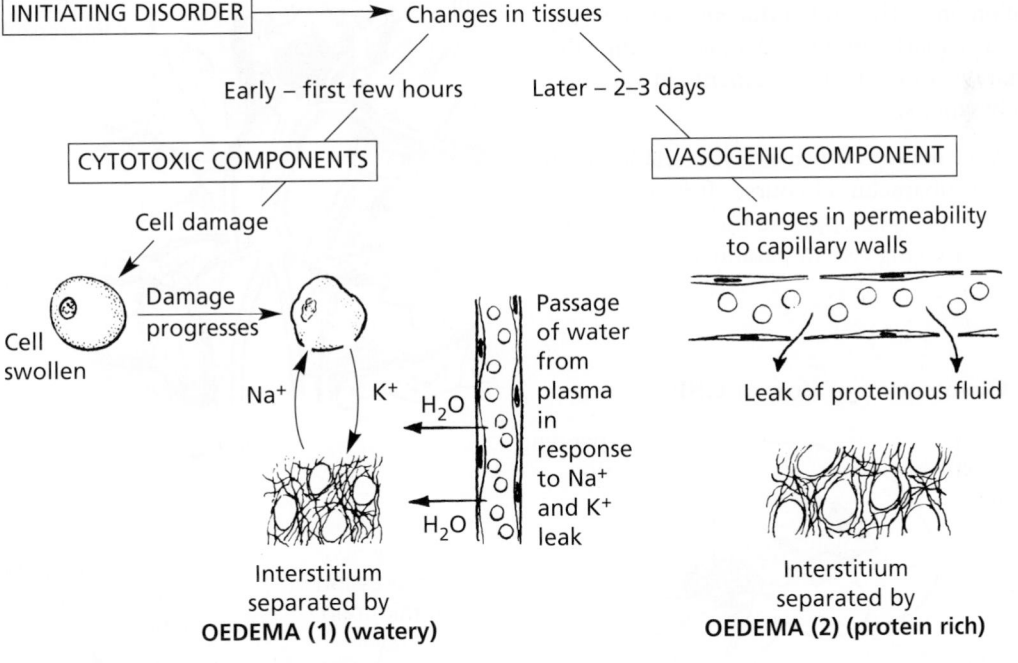

**Interstitium separated by OEDEMA (1) (watery)**

**Interstitium separated by OEDEMA (2) (protein rich)**

*Notes*

(a) Components (1) and (2) overlap.

(b) The oedema fluid tends to spread in the white matter.

(c) The severity of oedema formation is very variable and unpredictable clinically.

(d) In clinical practice, therapy has two aspects:

    1. Treatment of the initiating disorder by any appropriate means.

    2. Minimising the formation of oedema by the use of

        (i) osmotic agents, e.g. urea or mannitol;

        (ii) steroids.

# INCREASED INTRACRANIAL PRESSURE – SECONDARY COMPLICATIONS

1. **Vascular damage**
   (a) Compression of the central retinal
       vein causes PAPILLOEDEMA, an
       important clinical sign of raised ICP.
       *Note*: Axonal flow in the optic nerve
       is reduced, contributing to swelling
       of the optic disc.
   (b) Stretching and compression of blood vessels
       may cause haemorrhage and infarction
       quite remote from the initiating lesion –
       secondary midbrain and calcarine infarction
       and haemorrhage are common.

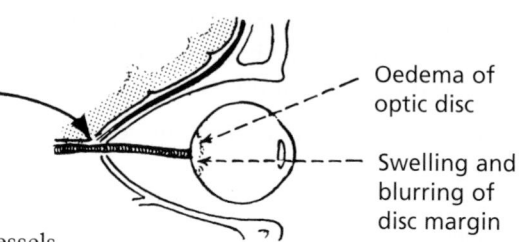

Oedema of
optic disc

Swelling and
blurring of
disc margin

2. **Intracranial nerve damage**

Oculomotor (III) and abducens (VI) nerves
are particularly prone to damage, giving rise
to paralysis of ocular movements in varying
combinations.

The VIth nerve is especially vulnerable due to
its long subarachnoid course. It is often the
nerve on the side opposite the lesion which is
stretched giving rise to paradoxical signs.

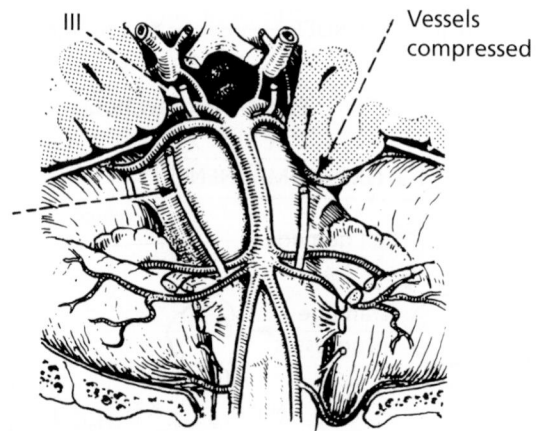

III

Vessels
compressed

3. **Obstruction of flow of CSF**

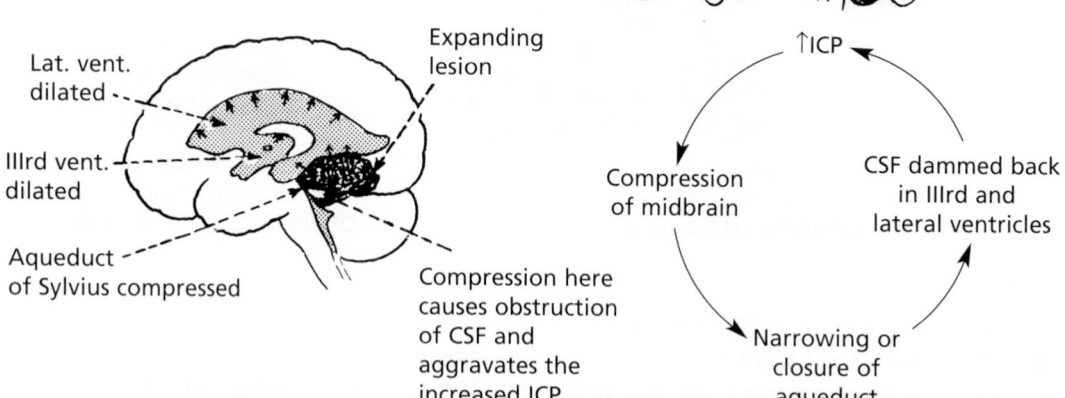

Lat. vent.
dilated

IIIrd vent.
dilated

Aqueduct
of Sylvius compressed

Expanding
lesion

Compression here
causes obstruction
of CSF and
aggravates the
increased ICP

↑ICP

Compression
of midbrain

CSF dammed back
in IIIrd and
lateral ventricles

Narrowing or
closure of
aqueduct

4. **Changes in the skull bones**

Long continued ICP causes bone erosion and thinning visible on X-ray.

(a) Erosion of posterior clinoid processes of sphenoid bone.
(b) In children, before the skull is fully ossified, the inner table is thinned at the sites of
    convolutional pressure giving a striking X-ray appearance.

# CIRCULATORY DISTURBANCES

(1) Hypoxia and ischaemia and (2) intracranial haemorrhage are the important and common mechanisms causing brain damage.

## ACUTE HYPOXIC DISORDERS

*Blood supply:*
20% of cardiac output is delivered via carotid and vertebral arteries

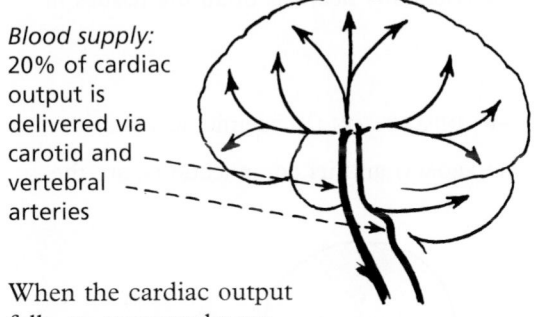

When the cardiac output falls, an autoregulatory vascular control mechanism protects the cerebral blood supply the arterial blood pressure (BP) must be kept above 50 mmHg.

*Neuronal aerobic metabolism of glucose*

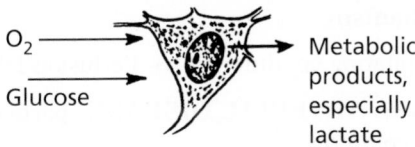

There are no reserves of $O_2$ or glucose in the brain, therefore a constant delivery via arterial blood is necessary.

Neurones are very susceptible to hypoxia (and hypoglycaemia); with complete $O_2$ deprivation neuronal **necrosis** occurs in 5–7 minutes (at normal temperatures).

The following flow diagram illustrates the factors which influence availability of $O_2$ and the conditions giving rise to hypoxia.

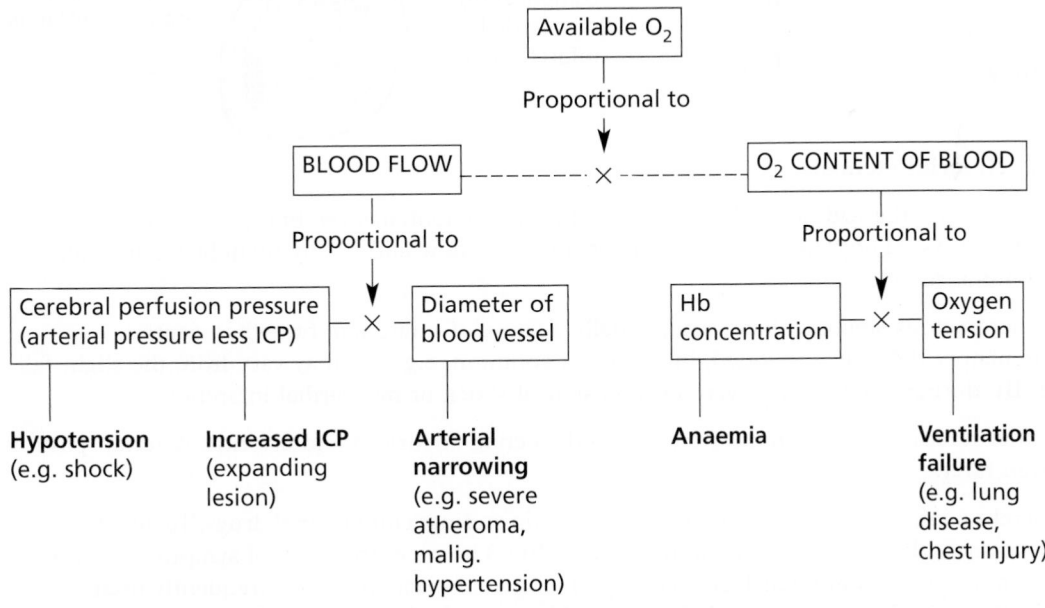

These conditions, singly or together, can be responsible for cerebral hypoxia.

# CEREBRAL INFARCTION

This condition, the commoner of the two main types of stroke (the other is spontaneous intracerebral haemorrhage), is caused by failure of the supply of oxygen (and glucose) to maintain the viability of the tissues in the territory of a cerebral arterial branch. This is not always due to simple local arterial occlusion, and very often a component of central circulatory deficiency is contributory. The lesion is essentially necrosis of all the tissues in the affected territory.

### Mechanism

Precipitating condition ⟶ Perfusion failure ⟶ INFARCTION (ischaemic necrosis)

**LOCAL ARTERIAL DISEASE** (particularly ATHEROMA) and its complications, are the most common.

### 1. Arterial occlusions

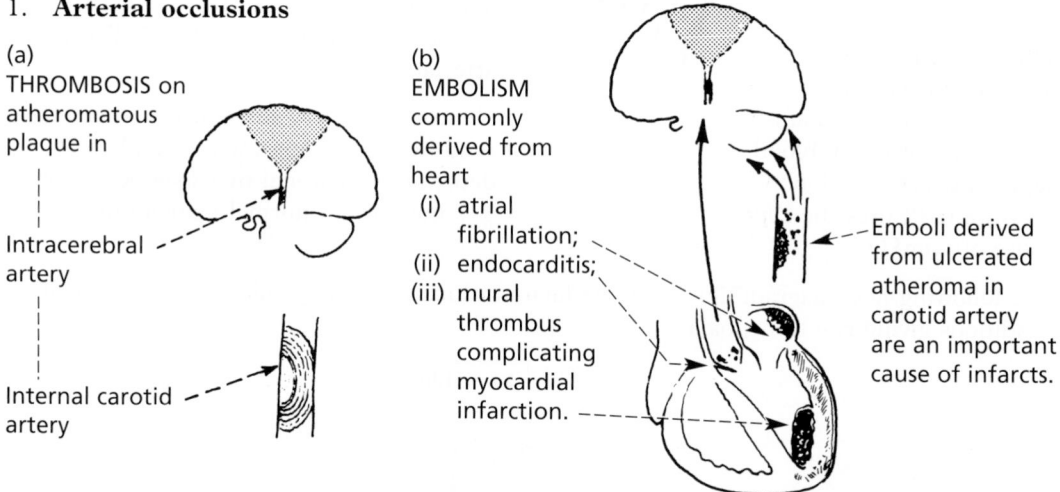

(a)
THROMBOSIS on atheromatous plaque in

Intracerebral artery

Internal carotid artery

(b)
EMBOLISM commonly derived from heart
(i) atrial fibrillation;
(ii) endocarditis;
(iii) mural thrombus complicating myocardial infarction.

Emboli derived from ulcerated atheroma in carotid artery are an important cause of infarcts.

### 2. Arterial stenosis

ATHEROMA – the widespread loss of arterial lumen potentiates cerebral perfusion deficiency in two ways: (1) by distributing the normal arterial flow and (2) by prejudicing anastomotic communications.

Atheromatous stenosis alone is not usually a cause of infarction, but when central circulatory deficiency is added, infarction is common, e.g. this may vary from the slight fall in BP during sleep to the severe hypotension of shock or myocardial infarction.

Other rarer causes of arterial stenosis are dissecting aneurysm and arteritis. Arterial spasm is even rarer.

Cerebral infarction can now be treated by administering 'clot busting' drugs. To avoid permanent damage these need to be given within 3 hours of the onset of symptoms. Tissue plasminogen activator which converts plasminogen to plasmin is most frequently used. Cerebral bleeding is a potential side effect. Alternatively thrombus can be surgically removed using mechanical embolectomy. If the carotid artery is stenosed then endarterectomy may reduce the risk of recurrence when performed after cerebral infarction. The success of these treatments is variable but has revolutionised the outcome of ischaemic stroke.

# CEREBRAL INFARCTION

## SITES

While infarcts may occur anywhere in the brain, depending on the vagaries of the precipitating arterial lesions, certain sites are more commonly affected.

1. In cases of local arterial occlusion, **internal structures supplied by 'end' arterial branches** are particularly vulnerable. The cortex is often protected in variable degrees by anastomoses of other cerebral arteries. This is illustrated in the territory of the middle cerebral artery.

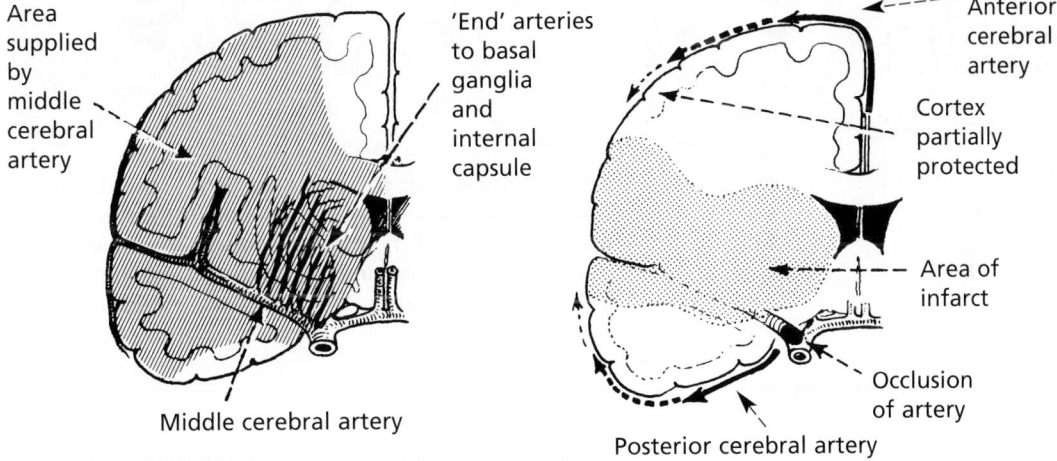

Area supplied by middle cerebral artery

'End' arteries to basal ganglia and internal capsule

Anterior cerebral artery

Cortex partially protected

Area of infarct

Occlusion of artery

Middle cerebral artery

Posterior cerebral artery

2. **Boundary zones** (see p. 96)

The cortex in particular is damaged in boundary zone infarction. In these cases, central circulatory deficiency is an important component, e.g. hypotension.

# BRAIN DAMAGE DUE TO CARDIAC ARREST

This is characterised by widely distributed selective neuronal necrosis – the neurones are more susceptible to hypoxia than the supporting cells.

**Affected areas** –   Total cortical necrosis
            or
            most sensitive zones – Hippocampus
                        – Layers III, V, VI of cortex
                        – Within sulci
                        – Purkinje cells of cerebellum.

*Note:* (a) These changes do not become apparent unless the patient survives at least 12 hours after the arrest.
    (b) Similar types of neuronal damage can be seen in severe acute hypoglycaemia, carbon monoxide or barbiturate poisoning.

# CEREBRAL INFARCTION

The diagram below illustrates the evolution of an infarct, e.g. in the territory of the middle cerebral artery. Up to 24 hours there is virtually no visible change.

| 18–24 hrs | After 24 hours | After a few days | After weeks/months |
|---|---|---|---|
| **Gross appearances** | | | |
| | Less difficult to see | Line of demarcation seen | Demolition + scarring |

**Very difficult to see**

Slight swelling — Blurring of white/grey junction

Necrotic tissue. Soft to touch; usually pale but may be congested if blood has permeated in (haemorrhagic infarct)

Cyst with pale or yellowish fluid — Shrinkage of scarred area: compensatory dilatation of ventricle

**Microscopic appearances**

Early neuronal damage → Necrosis of neurones

**Early neuronal damage**

Organisation of infarct begins; macrophages appear; capillary sprouting; oedema diminishing

Organisation well established; neurones disappear; numerous macrophages; gliosis

**Clinical associations**

**FUNCTIONAL LOSS**

Effects are maximal in the early stages when oedema and circulatory disturbance in the adjacent tissues augment the functional loss caused by infarct. Larger infarcts may be associated with loss of consciousness.

The prognostic assessment of final functional loss cannot be made until the changes have subsided and any possible functional compensations have been established. This takes many weeks. Complete clinical recovery may follow small infarcts. Prompt thrombolytic therapy with tissue plasminogen activator can limit the degree of permanent disability.

# CEREBRAL HAEMORRHAGE

Spontaneous intracranial bleeding is the second main type of stroke. In the great majority of cases there is localised arterial disease aggravated by hypertension. A small number are associated with cerebral tumours, systemic bleeding diathesis or arteriovenous malformations.

In most hypertensives over middle age, **microaneurysms** are found in the very small cerebral arteries. It is believed that rupture of one of these aneurysms is the immediate cause of intracerebral haemorrhage.

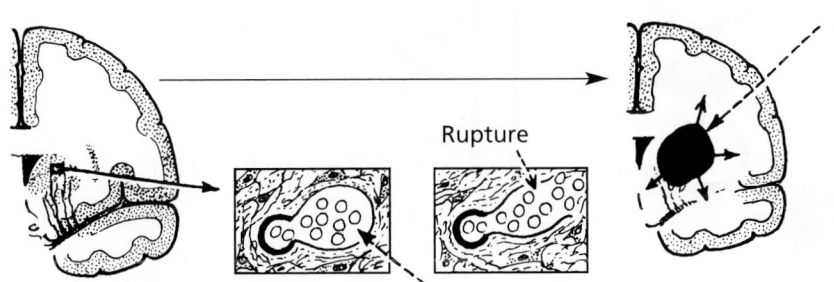

Rupture

**Haematoma** forms. Commonest site is branches of middle cerebral artery to basal ganglia and internal capsule; also occurs in pons and cerebellum.

Thin-walled microaneurysm

**Progress**
The onset is usually sudden with headache and, because of the high blood pressure, progress is rapid and the haemorrhage large.

↓

Associated raised ICP effects

↓

Death in many cases

When the bleeding is limited, there is survival with varying residual paralysis.

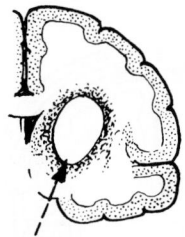

**Final outcome**
Cystic space containing yellow-brown fluid walled off by gliosis.

Apoplectic cyst

*Note*: Intracerebral bleeding may track irregularly and often reaches the subarachnoid space and ventricles.

# SUBARACHNOID HAEMORRHAGE

This is commonly but not exclusively the result of rupture of a 'berry' aneurysm at or near the circle of Willis. The basic abnormality is a congenital weakness of the elastic tissues in the arterial wall; only rarely is an aneurysm present at birth, and while subarachnoid haemorrhage does occur in young people, the incidence increases with age. Hypertension is an important contributing factor.

**Sites** – often multiple, near arterial junctions.

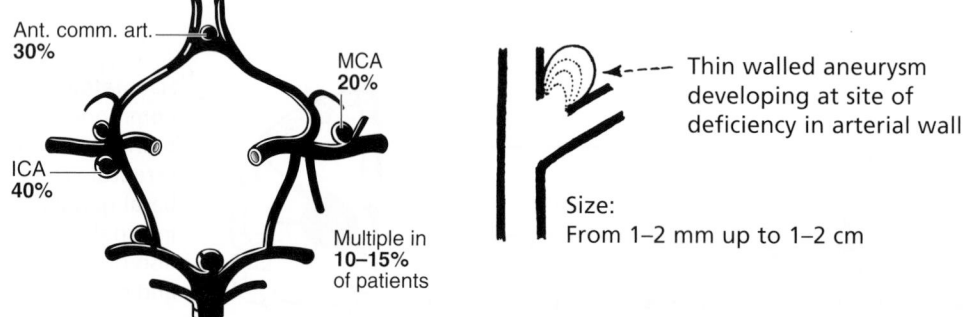

Ant. comm. art.
**30%**

MCA
**20%**

ICA
**40%**

Multiple in
**10–15%**
of patients

Thin walled aneurysm developing at site of deficiency in arterial wall

Size:
From 1–2 mm up to 1–2 cm

Not all aneurysms rupture; they are found incidentally at autopsy.

Massive haemorrhage may be preceded by one or more small leaks – marked by headache without functional loss.

## Progress

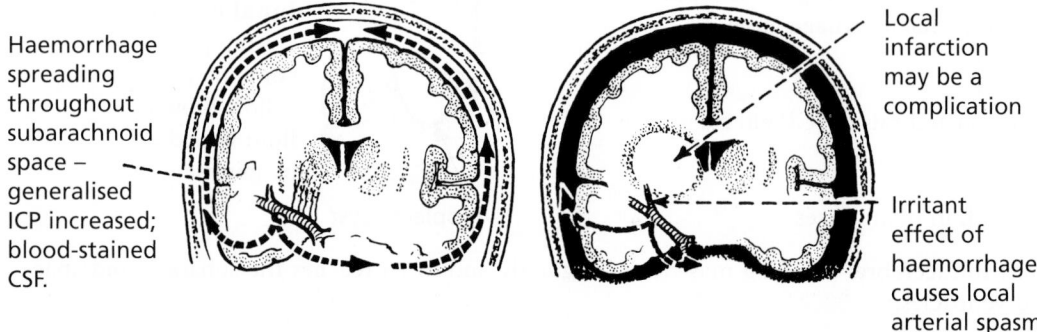

Haemorrhage spreading throughout subarachnoid space – generalised ICP increased; blood-stained CSF.

Local infarction may be a complication

Irritant effect of haemorrhage causes local arterial spasm

*Note*: The aneurysm may rupture directly into the brain and mimic an intracerebral haemorrhage.

## CSF findings

1–24 hours — Blood stained; blood content constant in sequential samples (distinguishes blood derived from a traumatic tap).
— Centrifuge supernatant – may be pink due to haemolysis.

24 hours onwards — Supernatant shows xanthochromia (yellow colour due to presence of blood degradation products).

Other causes of cerebral haemorrhage of either type are vascular malformations and coagulation disorders.

# HEAD INJURY

Head injuries of varying severity are common nowadays, particularly as a consequence of road traffic accidents. Immediate damage is caused by two main mechanisms which overcome the protection of the vulnerable cerebral tissues provided by the skull and the CSF 'water cushion'.

## 1. Direct blows to the head (e.g. missile head injury)

Usually cause injury to the soft tissues of the scalp and often fracture of the skull with contusion or laceration of the underlying brain.

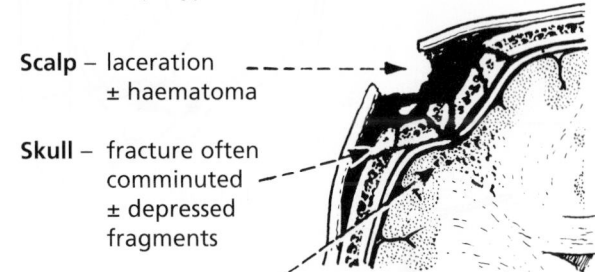

**Scalp** – laceration
± haematoma

**Skull** – fracture often comminuted ± depressed fragments

**Brain** – contusion, laceration or haematoma

## 2. Non-missile head injury

Since the head is usually freely moveable on the neck, the sudden application of forces derived from **acceleration, deceleration** and, particularly, **rotation** of the head often causes serious brain injury.

### (a) Skull fractures

(i) *Skull damage*

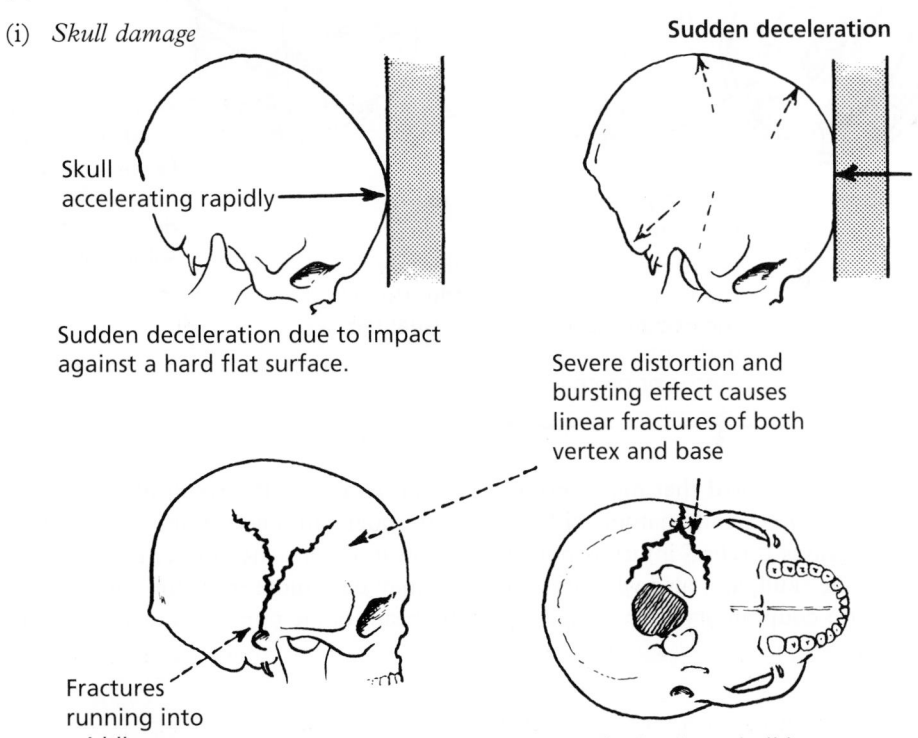

Skull accelerating rapidly

**Sudden deceleration**

Sudden deceleration due to impact against a hard flat surface.

Severe distortion and bursting effect causes linear fractures of both vertex and base

Fractures running into middle ear ——————————→ Continuing into skull base

# HEAD INJURY

### Acceleration/deceleration injury

(ii) *Brain damage*

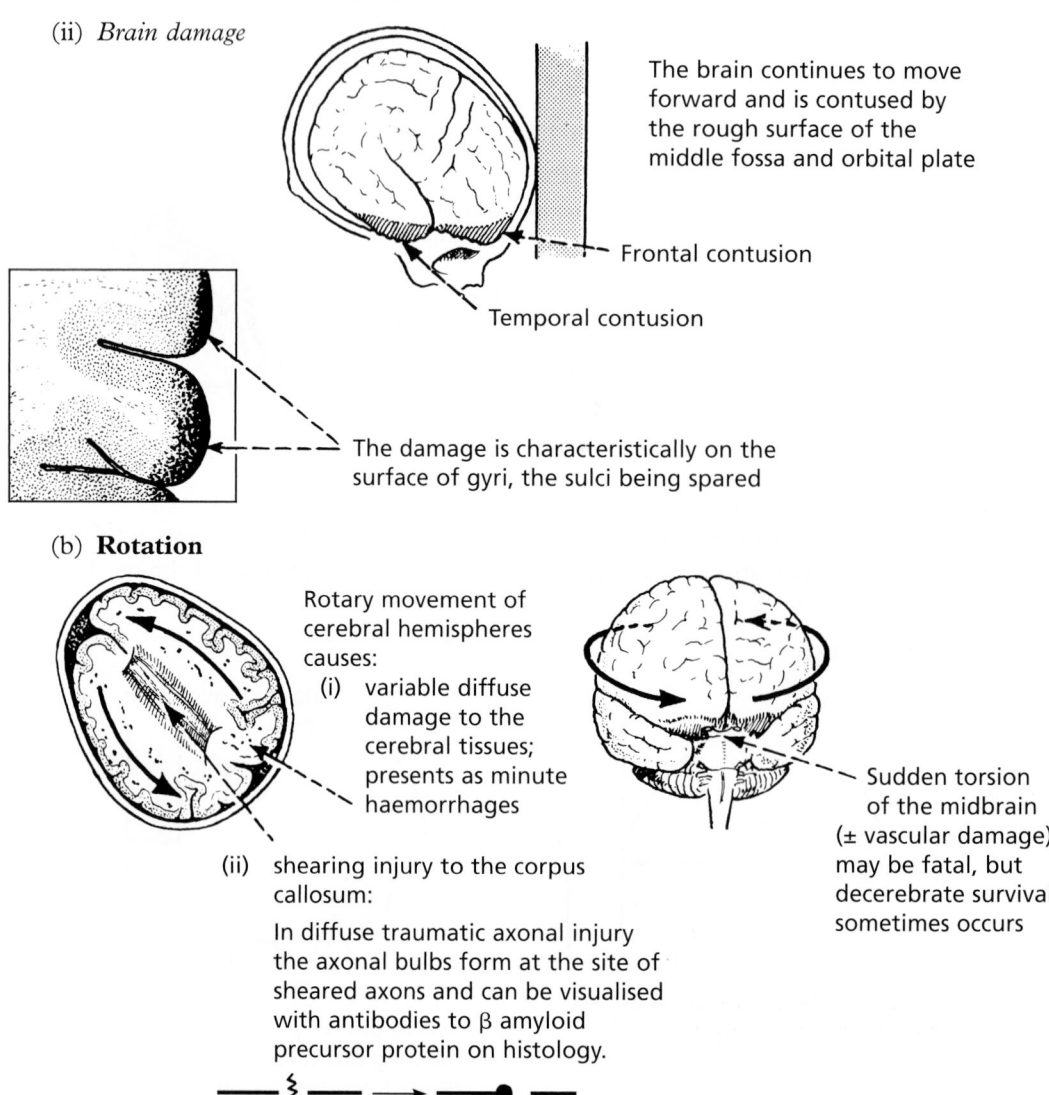

The brain continues to move forward and is contused by the rough surface of the middle fossa and orbital plate

— Frontal contusion

Temporal contusion

The damage is characteristically on the surface of gyri, the sulci being spared

(b) **Rotation**

Rotary movement of cerebral hemispheres causes:
  (i) variable diffuse damage to the cerebral tissues; presents as minute haemorrhages

(ii) shearing injury to the corpus callosum:

In diffuse traumatic axonal injury the axonal bulbs form at the site of sheared axons and can be visualised with antibodies to β amyloid precursor protein on histology.

Sudden torsion of the midbrain (± vascular damage) may be fatal, but decerebrate survival sometimes occurs

*Note:* It will be appreciated that more serious cerebral damage is the result of interaction of complex physical forces and anatomical features. An understanding of these mechanisms explains why serious cerebral injury is not uncommon in the absence of damage to the scalp or fracture of the skull, and also why brain damage may be remote from the site of impact: so-called 'contre-coup' injury is sustained when the brain tissue opposite the site of impact is contused.

# HEAD INJURY

## DELAYED COMPLICATIONS

In addition to damage sustained immediately at the time of impact, certain serious complications may supervene over the next hours or few days.

1. **Haemorrhages**

    (a) **Extradural haematoma**
    This type of haemorrhage classically occurs as a complication of linear fracture of the skull vault when the middle meningeal artery is torn.

    Artery torn at site of fracture     Haemorrhage gradually strips dura from bone     A large, saucer-shaped haematoma forms

    The classic clinical association is a direct blow to the head from which recovery is rapid. After a lucid interval of varying duration up to several hours, signs of increased intracranial pressure supervene. This chain of events is explained by the time taken for the haemorrhage to accumulate by stripping the dura from the skull.

    (b) **Subdural haematoma.** This may occur at any site and is often extensive because of the loose attachment of the dura and arachnoid membranes. It is usually due to rupture of small bridging veins.

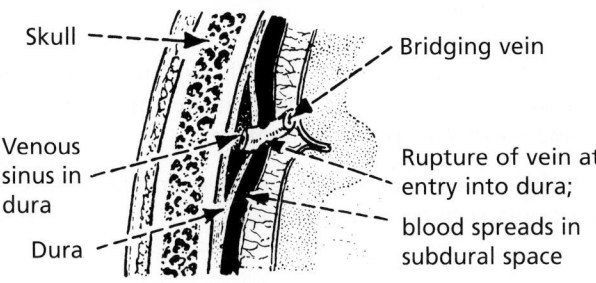

    Skull — Bridging vein

    Venous sinus in dura — Rupture of vein at entry into dura; blood spreads in subdural space

    Dura —

    These acute subdural haematomas are often associated with subarachnoid haemorrhage and cerebral contusions.

    (c) **Intracerebral haematomas** occur in association with cortical contusions particularly in the temporal and frontal lobes (burst lobe); but also at random deep within the hemispheres due to shearing at the time of impact. Large haematomas are uncommon.

# HEAD INJURY

2.  **Cerebral oedema** is an important complication.

    Increased intracranial pressure ⟶ Cerebral hypoxia.

3.  **External leakage of CSF** (and blood) from the ear and nose may complicate fractures of the skull base. This complication may be of long duration and is always a potential entry for infection.

4.  **Local infection** may complicate compound fractures and progress to meningitis.

## LATE COMPLICATIONS

1.  **Epilepsy**

    Head injury is an important cause of epilepsy. The risk is highest in severe missile head injury and may be related to ischaemic brain damage.

2.  **Chronic subdural haematoma**

    A thick layer of fluid and partially clotted blood gradually accumulates between the dura and arachnoid membranes which show considerable reactive thickening.

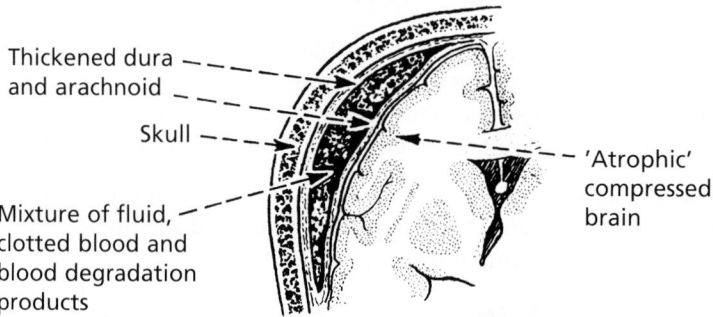

The precise cause is not known; most cases occur in alcoholics or in elderly people already suffering from cerebral atrophy, and it is possible that the small bridging veins are unduly stretched and become more susceptible to damage.

The clinical signs are usually insidious in onset and progressive, and in many cases there is a history of either no or only very trivial injury.

# AGEING AND DEMENTIA

## NORMAL BRAIN AGEING

With normal ageing the brain becomes atrophic, but the morphological changes described below are not necessarily accompanied by loss of intellect.

### Changes in old age

**Gross** as seen naked-eye at autopsy

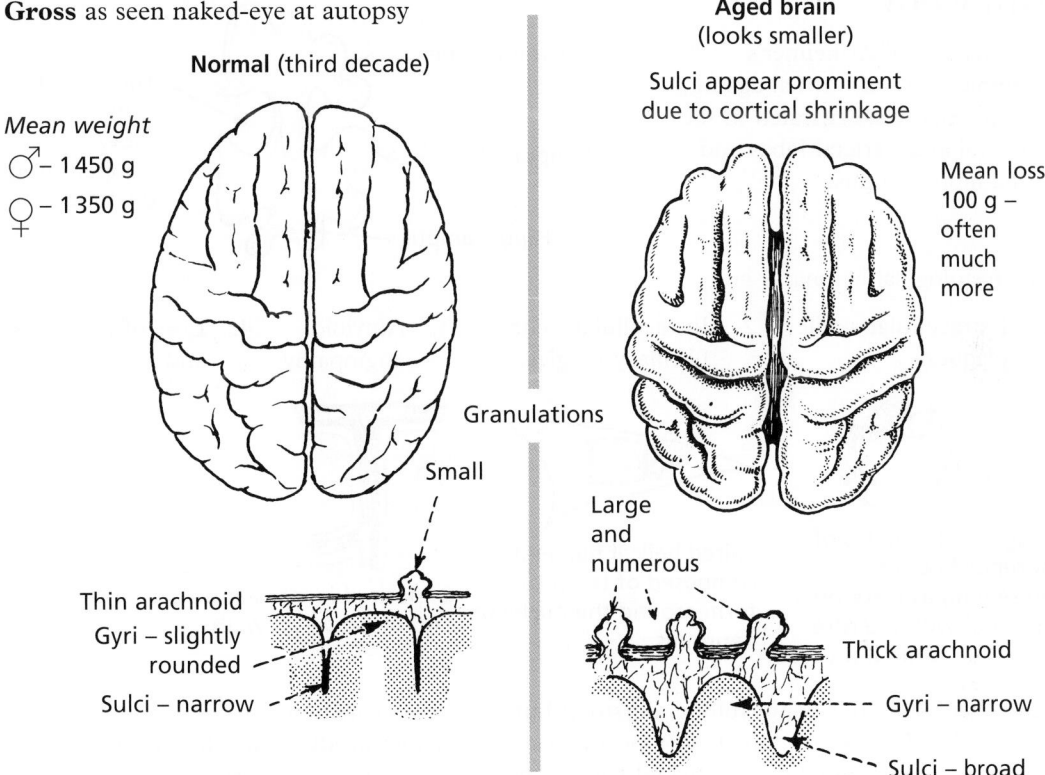

**Normal** (third decade)

*Mean weight*
♂ – 1450 g
♀ – 1350 g

**Aged brain**
(looks smaller)

Sulci appear prominent
due to cortical shrinkage

Mean loss
100 g –
often
much
more

Granulations

Small

Large
and
numerous

Thin arachnoid
Gyri – slightly
rounded
Sulci – narrow

Thick arachnoid

Gyri – narrow

Sulci – broad

There is compensatory enlargement of the lateral ventricles.

### Dementia

Dementia is defined as 'an acquired progressive global impairment of intellect, memory and personality, without impairment of consciousness'. Around 5% of the population over 65 years of age are affected, and the proportion rises to over 20% of those over 80 years of age.

Main causes are:

1. Alzheimer's disease 70%
2. Multi-infarct dementia 10–15%
3. Lewy body dementia 10–20%

Rare causes include:

1. Genetic disorders (Huntington disease, Pick disease).
2. Infections (Creutzfeld-Jacob disease, see p. 599, AIDS).

# ALZHEIMER'S DISEASE

This disease accounts for around 70% of cases of dementia. While typically a disease of the elderly, especially females, it is also seen in patients under 60 years, in whom there is often a family history (although only about 5% of cases are familial). Almost all patients with Down syndrome who survive to 50 years develop Alzheimer's (suggesting that chromosome 21 is important).

## PATHOLOGY

The changes of Alzheimer's resemble those of normal ageing, but are greatly exaggerated in the temporal and parietal lobes and in the hippocampus.

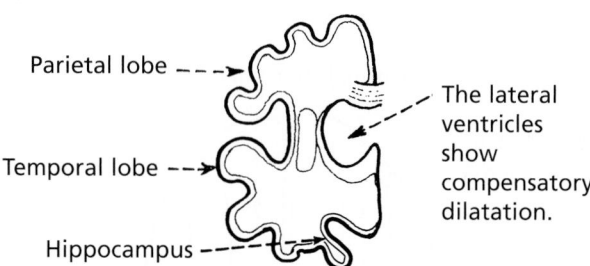

Parietal lobe
Temporal lobe
Hippocampus
The lateral ventricles show compensatory dilatation.

The histological hallmarks are:

1. Extracellular senile plaques.

2. Intracellular neuro fibrillary tangles.

3. Amyloid angiopathy.

4. Loss of neurones and synapses.

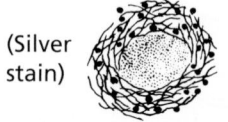

(Silver stain)

Tangled aggregates of distended neurites presenting as black dots and rods with a centre core of amyloid β-protein.

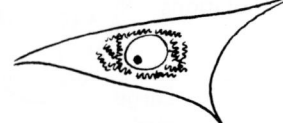

Paired helical filaments composed of tau protein form around the nuclei of neurones.

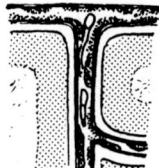

Deposited in meninges and blood vessel walls.

**Pathogenesis** – this is not fully understood but the theories include:

1. *Amyloid Hypothesis* – this theory postulates that amyloid products are the cause of the disease. Accumulation of amyloid triggers neuronal degeneration, disrupts calcium homeostasis, induces apoptosis and builds up in mitochondria where it inhibits enzyme function. The amyloid hypothesis is supported by genetic factors (see below).

2. *Inflammatory Hypothesis* – this theory postulates that when normal brain tissue is disrupted as a result of inflammation, this can cause misfolding and, subsequently, accumulation of amyloid. The effects may accumulate over many years as an acceleration of normal cellular senescence. Individuals who take anti-inflammatory drugs have a lower risk of Alzheimer's disease.

**Genetic factors** – several genes are involved

1. Amyloid precursor protein (chromosome 21) – early onset Alzheimer's.
2. Presenilin 1 and 2 (chromosome 14 and 1) – proteins involved in binding amyloid precursor proteins.
3. Apolipoprotein E – the E4 allele is associated with late onset disease.
   – it may determine the age of onset.
   – 40–80% of the those with Alzheimer's disease have at least one Apo E4 allele.
4. α-2 macroglobulin – may be involved in clearance of amyloid proteins.

# DEMENTIA

## MULTI-INFARCT DEMENTIA

This form of dementia is associated with vascular disease – with infarcts often in the middle cerebral arterial distribution. The volume of brain loss appears to be important.

Loss of >100 mL of brain correlates with dementia.

Hypertension is an important underlying factor. A stepwise progression is typical.

## LEWY BODY DEMENTIA

This disorder accounts for 10–20% of dementias. Clinically there are overlapping features with Parkinson's disease. There is widespread neuronal loss in the cerebral cortex. Characteristic Lewy bodies are identified in surviving neurones. Known components of Lewy bodies include alpha synuclein and ubiquitin.

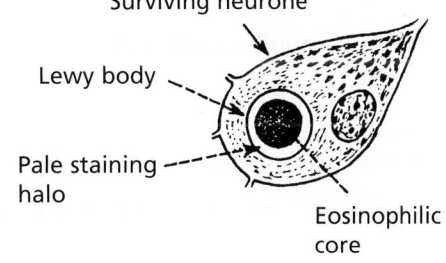

Surviving neurone

Lewy body

Pale staining halo

Eosinophilic core

## PICK DISEASE

This uncommon form of dementia has a strong familial (autosomal dominant) component. There is typically severe atrophy of the temporal and frontal lobes. The histological marker in the surviving neurones is the Pick body.

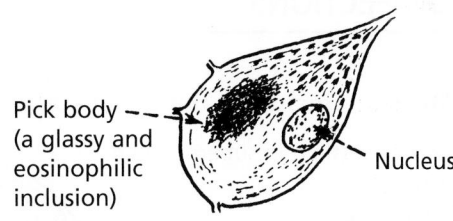

Pick body – – (a glassy and eosinophilic inclusion)

Nucleus

## HUNTINGTON DISEASE

This is an uncommon autosomal dominant condition beginning in the third or fourth decade and characterised by psychiatric disorders, progressive dementia and in some patients bizarre writhing movements (chorea).

### Pathology

The caudate nucleus is severely atrophic. The genetic locus is on chromosome 4 and consists of a trinucleotide repeat with up to 34 copies in unaffected patients. In Huntington disease the number of repeats increases with each successive generation resulting in earlier onset of symptoms (genetic anticipation). Genetic screening is available.

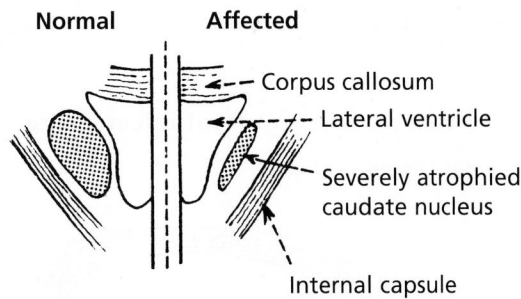

Normal    Affected

Corpus callosum

Lateral ventricle

Severely atrophied caudate nucleus

Internal capsule

## PUNCH DRUNK SYNDROME (DEMENTIA PUGILISTICA)

Professional boxers may develop dementia due to neuronal damage caused by repeated blows to the head.

# INFECTIONS

Compared with the high incidence of infection generally, infection of the CNS is uncommon. The pathological effects may be slight and wholly recoverable as in some virus infections, or severe, leading to permanent damage or death.

Anatomically, infections fall into two main groups which tend to remain separated due to the intervention of the **pial** barrier (see p. 569).

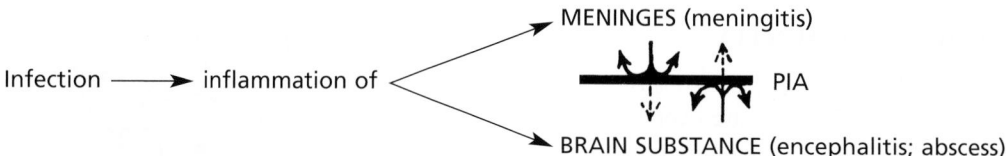

Infection ⟶ inflammation of ⟨ MENINGES (meningitis)

PIA

BRAIN SUBSTANCE (encephalitis; abscess)

Infections will be considered in three broad aetiological groups:

(1) bacterial, (2) viral and (3) miscellaneous types.

# BACTERIAL INFECTIONS

1. **Most commonly by the blood stream**

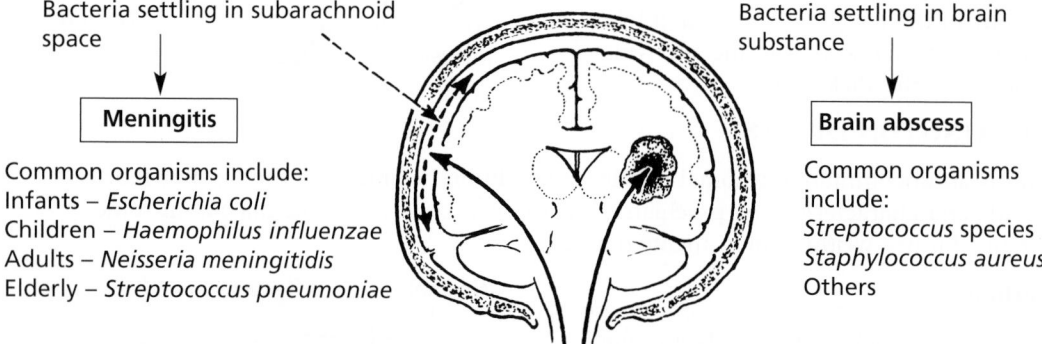

Bacteria settling in subarachnoid space

**Meningitis**

Common organisms include:
Infants – *Escherichia coli*
Children – *Haemophilus influenzae*
Adults – *Neisseria meningitidis*
Elderly – *Streptococcus pneumoniae*

Bacteria settling in brain substance

**Brain abscess**

Common organisms include:
*Streptococcus* species
*Staphylococcus aureus*
Others

2. **From an adjacent local infected site** – these are pyogenic infections.

   (a) *Fracture of skull*

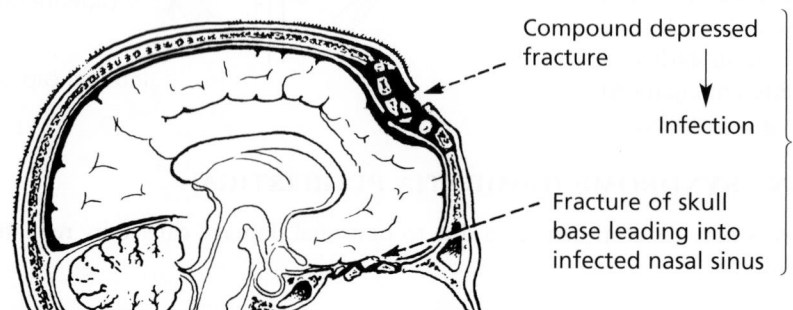

Compound depressed fracture

↓

Infection

Fracture of skull base leading into infected nasal sinus

(1) Extradural abscess

(2) Subdural abscess (empyema)

(3) Meningitis

# BACTERIAL INFECTIONS

(b) *Middle ear and mastoid disease*

In untreated purulent otitis media, three serious complications may arise from spread of the inflammation.

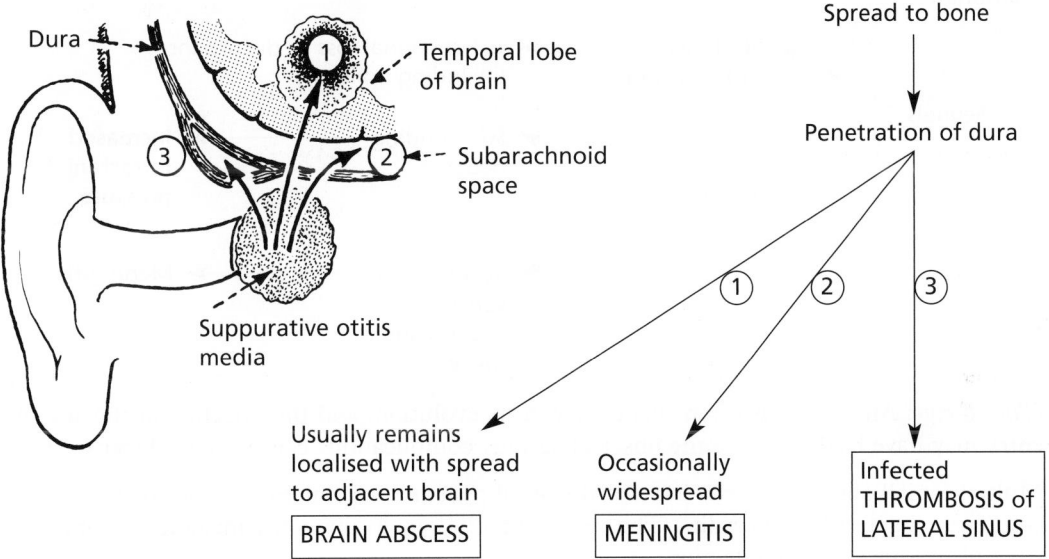

## PYOGENIC MENINGITIS

The whole subarachnoid space contains purulent exudate which is maximal in sulci and around the brain base cisternae.

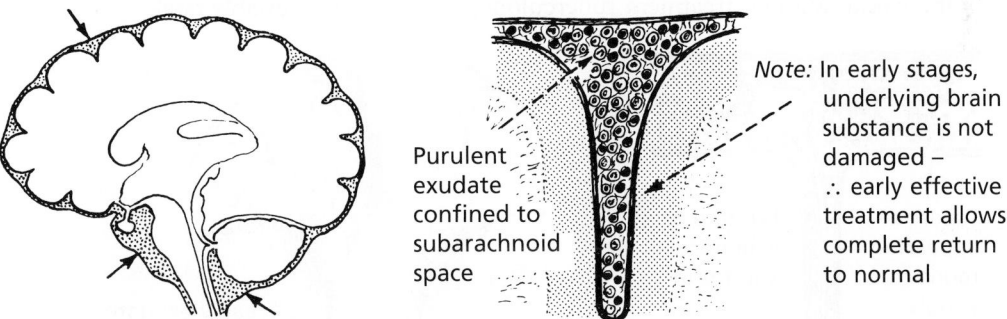

In untreated or ineffectively treated patients who survive, complications include cranial nerve damage, hydrocephalus and variable brain damage.

The CSF in the acute stage contains neutrophils and the infecting organism can usually be demonstrated.

# BACTERIAL INFECTIONS

### PYOGENIC BRAIN ABSCESS

The abscesses resulting from direct spread of adjacent infection or by blood-borne infection – as seen particularly in bronchiectasis – are often well circumscribed by a pyogenic membrane.

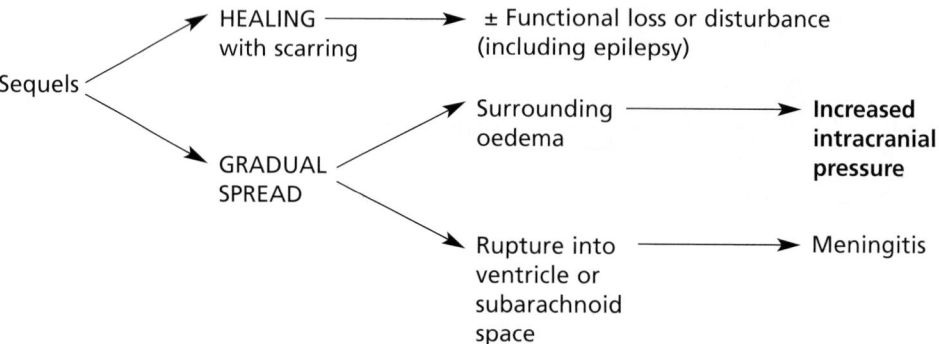

*Clinical note*: An abscess is often silent early in its evolution, and the infection at the site of entry may have healed before the onset of serious complications causes clinical signs.

Multiple small abscesses occur in staphylococcal pyaemia and microabscesses may complicate bacterial endocarditis. The cerebral pathology in these circumstances is only one facet of serious systemic infection.

### TUBERCULOSIS

Infection of the nervous system is always secondary to disease elsewhere and may be a component of miliary tuberculosis. It may complicate AIDS and remains prevalent in many parts of the world. Without treatment tuberculous meningitis is invariably fatal.

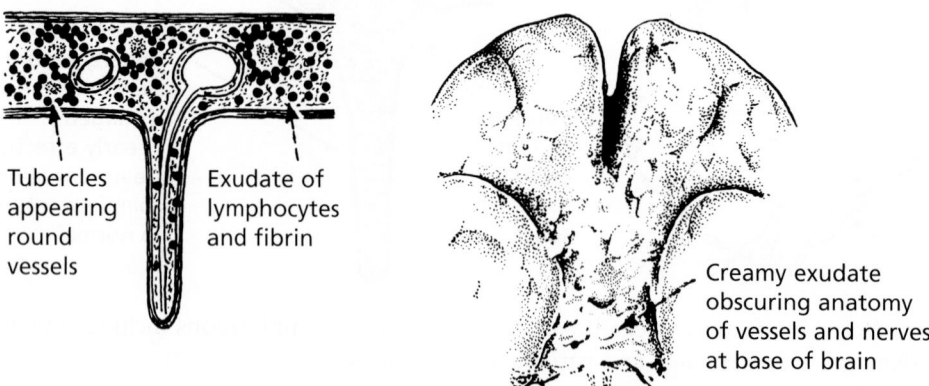

**TUBERCULOMA.** These localised tuberculous cerebral abscesses are now very rare.

**SYPHILIS.** Neurological syphilis is rare nowadays. The main pathological lesions are described on page 115.

# VIRUS INFECTIONS

Compared with the incidence of virus infections in general, infection of the CNS is rare, even with viruses having an affinity for the CNS – **NEUROTROPIC VIRUSES**.

There are three broad groups:

1. **Acute**
   Cell lysis occurs towards the end of the viraemic phase of infection. This is the common type of disease. Herpes simplex, mumps, poliovirus and togaviruses are examples.

2. **Persistent**
   Viruses which usually cause damage outside the CNS behave uncharacteristically and cause continuing and active disease of the CNS over a long period (months – years). Measles, rubella and JC papovavirus are examples.

3. **Latent** virus infection is seen in herpes zoster and possibly plays a role in the demyelinating diseases.

   Virus infection also has a possible role in oncogenesis within the CNS.

## Routes of infection

Most viruses arrive at the CNS via the blood, but the factors which potentiate the establishment of disease within the CNS are poorly understood.

## Primary portal of entry

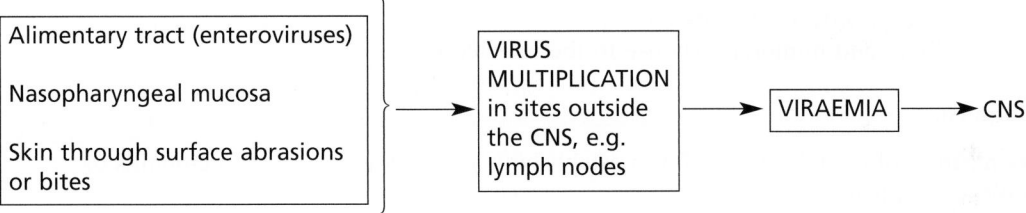

In rabies, the virus travels from the wound up the peripheral nerves to the CNS; a similar mechanism may be involved in herpes simplex encephalitis.

# VIRUS INFECTIONS

## BASIC PATHOLOGICAL EFFECTS

(a) **VIRAL MENINGITIS** is the commonest form of meningitis; the disease is usually mild and only the meninges are affected. Recovery is usually complete.

(b) In more severe cases, the brain substance is also damaged in varying degree **ENCEPHALITIS** (meningoencephalitis).

The meninges (CSF) contain increased protein, normal sugar and a mononuclear cellular infiltrate (particularly **lymphocytes**, plasma cells and large mononuclear cells).

In the brain the characteristic changes are:

1. PERIVASCULAR CUFFING (same infiltrate as meninges).

2. ACUTE NEURONAL DAMAGE up to complete lysis with accompanying neuronophagia and inflammatory changes. In some conditions, surviving neurones contain cytoplasmic and/or nuclear inclusions. Specific viral inclusions, e.g. HSV and CMV, may be detected by immunohistochemistry.

To these basic changes, damage to myelin and glial tissue may be added, and small focal haemorrhages may be seen. The damage is effected in two ways:

1. By the direct effects of virus on cells.
2. By cellular and humoral response to the infected cell.

## Diagnosis

Examination of the CSF is helpful in establishing a diagnosis of aseptic meningitis or meningoencephalitis.

*Note*: The findings in tuberculous meningitis are very similar except that in tuberculous meningitis the CSF **sugar is low**.

The specific virus aetiology is more difficult to establish. PCR of CSF is useful for some viruses (esp. HSV). In severe cases brain biopsy may be required.

## Clinical associations and progress

In viral meningitis, the illness is mild with fever, headache and neck stiffness being the main signs. Recovery is almost always complete.

In meningoencephalitis, signs of cerebral 'irritation' and neuronal damage are seen, e.g. mental confusion, delusion, stupor, convulsions and coma, and there may be localising signs. In mild cases, recovery is complete, but in more severe cases residual paralysis and other signs indicative of permanent brain damage may follow. Death in coma with respiratory failure occurs in very severe cases.

# VIRUS INFECTIONS

## HERPES SIMPLEX VIRUS (HSV) ENCEPHALITIS

This is the commonest form of severe acute viral encephalitis and is almost always due to Herpes Simplex Virus Type 1. It occurs in two forms:

1. In infancy, as part of a generalised HSV infection.
2. In adults, due to reactivation of the virus in the trigeminal ganglion.

Most cases are sporadic but immunosuppression increases the risk. The temporal lobes are most affected. Early treatment with antiviral drugs has now greatly reduced the previous high mortality.

## HERPES ZOSTER (see also p. 120)

This is a disease of adults, presenting as a painful vesicular rash, usually unilateral and affecting one or a few adjacent dermatomes only. It is due to recurrence of a latent varicella (chickenpox) infection.

**Mechanism**

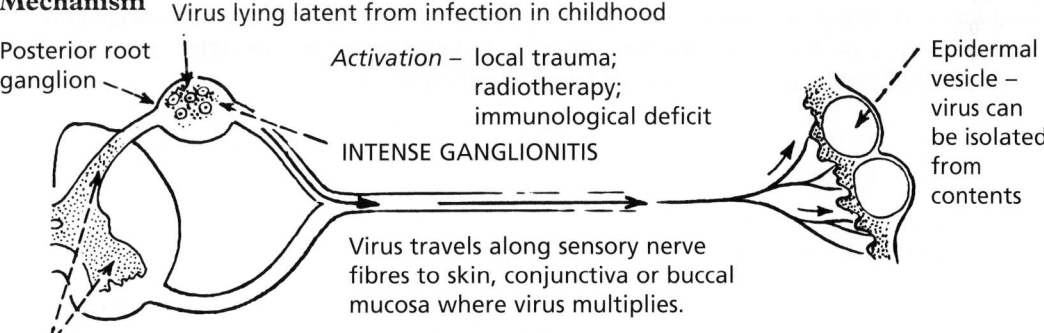

Virus lying latent from infection in childhood

Posterior root ganglion

*Activation* – local trauma; radiotherapy; immunological deficit

INTENSE GANGLIONITIS

Virus travels along sensory nerve fibres to skin, conjunctiva or buccal mucosa where virus multiplies.

Epidermal vesicle – virus can be isolated from contents

Minor secondary degenerative changes in cord

**Sequels**
1. An occasional sequel is intense pain with varying paraesthesiae and anaesthesia long after the acute phase has healed.
2. In cases of Vth nerve herpes, serious damage to the eye may result.

## RABIES

The rabies virus shows marked neurotropism and can infect most mammals. Various wild carnivores (fox, jackal, skunk, vampire bats) are the natural reservoir. Many human cases are contracted from dogs.

**Mechanism**

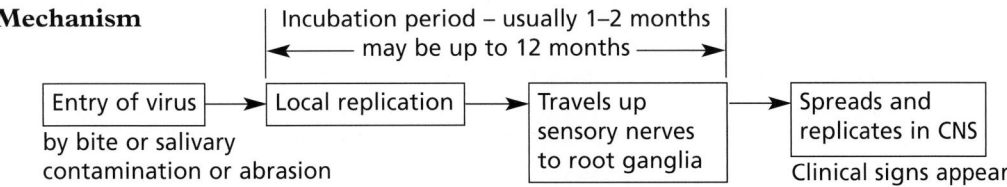

Incubation period – usually 1–2 months
may be up to 12 months

Entry of virus by bite or salivary contamination or abrasion → Local replication → Travels up sensory nerves to root ganglia → Spreads and replicates in CNS

Clinical signs appear

# VIRUS INFECTIONS

An unremitting encephalitis particularly affecting the grey matter is established. Diagnostic Negri bodies (virus inclusions) are found at autopsy in the pyramidal cells of the hippocampus and the Purkinje cells of the cerebellum.

Clinically, the encephalitis presents with extreme excitation of the sensory system. The classical hydrophobia (fear of water) is due to serious disturbance of the swallowing mechanism with muscular spasm. Without supportive therapy death occurs and is due to respiratory muscle spasm or paralysis.

## ENTEROVIRUSES

These are small RNA viruses (picornavirus group) and include POLIOVIRUSES, COXSACKIE VIRUSES and ECHOVIRUSES.

Infection is acquired by ingestion of faecally contaminated material followed by proliferation in the intestine. In only a small minority of infected cases does the virus pass the blood-brain barrier and cause disease of the CNS.

In addition to aseptic meningitis, the POLIOVIRUSES (and very occasionally Coxsackie and Echo viruses) cause the classic paralytic disease, **ANTERIOR POLIOMYELITIS**. Vaccination has dramatically reduced the global incidence of poliomyelitis.

# VIRUS INFECTIONS

## Pathological changes

The pathological changes are reflected in three clinical stages: (1) acute, (2) recovery and (3) permanent residual disability.

**(1) Acute** (up to 2 weeks)

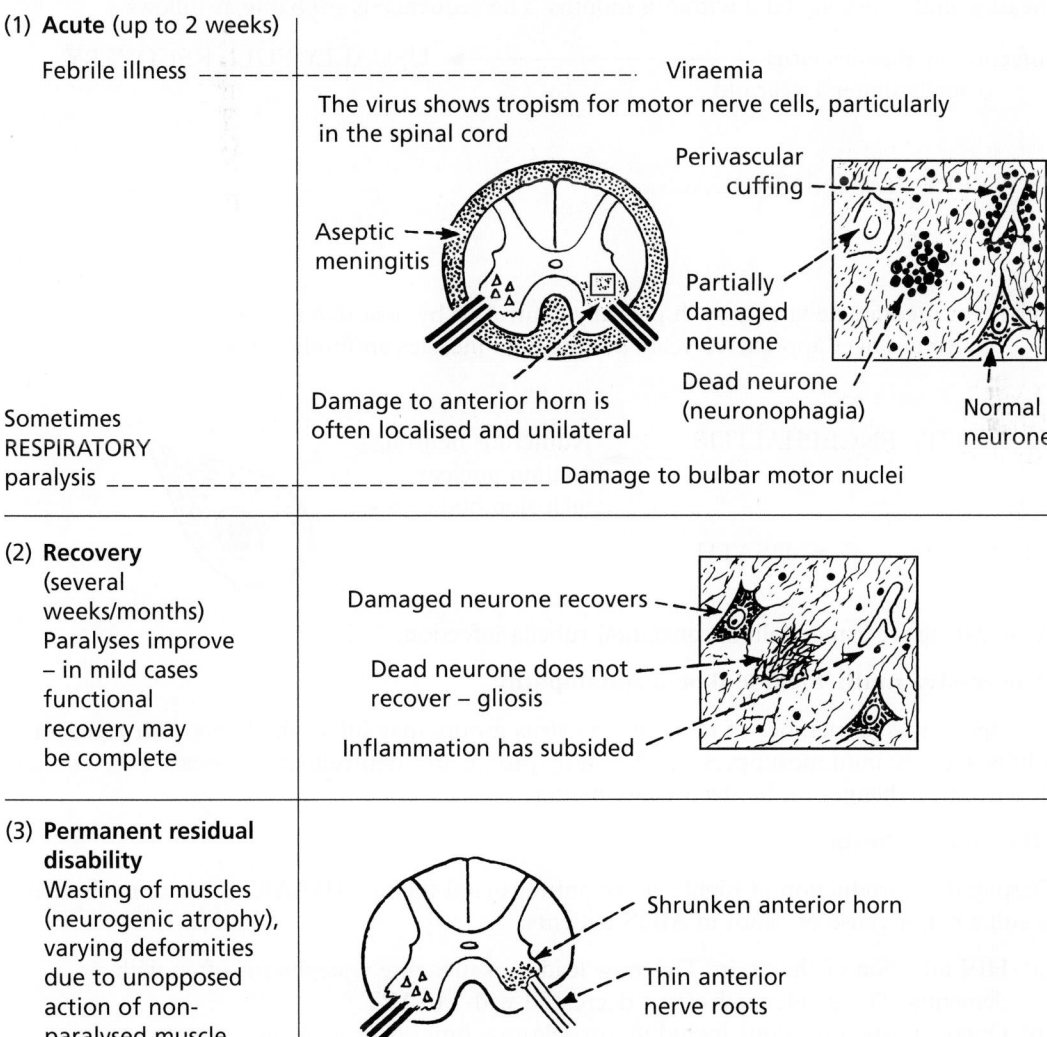

Febrile illness —————————————————————— Viraemia

The virus shows tropism for motor nerve cells, particularly in the spinal cord

Perivascular cuffing

Aseptic meningitis

Partially damaged neurone

Dead neurone (neuronophagia)

Normal neurone

Damage to anterior horn is often localised and unilateral

Sometimes RESPIRATORY paralysis ————————————————— Damage to bulbar motor nuclei

**(2) Recovery**
(several weeks/months)
Paralyses improve
– in mild cases
functional
recovery may
be complete

Damaged neurone recovers

Dead neurone does not recover – gliosis

Inflammation has subsided

**(3) Permanent residual disability**
Wasting of muscles (neurogenic atrophy), varying deformities due to unopposed action of non-paralysed muscle

Shrunken anterior horn

Thin anterior nerve roots

# VIRUS INFECTIONS

### PERSISTENT VIRUS INFECTIONS

**Subacute sclerosing panencephalitis** is a very rare disorder due to reactivation of latent measles virus. It affects children and young adults, often several years after uncomplicated measles, and is usually fatal within 6 months. The sequence is probably as follows:

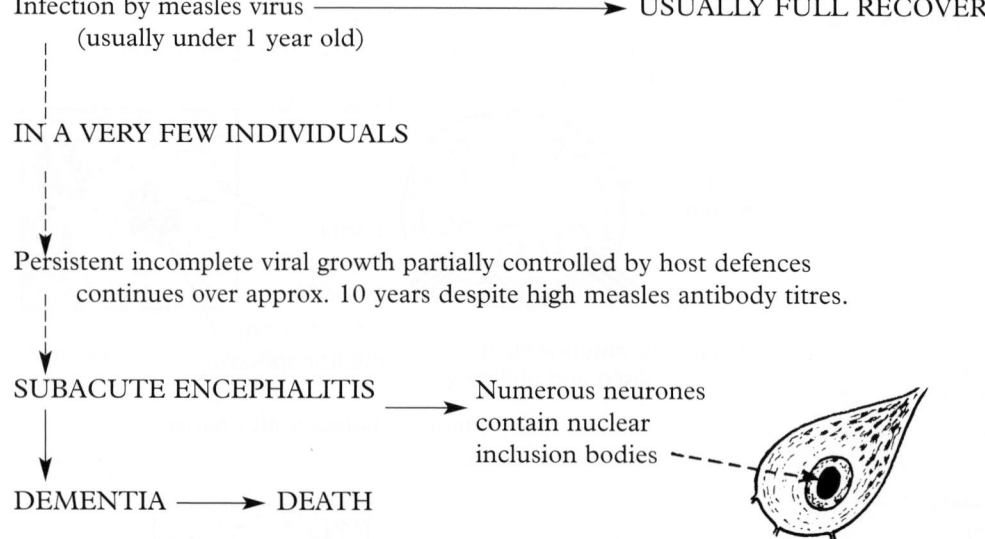

Infection by measles virus ⟶ USUALLY FULL RECOVERY.
(usually under 1 year old)

IN A VERY FEW INDIVIDUALS

Persistent incomplete viral growth partially controlled by host defences continues over approx. 10 years despite high measles antibody titres.

SUBACUTE ENCEPHALITIS ⟶ Numerous neurones contain nuclear inclusion bodies

DEMENTIA ⟶ DEATH

A similar disorder may follow congenital rubella infection.

### Progressive multi-focal leukoencephalopathy

JC papovavirus, a member of the polyoma virus group, may infect the oligodendrocytes of adults who are immunosuppressed. A rapidly progressive demyelinating disease follows with degenerative changes in the deep white matter.

### HIV and the brain

Despite the introduction of highly active antiretroviral therapy (HAART), brain involvement is still a major cause of death in AIDS patients.

(a) HIV infection of the brain. This may lead to a subacute encephalitis often with dementia. The incidence has not decreased with HAART.
(b) Opportunistic infections including toxoplasma, fungi (*Cryptococcus*), viruses (*Cytomegalovirus*).
(c) Tumours – especially cerebral lymphoma.

The incidence of (b) and (c) has decreased dramatically with HAART.

# PRION DISEASES

Also known as the transmissible spongiform encephalopathies, this group of diseases is caused by abnormal, distorted PRIONS. A prion is a small protein molecule found in the brain cell membrane. Normal cellular prion protein is termed $PrP^c$ whereas the distorted protein is termed $PrP^{sc}$ (originally referring to scrapie but now a generic term).

## THE PRION HYPOTHESIS

When a distorted prion molecule reaches the prions in the brain cell membrane of an individual, that molecule is able to act as a three-dimensional template to cause a normal prion molecule to adopt a similar distorted shape. This in turn can distort further proteins and so on.

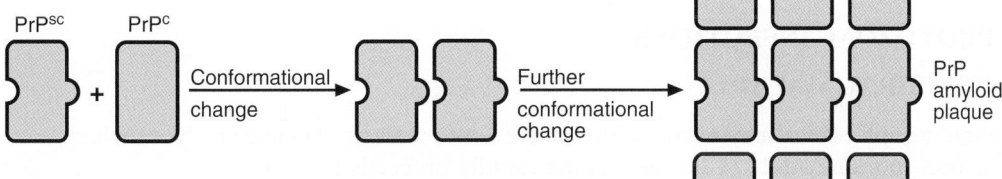

## PATHOLOGY

There are four characteristic histological features:

1. Spongiform change.
2. Neuronal loss.
3. Astrocytosis.
4. Amyloid plaque formation.

Vacuoles around neurones and in neuropil

Astrocytosis

These are most frequently observed in the cerebellum.

They can be detected by immunohistochemistry with antibodies to $PrP^{sc}$.

## TYPES OF PRION DISEASE

1. **Creutzfeld-Jacob Disease (CJD)**
   this may be: (i) **sporadic**, (ii) **acquired** through contact with infected material, e.g. pituitary derived hormones, corneal grafts or (iii) **familial** due a point mutation of the PrP gene. Spongiform change is the most consistent histological features. Plaques occur in around 10% of cases.

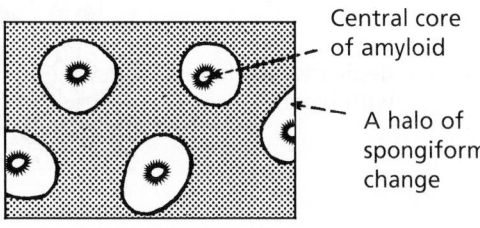

Central core of amyloid

A halo of spongiform change

2. **Variant CJD** – This occurs in younger patients with early psychiatric symptoms and a longer clinical course. The strain of PrP responsible for vCJD is identical to a bovine spongiform encephalopathy (BSE) and is caused by ingestion of products from infected cattle. In contrast with CJD florid plaques are a histological hallmark. Also, unlike CJD, PrP may be detected in lymphoid tissue.
3. **Other** – includes KURU (historical) due to ingestion of human brain by cannibalism in New Guinea and GERSTMANN-STRAUSSLER-SCHEINKER disease, a familial dementia.

# MISCELLANEOUS INFECTIONS AND INFESTATIONS

### 1. FUNGAL INFECTIONS

(a) **Primary infections**. In healthy adults, fungal infections are rare. Occasionally in the presence of heavy exposure to fungus, localised infection, often clinically insignificant, may occur, and in very rare cases CNS infection is a complication. In CRYPTOCOCCOSIS (*Cryptococcus neoformans*), the fungus exhibits neurotropism and occasionally causes meningitis in otherwise healthy subjects.

(b) **Opportunistic infections** are becoming more common nowadays due to the use of immunosuppressive therapy and the increasing prevalence of AIDS. Various fungi including *Candida, Aspergillus, Nocardia* may cause serious cerebral damage. The incidence is decreasing in AIDS patients due to HAART.

### 2. PROTOZOAL INFECTIONS

### (a) CEREBRAL MALARIA

Cerebral complications may occur in the severe acute malaria (falciparum type) which affects non-immune adults. Clinically, coma rapidly proceeds to death.

*Mechanism*

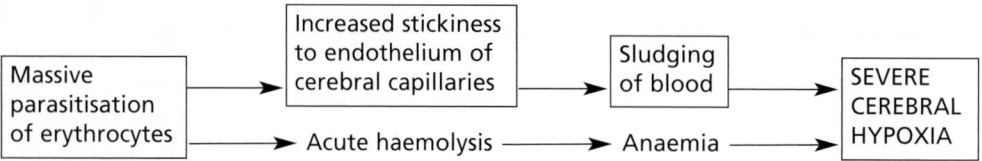

At autopsy the brain is swollen (oedema) and there may be petechial haemorrhages. Histologically, the capillaries are congested and malarial parasites and pigment are easily seen.

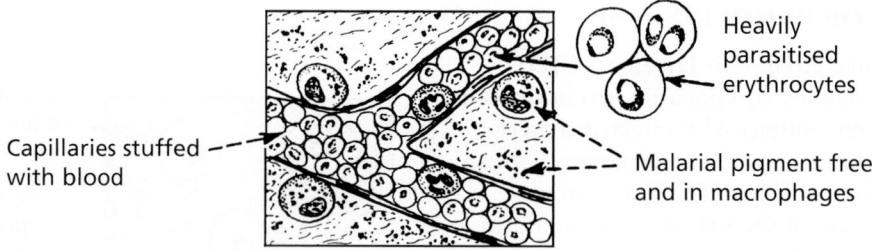

# MISCELLANEOUS INFECTIONS AND INFESTATIONS

## (b) TOXOPLASMOSIS

Although infection by *Toxoplasma gondii* is common, serious nervous tissue damage is rare and is seen in two main circumstances. In both, it occurs as part of a systemic infection.

(i) In **congenital toxoplasmosis**, the infection is acquired by the fetus during a primary maternal infection.

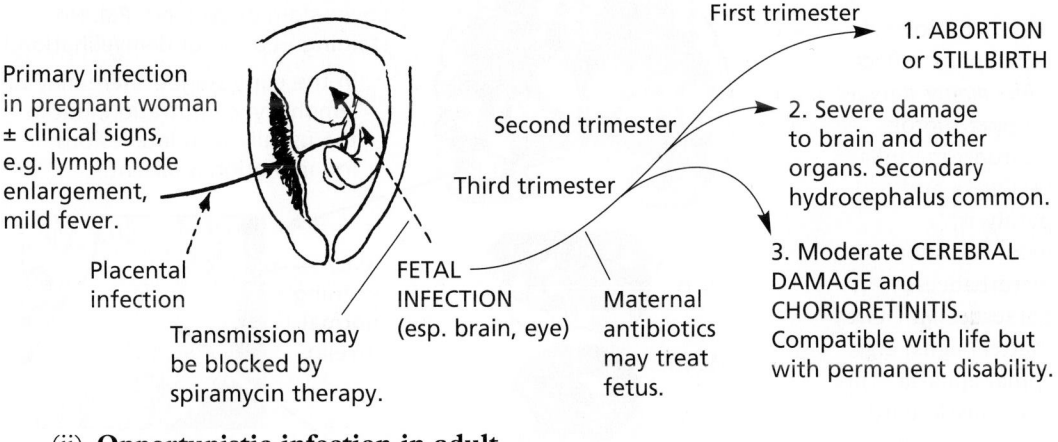

(ii) **Opportunistic infection in adult**.

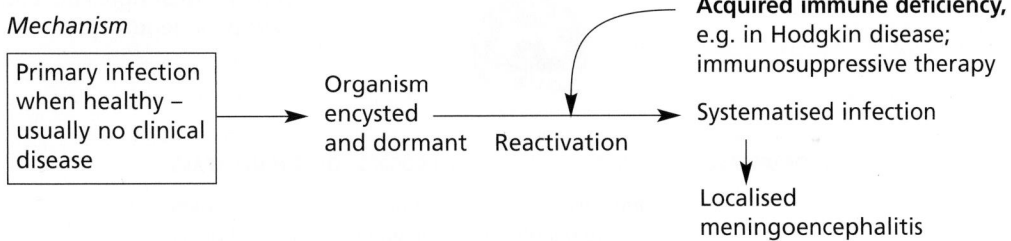

## (c) TRYPANOSOMIASIS (AFRICAN SLEEPING SICKNESS)

*Trypanosoma brucei* infection is transmitted to humans from animal reservoirs by the Tsetse fly. The organism is neurotropic and a meningoencephalitis results. The infection is associated with excessive IgM production in CSF. The 'cuffing' infiltrate has a high component of plasma cells and also 'Mott' cells – plasma cells distended by eosinophilic globules (denatured Ig).

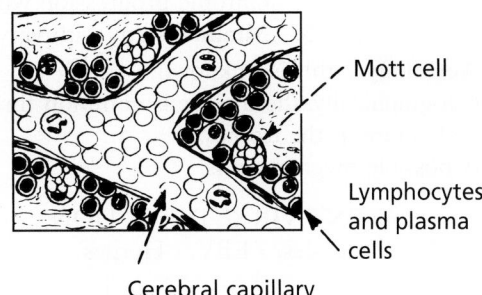

## 3. METAZOAL INFESTATION

### Cysticercosis

The larvae of *Taenia solium* may encyst in the brain and can be the cause of epilepsy.
**Hydatid cyst** – also occurs in the brain (see p. 392).

# DEMYELINATING DISEASES

### MULTIPLE SCLEROSIS (MS)

This is the commonest demyelinating disease – where the myelin sheath breaks down, leaving the axons healthy but with serious effects on their function. Multiple sclerosis is a chronic disease of young adults.

### Clinical associations

The neurological signs: pons reflect *white matter damage* – upper motor neurone; medulla weakness and paralysis; incoordination; visual disturbances; paraesthesia. ('Grey matter' signs, e.g. spinal aphasia – fits and muscle cord atrophy are rare.)

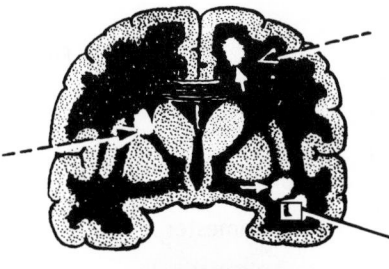

(Normal myelin stained black with Loyez stain or Weigert–Pal. No staining in areas of demyelination.)

In the early stages, there may be lymphocytic infiltration, but in the usually seen late lesions inflammation is absent.

Pons

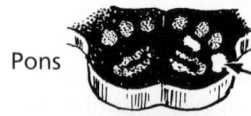

Medulla

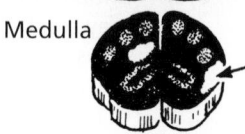

Spinal cord

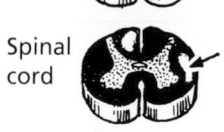

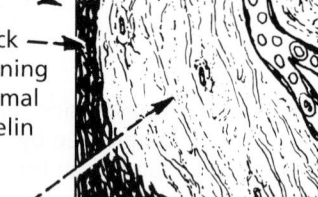

Black staining normal myelin

Plaque – no myelin; axons remain; glial fibres increased; few oligodendrocytes.

| COURSE OF DISEASE | ONSET | PROGRESS OVER MANY YEARS |
|---|---|---|
| | Often acute; may be unnoticed | Remission … relapse … remission → incremental deterioration → death |

Variants are:  1.  Acute severe disease – rapid progress to death.
2.  Chronic progression without remission.
3.  Minimal signs with very long remissions.

**Aetiology** – this is unknown.
Geographically, the disease is common throughout temperate Europe and North America and is rare in the tropics.
A possible mechanism is:

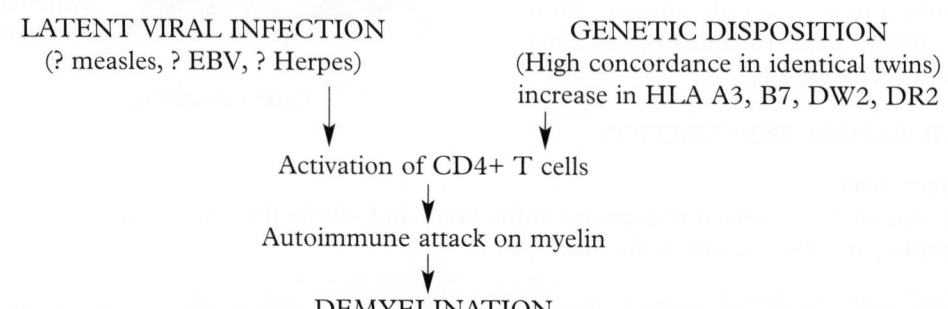

LATENT VIRAL INFECTION
(? measles, ? EBV, ? Herpes)

GENETIC DISPOSITION
(High concordance in identical twins)
increase in HLA A3, B7, DW2, DR2

Activation of CD4+ T cells

Autoimmune attack on myelin

DEMYELINATION

# DEMYELINATING DISEASES

## ACUTE DISSEMINATED ENCEPHALOMYELITIS

An acute encephalitis in which demyelination is a prominent and characteristic feature is a very rare sequel to many natural viral diseases such as mumps, measles, chickenpox and rubella and to vaccination, historically against smallpox and rabies.

Clinically, there is fever, headache, vomiting and drowsiness followed by coma. There may be clinical evidence of focal neurological damage. Pathological changes are widespread in the brain and cord and rapidly progressive.

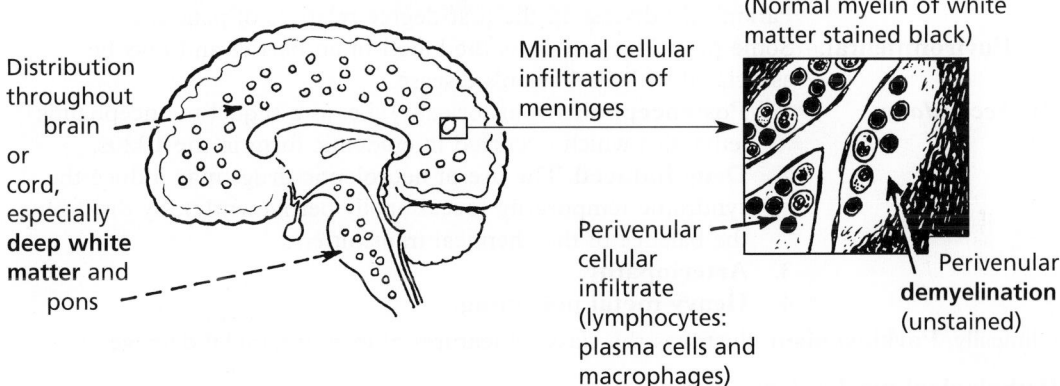

Distribution throughout brain or cord, especially **deep white matter** and pons

Minimal cellular infiltration of meninges

(Normal myelin of white matter stained black)

Perivenular cellular infiltrate (lymphocytes: plasma cells and macrophages)

Perivenular **demyelination** (unstained)

In **ACUTE HAEMORRHAGIC LEUKOENCEPHALITIS**, to these are added actual petechial haemorrhages from damaged vessels, particularly in the white matter; not all cases follow virus infection.

**Mechanism.** It is thought that in these disorders the damage to the myelin is not the result of direct virus attack but is an *auto-immune* reaction in which the antigen is a component of myelin and the virus in some unknown way acts as a trigger.

## DISEASES DUE TO ABNORMAL MYELIN

In this group of rare 'leukodystrophies', the molecular structure of myelin is abnormal usually due to abnormal or deficient enzyme action. Most cases are genetically determined, present in early life and progress fairly rapidly.

Abnormal metabolites which can be specifically identified accumulate in macrophages, glial cells and sometimes neurones.

e.g.
1. In **metachromatic leukodystrophy**, the accumulation of a *sulphatide* gives a metachromatic staining reaction and characteristic Electron microscopic appearance.
2. In **Krabbe disease** there are typical multinucleated histiocytes (called globoid cells) containing *cerebroside*.

# PARKINSON'S DISEASE

This is a disease of the extrapyramidal system which links the higher motor centres and effector motor cells of the spinal cord. Important neurotransmitters are DOPAMINE and γ-aminobutyric acid (GABA).

**Aetiology** – The disease occurs in two main circumstances:

(a) *Idiopathic*:     The majority of cases occurring in the elderly population (1% of over 60s) are idiopathic and the cause remains unclear. Genetic and environmental factors may be involved.

    **Genetic**:     There is a two to three times increased risk of the development of Parkinson's disease in the first-degree relatives of patients.

    **Environmental**:   Some pesticides can cross the blood-brain barrier and may be associated with Parkinson's disease.

(b) *Secondary*:     1. **Postencephalitic** (historically), i.e. as a sequel to encephalitis lethargica which occurred in epidemic form in the 1920s.

                2. **Drug induced**. The use of neuroleptic drugs may induce the syndrome temporarily (occasionally permanently), by disturbing the balance of the chemical transmitters.

                3. **Arteriopathy**.

                4. **Heavy metal poisoning**.

Clinically, **Parkinsonism** illustrates the classical features of extrapyramidal damage.

**Pathological mechanism**

In all cases of long-standing Parkinsonism of any type, degenerative changes are seen in the extrapyramidal nuclei. In particular, there is depigmentation of the substantia nigra.

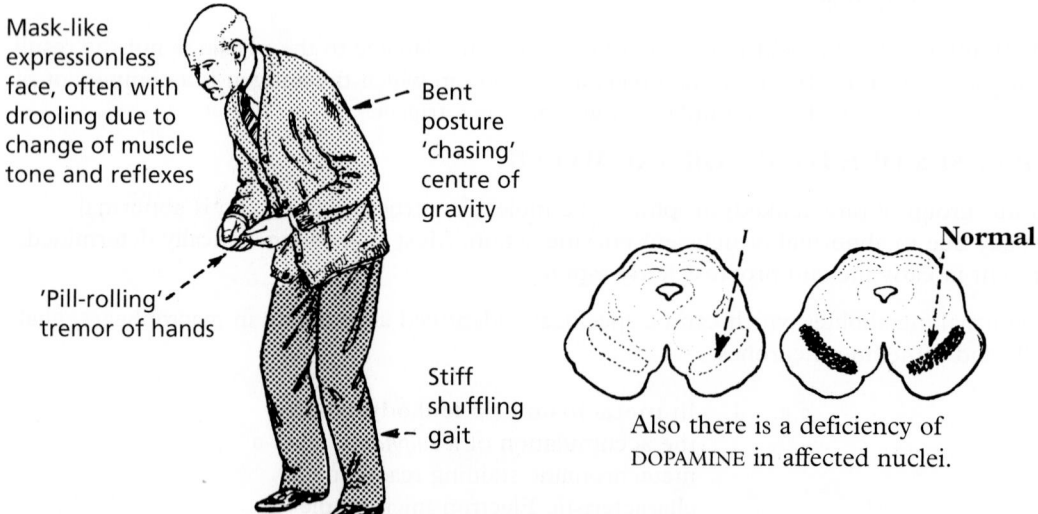

Mask-like expressionless face, often with drooling due to change of muscle tone and reflexes

'Pill-rolling' tremor of hands

Bent posture 'chasing' centre of gravity

Stiff shuffling gait

**Normal**

Also there is a deficiency of DOPAMINE in affected nuclei.

Histologically, there is loss of neurones, and the surviving nerve cells contain inclusions known as Lewy bodies (p. 589).

Other extrapyramidal disorders include the choreas, of which there are two main types.

**Sydenham chorea** occurs in children with rheumatic fever, while chorea is a manifestation in some patients with **Huntington disease**.

# MISCELLANEOUS DISORDERS

## NUTRITIONAL AND METABOLIC DISORDERS (ENCEPHALOPATHIES)

In the last analysis, all disorders in this group are mediated by disturbed neuronal metabolism, so that exact classification may present some difficulty. However, it is convenient to consider them in two broad groups.

## 1. NUTRITIONAL DEFICIENCY

The vitamins of the B group are important coenzymes in several intracellular oxidative pathways. Deficiency, which may arise from primary malnutrition but more commonly in association with alcohol abuse, is the cause of degenerations of the brain, spinal cord and peripheral nerves.

### Wernicke encephalopathy

Clinically, this condition presents with disturbances of consciousness, ataxia and visual disturbances, and without prompt treatment progresses to death in coma. In Western countries, chronic alcoholism is usually present; often a particularly heavy bout of drinking precipitates the condition.

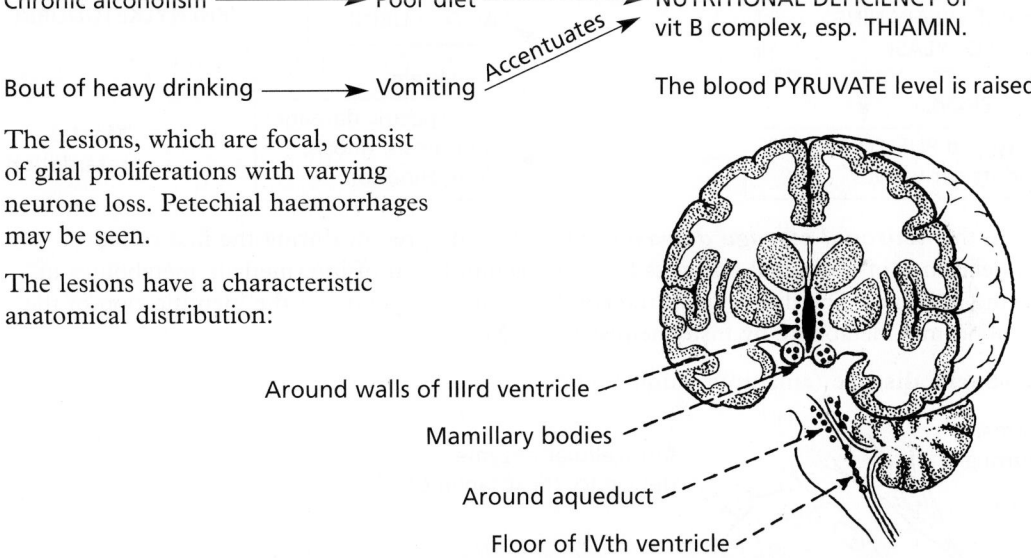

Chronic alcoholism ⟶ Poor diet ⟶ NUTRITIONAL DEFICIENCY of vit B complex, esp. THIAMIN.

Bout of heavy drinking ⟶ Vomiting *Accentuates*

The blood PYRUVATE level is raised.

The lesions, which are focal, consist of glial proliferations with varying neurone loss. Petechial haemorrhages may be seen.

The lesions have a characteristic anatomical distribution:

Around walls of IIIrd ventricle

Mamillary bodies

Around aqueduct

Floor of IVth ventricle

Prompt treatment with thiamin minimises the damage, but if treatment is omitted or delayed, permanent damage results. The patient may have a persistent Korsakoff psychosis. At autopsy, there is visible shrinkage of the mamillary bodies.

# MISCELLANEOUS DISORDERS

### 2.  METABOLIC DISORDERS

In the following examples, the metabolic defect causes neurological disorder, but in addition, other organs are seriously disturbed.

(a) *Aminoacidopathies*

A wide variety of hepatic enzyme defects in the complex metabolism of amino acids has now been described. When neurological damage occurs, it is essentially non-specific and developing in the immediate postnatal period, a critical time in the development of the brain which leads to *mental retardation*.

**Phenylketonuria** is an example.

The importance of this disease is that the effects can be prevented by dietary restriction of phenylalanine-containing substances, provided the treatment is begun within 60 days of birth.

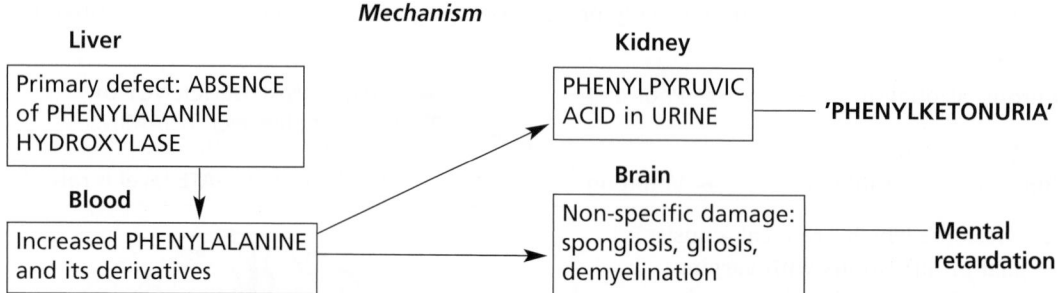

*Mechanism*

| Liver | Kidney |
|---|---|

**Liver**

Primary defect: ABSENCE of PHENYLALANINE HYDROXYLASE

**Blood**

Increased PHENYLALANINE and its derivatives

**Kidney**

PHENYLPYRUVIC ACID in URINE ──── **'PHENYLKETONURIA'**

**Brain**

Non-specific damage: spongiosis, gliosis, demyelination ──── **Mental retardation**

(b) In the *neuronal storage diseases*, which usually present during the first decade, deficiency of lysozomal enzymes leads to accumulation of intermediate metabolites in the neurones. The diagnosis of the condition often depends on the identification of the abnormal metabolite by histochemistry or EM.

**Tay-Sachs disease** (amaurotic familial idiocy) is an illustrative example.

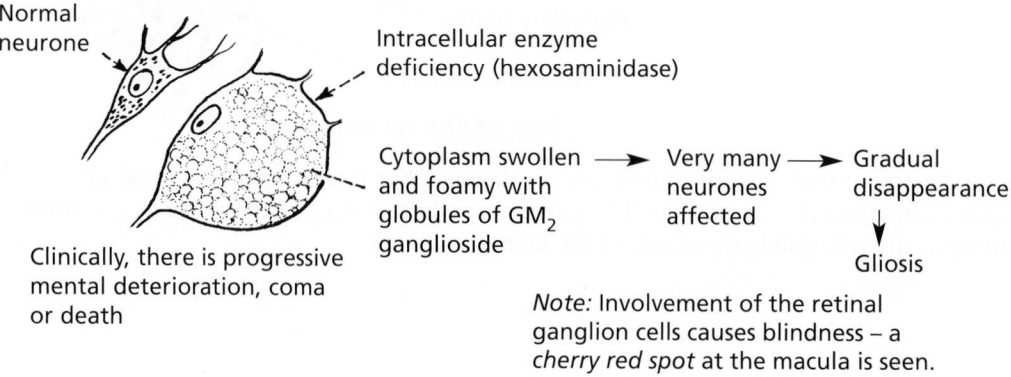

Normal neurone

Intracellular enzyme deficiency (hexosaminidase)

Cytoplasm swollen and foamy with globules of $GM_2$ ganglioside ──► Very many neurones affected ──► Gradual disappearance ↓ Gliosis

Clinically, there is progressive mental deterioration, coma or death

*Note:* Involvement of the retinal ganglion cells causes blindness – a *cherry red spot* at the macula is seen.

In these disorders, other organs may be mildly affected by the enzyme defect but the neurological effects are predominant.

# DISEASES OF THE SPINAL CORD

In purely spinal lesions, basic disease processes have important anatomical and functional implications. Lack of space for expansion produces important compression effects. Examples are:

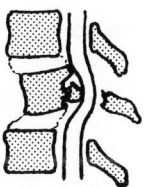 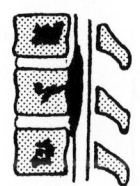 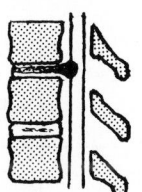 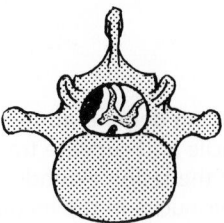

Fracture/ dislocation of vertebra

Tumour (usually secondary) in vertebrae growing into canal

Prolapse of intervertebral disc

Tumour of meninges or nerve sheath

**Effects**

**Normal**

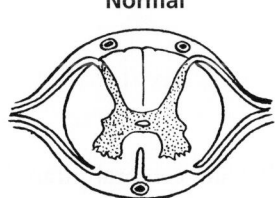

Cord, nerve roots and blood vessels loosely suspended in CSF 'water bath'

Compression

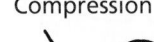 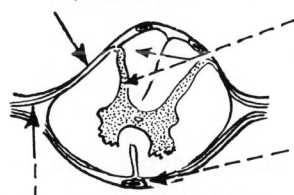

(1) *Damage to neurones and nerve tracts*
May be focal but is often transverse and complete

(2) *Vascular compression*
Impairment of circulation may cause infarction; this is important particularly in traumatic cases

(3) *Damage to nerve roots* (radiculitis); a common complication of spondylosis

At the level of the lesion, there is loss of the sensory and motor connections which constitute the spinal reflex.

In addition, severance of the longitudinal tracts cuts off the cerebral connections to all parts below the lesion.

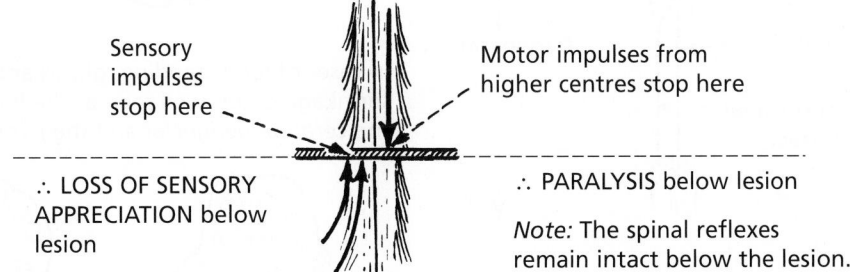

Sensory impulses stop here

Motor impulses from higher centres stop here

∴ LOSS OF SENSORY APPRECIATION below lesion

∴ PARALYSIS below lesion

*Note:* The spinal reflexes remain intact below the lesion.

# DISEASES OF THE SPINAL CORD

### ASCENDING AND DESCENDING DEGENERATIONS

The long tract fibres which are cut off from their neurones progressively degenerate.

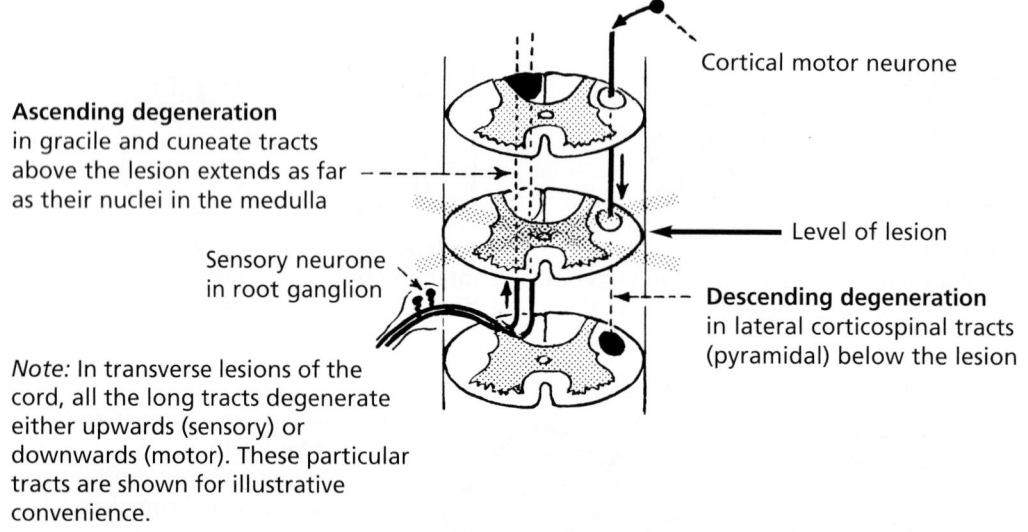

**Ascending degeneration**
in gracile and cuneate tracts
above the lesion extends as far
as their nuclei in the medulla

Sensory neurone
in root ganglion

*Note:* In transverse lesions of the
cord, all the long tracts degenerate
either upwards (sensory) or
downwards (motor). These particular
tracts are shown for illustrative
convenience.

Cortical motor neurone

Level of lesion

**Descending degeneration**
in lateral corticospinal tracts
(pyramidal) below the lesion

The commonest example of **descending degeneration** is seen following cerebral infarction
involving the internal capsule; the degeneration extends from the lesion along the
corticospinal axons to their terminations in the anterior horn.

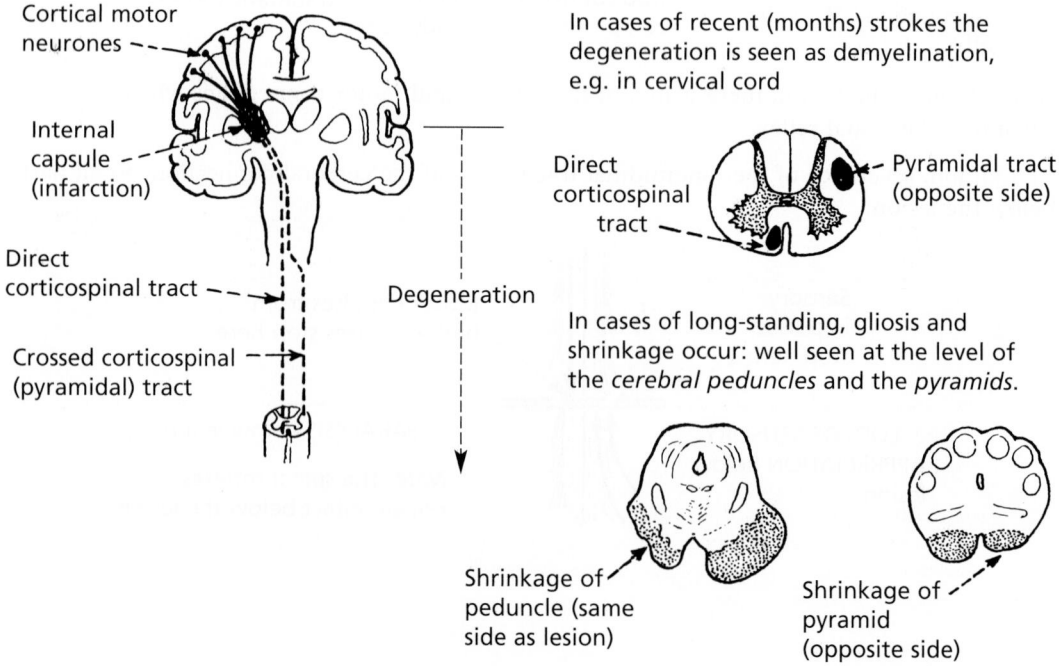

Cortical motor
neurones

Internal
capsule
(infarction)

Direct
corticospinal tract

Crossed corticospinal
(pyramidal) tract

Degeneration

In cases of recent (months) strokes the
degeneration is seen as demyelination,
e.g. in cervical cord

Direct
corticospinal
tract

Pyramidal tract
(opposite side)

In cases of long-standing, gliosis and
shrinkage occur: well seen at the level of
the *cerebral peduncles* and the *pyramids*.

Shrinkage of
peduncle (same
side as lesion)

Shrinkage of
pyramid
(opposite side)

# DISORDERS OF MOTOR PATHWAYS

The concept of upper and lower motor neuronal activity, based on anatomical and physiological evidence, has great clinical value in diagnosis.

The **upper motor neurones** (UMNs) synapse with the **lower motor neurones** (LMNs)

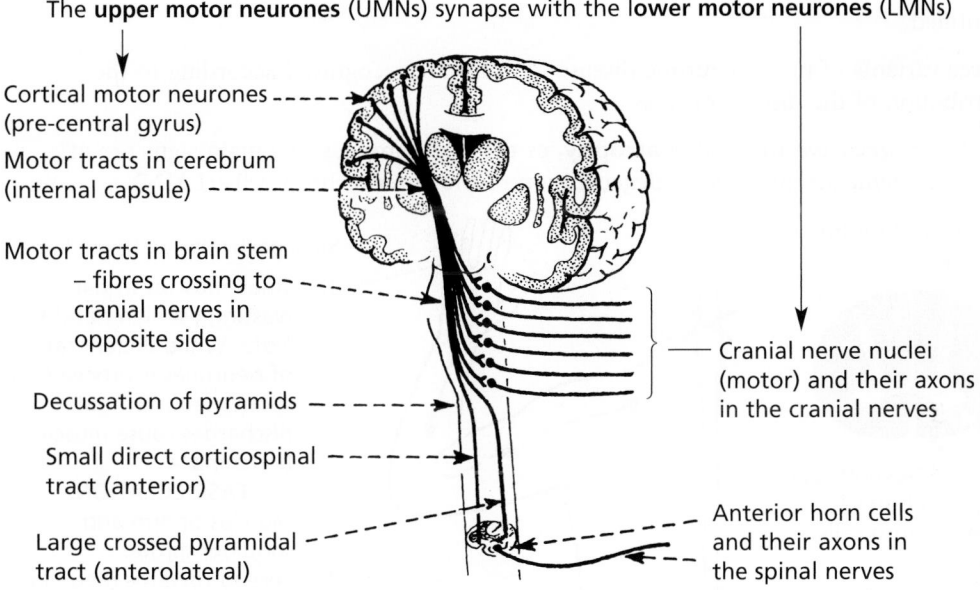

Cortical motor neurones (pre-central gyrus)

Motor tracts in cerebrum (internal capsule)

Motor tracts in brain stem – fibres crossing to cranial nerves in opposite side

Decussation of pyramids

Small direct corticospinal tract (anterior)

Large crossed pyramidal tract (anterolateral)

Cranial nerve nuclei (motor) and their axons in the cranial nerves

Anterior horn cells and their axons in the spinal nerves

It will be appreciated that in its long course from the cerebral cortex to the anterior horn, the upper motor neurone is susceptible to damage from a variety of disease processes acting at various sites. The lower motor neurone may be damaged in the cord or in the peripheral nerve. Important illustrative examples are:

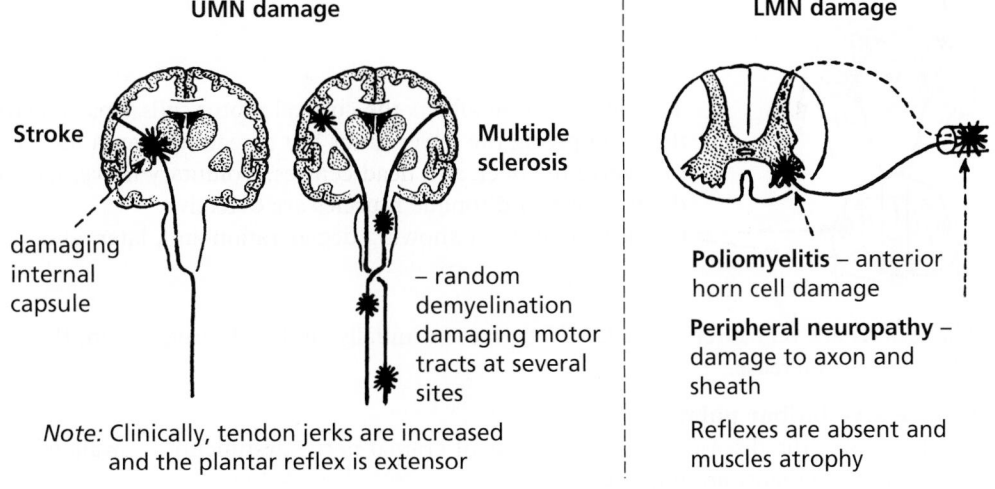

UMN damage

Stroke

damaging internal capsule

Multiple sclerosis

– random demyelination damaging motor tracts at several sites

*Note:* Clinically, tendon jerks are increased and the plantar reflex is extensor

LMN damage

**Poliomyelitis** – anterior horn cell damage

**Peripheral neuropathy** – damage to axon and sheath

Reflexes are absent and muscles atrophy

# MOTOR NEURONE DISEASE

This is a disease of unknown aetiology occurring predominantly in adult males. In a few cases motor neurone disease is familial and is caused by a mutation in the gene encoding a free radical scavenger, superoxide dismutase 1. Other susceptibility genes have been identified.

Three variants of motor neurone disease (MND) are recognised according to the distribution of the disease process.

1.  In **progressive muscular atrophy**, as the name implies, the main signs are of neurogenic atrophy due to degeneration of the anterior horn cells (LMN).

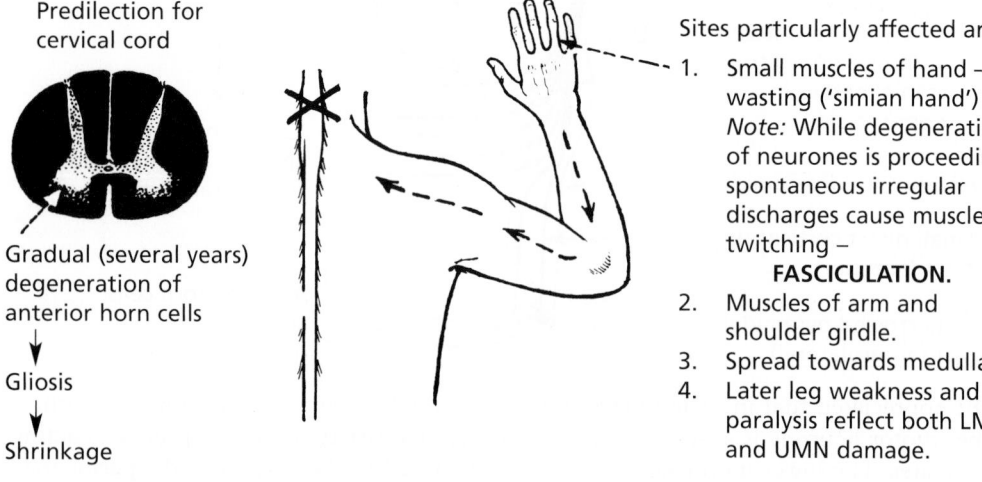

Predilection for cervical cord

Gradual (several years) degeneration of anterior horn cells

↓

Gliosis

↓

Shrinkage

Sites particularly affected are:

1.  Small muscles of hand – wasting ('simian hand') *Note:* While degeneration of neurones is proceeding spontaneous irregular discharges cause muscle twitching – **FASCICULATION.**
2.  Muscles of arm and shoulder girdle.
3.  Spread towards medulla.
4.  Later leg weakness and paralysis reflect both LMN and UMN damage.

2.  In **amyotrophic lateral sclerosis** there is both UMN and LMN damage: 'lateral sclerosis' indicates the degeneration of the pyramidal tracts.

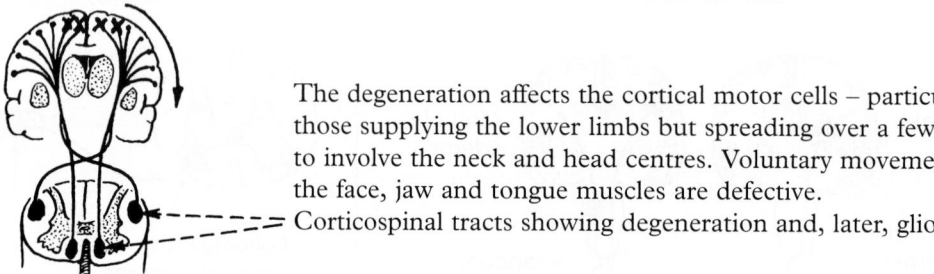

The degeneration affects the cortical motor cells – particularly those supplying the lower limbs but spreading over a few years to involve the neck and head centres. Voluntary movements of the face, jaw and tongue muscles are defective.

Corticospinal tracts showing degeneration and, later, gliosis.

The lesions are very rarely pure UMN type even initially, and with progression, the LMN lesions increase.

3.  **Progressive bulbar palsy**

In a few cases, the disease begins with signs of cranial nerve dysfunction – swallowing and facial movements are impaired.

### Progress

In MND after a long progressive illness the stage is reached when the bulbar degeneration is severe enough to prevent elimination of secretions from the respiratory tract. Death is usually due to aspiration bronchopneumonia or respiratory failure.

# MIXED MOTOR AND SENSORY DISORDERS

## SUBACUTE COMBINED DEGENERATION OF CORD

Due specifically to vitamin $B_{12}$ deficiency. If replacement therapy is begun early enough, there is restoration to normal.

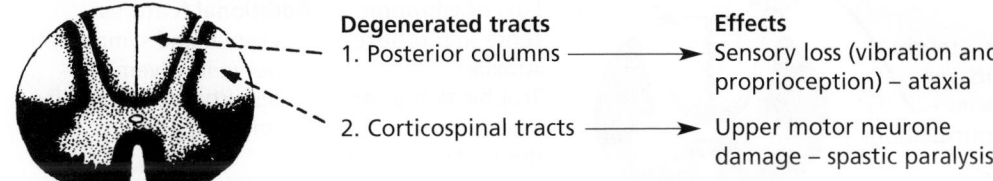

**Degenerated tracts**

1. Posterior columns ⟶

2. Corticospinal tracts ⟶

**Effects**

Sensory loss (vibration and proprioception) – ataxia

Upper motor neurone damage – spastic paralysis

## SYRINGOMYELIA

In this condition, a glial-lined cystic space gradually expands within the cord, usually in the cervical region. The pathogenesis is not certain, but it is suggested that the lesion is essentially an expansion of the central canal associated with a mild developmental abnormality of the distal end of the IVth ventricle. Some cases follow spinal trauma.

**Effects**

Damage to sensory fibres decussating in the cord. Loss of temperature and touch in local segments (**dissociated anaesthesia**).

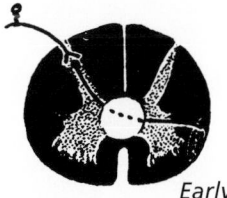

*Early*

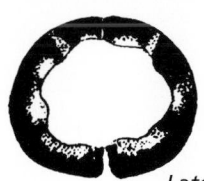

*Late*

Destruction of grey matter and gradual affection of long tracts. Loss of local reflexes. Severe sensory loss. Spastic paralysis.

## SPINOCEREBELLAR DEGENERATIONS

This is a large group of related disorders, usually familial, in which there is motor and sensory degeneration particularly affecting gait, posture, equilibrium and movement. There is sometimes optic nerve and retinal damage and intellectual disturbance.

Friedreich ataxia is the most common hereditary ataxia and is caused by expansion of a trinucleotide triplet repeat in the FRATAXIN gene on chromosome 9. Deficiency of frataxin leads to mitochondrial respiratory chain dysfunction. In addition to the effects of spinocerebellar degeneration there may be cardiomyopathy with arrhythmia.

## SENSORY DISORDERS

In **TABES DORSALIS**, a tertiary manifestation of syphilis in which the lumbar cord is commonly affected, there is degeneration of the posterior nerve roots and columns.

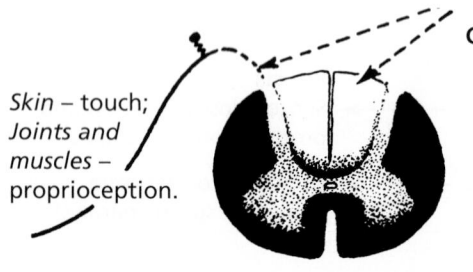

*Skin* – touch;
*Joints and muscles* – proprioception.

**Clinically**
Loss of vibration sense and reflexes;
Ataxia;
Trophic skin ulcers;
Severe joint derangement
(Charcot, p. 650).

**Additional features**
Cranial and sympathetic nerve involvement – disturbance of pupillary reflex;

Painful visceral crises.

# THE PERIPHERAL NERVES/THE NEUROPATHIES

There are three main reactions that occur in peripheral nerves.

1.  Traumatic damage followed by regeneration or formation of a traumatic neuroma.
2.  Damage to axons and myelin sheath.
    (a) Axonal degeneration

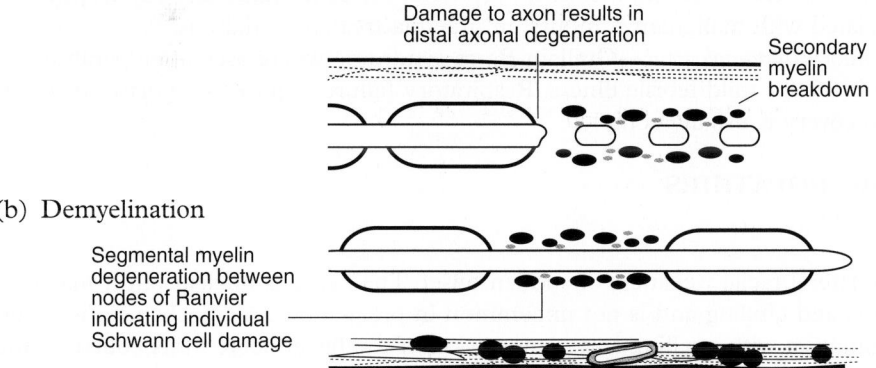

3.  Damage to supporting structures, e.g. blood vessels or epi-, peri- or endoneurium.

## CLINICAL MANIFESTATIONS OF PERIPHERAL NERVE DISORDERS

1.  ***Mononeuropathy***: single nerve damage by compression, e.g. compression of median nerve in carpal tunnel syndrome, compression of nerve root by prolapsed intervertebral disc.
2.  ***Mononeuritis multiplex***: where several nerves are involved, e.g. arteritis with inflammation of vasa nervorum leading to ischaemia.

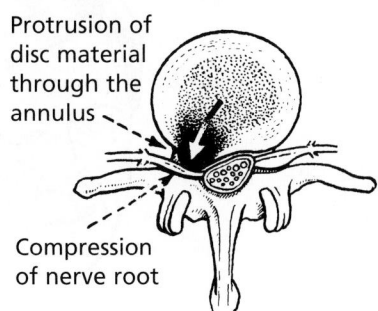

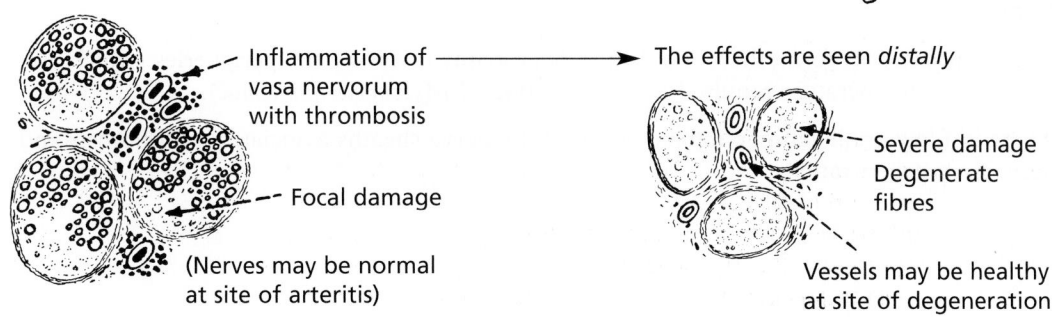

# THE NEUROPATHIES

3. ***Polyneuropathy***: where there is extensive and symmetrical disturbance of function, often peripheral in distribution and especially affecting the legs. There are many causes:
*Toxic* – diphtheria; lead; arsenic; drugs used in medicine.
*Deficiency states* – particularly vitamin B complex deficiency causing Beri-Beri.
*Metabolic disorders* – diabetes mellitus; porphyria, metachromatic leukodystrophy, associated with malignant tumours, in uraemia treated by dialysis.
*Inflammatory/Immunological* – Guillain-Barré syndrome where ascending paralysis occurs usually after a mild febrile illness. Respiratory failure requires supportive treatment but recovery is usually complete.

## OTHER NEUROPATHIES

### Bell palsy

This is a unilateral facial weakness of sudden onset. The cause is unclear but it may occur with draughts and chilling and is not uncommon in pregnancy. The mechanism is thought to be inflammation with swelling and compression of the facial nerve in its course in the bone adjacent to the internal auditory meatus. Progress: 75% of cases recover in about 4–8 weeks.

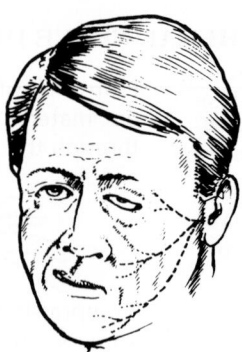

Note drooping and loss of facial expression on paralysed side. Facial muscles pull across the mid line – mouth is distorted.

### Leprosy

In the lepromatous form, there is a diffuse neuropathy involving the peripheries (which are at the lower temperature required for proliferation of *Mycobacterium leprae*).

There is a low grade chronic inflammation of the nerve sheaths associated with fibrosis and nerve fibre degeneration.

# HYDROCEPHALUS

In hydrocephalus, the volume of the CSF is increased and the ventricles are dilated. In the majority of cases, there is an increase in intracranial pressure. Three possible **mechanisms** are considered.

1. **Overproduction of CSF**

   The choroid plexus will secrete more CSF to compensate for any external leak, but overproduction is not a cause of hydrocephalus.

2. **Obstruction to the flow of CSF is the common mechanism.**

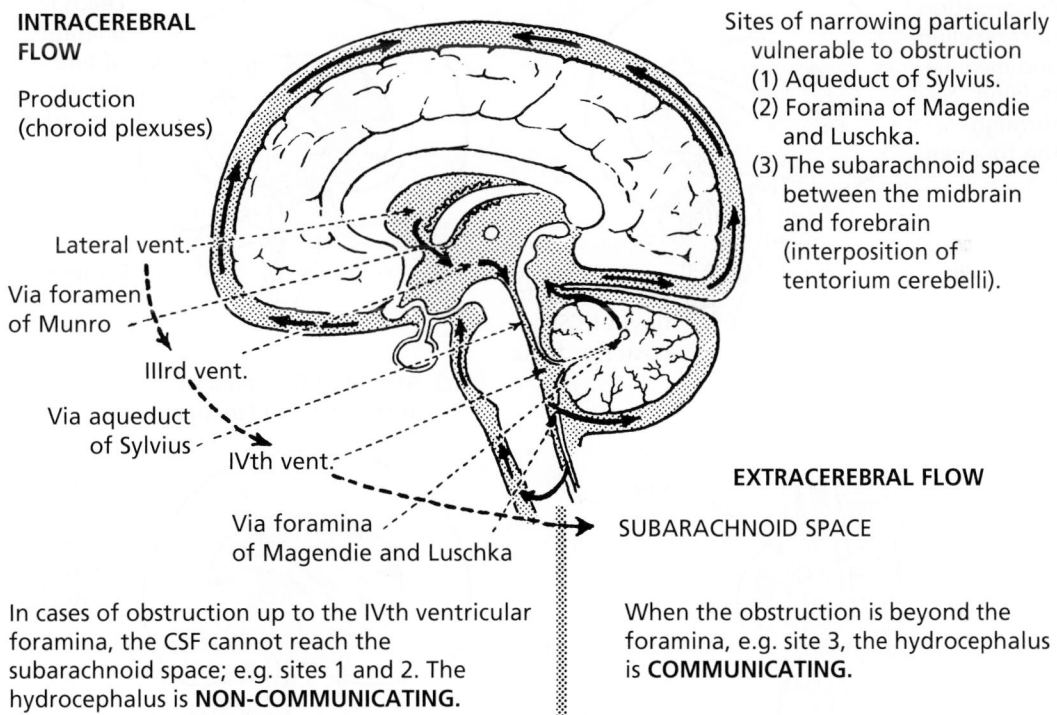

**INTRACEREBRAL FLOW**

Production (choroid plexuses)

Lateral vent.

Via foramen of Munro

IIIrd vent.

Via aqueduct of Sylvius

IVth vent.

Via foramina of Magendie and Luschka

Sites of narrowing particularly vulnerable to obstruction
(1) Aqueduct of Sylvius.
(2) Foramina of Magendie and Luschka.
(3) The subarachnoid space between the midbrain and forebrain (interposition of tentorium cerebelli).

**EXTRACEREBRAL FLOW**

SUBARACHNOID SPACE

In cases of obstruction up to the IVth ventricular foramina, the CSF cannot reach the subarachnoid space; e.g. sites 1 and 2. The hydrocephalus is **NON-COMMUNICATING.**

When the obstruction is beyond the foramina, e.g. site 3, the hydrocephalus is **COMMUNICATING.**

3. **Defective absorption of CSF** is a rare mechanism.

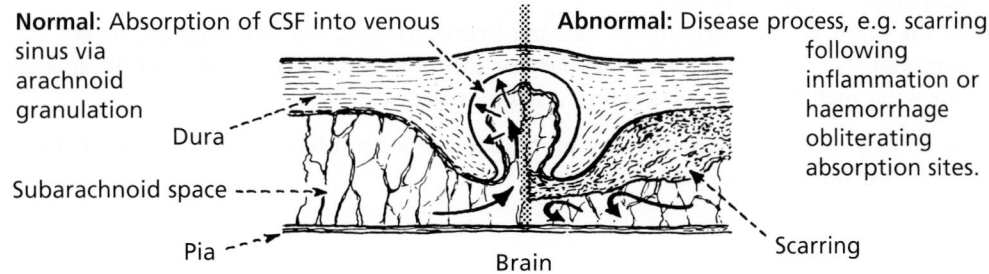

**Normal:** Absorption of CSF into venous sinus via arachnoid granulation

Dura

Subarachnoid space

Pia

Brain

**Abnormal:** Disease process, e.g. scarring following inflammation or haemorrhage obliterating absorption sites.

Scarring

# HYDROCEPHALUS

### CAUSES

The diseases causing hydrocephalus fall into two groups:

1. **Congenital (developmental) abnormalities**
   The common conditions are:

   (a) *The Arnold–Chiari malformation*

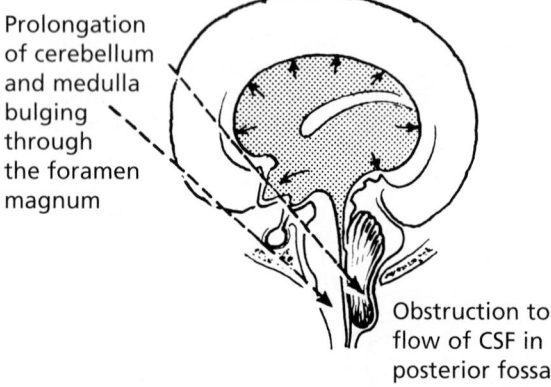

Prolongation
of cerebellum
and medulla
bulging
through
the foramen
magnum

Obstruction to
flow of CSF in
posterior fossa

Associated with
spina bifida, usually
*meningomyelocele*

Dura
deficient

Arachnoid and
nervous tissue
lying under
bulging skin

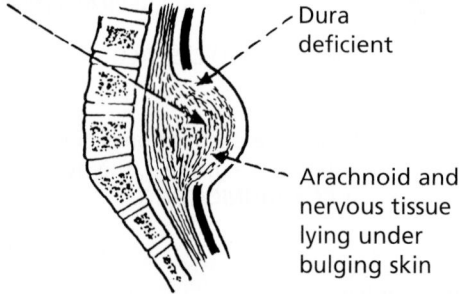

   (b) *Congenital stenosis or atresia of aqueduct of Sylvius*

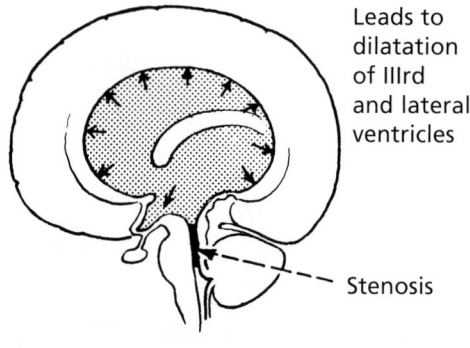

Leads to
dilatation
of IIIrd
and lateral
ventricles

Stenosis

   (c) *Atresia of foramina of Magendie and Luschka*

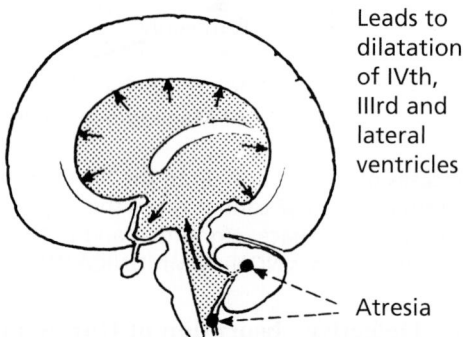

Leads to
dilatation
of IVth,
IIIrd and
lateral
ventricles

Atresia

2. **Acquired hydrocephalus**
   Of the many possible conditions causing hydrocephalus, the following are most common: (a) cerebral tumour (primary or secondary) and (b) scarring of the meninges following meningitis or subarachnoid haemorrhage.

   As already explained, whether any particular disease produces hydrocephalus depends largely on the site affected.

# HYDROCEPHALUS

## EFFECTS

**In the infant and young child**, the pliable skull expands to accommodate the enlarging brain – but these extreme changes do not occur if an effective shunt is inserted.

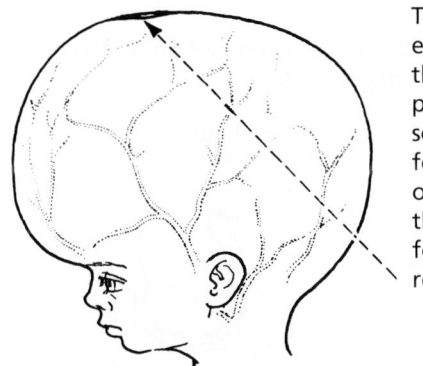

There is great enlargement of the head with prominent scalp veins, and forehead overhanging the eyes. The fontanelle remains open.

Clinically mental deficiency is common.

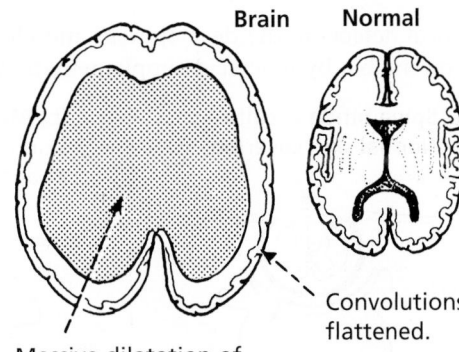

Convolutions flattened.

Massive dilatation of ventricles with marked thinning and stretching of brain.

In the **older child and adult**, enlargement of the brain is prevented by the inability of the skull to expand. The main change is dilatation of the ventricles associated with the effects on the brain of increased intracranial pressure.

## SPECIAL TYPES OF HYDROCEPHALUS

1.  In cases of generalised cerebral atrophy, the ventricular system enlarges to compensate for the loss of cerebral tissue. This also happens locally when cerebral tissue is lost, e.g. following infarction.

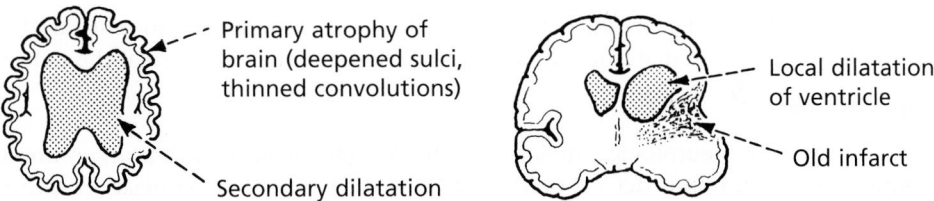

Primary atrophy of brain (deepened sulci, thinned convolutions)

Secondary dilatation

Local dilatation of ventricle

Old infarct

No increase in pressure is involved and the pathological and clinical effects wholly reflect the primary loss of cerebral tissue. The condition is sometimes called **secondary hydrocephalus**.

2.  **Normal pressure hydrocephalus**

    In this rare condition, progressive mental deterioration (dementia) and disturbances of gait and micturition are associated with ventricular dilatation. CSF pressures are usually at the high end of the normal range. The exact mechanism is not understood but it is thought to be a form of communicating hydrocephalus with unpaired CSF reabsorption at the arachnoid granulations. The diagnosis has assumed importance because in some cases CSF shunt procedures have arrested the progress. The aetiology is obscure.

# DEVELOPMENTAL ABNORMALITIES

Developmental abnormalities of the brain and cranium are relatively common. They range from anencephaly (absence of brain) to minor malformations, e.g. meningocele and encephalocele. There may be associated congenital defects elsewhere in the body.

## NEURAL TUBE DEFECTS

Local defects in the development and closure of the neural tube are common and largely preventable by folic acid supplementation in pregnancy. They include:

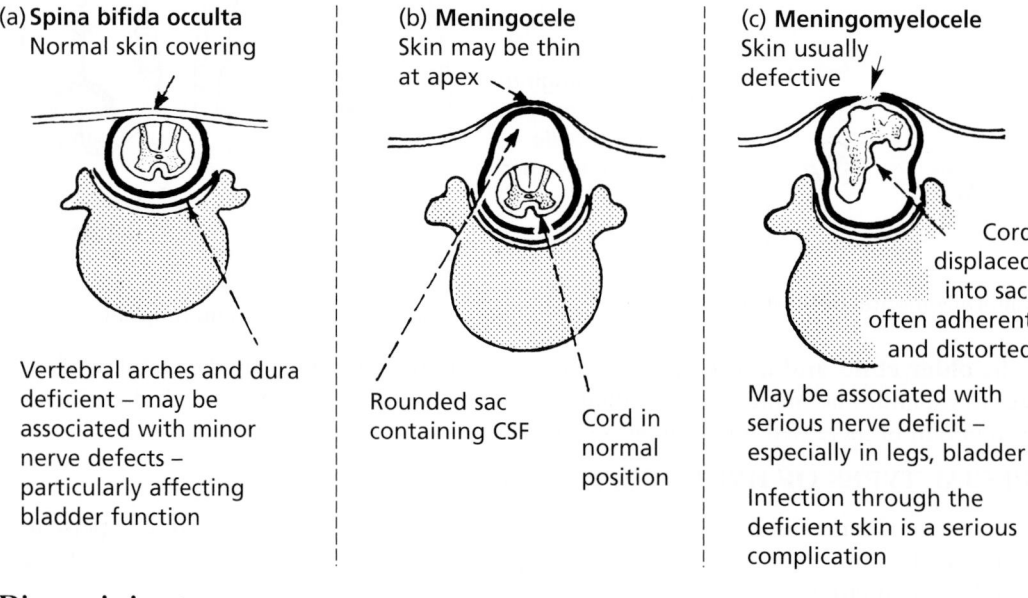

(a) **Spina bifida occulta**
Normal skin covering

Vertebral arches and dura deficient – may be associated with minor nerve defects – particularly affecting bladder function

(b) **Meningocele**
Skin may be thin at apex

Rounded sac containing CSF

Cord in normal position

(c) **Meningomyelocele**
Skin usually defective

Cord displaced into sac: often adherent and distorted

May be associated with serious nerve deficit – especially in legs, bladder

Infection through the deficient skin is a serious complication

### Diagnosis in utero

$\alpha$-fetoprotein leaks through the defective skin covering and increased amounts are found in the amniotic fluid and in maternal blood. Ultrasonography may also reveal the defect.

### Complications

In addition to severe neurological deficits which are aggravated by infection, an important complication even in minor defects is **HYDROCEPHALUS** due to an association with the Arnold-Chiari Malformation (p. 616).

# TUMOURS OF THE NERVOUS SYSTEM

The following scheme illustrates the various non-specific clinicopathological effects of a tumour within the skull.

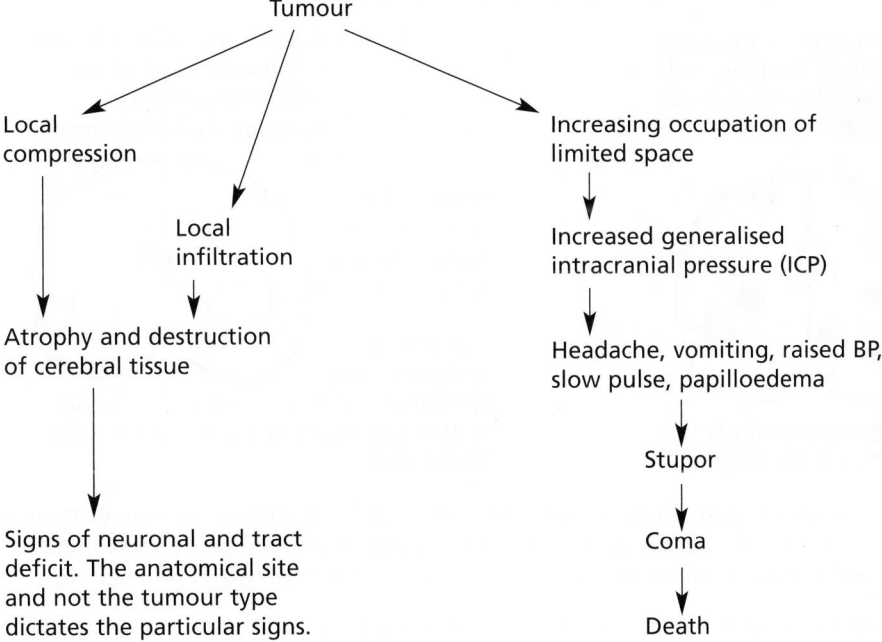

An important factor which materially influences the relative importance of each of these effects is the rate of tumour growth.

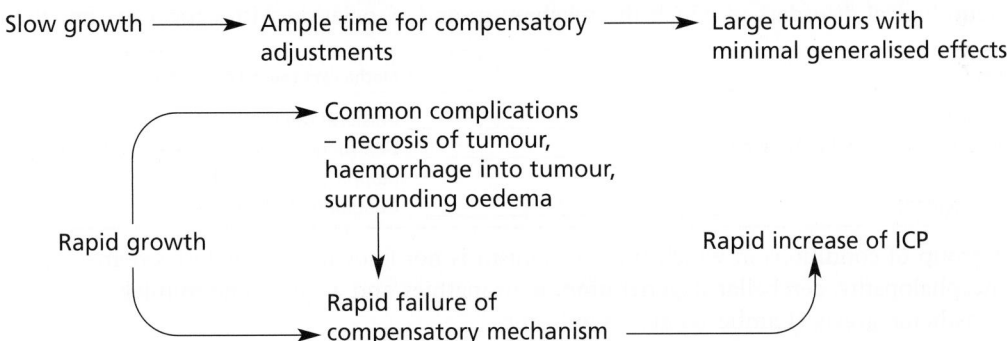

Tumours will be considered in a simplified form under the following broad headings:

1. Secondary neoplasms.
2. Neoplasms of neuroectodermal origin.
3. Neoplasms arising in supporting tissue (mesodermal).
4. Neoplasms and swellings of developmental origin.
5. Neoplasms of nerve sheaths.

# SECONDARY BRAIN TUMOURS

In the general population the incidence of metastatic cerebral tumour is much higher than that of primary cerebral neoplasm. The two most common primary sites are lung and breast, but any malignant tumour can metastasise to the brain.

The common presentation is in the form of multiple, well-delineated spherical nodules, randomly distributed.

A less common distribution is by permeation of the subarachnoid space – **meningeal carcinomatosis.**

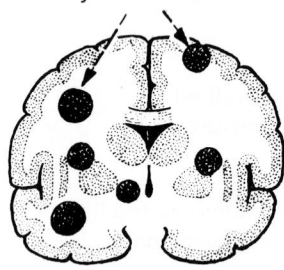

Only occasionally is there a single nodule.

Brain surface covered by a layer of tumour tissue ------→

Carcinoma, leukaemia and lymphoreticular neoplasms may spread in this way (malignant cells may be seen in the CSF).

Secondary tumours may cause serious spinal damage by destroying the integrity of the vertebrae although the vertebral discs usually remain intact (compared with spinal TB). The prostate and cervix, in addition to lung, breast and kidney, are usual primary sites.

In contrast to tumours causing neurological damage by their physical presence and growth, less commonly *non-metastatic effects of cancer* are seen.

There is a wide range of disorders which are conveniently divided into two groups:

1. Neurological disorders in which the mechanism and association with cancer are known:

| Examples | | Mechanism caused by cancer |
|---|---|---|
| Opportunistic infections | | Immune depression |
| Metabolic and hormonal imbalance | | Destruction of organs, e.g. liver, kidney |
| | | Inappropriate secretion |
| Vascular accidents | | Coagulation disorders |

2. A group of conditions in which the mechanism is not known. This includes dementia, encephalopathy, cerebellar degeneration, neuropathies and a syndrome mimicking myasthenia gravis (Lambert-Eaton syndrome).

# PRIMARY BRAIN TUMOURS

## GLIOMAS

### Astrocytoma

This is a low grade tumour derived from astrocytes and occurring most frequently in the cerebrum of young adults.

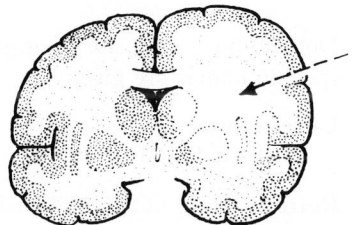

The tumour which has ill-defined margins grows irregularly into the surrounding brain tissue and only latterly causes increased ICP

Note enlargement of hemisphere by ill defined growth.

Because they have ill-defined margins, astrocytomas are difficult to eradicate and slowly but inexorably grow and eventually cause death. Many eventually transform to a high grade tumour (anaplastic astrocytoma or glioblastoma). The rare pilocytic astrocytoma occurs in the cerebellum or optic nerve of children and carries a good prognosis.

### Glioblastoma

This is the commonest glial tumour and may occur de novo or following a history of low-grade astrocytoma. This is a highly malignant tumour and the cells are pleomorphic, with mitoses, necrosis and a striking proliferation of blood vessels.

The prognosis of these patients is very poor.

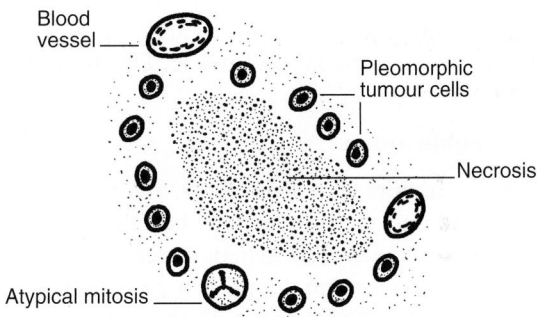

### Oligodendroglioma

These tumours, derived from oligodendroglia, tend to occur in the cerebrum of adults and may present clinically with epilepsy. They are usually slow growing and often show calcification. Cytogenetic studies have shown that tumours with loss of heterozygosity for 1p and 19p are chemosensitive and therefore have a better prognosis.

### Ependymoma

These are also rare and arise from the lining of the ventricles and central spinal cord. They may block the flow of CSF and cause hydrocephalus.

*Note:* The above gliomas very rarely metastasise outside the nervous system.

# TUMOURS OF THE NERVOUS SYSTEM

### TUMOURS OF NEURONAL TYPE CELLS

Fully differentiated neurones can neither multiply nor give rise to neoplasms. Tumours of this type, derived from primitive nerve precursors (blast cells), are seen in infancy and childhood before completion of differentiation.

They display a basic histological pattern.

Closely aggregated small cells with hyperchromatic round or oval nuclei and scanty cytoplasm

Rosettes, the centres of which are formed by rudimentary nerve fibres, are often seen and represent a step towards differentiation

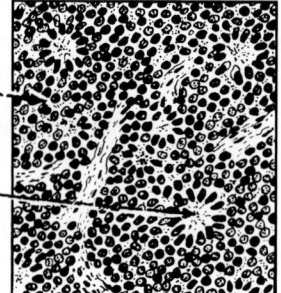

Depending on the site of origin, specific names are given:

**Cerebellum:**
    MEDULLOBLASTOMA

**Retina:** RETINOBLASTOMA

**Sympathetic ganglia (including adrenal medulla):**
    NEUROBLASTOMA and GANGLIONEUROMA

### Medulloblastoma

This highly malignant tumour arises in and spreads over the surface of the cerebellum, often invading the IVth ventricle. Diffuse tumour nodules may develop on surfaces bathed by CSF.

### Retinoblastoma

These tumours arise from the retina in children under 3 years. Around 40% of cases are inherited and the tumour may be bilateral. The remaining cases arise sporadically and are usually unilateral. The genetic mechanism involves inactivation of the retinoblastoma gene (RB gene), a tumour suppressor gene situated on the short arm of chromosome 13 (13q14). Untreated the tumour may fill the eye and spread locally into the brain via the optic nerve or systemically after invasion of the choroid. Modern therapy is curative in around 90% of cases. Some inherited cases also develop pinealoblastoma (so-called 'trilateral retinoblastoma').

### Neuroblastoma

These tumours arise from the precursor cells of the autonomic system; the majority occur in the adrenal medulla. They grow rapidly to become large, soft, haemorrhagic and necrotic retroperitoneal masses soon metastasising to lymph nodes, liver and bones.

### Ganglioneuroma

In some cases, neuronal differentiation proceeds, and mature ganglion cells appear and nerve fibres are formed. In some instances, differentiation is complete; such tumours are found in adult life particularly in the mediastinum where they may grow slowly, eventually causing signs due to their size, but never metastasising. With intermediate degrees of differentiation the name ganglioneuroblastoma is used.

# TUMOURS OF THE NERVOUS SYSTEM

## Meningiomas

These are thought to arise from arachnoid granulations and so are found most commonly adjacent to venous sinuses. They account for 15–20% of intracranial tumours. They are slow growing and essentially 'benign'. A few more aggressive tumours may metastasise.

A smooth firm lobulated tumour arising from a broad base adjacent to the sagittal sinus

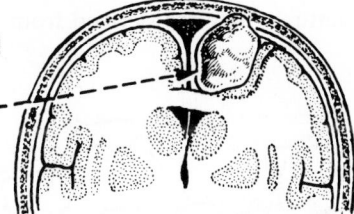

The effects are due to local compression of nervous tissues.

The skull may be eroded.

Growth to large size is usually slow so that the compensating mechanisms prevent increased intracranial pressure. Occasional meningiomas arise in the spine.

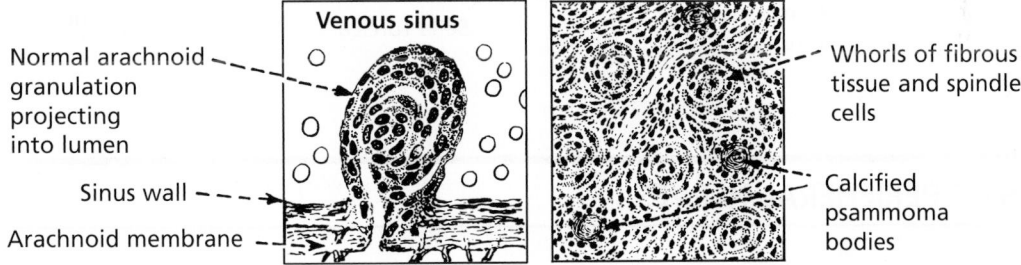

Normal arachnoid granulation projecting into lumen

Sinus wall

Arachnoid membrane

**Venous sinus**

Whorls of fibrous tissue and spindle cells

Calcified psammoma bodies

The histological appearances are variable depending on the relative amounts of cells and collagen, and they mimic in varying degree the arachnoid granulations. Concentric calcified structures (psammoma bodies) are often seen.

## Other mesodermal tumours

True vascular neoplasms are rare, but vascular HAMARTOMAS are fairly common and are a cause of intracranial haemorrhage and epilepsy. These lesions show great variation in site, size and complexity.

Primary microglial and lymphoid tumours are rare; the latter may be intrinsic to the CNS or be metastatic from a primary tumour outside the CNS. Primary cerebral lymphomas are commonly associated with Epstein–Barr virus and are an important complication of AIDS.

The incidence of CNS lymphomas is apparently increasing. This may be due to better diagnosis and/or to the more common use of therapeutic immunosuppression.

# TUMOURS OF THE NERVOUS SYSTEM

### Craniopharyngioma

This is a benign epithelial tumour arising in suprasellar areas. Similar benign cysts also occur.

### Germ cell tumours

These occasionally arise in midline structures: they are derived from embryologically misplaced germ cells.

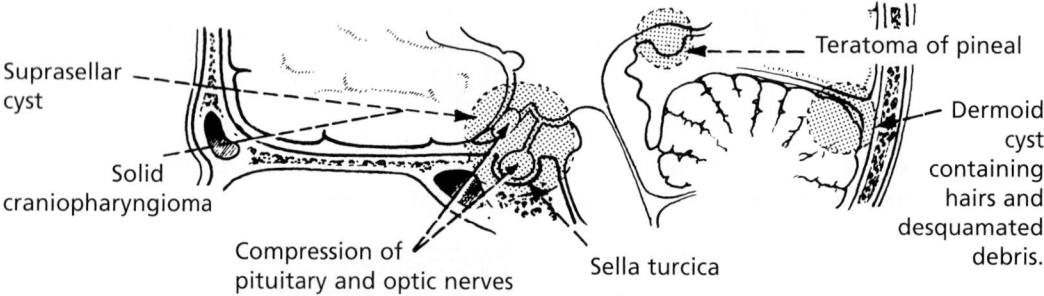

Suprasellar cyst

Solid craniopharyngioma

Compression of pituitary and optic nerves

Sella turcica

Teratoma of pineal

Dermoid cyst containing hairs and desquamated debris.

# TUMOURS OF PERIPHERAL NERVES

These tumours arise in nerve roots within the skull and spine, or in the peripheral nerves. Nomenclature is based on the tissue of origin.

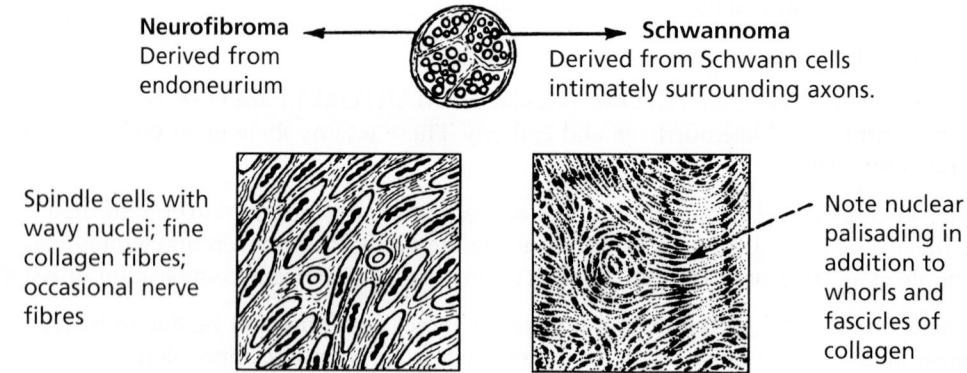

Neurofibroma
Derived from endoneurium

Schwannoma
Derived from Schwann cells intimately surrounding axons.

Spindle cells with wavy nuclei; fine collagen fibres; occasional nerve fibres

Note nuclear palisading in addition to whorls and fascicles of collagen

*Note*: Since neurones do not give rise to these neoplasms, the term neuroma is not used. Traumatic neuroma indicates proliferating nerve endings following injury and is not a true neoplasm (see p. 68).

Nerve sheath tumours may be single or multiple; their effects are due to compression of adjacent neural tissue and are seen best within the skull or spinal cord.

# TUMOURS OF THE NERVOUS SYSTEM

## SCHWANNOMA

**Acoustic Neuroma** is a good example. This tumour arises from the VIIIth nerve in the cerebellopontine angle. Although this tumour is benign, it grows around adjacent structures and has an irregular surface so that it may be difficult to remove.

The tumour exerts its effects by compression – distortion of the VIIIth nerve (tinnitus → deafness) and adjacent nerves. Pressure on IVth ventricle → hydrocephalus → increased intracranial pressure.

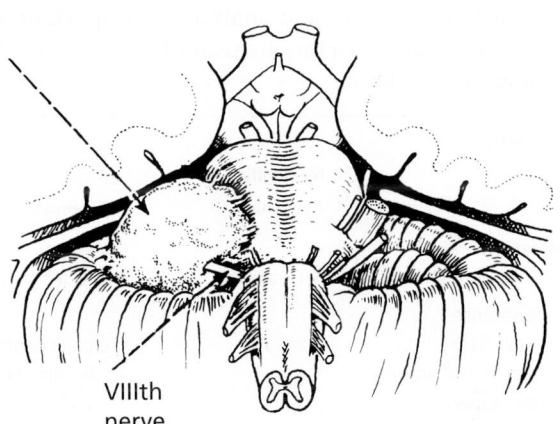

VIIIth nerve

These tumours are rarely multiple as part of neurofibromatosis Type 2 (associated with NF2 gene on chromosome 22).

### Neurofibromas

These may be solitary or, in neurofibromatosis, multiple and affect peripheral nerves over a wide area or occupy a single group of nerves. They form either rounded nodules or fusiform swellings and may be cosmetically disfiguring.

**Multiple neurofibromas** occur in neurofibromatosis Type 1. This is an autosomal dominant condition caused by a mutation in the NF-1 gene on chromosome 17. Plexiform neurofibroma, which involves a group of nerves forming complex thickening, is considered pathognomonic of neurofibromatosis Type 1.

Unlike schwannomas, a small but significant proportion of neurofibromas undergo transformation to malignant peripheral nerve sheath tumours. The risk is highest when associated with NF-1.

# CEREBROSPINAL FLUID

Although the CSF and extracellular fluid of the CNS are essentially similar in composition, changes in the CSF are not reliable indicators of disease within the brain parenchyma.

However, since the CSF reflects conditions in the subarachnoid space, in clinical practice detailed examination and analysis are important and are mandatory in suspected meningitis. The important observations using CSF obtained by lumbar puncture are grouped under headings as follows.

| NORMAL | IN DISEASE | | | |
|---|---|---|---|---|
| | Meningitis | | Virus Infection | |
| | Pyogenic | Tuberculous | Meningoencephalitis | Miscellaneous |
| **Pressure**<br>60–180 mm H$_2$O | ↑ Over 200 | ↑ Over 200 | ↑ High | ↓ Below spinal block |
| **Appearance**<br>Crystal clear<br>*(for blood staining see below) | Turbid | Opalescent: may be fine fibrin web | Opalescent | - |
| **Cell Content**<br>0–4 mononuclears/μL | +++<br>>1000 Neutrophils | +++<br>Lymphocytes | ±+<br>Lymphocytes | - |
| **Biochemistry**<br>Protein 0.2–0.4 g/L | ↑ 1–10 g/L | ↑ 1–3 g/L | ↑ 0.5–2 g/L | Very high in spinal block |
| Glucose<br>50–80 mg/100 mL<br>(2.8–4.4 mmol/L) | greatly↓ or absent | Low 20–30 mg | Normal | Normal |

*When the CSF is blood-stained, it is important to distinguish between contamination due to trauma caused by the tap and true intracranial haemorrhage.

| | CONTAMINATION | TRUE HAEMORRHAGE |
|---|---|---|
| **Supernatant after centrifugation** | Clear | Yellow due to bilirubin (red cell degeneration) |
| **Cell count – leucocyte:RBC ratio** | Normal | Increased |

**Microbiology.** Identification of organisms is very important.

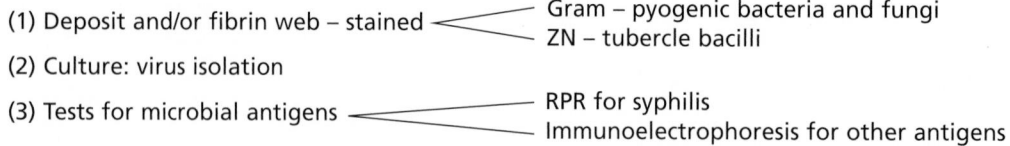

(1) Deposit and/or fibrin web – stained ——— Gram – pyogenic bacteria and fungi
ZN – tubercle bacilli

(2) Culture: virus isolation

(3) Tests for microbial antigens ——— RPR for syphilis
Immunoelectrophoresis for other antigens

# THE EYE

## CATARACT

The normal lens consists of soluble crystalline proteins encased within elongated lens fibre cells surrounded by an elastic lens capsule. There is also a layer of lens epithelium beneath the anterior capsule. The metabolism of the lens depends on diffusion of nutrients from the aqueous. In cataract the lens is opaque either because of disorganisation of the fibre membranes at a microscopic level or of the lens proteins at a molecular level. Cataract is one of the most common and treatable causes of blindness worldwide.

### Aetiology of cataracts

**Developmental**: due to congenital malformation or toxic damage to lens fibres, e.g. Rubella.

**Trauma**: in blunt trauma, resulting shock waves may rupture lens fibres. In penetrating trauma, rupture of the lens capsule leads to fibre disruption and alterations in fluid content.

**Inflammation**: inflammatory mediators alter the constituents of the aqueous.

**Metabolic disease**: hypocalcaemia and diabetes alter the constituents of the aqueous.

**Senile**: due to degradation of lens proteins in the oldest central part of the lens.

## GLAUCOMA

This is a common cause of blindness in the Western world. Glaucoma occurs when intraocular pressure (IOP) rises to an extent which causes damage to tissues within the eye.

### Normal

IOP is maintained by a balance between aqueous production by the ciliary body and outflow via the trabecular meshwork (TM) and canal of Schlemm.

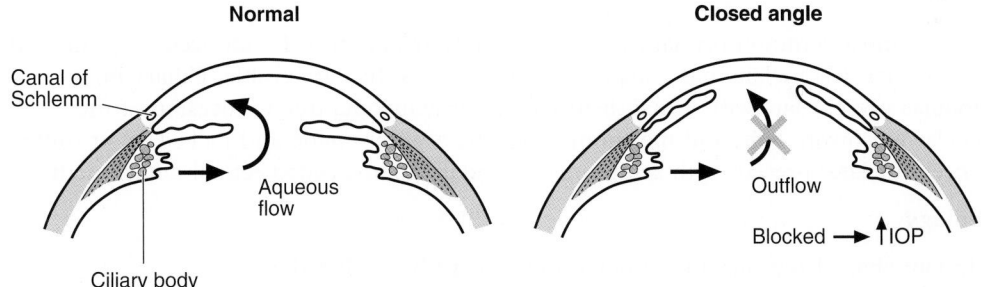

### Types

### *Open Angle*

(a) Primary – acquired disease due to increased resistance in the TM.
(b) Secondary – due to blockage of the TM by tumour cells, leaked lens protein, etc.

# THE EYE

### *Closed Angle*

(a) Primary – the iris root becomes opposed to the TM. This is in part due to anatomical variations in the anterior segment. It is, for example, more common in East Asian and Inuit groups with a shallower anterior chamber.

(b) Secondary – due to intraocular neovascularisation, e.g. diabetes, ocular ischaemia.

**Congenital** – due to malformation of the TM.

### *Effects of Increased IOP*

Corneal oedema
Iris ischaemia
Ciliary body atrophy
Cataract
Retinal atrophy
Cupping of optic disc
Enlargement of the eye in children
    (buphthalmos = ox eye)

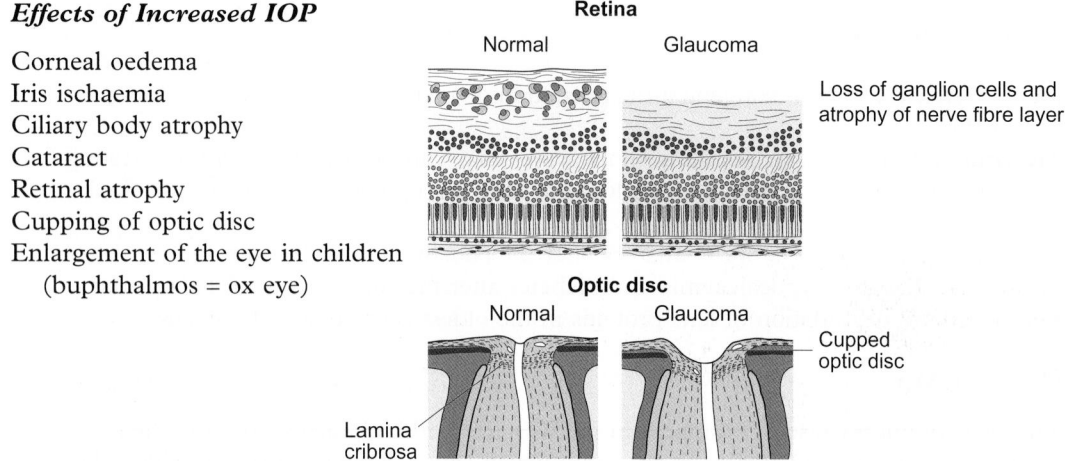

## TUMOURS

Retinoblastoma is the most common primary intraocular tumour of childhood. This is discussed on page 622.

### Melanoma

This is the most common primary intraocular tumour in adults. It can occur anywhere in the uveal tract. Iris melanomas usually present early, as they are visible. Ciliary body melanomas present late with visual disturbances or glaucoma due to invasion of the trabecular meshwork. Choroid melanomas may be asymptomatic and picked up at routine eye checks or later present with symptoms secondary to associated retinal detachment.

### Pathology

Mushroom-shaped tumour due to horizontal spread beneath retina.
Spindle cells (better prognosis).
Epithelioid cells (poorer prognosis).
The majority of tumours are mixed cell type.
Cytogenetics-loss of one copy of chromosome 3 (monosomy 3) carries a poor prognosis.

# THE EYE

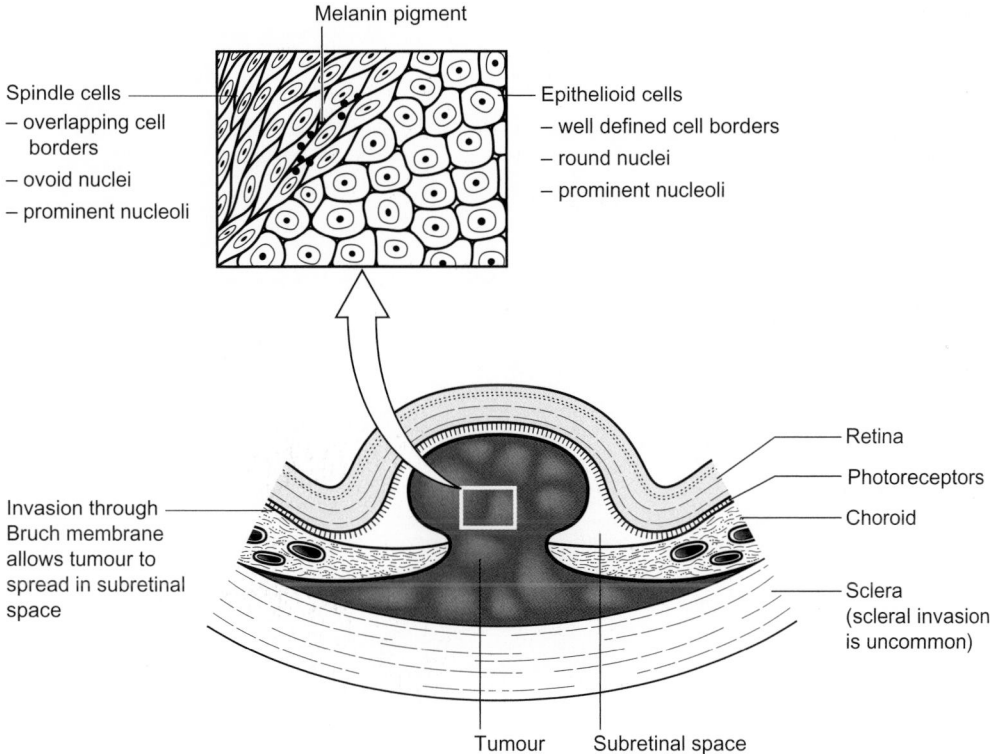

## Secondary tumours

Metastasis is the commonest type of intraocular malignancy. These usually occur in the choroid and the most common primary sites are breast and lung.

# MUSCULO-SKELETAL SYSTEM

## OBJECTIVES

1. To understand the basic structure and function of both bone and synovial joints.
2. To have a knowledge of the pathology of osteoporosis and the other main metabolic bone diseases.
3. To have a knowledge of the main tumour types affecting the musculoskeletal system.
4. To understand the pathology underpinning the major joint disorders.
5. To have a basic knowledge of skeletal muscle structure and function and how disorders of muscle are investigated.
6. To understand the pathogenesis of the muscular dystrophies.

# BONE

There are two different forms of normal adult bone, both with a lamellar (layered) structure.

### 1. COMPACT BONE

Seen in long bone shafts and forms the dense outer shell (cortex). – – – – – –→

The basic units of compact bone are Haversian systems (osteons) arranged in vertical columns.

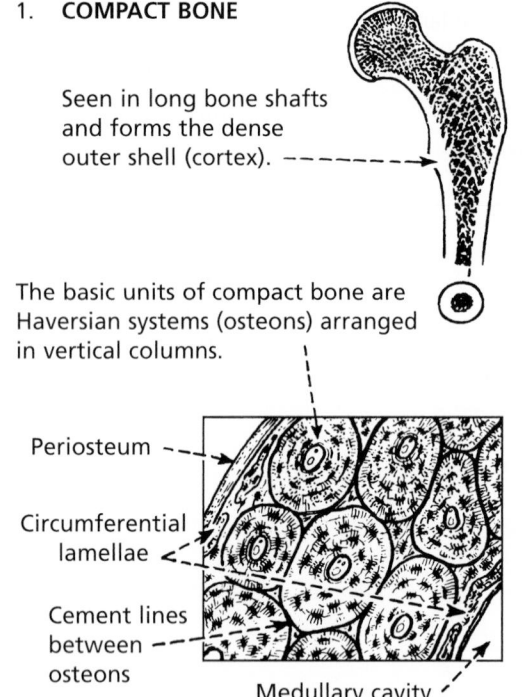

Periosteum – –

Circumferential lamellae <

Cement lines between – – osteons

Medullary cavity

### 2. CANCELLOUS BONE

Found within medullary cavities along with bone marrow. The major form in vertebral and in flat bones such as the pelvis.

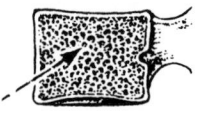

Haemopoietic marrow

The basic unit of cancellous bone is the trabecula, arranged along lines of stress.

*Note:* Cancellous bone comprises 20% of bone mass but 80% of bone turnover due to its large surface area.

# BONE

**WOVEN BONE** (non-lamellar) is a primitive form laid down in foetal development. In adult life, this type is seen in bone repair and bone-forming tumours. It can be remodelled to be replaced by lamellar bone.

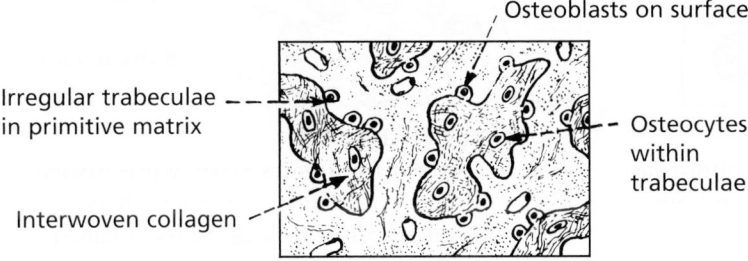

Osteoblasts on surface

Irregular trabeculae in primitive matrix

Interwoven collagen

Osteocytes within trabeculae

## Bone and calcium

Bone acts as a reservoir for calcium, which is maintained within a narrow range (2.1–2.6 mmol/L). Hypocalcaemia stimulates the parathyroid glands to produce parathyroid hormone (PTH) which promotes bone resorption, calcium absorption from the gut and reabsorption of calcium from the kidney. As the serum calcium rises, PTH production is switched off.

# BONE TURNOVER

Bone is a dynamic tissue. It is formed by osteoblasts and removed by osteoclasts.

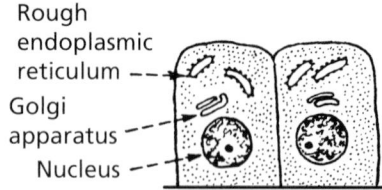

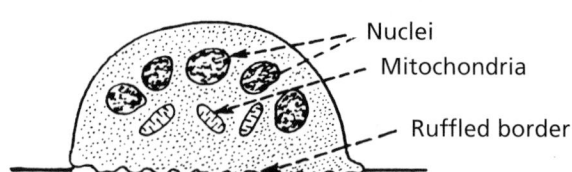

## OSTEOBLASTS

- Derived from osteoprogenitor cells.
- Produce Type I collagen and other proteins.
- Secrete alkaline phosphatase – a marker of bone formation.
- Stimulated by mechanical stress, androgens, cytokines, e.g. TGF-β.

## OSTEOCLASTS

- Derived from bone marrow precursors.
- Produce acid and enzymes such as Cathepsin K which degrades collagen.
- Stimulated by cytokines e.g. IL-1, IL-6 (indirectly by PTH).
- Inhibited by oestrogens.

The activities of the two cell types are closely 'coupled' in the normal process of bone turnover. In the adult, 10% of the skeleton is replaced annually. The process has *activating* and *inhibitory* arms.

## ACTIVATION

Osteoblasts bear RANKL (**R**eceptor **A**ctivator of **N**F-κB **L**igand).

Binds to RANK

Proliferation and differentiation into osteoclasts

## INHIBITION

Under other circumstances osteoblasts and other cells produce osteoprotegerin (OPG), a soluble molecule which blocks activation through RANK.

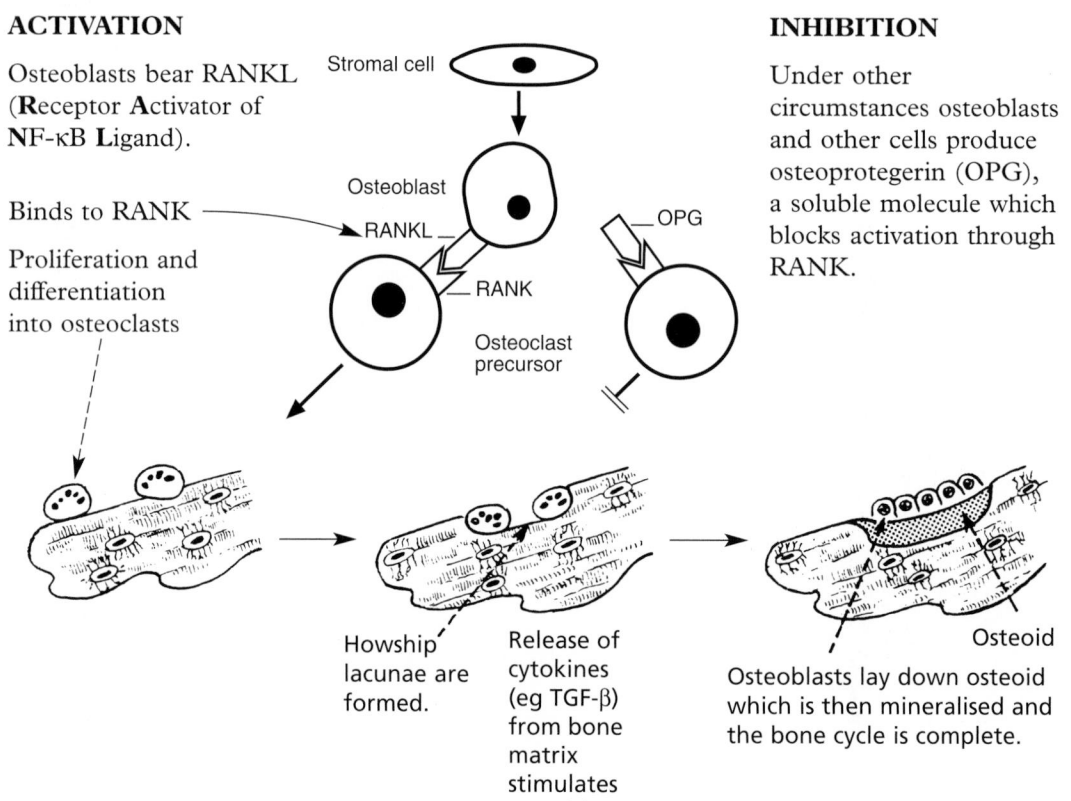

Howship lacunae are formed.

Release of cytokines (eg TGF-β) from bone matrix stimulates osteoblasts.

Osteoid

Osteoblasts lay down osteoid which is then mineralised and the bone cycle is complete.

# METABOLIC BONE DISEASE

## 1. OSTEOPOROSIS

**OSTEOPOROSIS** is the commonest disorder of bone. It is defined as a systemic disease characterised by:

(1) low bone mass;
(2) Microarchitectural deterioration of bone; with
(3) an increase in bone fragility and susceptibility to fracture.

A patient is said to have osteoporosis if BONE MINERAL DENSITY is >2.5 standard deviations below the mean of normal young subjects.

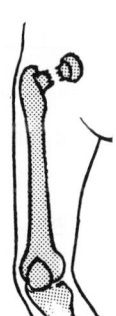

**Clinical features** – osteoporosis becomes more common with increasing age and is more common in women, especially after the menopause.

1. It causes bone fractures (collapse) of vertebral bodies with loss of height and kyphosis.
2. Fracture of the femoral neck or other long bones (especially Colles' fracture of distal radius).

*Note*: In osteoporosis, routine serum biochemical tests – particularly the calcium levels – are within the normal range.

### Pathology

The changes in the vertebral bodies are shown.

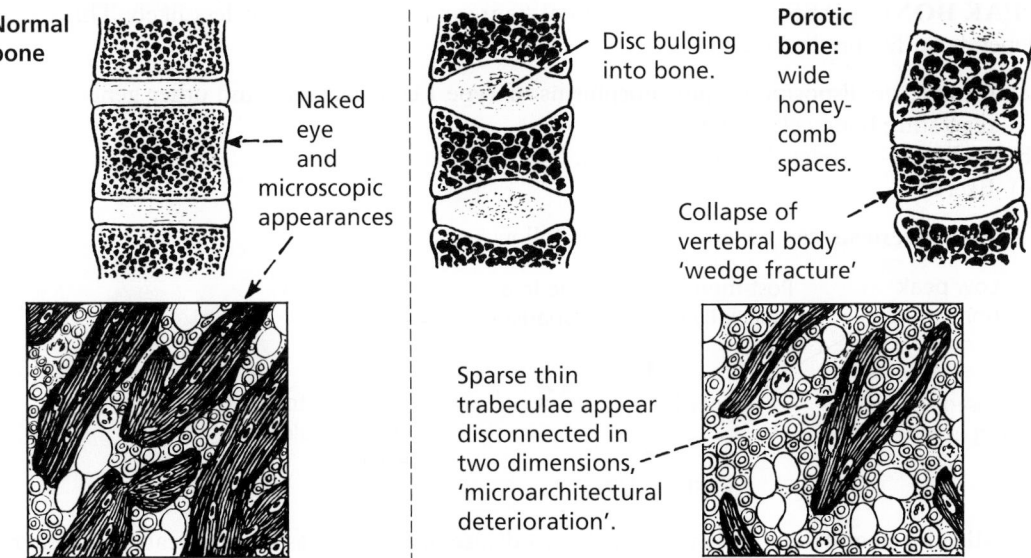

Normal bone

Naked eye and microscopic appearances

Disc bulging into bone.

Porotic bone: wide honey-comb spaces.

Collapse of vertebral body 'wedge fracture'

Sparse thin trabeculae appear disconnected in two dimensions, 'microarchitectural deterioration'.

*Note*: The bone has a normal calcium content.

# METABOLIC BONE DISEASE

### Pathogenesis

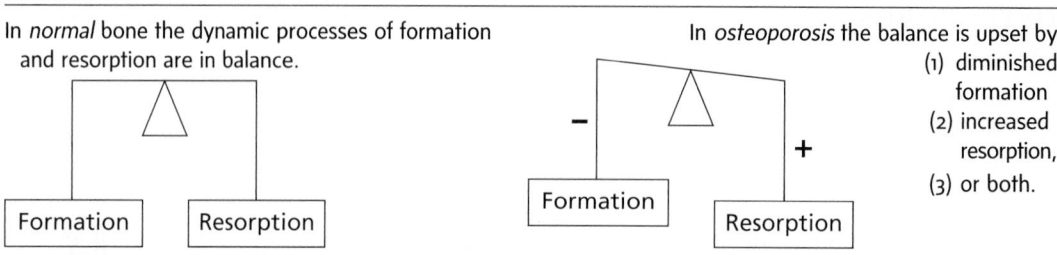

In *normal* bone the dynamic processes of formation and resorption are in balance.

Formation | Resorption

In *osteoporosis* the balance is upset by
(1) diminished formation
(2) increased resorption,
(3) or both.

Formation — Resorption +

Bone mass decreases with age in both sexes as osteoblastic activity falls.

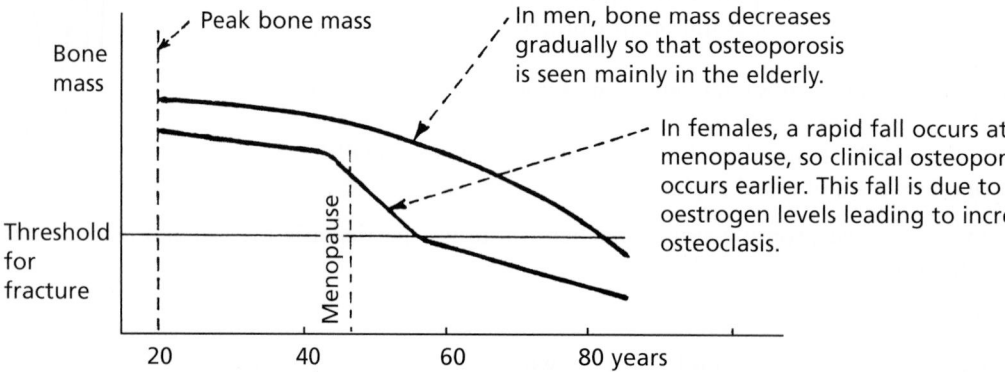

Peak bone mass

In men, bone mass decreases gradually so that osteoporosis is seen mainly in the elderly.

In females, a rapid fall occurs at menopause, so clinical osteopor occurs earlier. This fall is due to oestrogen levels leading to incre osteoclasis.

Bone mass

Threshold for fracture

Menopause

20    40    60    80 years

**PEAK BONE MASS** is key – a high initial figure makes osteoporosis less likely. This depends on factors including:

(a) Genetic predisposition – polymorphisms of Type I collagen gene and other genes regulating bone cell activity.
(b) Nutrition – especially calcium intake.
(c) Exercise.

The **pathogenesis** can be summarised as follows:

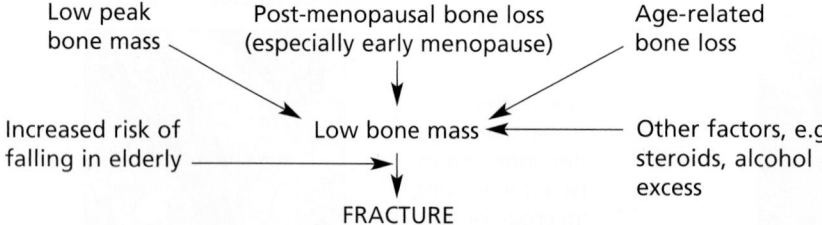

Low peak bone mass

Post-menopausal bone loss (especially early menopause)

Age-related bone loss

Increased risk of falling in elderly

Low bone mass

Other factors, e.g steroids, alcohol excess

FRACTURE

**Localised osteoporosis** is commonly due to disuse and is seen as a complication of other disorders, e.g. local IMMOBILISATION following fracture; limb paralysis; adjacent to severe joint disease with limitation of movement.

# METABOLIC BONE DISEASE

## 2. OSTEOMALACIA AND RICKETS

Osteomalacia and rickets are disorders of bone due to failure of mineralisation of newly formed osteoid, caused almost always by deficiency of vitamin D. The poorly calcified bones are soft, causing deformity or fracture.

**Osteomalacia** occurs in adult life and affects the osteoid which is being continually laid down in the normal remodelling of bone.

**Rickets** affects the growing child. As well as deformity and fractures, there is disturbance of growth plates. X-ray may show linear partial fractures of long bones which have failed to calcify (Looser zones).

### Causes of vitamin D deficiency:

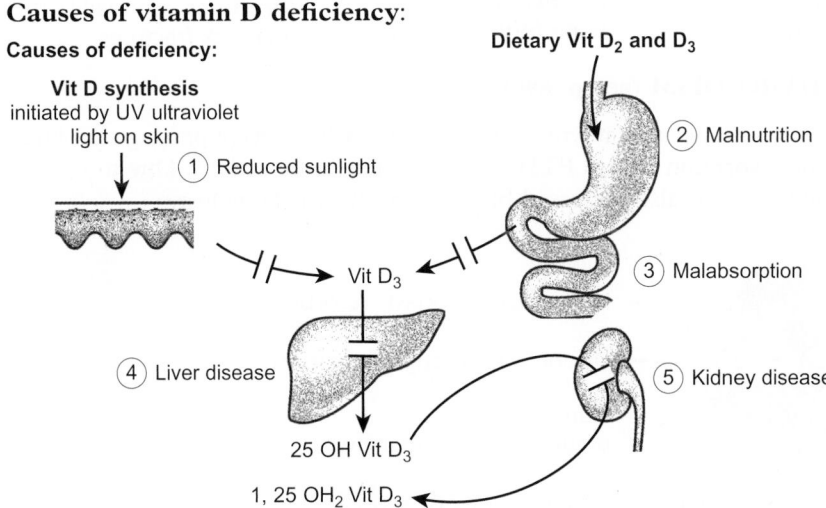

**Causes of deficiency:**

**Dietary Vit $D_2$ and $D_3$**

**Vit D synthesis** initiated by UV ultraviolet light on skin

(1) Reduced sunlight

(2) Malnutrition

Vit $D_3$

(3) Malabsorption

(4) Liver disease

(5) Kidney disease

25 OH Vit $D_3$

1, 25 $OH_2$ Vit $D_3$

### Pathology

The low levels of vitamin D result in reduced absorption of calcium from the gut, with resultant hypocalcaemia. There is also reduced phosphate absorption. This causes failure of bone calcification/mineralisation.

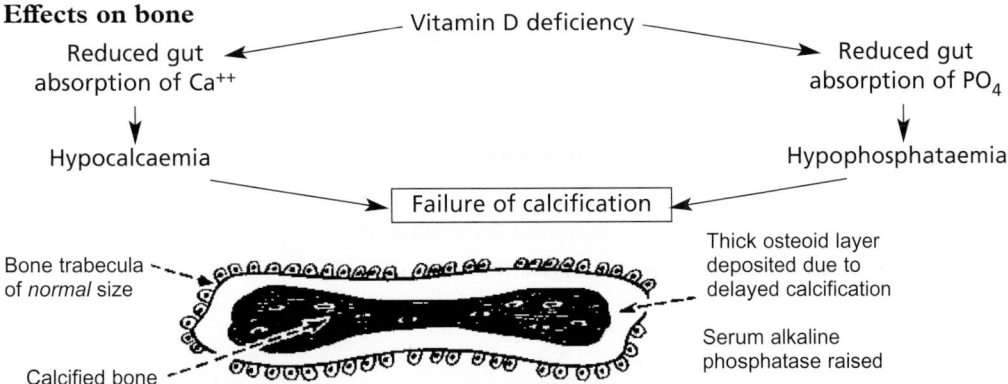

**Effects on bone**

Vitamin D deficiency

Reduced gut absorption of $Ca^{++}$

Reduced gut absorption of $PO_4$

Hypocalcaemia

Hypophosphataemia

Failure of calcification

Bone trabecula of *normal* size

Thick osteoid layer deposited due to delayed calcification

Serum alkaline phosphatase raised

Calcified bone

*Note*: The hypocalcaemia seen in osteomalacia stimulates an increase in PTH levels and mild hyperparathyroidism.

# METABOLIC BONE DISEASE

In **rickets** the growing ends of long bones are abnormal.

**Normal**  **Rickets**

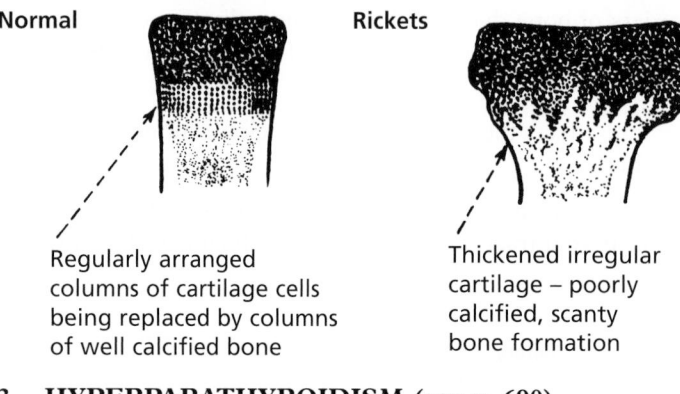

Regularly arranged columns of cartilage cells being replaced by columns of well calcified bone

Thickened irregular cartilage – poorly calcified, scanty bone formation

This results in stunting of growth and bowing of the lower limbs as well as muscle weakness.
In females, permanent deformities of the pelvis can cause serious difficulty during childbirth.
There is an increased risk of fractures, especially greenstick fractures.

## 3. HYPERPARATHYROIDISM (see p. 690)

Bone changes may be seen in hyperparathyroidism, especially when severe or long standing. There is increased bone resorption due to PTH-induced osteoclastic activity. Due to 'coupling', osteoblastic activity is also increased but the net effect is bone loss.

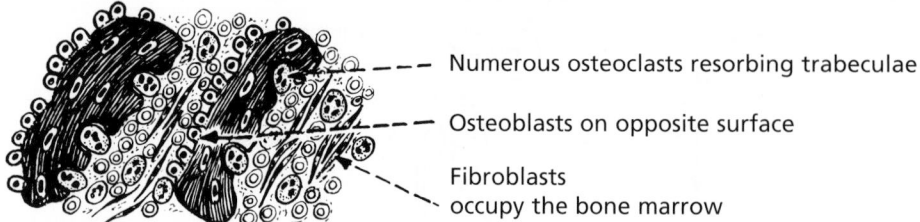

Numerous osteoclasts resorbing trabeculae

Osteoblasts on opposite surface

Fibroblasts occupy the bone marrow

These changes affect all bones. There may be marked loss of bone with numerous osteoclasts and haemosiderin pigment – the so-called 'brown tumour of hyperparathyroidism', which can mimic giant cell tumour.

## 4. RENAL OSTEODYSTROPHY

Bone disease is common in chronic renal failure. It is a combination of osteomalacia and hyperparathyroidism, together with loss of bone synthesis.

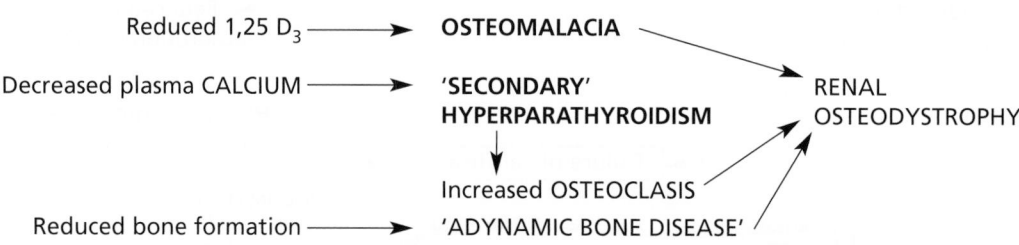

Reduced 1,25 $D_3$ ⟶ **OSTEOMALACIA**

Decreased plasma CALCIUM ⟶ **'SECONDARY' HYPERPARATHYROIDISM** ⟶ RENAL OSTEODYSTROPHY

Increased OSTEOCLASIS

Reduced bone formation ⟶ 'ADYNAMIC BONE DISEASE'

# METABOLIC BONE DISEASE

## 5. PAGET'S DISEASE OF BONE

This disease of unknown aetiology usually presents after the age of 50 years and is more common in males. It is fairly common (3% of autopsies), but only in its more severe form are there clinical symptoms. The disorder is focal: the bones particularly affected are the pelvis, vertebrae, skull and lower limbs. It has been suggested that viral infection (e.g. paramyxovirus, distemper) of osteoclasts is responsible. Genetic factors are also important.

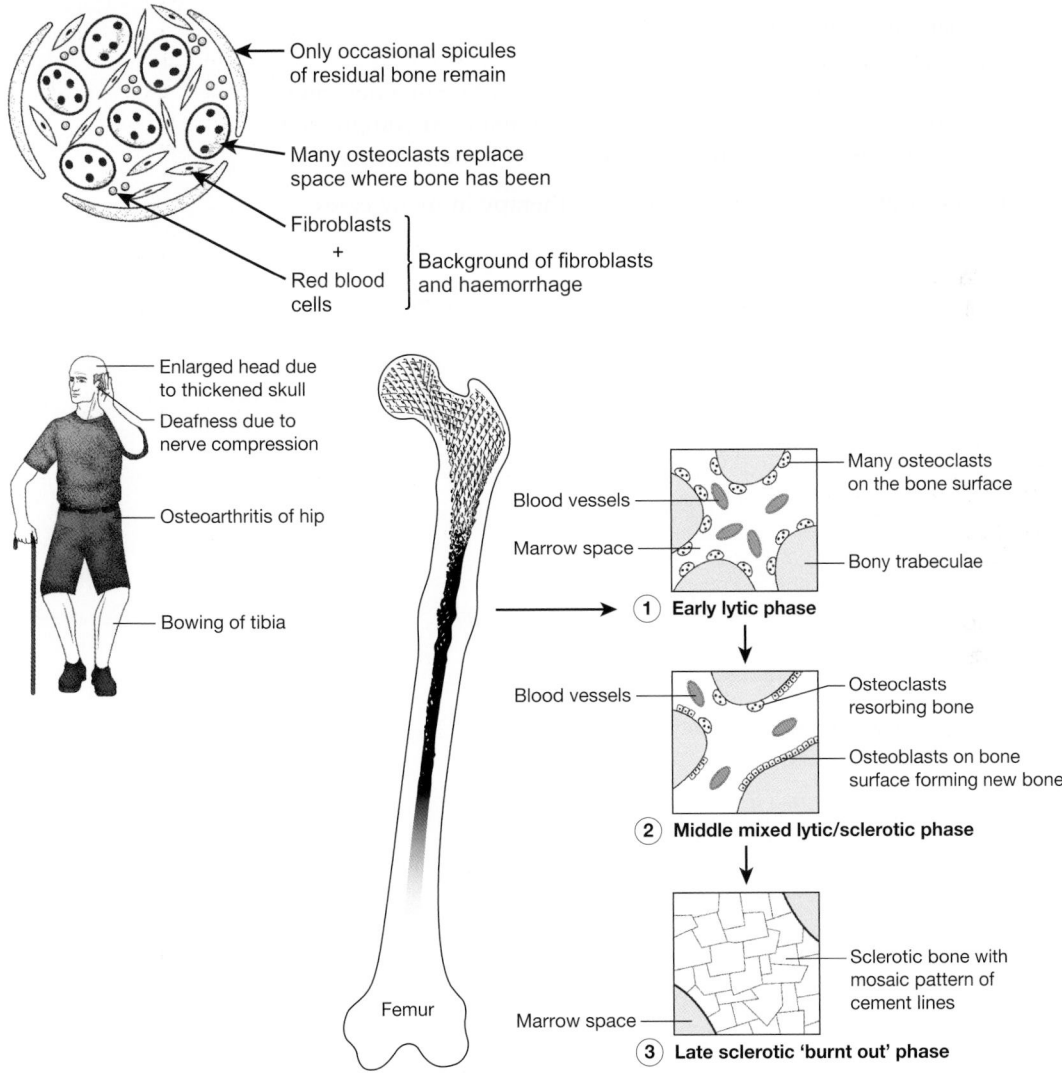

Only occasional spicules of residual bone remain

Many osteoclasts replace space where bone has been

Fibroblasts
+
Red blood cells
} Background of fibroblasts and haemorrhage

Enlarged head due to thickened skull

Deafness due to nerve compression

Osteoarthritis of hip

Bowing of tibia

Femur

Blood vessels

Marrow space

Many osteoclasts on the bone surface

Bony trabeculae

① **Early lytic phase**

Blood vessels

Osteoclasts resorbing bone

Osteoblasts on bone surface forming new bone

② **Middle mixed lytic/sclerotic phase**

Marrow space

Sclerotic bone with mosaic pattern of cement lines

③ **Late sclerotic 'burnt out' phase**

# METABOLIC BONE DISEASE

To begin with, there is a localised increase in **osteoclastic** activity causing bone resorption. This is followed by marked **osteoblastic** activity. There follows cycles of chaotic bone resorption and formation, so that irregular bone trabeculae with mosaic cement lines are formed. The bone is thickened and its structure is defective and weak. Biochemical changes reflect the cellular activity, i.e. *alkaline phosphatase* ↑(osteoblastic); *urinary hydroxyproline* ↑(collagen destruction).

Whilst it may be asymptomatic, the main clinical effects are:

- Bone pain and deformity.
- Pathological fracture.
- Osteoarthritis (due to abnormal stresses caused by bone deformity).
- Nerve compression leading to deafness or spinal cord compression.
- An increased risk (×30) of the development of bone sarcoma.

The use of bisphosphonates offers effective therapy in many cases.

# BONE – MISCELLANEOUS

## OSTEONECROSIS (AVASCULAR NECROSIS)

Interruption of its blood supply causes bone to undergo necrosis. This tends to occur with fractures at sites where the vascular supply is damaged. Fractures of the femoral neck and scaphoid bone are good examples.

Non-traumatic causes include corticosteroid therapy, alcoholism, sickle cell anaemia, Gaucher disease and, historically, in decompression in those working in increased atmospheric pressure (caisson disease).

Bone necrosis occurring at an articular surface often leads to degenerative arthritis.

**Fracture of femoral neck**      **Scaphoid**      **Humerus in tunnel worker**

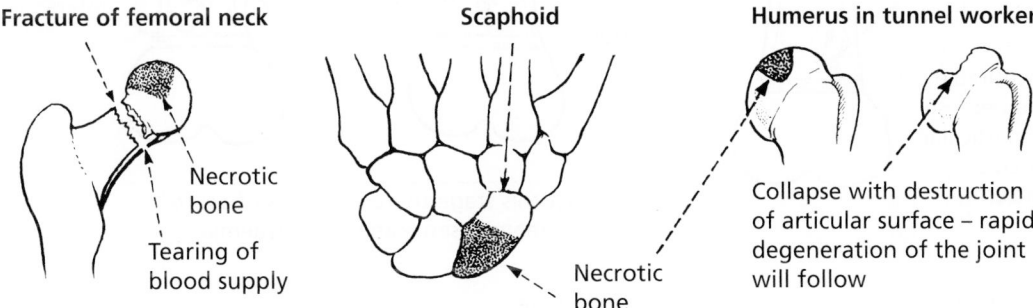

Necrotic bone

Tearing of blood supply

Necrotic bone

Collapse with destruction of articular surface – rapid degeneration of the joint will follow

*Note:* These areas of necrotic bone may appear radiodense due to disuse osteoporosis of the adjacent living bone.

In children and adolescents osteonecrosis occurs at several epiphyseal sites. The commonest is Perthes disease, in which necrosis of one or both femoral heads occurs in children aged 4–10 years (male:female = 5:1).

## FIBROUS DYSPLASIA OF BONE

This disorder may affect one (monostotic) or several (polyostotic) bones. On histology, well demarcated fibrous tissue containing small abnormal woven bone trabeculae is seen. Somatic mutations of the *GNAS1* gene, which encodes the α subunit of a stimulatory G-protein, are responsible. Whether the disease is polyostotic or monostotic depends on the stage of development of the embryo when the mutation occurs, a state known as mosaicism.

### Complications

Fracture or deformity of the weakened bone.

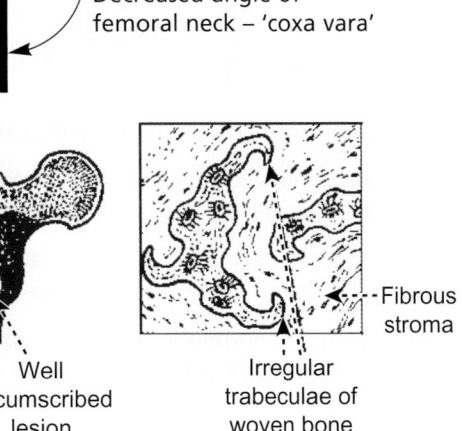

Decreased angle of femoral neck – 'coxa vara'

Well circumscribed lesion

Irregular trabeculae of woven bone

Fibrous stroma

# INFECTIONS OF BONE

### ACUTE OSTEOMYELITIS

This is classically caused by *Staphylococcus aureus* and affects the metaphyses of long bones in children. The incidence has been greatly reduced by the use of antibiotics which aborts the development of the disease. The bacteria are blood borne and settle in the cancellous bone of the metaphysis. The effects are dramatic and rapidly progressive.

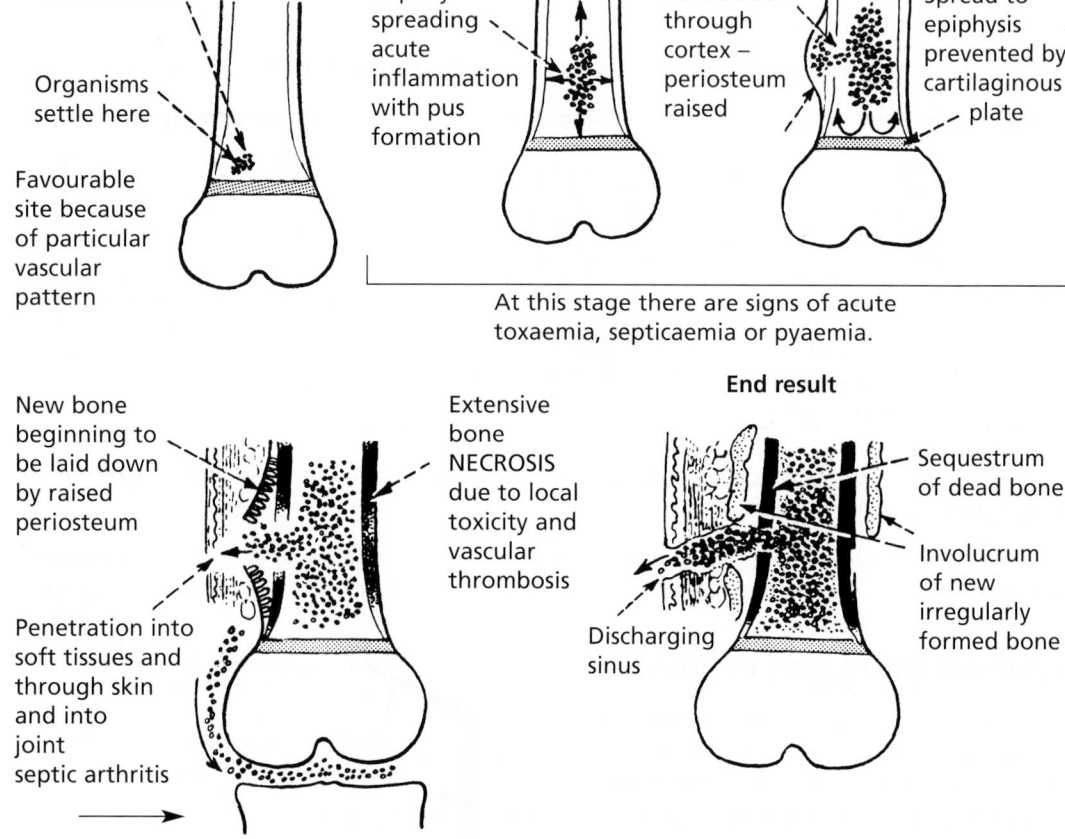

Bacteraemia

Organisms settle here

Favourable site because of particular vascular pattern

Rapidly spreading acute inflammation with pus formation

Penetration through cortex – periosteum raised

Spread to epiphysis prevented by cartilaginous plate

At this stage there are signs of acute toxaemia, septicaemia or pyaemia.

New bone beginning to be laid down by raised periosteum

Penetration into soft tissues and through skin and into joint septic arthritis

Extensive bone NECROSIS due to local toxicity and vascular thrombosis

**End result**

Discharging sinus

Sequestrum of dead bone

Involucrum of new irregularly formed bone

The presence of necrotic bone ensures that the inflammation continues.

The late complications are chronic osteomyelitis, disturbance of bone growth, **AMYLOID** disease may occur and occasionally squamous carcinoma arises in a sinus.

Other pyogenic bacteria can cause osteitis – the *Salmonella* group (esp. *Salmonella typhi*) and *Brucella*, the latter often causing a low-grade osteitis of the spine.

With inadequate antibiotic treatment, acute inflammatory processes may be converted into low-grade osteitis. Staphylococcal infection of the spine may present in adults in this way.

# INFECTIONS OF BONE

## TUBERCULOSIS

The incidence of bone and joint infection parallels that of the more common pulmonary infection. It is therefore low in developed countries but still significant elsewhere, and has risen in association with HIV infection.

The spine and growing ends of long bones, including the epiphyses, are affected by blood borne spread and the infection spreads to the adjacent joints.

Bone is destroyed and replaced by granulomatous inflammation with caseous necrosis. Spinal infection spreads into adjacent tissues and leads to 'cold abscess' formation.

Although the progress is much less rapid than in acute osteomyelitis, without adequate treatment serious damage to bones and joints occurs.

# DEVELOPMENTAL ABNORMALITIES

**Generalised abnormalities** are rare and usually inherited.

1. **ACHONDROPLASIA** is the commonest cause of dwarfism, with short, deformed limbs and a waddling gait. The bones at the skull base are underdeveloped.
   A mutation of the fibroblast growth factor receptor gene (*FGFR3*) is responsible, which causes constitutive activation and inhibits cartilage growth. Although inherited as an autosomal dominant trait, 80% of cases result from new mutations.

2. **OSTEOGENESIS IMPERFECTA** (brittle bone disease) is a congenital disorder characterised by thin brittle bones which fracture easily. It is important to distinguish this from 'non-accidental injury'. The basic defect is in the osteoblasts which fail to synthesise collagen properly, due to mutations affecting the Type I collagen genes on chromosomes 7 and 17. The severity of the disorder depends on the type of mutation, some cases being lethal in utero.

A long bone showing three fractures.

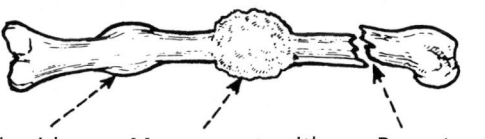

Old, with deformity    More recent, with exuberant callus    Recent, with displacement

Patients may have:
(a) Very thin sclerae which appear blue.
(b) Abnormal tooth development due to defective dentine formation.

# DEVELOPMENTAL ABNORMALITIES

3. **OSTEOPETROSIS** (marble bone disease of Albers-Schönberg) is a rare disorder in which there is impaired osteoclast function, in some cases due to deficiency of carbonic anhydrase. This results in failure of bone remodelling and abnormal conversion of cartilage to bone. The whole skeleton becomes dense and the bones thickened, but weakened.

*Complications* are: (a) Anaemia due to failure of development of the bone marrow cavity.
(b) Fractures.
(c) Cranial nerve compression.

Bone marrow transplantation provides functioning osteoclasts and reverses the skeletal abnormalities.

## CYSTS OF BONE

Simple bone cysts (unicameral/single chamber) have a thin fibrous lining and occur in the proximal humeral and femoral metaphyses of children. They often present with fracture.

Aneurysmal bone cysts (expanding blood-filled cysts in adolescents) are eccentric expanding blood-filled cysts presenting with swelling, pain or fracture.

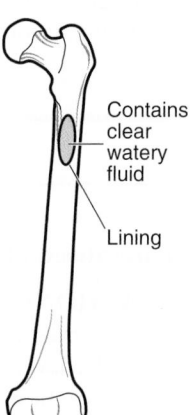

Contains clear watery fluid

Lining

# TUMOURS IN BONE

Primary bone tumours are rare. There are both benign and malignant forms, examples of which follow. In contrast, metastatic tumours and myeloma are common.

## OSTEOID OSTEOMA

This uncommon benign tumour has a striking clinical presentation and distinctive pathology.

**Clinical**: classically, an adolescent complains of well-localised, increasingly severe bone pain. Aspirin and non-steroidals give relief.

**Pathological**: the lesion is a small focus (nidus) of newly formed irregular trabeculae of osteoid or poorly calcified woven bone in a highly vascular stroma.

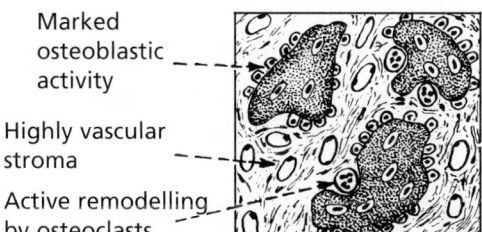

Marked osteoblastic activity

Highly vascular stroma

Active remodelling by osteoclasts

Radiologically a very small radiolucent nidus (<1.5 cm diameter) is surrounded by densely calcified bone

**Note:** Reaction in surrounding bone; sclerosis of adjacent cortex and periosteal bone thickening.

## GIANT CELL TUMOUR (OSTEOCLASTOMA)

This uncommon tumour presents in adult life (age 20–40 years), at the end of a long bone, especially adjacent to the knee. The tumour destroys bone and the cortex gradually expands, becoming egg-shell thin. Pathological fracture is common.

The histology is characteristic:

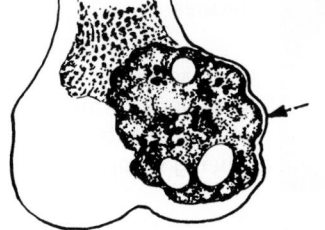

Lower end of femur showing expansion of cortex by partly cystic, partly solid haemorrhagic tumour

Numerous osteoclast-like giant cells and ovoid tumour cells in a vascular stroma

**Behaviour**: almost all giant cell tumours are benign. Most are cured by thorough removal: approximately 20% recur; well under 5% become malignant and metastasise to the lungs. If a tumour is irresectable it may be treated with the monoclonal antibody denosumab which targets RANKL protein, an essential component of osteoclast function. This is an example of biological therapy.

## EOSINOPHILIC GRANULOMA (at the benign end
of the spectrum of Langerhans histiocytosis) usually presents as single osteolytic radiolucent lesions of bone in children. Vertebral collapse and pathological fractures are sometimes seen.

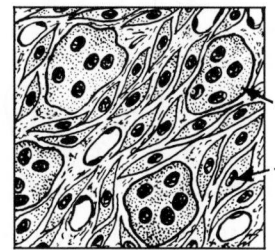

Eosinophils

Langerhans cells

Multinucleate giant cells

The prognosis is usually good.
The histological appearances are typical.

# TUMOURS IN BONE

### MALIGNANT TUMOURS

Primary malignant tumours of bone are not common, but they are important as many arise in young people and are highly malignant. Some arise in older people with pre-existing bone disorders, e.g. Paget's disease, previous irradiation.

### Osteosarcoma

This is a highly malignant bone-forming tumour. It affects two distinct age groups and there is a preponderance of males over females.

| YOUNG AGE GROUP – MAJORITY OF CASES (10–25 YEARS) | ELDERLY SUBJECTS (OVER 60 YEARS) |
|---|---|
| The tumour usually arises near the end of a limb long bone (particularly around the knee). | In 50% of this group, Paget's disease is associated. Long bones, vertebrae and the pelvis are often affected, and tumours may be multicentric in origin. |

The 'classic' tumour in an adolescent begins in the metaphysis of the medullary cavity. Most patients complain of bone pain, and when the tumour penetrates the cortex there may be a soft tissue swelling.

Tumour begins here: spread through cortex has occurred

Periosteum stripped from bone

Spicules of reactive bone forming

The clinical signs are pain and swelling of the lower thigh

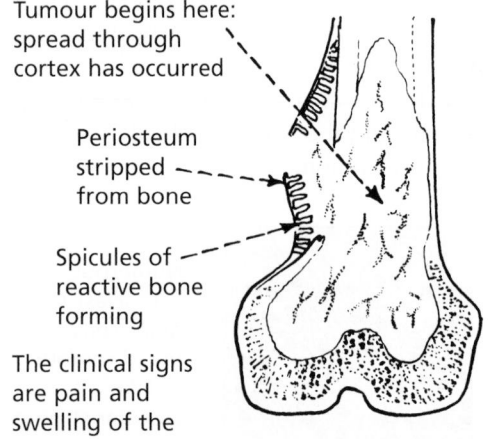

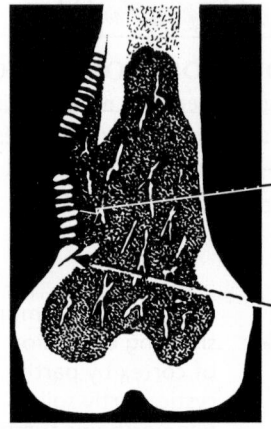

The radiological counterpart is a patchily radiolucent tumour

Sun-ray appearance due to new bone spicules

Codman triangle (new bone forming where periosteum is being stripped)

*Note:* At this stage lung metastases may be present.

Histologically, varying amounts of osteoid, woven bone and sometimes islands of primitive cartilage are seen. The tumour cells are pleomorphic and mitotically active. With modern chemotherapy 60–70% of patients survive for 5 years.

# TUMOURS IN BONE

## Chondrosarcoma

This is a malignant cartilage-forming tumour. It shows a much slower growth pattern and affects the age group 40–70 years. It can arise de novo or on a background of pre-existing multiple enchondromatosis in a small number of cases. The tumours arise particularly in the limb girdles and proximal long bones and consist of lobules of cartilage. Progressive local extension is usual. Metastases, usually to the lung, are rare.

## Ewing sarcoma

This rare malignant tumour affects the young (age 5–20 years) and arises in long bones, pelvis, ribs and scapulae. It is very aggressive, metastasising early to lungs and other bones.

The tumour cells are small and uniform. Fever and an elevated white count are common and may mimic osteomyelitis. The histological appearances may mimic lymphoma.

Sheets of uniform darkly staining tumour cells. The cells have very little cytoplasm. ⟶

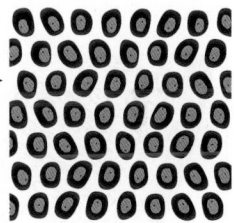

Ewing sarcoma is a primitive neuro-ectodermal tumour associated with translocation and fusion of genes, typically the *EWSR1* and *FLI1* genes, on chromosomes 11 and 22. With chemotherapy, survival is similar to that of osteosarcoma.

## Lymphoid tumours

Lymphoma and myeloma (see p. 470) may arise in bone, causing bone destruction.

## SECONDARY TUMOURS IN BONE

THIS IS BY FAR THE MOST COMMON TYPE OF TUMOUR IN BONE.

Tumours which show a predilection for spread to bone are carcinoma of the PROSTATE, BREAST, LUNG, KIDNEY and THYROID. Metastases are usually multiple. The incidence of bone secondaries ESPECIALLY IN THE SPINE is very high when these tumours become widespread. Occasionally latent renal and thyroid cancers present as a single bony metastasis with pathological fracture.

Metastases are usually osteolytic with extensive destruction of bone. In a minority of cases, osteoblastic activity is stimulated by the presence of the tumour so that dense reactive bone is formed. Osteosclerotic secondaries of this type are seen, particularly in cancers of the PROSTATE and BREAST.

# JOINT DISEASE

The diagram illustrates the structure of a **synovial joint**.

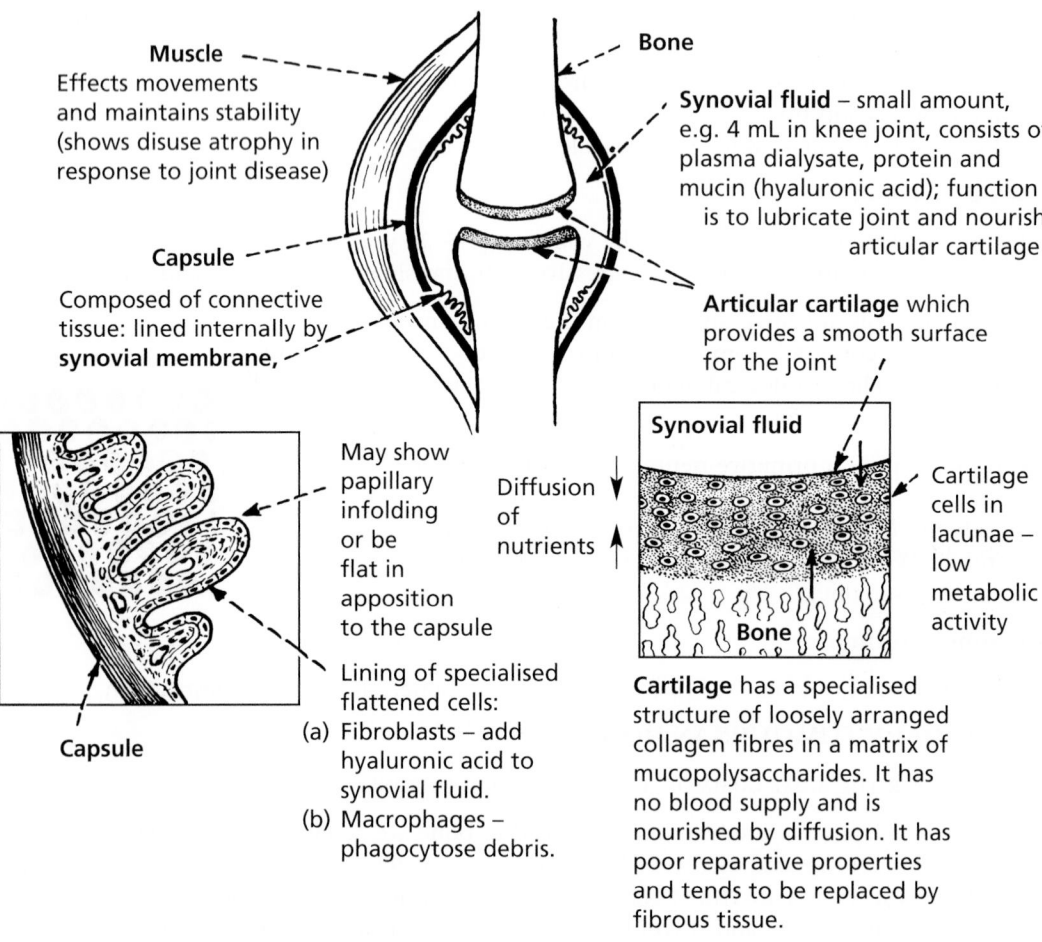

**Muscle**
Effects movements and maintains stability (shows disuse atrophy in response to joint disease)

**Bone**

**Synovial fluid** – small amount, e.g. 4 mL in knee joint, consists of plasma dialysate, protein and mucin (hyaluronic acid); function is to lubricate joint and nourish articular cartilage

**Capsule**
Composed of connective tissue: lined internally by **synovial membrane,**

**Articular cartilage** which provides a smooth surface for the joint

**Capsule**

May show papillary infolding or be flat in apposition to the capsule

Diffusion of nutrients ↓↑

Lining of specialised flattened cells:
(a) Fibroblasts – add hyaluronic acid to synovial fluid.
(b) Macrophages – phagocytose debris.

Synovial fluid

Cartilage cells in lacunae – low metabolic activity

Bone

**Cartilage** has a specialised structure of loosely arranged collagen fibres in a matrix of mucopolysaccharides. It has no blood supply and is nourished by diffusion. It has poor reparative properties and tends to be replaced by fibrous tissue.

The two most common joint diseases illustrate how the individual components of a joint may be initially affected:

| | |
|---|---|
| **Rheumatoid arthritis** essentially an inflammation of **synovial membrane** | **Osteoarthritis** essentially a degeneration of **articular cartilage** |

As the diseases progress, other secondary effects are added and may obscure the basic pathology.

# JOINT TRAUMA

Trauma is very variable in its severity and effects.

At one end of the scale a single incident of 'sprain' or 'strain' involves only minor soft tissue damage with minimal associated haemorrhage. In these circumstances the healing capacity of joints is rapid and complete.

With mild degrees of trauma, particularly if repeated, the synovial membrane shows non-specific reactive changes which include hyperaemia and a mild chronic inflammatory cellular infiltrate. There is often a joint **effusion**.

Serious damage to joints include:

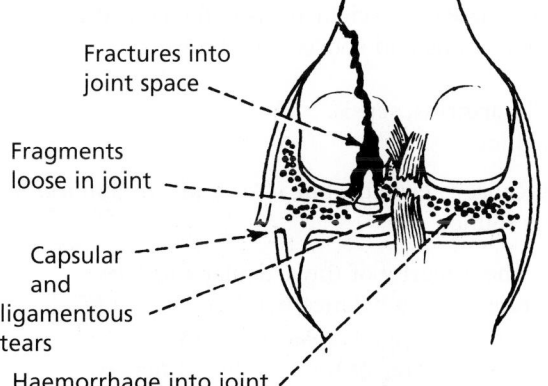

Fractures into joint space

Fragments loose in joint

Capsular and ligamentous tears

Haemorrhage into joint

Possible sequels are:
1. The articular surface is permanently deformed (ineffective repair of cartilage).
2. Loose body continues to cause traumatic damage to cartilage.
3. Ligaments may not heal or are united by poor scar tissue.

The medial meniscus of the knee is susceptible to tears:

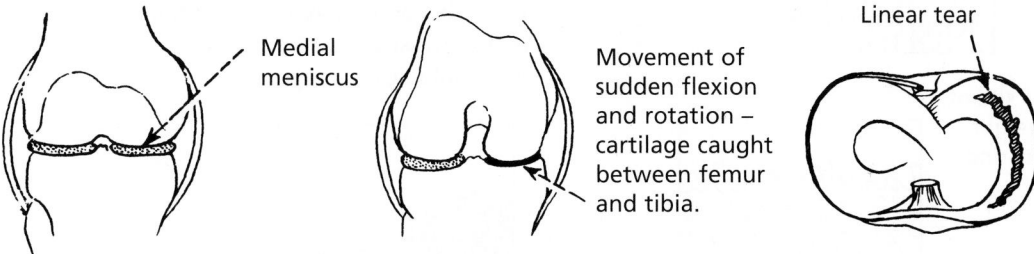

Medial meniscus

Movement of sudden flexion and rotation – cartilage caught between femur and tibia.

Linear tear

Locking of the joint and effusion are common.

Apart from damage directly attributable to trauma, the most important consequence is an increased risk of osteoarthritis due to damage to the articular cartilage.

# OSTEOARTHRITIS (OA)

### OSTEOARTHRITIS (OA)

**This** is the commonest disorder of joints and the commonest cause of chronic disability after middle age. The basic pathology is degeneration of the articular cartilage. The main clinical features are pain and stiffness.

The disorder is divided into two main groups. In both types the basic pathological processes are the same.

1. In **secondary OA** there is a clear association with some predisposing condition which may be virtually any abnormality of a joint. Of particular importance are:
   a) Abnormality of the articular surfaces (e.g. following injury).
   b) Abnormal stresses on the joint (e.g. the increased weight-bearing demanded by obesity; association with particular occupations and sports), or abnormal alignments.
   c) Previous inflammation, e.g. rheumatoid arthritis, sepsis.
   This type often affects a single predisposed joint.

2. In **primary OA** no obvious predisposing cause is evident, but often runs in families. In some, mutation of Type II collagen gene is found.

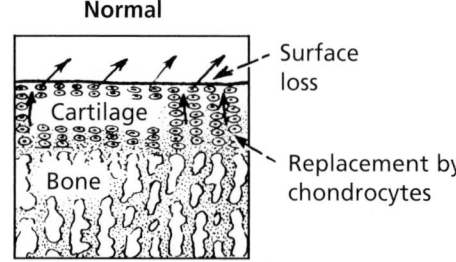

**Normal**

Surface loss

Cartilage

Replacement by chondrocytes

Bone

The integrity of the articular cartilage represents a balance between 'wear and tear' losses and replacement by chondrocytes of the specialised matrix.

The earliest change in OA is in the chemical composition of the matrix, which becomes softer. This is followed by progressive characteristic morphological changes.

**At site of weight bearing**

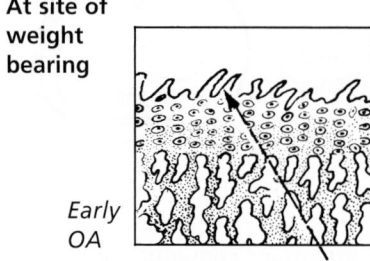

*Early OA*

Flaking and fibrillation of surface

*Later OA*

Areas of cystic degeneration

Loss of cartilage; exposure of bone which becomes hard and polished (eburnated)

# OSTEOARTHRITIS (OA)

**At edge of joint**

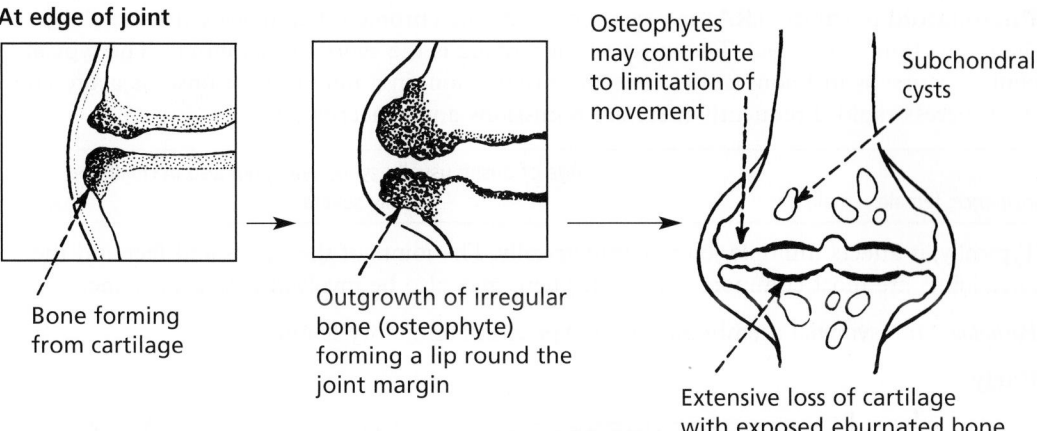

Bone forming from cartilage

Outgrowth of irregular bone (osteophyte) forming a lip round the joint margin

Osteophytes may contribute to limitation of movement

Subchondral cysts

Extensive loss of cartilage with exposed eburnated bone

In this type the larger weight-bearing joints and the spine in particular are susceptible. The interphalangeal joints may also bear osteophytic outgrowths (Heberden and Bouchard nodes).

The synovial membrane may show mild, non-specific inflammation and effusion may occur, but these changes are secondary.

OA is the main indication for hip and knee replacement surgery.

A particularly severe form (Charcot joint) is seen when the nerve supply to a joint is defective – neuropathic arthropathy.

## GOUT

Patients with gout develop acute arthritis, often of the great toe. Gout is caused by excessive uric acid which is a product of purine (DNA) breakdown. In gout, there is hyperuricaemia (serum uric acid >7 mg/dL). Periodically, urate crystals are deposited within the affected joint, at first in the articular cartilage, but chronically in the adjacent bone and soft tissues, forming masses known as tophi. Joint aspiration shows characteristic appearances.

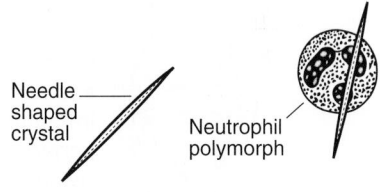

Needle shaped crystal

Neutrophil polymorph

**PSEUDO-GOUT**. In this condition of the elderly, rhomboid crystals of calcium pyrophosphate are deposited in the joint, evoking an inflammatory reaction. Larger joints such as the knee tend to be affected. A chronic degenerative arthritis may supervene or co-exist. The radiological appearances are known as chondrocalcinosis.

# RHEUMATOID ARTHRITIS (RA)

**Rheumatoid arthritis (RA)** is a common systemic chronic inflammatory disease (1–3% of the population in Europe). The most affected tissue is the synovial membrane. The typical clinical course is insidious in its onset and progression; in a minority the onset is acute and the progress rapid. Frequently there are remissions and exacerbations.

| | |
|---|---|
| *Incidence*: female > male 3:1 | *Age of onset*: usually 35–55 years, but also in childhood – usually severe. |

Typically, it affects multiple joints symmetrically. The joints of the hands and feet and the knee joints are most commonly affected. There may also be involvement of the spine.

*Pathology*: the synovial membrane shows typical inflammatory features.

## Early

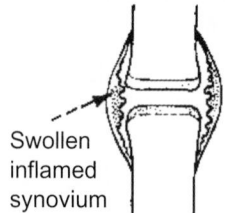

Swollen inflamed synovium

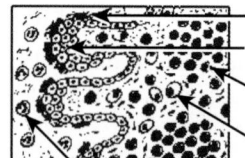

Fibrinous exudate

Villiform hyperplasia

Intense infiltration with lymphocytes and plasma cells

Fluid contains fibrin and neutrophils

Signs of inflammation with swelling over joints

A raised ESR and normochromic anaemia are evidence of the systemic illness.

## Intermediate

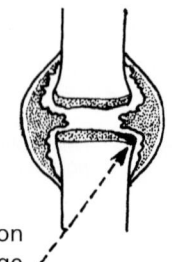

Laxity of capsule and soft tissue – inflammation in periarticular tissues

Destruction of cartilage by enzymatic action and granulation tissue spreading over the articular surface (pannus)

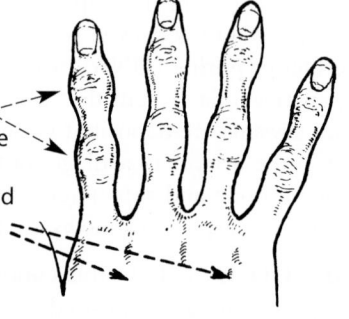

Joints swollen + marked muscle wasting (interosseous and thenar muscles)

## Late

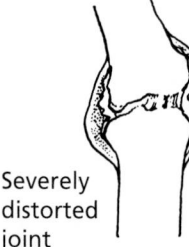

Severely distorted joint

Inflammation usually less marked – fibrous adhesions across joint – may be irregular bony union

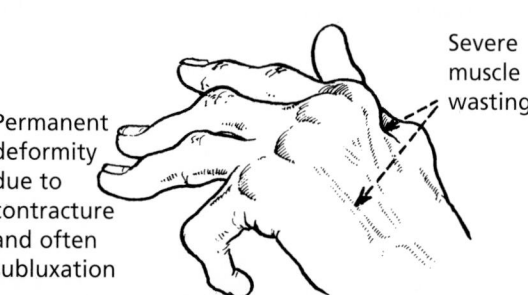

Permanent deformity due to contracture and often subluxation

Severe muscle wasting

# RHEUMATOID ARTHRITIS (RA)

RA is an auto-immune disease, with no single provoking factor. A possible hypothesis is:

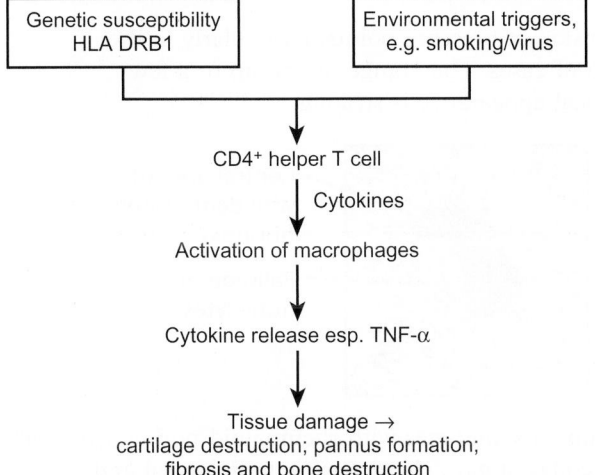

Joint destruction is due to a complex cascade of cytokines, inflammatory cell interaction, and alteration of activity of chondrocytes, osteoblasts and osteoclasts.

Modern biologic therapy directed against TNF-α suppresses disease activity and stops joint destruction.

### Rheumatoid factors

These are antibodies, mainly of IgM and IgG class, which are directed against the patient's IgG. They may form immune complexes which may contribute to the joint inflammation. A more recently recognized antibody is anti-cyclic citrullinated peptide (anti-CCP). Patients in whom auto-antibodies can be found in the serum are described as seropositive. Around 85% of RA patients are seropositive.

## RHEUMATOID ARTHRITIS (RA)

The systemic nature of the disease is illustrated by inflammatory processes affecting the connective tissues at other sites.

1. Rheumatoid nodules occur under the skin at pressure points, particularly in the forearms and elbow joints in one-fifth of cases. They range in size up to a few centimetres in diameter. The histological appearance is striking.

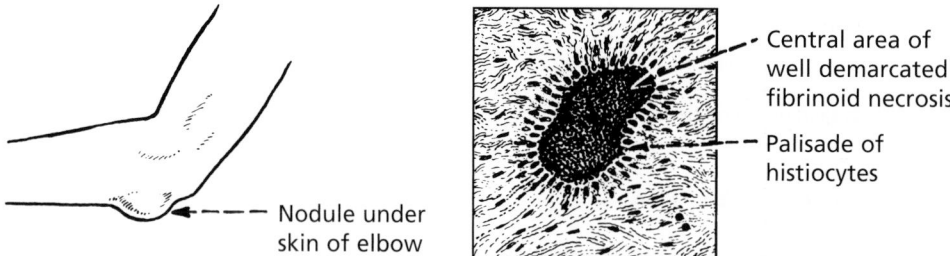

Nodule under skin of elbow

Central area of well demarcated fibrinoid necrosis

Palisade of histiocytes

2. The lung may show interstitial pneumonia sometimes with rheumatoid nodules. In coal miners, the mixture of coal dust and collagen gave characteristic radiological and pathological appearances – Caplan nodules.
3. Necrotising arteritis is a serious complication in a few cases.
4. A mild interstitial myocarditis, polymyositis or neuritis may be seen in some cases. Serosal inflammation, e.g. pericarditis and pleurisy, are common.
5. Particularly in juvenile RA, lymphadenopathy is common and splenomegaly may cause hypersplenism – so-called 'Felty syndrome'.
6. Amyloid disease – may complicate long-standing RA.

# SERO-NEGATIVE ARTHRITIS

**Ankylosing spondylitis (AS)** is an arthritis affecting particularly the sacroiliac, costovertebral and vertebral joints, but peripheral arthritis is also seen.

*Incidence*: 0.05% of population male:female 3:1.

*Age of onset*: young adults progressing into middle age. Rheumatoid factor negative.

The disorder is, like RA, an active chronic arthritis, but differs in that it may cause osseous ankylosis (bony union), so that no movement of the affected joints is possible.

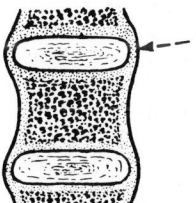

Bony union on the periphery of the intervertebral discs gives the characteristic radiological appearance – bamboo spine.

Aortitis leading to aortic incompetence and uveitis may be seen.

**Psoriatic arthritis** affects the axial and peripheral joints. Typically the distal interphalangeal joints are involved and the adjacent nails are affected.

**Reactive arthritis (formerly known as Reiter syndrome)** is a syndrome of polyarthritis, urethritis and uveitis following infections, e.g. *Chlamydia*, *Yersinia* and *Salmonella*. The detailed mechanisms are unclear.

**HLA association**. AS, psoriatic arthritis and reactive arthritis are associated with HLA-B27 (>95% in AS). Genetic susceptibility is an important factor predisposing to the arthritis.

| | OSTEOARTHRITIS | RHEUMATOID ARTHRITIS |
|---|---|---|
| **Type of disorder** | Degenerative | Inflammatory |
| **Site of initial damage** | Articular cartilage | Synovial membrane |
| **Age** | Late middle age + | Third decade (any age) |
| **Joints affected** | Large, weight-bearing, often single, pre-existing local factors in some cases | Small joints of hands and feet, multiple |
| **Systemic disease** | None<br>ESR – normal<br>Rheumatoid factor – absent | ++<br>ESR ↑<br>Rheumatoid factor positive<br>Secondary anaemia |

# INFECTIONS OF JOINTS

### 1. Acute infective arthritis

(a) Primary pyogenic haematogenous infection is now rare. It remains, however, a serious complication in joints already damaged. *S. aureus* is the common infecting organism.

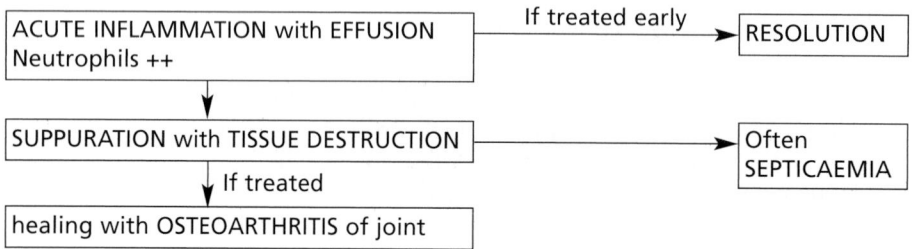

The essential changes are:

(b) Arthritis complicating **gonorrhoea** and **brucellosis**.

In both of these conditions, a polyarthritis may occur in the acute phase and, in a small number, continues as a low-grade arthritis. The spine particularly is affected in brucellosis.

### 2. Tuberculous arthritis

In Western countries the incidence is low: a few cases arise, complicating reactivated pulmonary tuberculosis in the elderly. If untreated, there is a low-grade chronic inflammation with effusion and progressive destruction of tissues.

The diagnosis requires culture of joint fluid and/or biopsy when the typical histology of tuberculosis is seen.

### 3. Lyme disease

is a polyarthritis due to the spirochete *Borrelia burgdorferi,* transmitted by bites from deer ticks.

# JOINT AND SOFT TISSUES – MISCELLANEOUS

## Pigmented villonodular synovitis (PVNS) (tenosynovial giant cell tumour)

This may affect any synovial tissue, but the knee and hip joints are most commonly involved.

It typically affects people aged 20–50 years. The synovial membrane shows proliferation of brown pigmented large villi or rounded nodules.

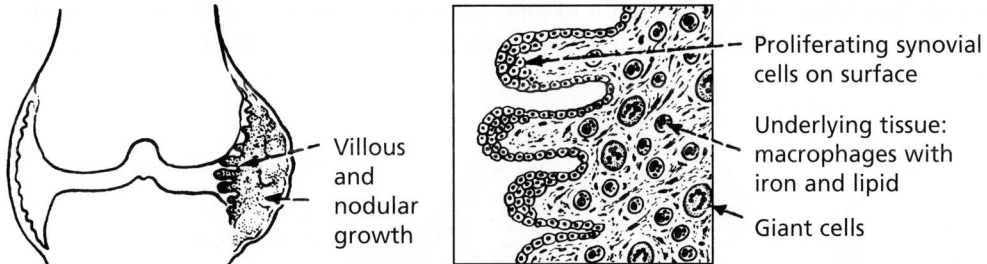

Villous and nodular growth

Proliferating synovial cells on surface

Underlying tissue: macrophages with iron and lipid

Giant cells

It is now thought to be neoplastic **but to all intents it never metastasises**.

The giant cell tumour of tendon sheath is now considered to be a solitary variant of PVNS.

Similar but well-defined nodules are common in the fingers and toes.

## SOFT TISSUE TUMOURS

These are dealt with on pages 166 and 167: 172–174.

## LOOSE BODIES IN JOINTS

Loose bodies are usually found in diseased or damaged joints and their presence tends to aggravate any existing disease. Clinically, there is often recurrent 'locking' of the joint.

**Degenerative**
Melon seed bodies ⎱ Products
Fragments of osteophytes ⎰ of arthritis

**Traumatic**
Fragments derived from fractures: tearing of cartilage

**Synovial chondromatosis** – numerous polypoidal projections of cartilage formed by metaplasia within the synovium

# PARA-ARTICULAR TISSUES – MISCELLANEOUS

### Bursae

These are synovial-lined spaces usually overlying bony prominences, e.g. the olecranon and patella, and often connected with adjacent joint spaces. They may become inflamed (bursitis).

### Ganglion

This is a swelling which forms in relation to joint synovium or more usually tendon sheath, due to myxoid degeneration. It is not lined by synovium. Ganglia are classically seen around the wrist.

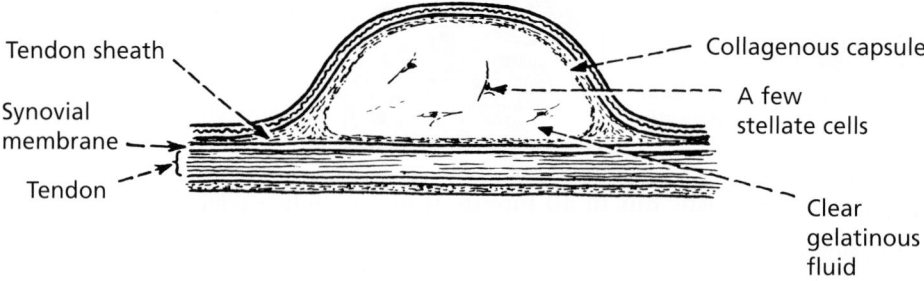

This type of myxoid cystic degeneration may occur at other less prominent sites, e.g. within the cartilaginous menisci of the knee.

**Dupuytren's contracture**. See page 124.

# COLLAGEN DISEASES

This term describes a group of multisystem diseases, many auto-immune in origin.

The group includes RA; systemic lupus erythematosus (SLE); systemic sclerosis; polyarteritis nodosa (PAN) and dermatomyositis.

## Systemic lupus erythematosus (SLE)

SLE is a chronic relapsing and resulting disease characterised by damage to multiple organs but especially the skin, joints, kidneys and central nervous system. It is much commoner in females.

SLE is an auto-immune disorder. There are antibodies directed against cellular constituents, e.g. anti-nuclear, anti-DNA. These auto-antibodies damage tissue by a Type III hypersensitivity reaction (p. 102).

Organs affected:

Kidney – often there is glomerulonephritis.
Skin – erythema of the bridge of the nose and cheeks (malar rash); made worse by sunlight.
Joints – synovitis.
Brain – focal neurological signs may develop due to vasculitis.
Heart – pericarditis, myocarditis, endocarditis (Libman–Sacks).
Lungs – pleuritis.

## Systemic sclerosis (scleroderma)

This is a rare, slowly progressive disease in which there is gradual fibrosis of various organs including the skin (face and hands), gastrointestinal tract, heart and lungs. It is associated with Raynaud disease. The basic abnormality is in the small blood vessels, which show sclerosis with intimal thickening. The change is associated with fibrosis of the surrounding tissues. Auto-antibodies, typically against nuclear components, are often found.

In collagen diseases, the basic mechanisms are inflammatory and are mediated by auto-immune processes. The inflammatory damage is very variable in its severity, its site of predilection and even its local effects. Multiple factors, of which inherited susceptibility and resistance are important, are involved. The following diagram illustrates the basic mechanisms.

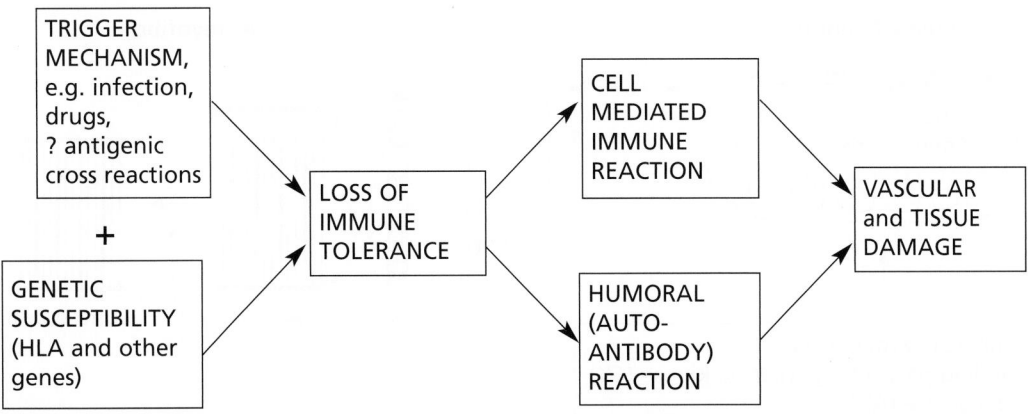

# COLLAGEN DISEASES

### Anatomy

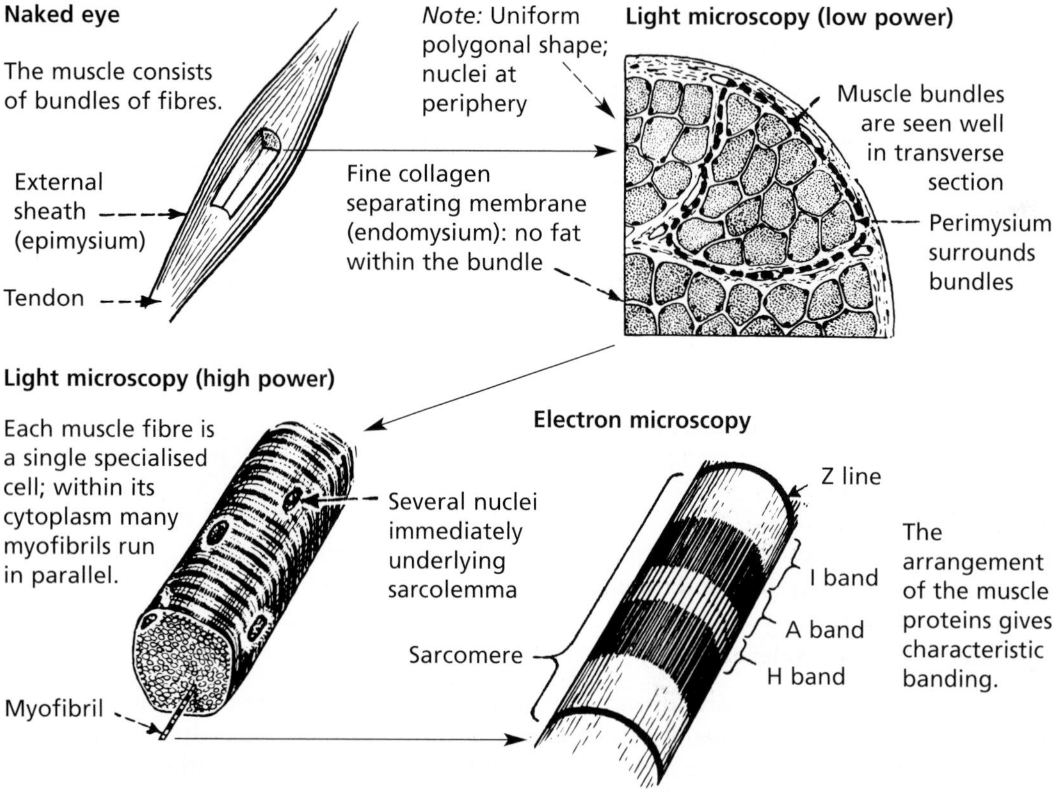

**Naked eye**

The muscle consists of bundles of fibres.

External sheath (epimysium) - - - →

Tendon - - →

*Note:* Uniform polygonal shape; nuclei at periphery

Fine collagen separating membrane (endomysium): no fat within the bundle

**Light microscopy (low power)**

Muscle bundles are seen well in transverse section

Perimysium surrounds bundles

**Light microscopy (high power)**

Each muscle fibre is a single specialised cell; within its cytoplasm many myofibrils run in parallel.

Several nuclei immediately underlying sarcolemma

Sarcomere

Myofibril - -

**Electron microscopy**

Z line

I band

A band

H band

The arrangement of the muscle proteins gives characteristic banding.

# SKELETAL MUSCLE

## MUSCLE CONTRACTION

The basic mechanism is as follows:

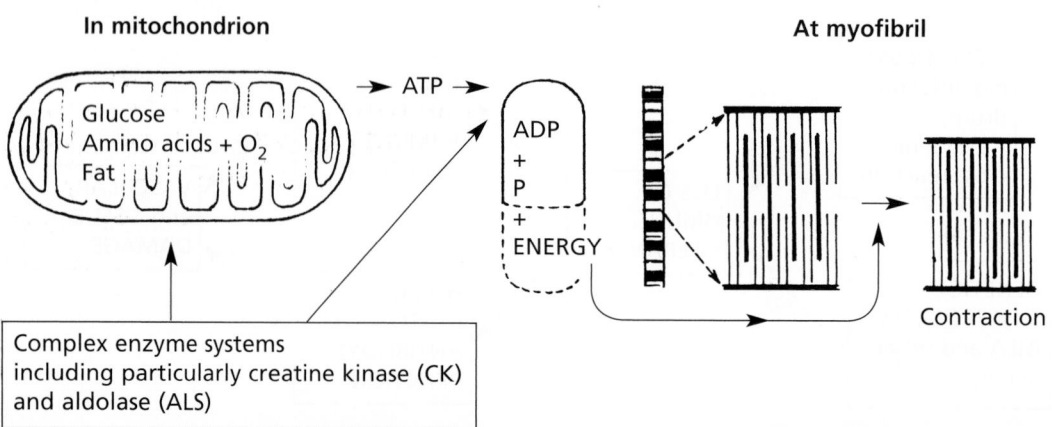

**In mitochondrion**

Glucose
Amino acids + $O_2$
Fat

→ ATP →

ADP
+
P
+
ENERGY

**At myofibril**

Contraction

Complex enzyme systems including particularly creatine kinase (CK) and aldolase (ALS)

# SKELETAL MUSCLE

There are three types of muscle fibre, related to differences in functional activity.

| | TYPE OF CONTRACTION | LOCATION | MYOGLOBIN | MITOCHONDRIA | METABOLISM |
|---|---|---|---|---|---|
| **Type I** (red muscle) | SLOW twitch, FATIGUE RESISTANT | POSTURAL MUSCLES | +++ | +++ | AEROBIC |
| **Type IIa** (red muscle) | FAST twitch, FATIGUE RESISTANT | e.g. in LEGS of SPRINTERS | +++ | +++ | AEROBIC |
| **Type IIb** (white muscle) | FAST twitch, FATIGUABLE | ARM MUSCLES | + | + | ANAEROBIC |

*Note*: Most muscles are a mixture of the three fibre types, but the proportion varies according to the function of the muscle.

In section, the three fibre types are identified by their ATPase activity.

Normal muscle stained H & E

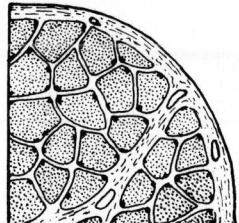

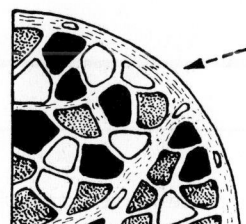

Normal muscle stained for ATPase activity

Type I = black
Type IIa = white
Type IIb = stipple
Note random mosaic pattern.

Muscle fibre function is not intrinsic but is conditioned by its type of nerve supply: any single anterior horn cell innervates fibres of only one type.

## MUSCLE INNERVATION

The motor unit consists of: a single lower motor neurone (**LMN**) – and the muscle fibres it supplies.

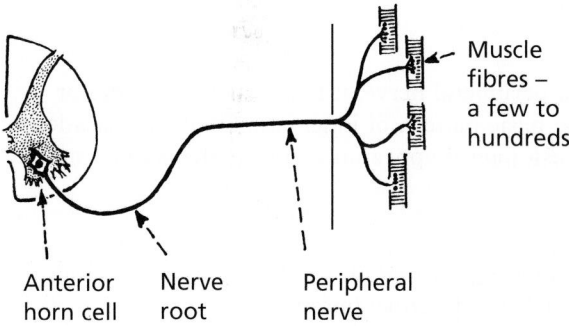

Anterior horn cell    Nerve root    Peripheral nerve

Muscle fibres – a few to hundreds

### Muscle spindles

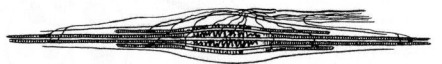

Muscle spindles are bundles of specialised fibres which control and refine muscle contraction and are important for proprioception. They are separately innervated from the surrounding fibres.

# ATROPHY AND HYPERTROPHY

**Generalised disuse atrophy** occurs as a result of prolonged immobilisation in bed. Local atrophy follows immobilisation due to joint disease or after bone fractures.

**Hypertrophy** of muscle tissue in response to increased work load is well seen in athletes.

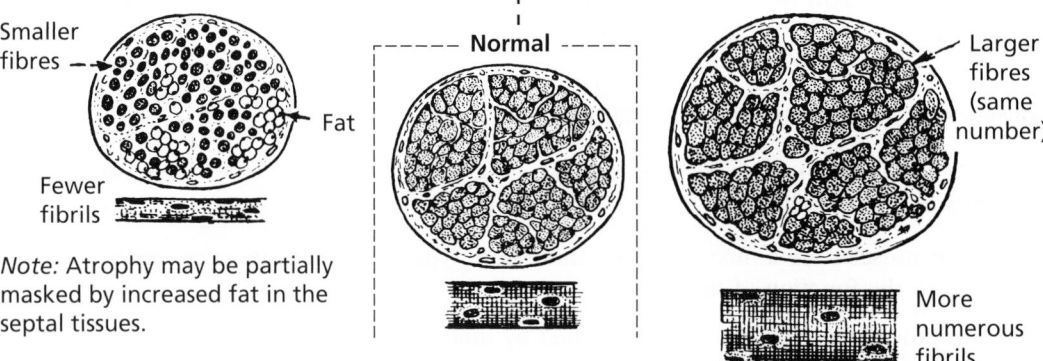

Smaller fibres

Fat

Fewer fibrils

*Note:* Atrophy may be partially masked by increased fat in the septal tissues.

Normal

Larger fibres (same number)

More numerous fibrils

# NEUROGENIC ATROPHY

This form of atrophy is seen when the nerve supply is damaged. The distribution of nerve fibres within the muscle is important and is represented diagrammatically in respect of two motor units: axon A and axon B.

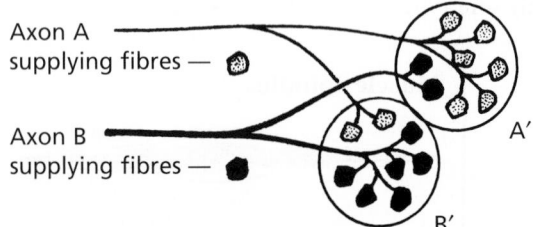

Axon A supplying fibres —

Axon B supplying fibres —

A′

B′

*Note:* While *axons A* and *B*, respectively, innervate the majority of fibres in bundles *A′* and *B′*, there is overlap between bundles. Since many axons supply a muscle the overlap is considerable.

Apart from complete traumatic section of a peripheral nerve, it is unusual for all motor fibres to a muscle to be destroyed. Both the basic pattern of innervation and the variations in nerve fibre damage are reflected in the histological appearances in the denervated muscle.

1. **Pattern of atrophy**

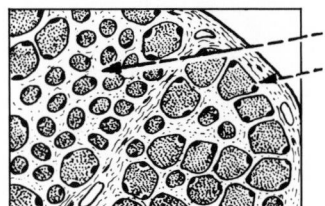

Groups of atrophic denervated fibres with adjacent groups of normal fibres.

# NEUROGENIC ATROPHY

### 2. Re-innervation

In an area of denervation, the terminal axonal branches of intact neurones sprout and can re-innervate the atrophic fibres. The effects of denervation and re-innervation are shown in a muscle bundle supplied by two axons, A and B.

**Denervation** of A

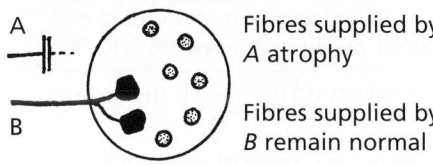

A

B

Fibres supplied by *A* atrophy

Fibres supplied by *B* remain normal

**Re-innervation** and **restoration** of fibre size

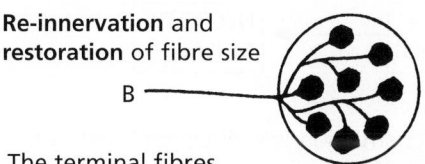

B

The terminal fibres of *B* now sprout and innervate the atrophic fibres which are restored to normal size.

# MYASTHENIA GRAVIS

The **MOTOR END-PLATE** is the specialised neuromuscular junction situated at the middle of each muscle fibre. The nervous impulse causes release of **ACETYLCHOLINE** at the specialised nerve endings – depolarisation at this site is the stimulus to contraction. The sarcolemma at this site contains **CHOLINESTERASE**.

In MYASTHENIA GRAVIS there are auto-antibodies which block the function of the postsynaptic acetylcholine receptors at the motor end-plate. This results in muscle weakness and early fatigue of the ocular and head and neck muscles particularly. It is commoner in women.

There is a strong association with THYMIC abnormalities. This may be *thymic germinal centre hyperplasia* or *thymoma*. These thymic lesions may alter tolerance to self-antigens and allow the formation of auto-antibodies.

# MUSCLE DAMAGE

## (a) Trauma and ischaemia

Trauma and ischaemia may combine to cause necrosis of a mass of muscle and the effects may be serious.

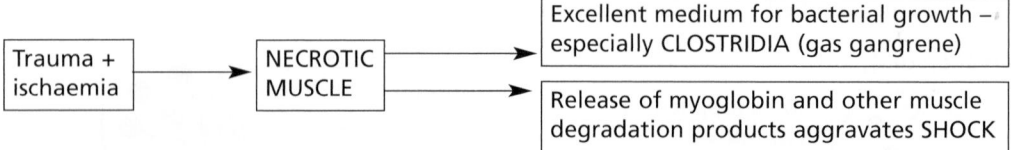

The latter situation is well exemplified in the CRUSH SYNDROME – classically seen in building collapse.

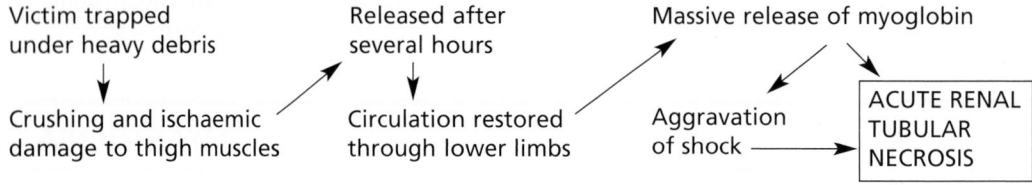

### Repair of muscle damage

The inflammatory response is followed by organisation with removal of the dead muscle. There are two possible results:

    (i) If the gap is not too great, regeneration effects restoration to normal.

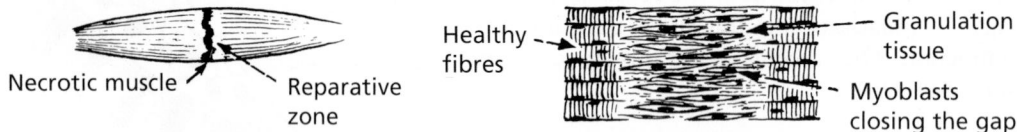

    (ii) If the gap is too great, scar tissue prevents the regeneration.

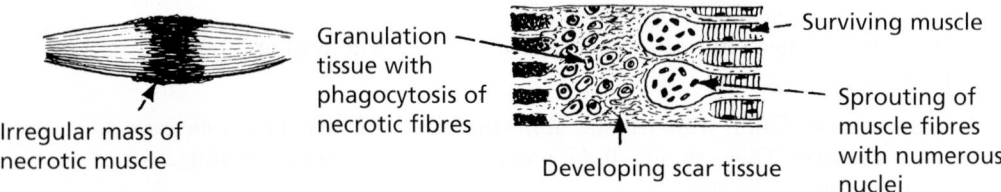

## (b) Inflammation

Pyogenic infections of muscle are uncommon but abscess formation may follow intramuscular injections.

### Viral myositis

A true myositis with focal necrosis of fibres, lymphocyte and macrophage infiltration can be caused by the Coxsackie group of viruses. The muscles of the upper thorax are particularly affected.

### Parasitic myositis

In trichinosis, the parasitic larvae encyst in the interstitial tissues within muscles. The adjacent muscle fibres become necrotic; focal calcification is often a late sequel.

# MUSCULAR DYSTROPHY

Muscular dystrophies are inherited diseases, causing muscle damage and weakness.

## Duchenne muscular dystrophy

This is the commonest and most serious form.

### Clinical features

Muscle weakness in early childhood; typically wheelchair-bound by 12 years of age and death by early adulthood.

### Pathology

The main features are

(1) muscle fibre necrosis and

(2) regeneration.

In time, fibres are atrophic and there is fibrosis and fatty replacement.

Biopsy shows:

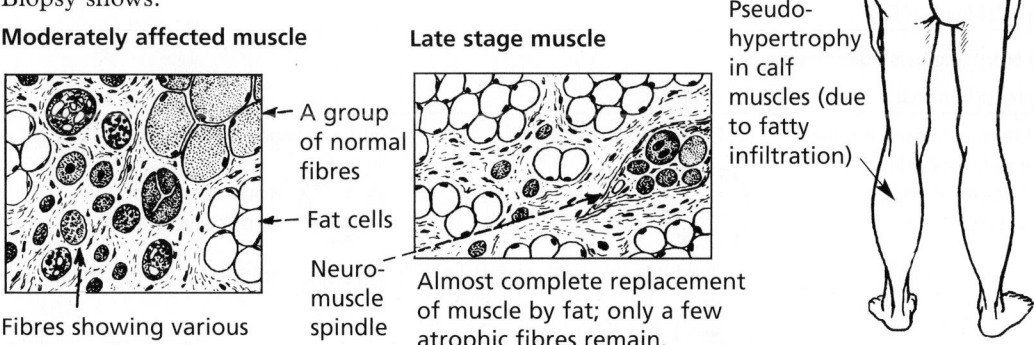

**Moderately affected muscle**

Fibres showing various degrees of atrophy

A group of normal fibres

Fat cells

Neuro-muscle spindle

**Late stage muscle**

Almost complete replacement of muscle by fat; only a few atrophic fibres remain.

Prominent winging of scapulae

Scoliosis (due to muscle weakness)

Pseudo-hypertrophy in calf muscles (due to fatty infiltration)

### Aetiology

This is an X-linked recessive disease occurring almost exclusively in boys. There are loss-of-function mutations of the dystrophin gene which lies on the short arm of chromosome X (Xp21).

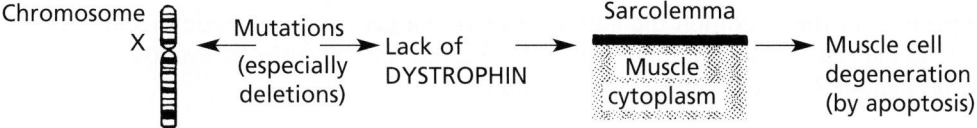

Chromosome X → Mutations (especially deletions) → Lack of DYSTROPHIN → Sarcolemma / Muscle cytoplasm → Muscle cell degeneration (by apoptosis)

Biopsy in early stages shows a lack of dystrophin using immuno-staining (anti-dystrophin antibodies).

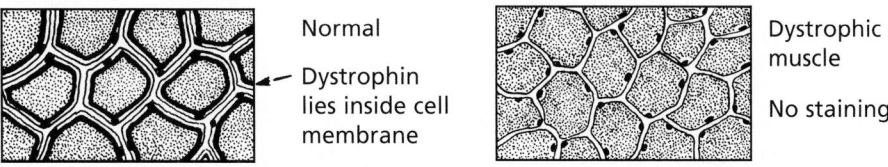

Normal

Dystrophin lies inside cell membrane

Dystrophic muscle

No staining

Genetic testing for mutations of the dystrophin gene on blood samples is now typically undertaken for diagnosis.

**Becker type** muscular dystrophy is a milder form caused by mutation in the dystrophin gene, resulting in diminished levels of the protein.

Other muscular dystrophies include the facio-scapulohumoral, limb girdle and myotonic dystrophy forms.

# INHERITED MYOPATHIES

### Specific metabolic defects

There is a group of genetic myopathies with specific biochemical or morphological abnormalities.

In some, the inborn error of metabolism is generalised and includes muscle. In others it is confined to the muscle fibre. Some examples will be given:

| **(1) Glycogen storage** | **(2) Lipid metabolism** | **(3) Ion channel myopathies (channelopathies)** |
|---|---|---|
| Type 2 (Pompe) – deficiency of acid maltase | Defect in free fatty acid transport into and utilisation within fibre: | Hyperkalaemic periodic paralysis – due to defect in gene encoding sodium |
| Type 5 (McArdle) – muscle phosphorylase | (a) carnitine palmityl transferase (CPT) | channel protein SCN4A. Potassium leaks out of cells. Patients suffer |
| Type 7 – phospho-fructokinase (PFK) | (b) muscle carnitine deficiency | muscle weakness and paralysis. |

**(4) Morphological abnormalities**

| **(a) Mitochondrial** | **(b) Others** | |
|---|---|---|
| Large or increased numbers of mitochondria – abnormal oxidative processes | (i) Central core myopathy<br>Central area is abnormal | (iii) Centronuclear myopathy<br>Rods of tropomysin under sarcolemma |
| | (ii) Rod body myopathy (nemaline)<br>Nucleus in middle of cell | (iv) Disproportion of fibre Types I and II |

These myopathies vary in age of onset, clinical presentation and prognosis.

A further rare autosomal dominant genetic abnormality of muscle is malignant hyperpyrexia. It is due to mutation involving the ryanodine receptor – a calcium release channel protein. In this condition the administration of a general anaesthetic precipitates acute muscle damage. Clinically, there is very high fever, muscle stiffness, cyanosis and acidosis. It is another example of a channelopathy.

# ACQUIRED MYOPATHIES

Inflammatory myopathies – polymyositis and dermatomyositis – are two similar inflammatory disorders of muscle.

**POLYMYOSITIS** – is an auto-immune disorder characterised by muscle pain and weakness, especially of proximal muscle groups. There is a T cell – mediated attack on muscle fibres by CD8+ cytotoxic T cells due to increased expression of MHC Class I on the myofibres. Treatment is with steroids or immunosuppressive drugs.

**DERMATOMYOSITIS** – has similar muscle changes and also skin lesions often on the face and hands. It is the most common inflammatory myopathy in children, where it presents in an isolated form. In adults, dermatomyositis may be a paraneoplastic phenomenon or there may be evidence of other connective tissue diseases, e.g. RA.

## Pathology

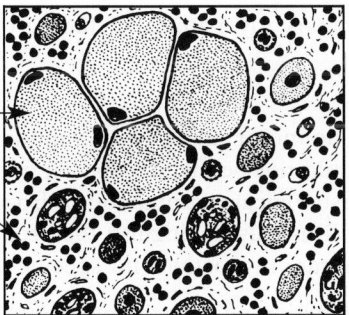

Muscle fibres show damage varying from atrophy to necrosis and some hypertrophied fibres are seen.

There is a lymphocytic infiltrate.

## OTHER MYOPATHIES

In any wasting disease, loss of muscle with weakness is seen.

### Primary condition

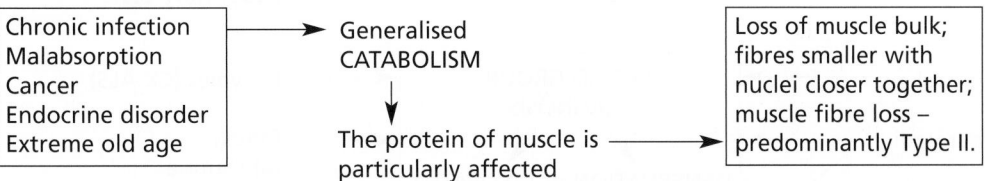

Chronic infection
Malabsorption
Cancer
Endocrine disorder
Extreme old age

Generalised CATABOLISM

The protein of muscle is particularly affected

Loss of muscle bulk; fibres smaller with nuclei closer together; muscle fibre loss – predominantly Type II.

Myopathy is seen in acromegaly, hyperthyroidism, hypothyroidism, hyperaldosteronism (due to hypokalaemia), hyperparathyroidism and in corticosteroid excess.

Other toxic myopathies include ethanol myopathy after binge drinking and drug-related myopathies associated with, e.g. statins, chloroquine and vincristine.

# MUSCLE DISEASES – DIAGNOSIS

Accurate diagnosis of muscular weakness and atrophy is important since there is considerable variation in prognosis and management of these disorders, although often there is no treatment.

A diagnosis is usually reached from a synthesis of the information obtained from investigations under three headings:

1.  **General clinical features,** e.g. *family history, age of onset, distribution of muscle weakness and rate of progress.*
2.  **Special investigation of neuromuscular electrical activity.** The rate of motor and sensory nerve conduction can be measured electrically.

The ELECTROMYOGRAM records the activity of groups of muscle fibres and even of individual fibres (usually fine needle electrodes). The pathological changes are reflected in variations of the electrical potential within the muscle during various types of activity.

These methods distinguish primary myopathies, including myotonias, from denervation atrophy.

3.  **Laboratory tests**
    (a) *MUSCLE BIOPSY.* The motor unit area of a moderately weak muscle is chosen (end-stage muscle should not be taken). Special precautions must be taken to minimise artefacts. Histological examination of frozen muscle, allowing histochemical tests, will usually distinguish the broad groups of disorders and identify the occasional rare myopathy with specific morphological features.

    Electron microscope examination and biochemical analysis may identify specific disorders.

    (b) *SERUM ENZYMES.* In the myopathies where muscle fibres are being destroyed, increased levels of creatine kinase (CK) and aldolase (ALS) are found.

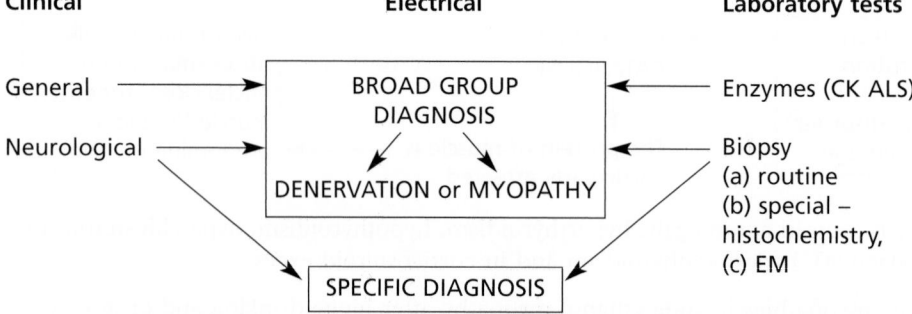

    (c) *GENETIC TESTING.* Advances in molecular genetics have eliminated the need for muscle biopsy in certain disorders such as Duchenne muscular dystrophy. This can be diagnosed by a simple blood test. Sequencing of DNA can be carried out to identify mutation of the dystrophin gene. Similarly, for myotonic dystrophy Type 1, the characteristic genetic abnormality on chromosome 19 can be detected.

# ENDOCRINE SYSTEM

## OBJECTIVES

**1.** To understand the aetiology and pathogenesis of diseases affecting the endocrine organs – pituitary, thyroid, adrenal, endocrine pancreas and parathyroid glands.

**2.** To have knowledge of the multiple endocrine neoplasia syndromes (MENS).

# ENDOCRINE DISEASES

Most endocrine glands are controlled by hormones produced in the anterior pituitary, themselves under control of substances produced in the hypothalamus. A variety of stimuli control pituitary and hypothalamic hormone release, especially feedback control from hormone levels from the target glands. Levels of pituitary hormones show a circadian rhythm.

**Endocrine diseases can be broadly classified as:**

*Hormone excess*
   – Primary overproduction by gland.
   – Secondary to excessive trophic hormone.

*Hormone deficiency*
   – Primary underproduction by gland, e.g. due to inflammation, post surgery.
   – Secondary to insufficient trophic hormones.

*Hormone resistance*
   – Target organ resistance.
   – Failure to activate hormone.

*Effects of non-functioning tumours*

   – Local pressure and invasion.
   – Metastatic disease.

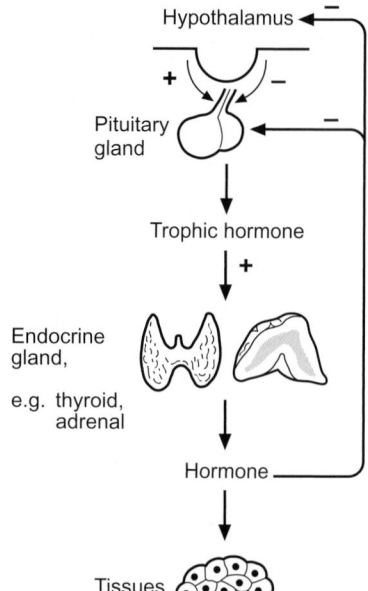

# PITUITARY GLAND

The pituitary gland is a bean-shaped gland at the base of the brain and has two parts: the anterior (adenohypophysis) and the posterior (neurohypophysis).

## Anterior pituitary (adenohypophysis)

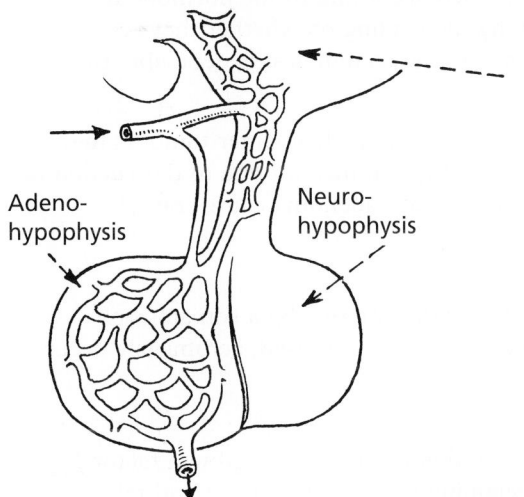

Adeno-hypophysis

Neuro-hypophysis

The blood supply is via a portal system from the hypothalamus. This brings peptides which stimulate or inhibit pituitary hormone production. The cells producing each hormone can be identified by immunohistochemistry (for stored hormone) or in situ hybridisation (for mRNA).

### Posterior pituitary

This is composed of neural tissue and secretes two hormones made in the hypothalamus (oxytocin and antidiuretic hormone).

**Thyrotrophs** produce thyroid stimulating hormone (TSH) which stimulates thyroid follicle cells. **Lactotrophs** produce prolactin which initiates and maintains lactation.

**Oxytocin**
– causes expulsion of milk during lactation;
– aids contraction of uterine smooth muscle during labour.

**Corticotrophs** produce adrenocorticotrophic hormone (ACTH) which stimulates glucocorticoid secretion.
**Antidiuretic hormone** (ADH) helps control water balance by altering the permeability of the renal collecting tubules. Deficiency leads to diabetes insipidus.

**Gonadotrophs** produce follicle stimulating hormone (FSH) which stimulates spermatogenesis, ovarian follicle development and luteinising hormone (LH) which controls Leydig cell function and promotes ovulation.

**Somatotrophs** produce growth hormone which stimulates liver and muscle protein synthesis and, indirectly through insulin-like growth factors (IGF-1), skeletal growth.

***Note***

1. ACTH (39 amino acids long) is synthesised as part of a large molecule pro-opiomelanocortin (POMC) from which other molecules including melanocyte-stimulating hormone (MSH) are derived.

2. Hypothalamic releasing hormones have been found for TSH (TRH); LH/FSH: (GnRH); ACTH (CRH) and GH (GHRH); somatostatin inhibits release of GH.

# PITUITARY HYPERFUNCTION

In most cases, this is associated with PITUITARY ADENOMA but rarely may be due to hyperplasia.

Pituitary adenomas are divided on the basis of size into MACROADENOMAS (>10 mm) and MICROADENOMAS (<10 mm). They can also be classified according to the hormone they secrete. They may be functional or non-functioning, depending on whether they secrete hormone. Activating mutations of the *GNAS* gene are the commonest genetic abnormality identified.

Small tumours present only if they produce excess hormones, while larger tumours may cause pressure effects (e.g. on optic chiasma) or with hypopituitarism due to destruction of normal pituitary. Occasionally haemorrhage into a pituitary adenoma causes raised intracranial pressure (PITUITARY APOPLEXY).

### Gigantism and acromegaly

These are both the result of excess production of growth hormone by a somatotroph adenoma. Gigantism arises in children before the epiphyses have fused; acromegaly occurs in adult life.

### Gigantism

The excess growth hormone stimulates hepatic secretion of insulin-like growth factor 1. There is excess skeletal growth with the bones retaining their normal shape and relative proportions. Fusion of epiphyses is delayed, but eventually occurs and the features of acromegaly appear.

### Acromegaly

There is overgrowth of bone and soft tissue.

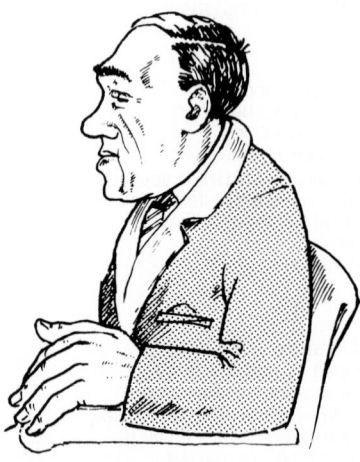

*Clinical signs*

Features coarsened: nose enlarged.
Prognathic (projecting jaw).
Irregular bone formation – interferes with joint function – leads to osteoarthritis.
Limbs enlarged.
Pain due to nerve compression is common. Glucose tolerance is diminished and diabetes occurs in 10%. High blood pressure (BP) with cardiac hypertrophy and extensive atheroma is common, and the patient may die in cardiac failure. There is a two- to three-fold increased risk of colonic cancer.

### PROLACTINOMAS

Prolactin secreting adenomas are often small. They are the most common type of hyperfunctioning adenoma. They cause amenorrhoea, infertility and occasionally galactorrhoea in younger women, but are usually asymptomatic in older women and men.

**CUSHING SYNDROME** is frequently due to an ACTH secreting adenoma when it is known as Cushing disease. The effects are described on page 682.

# HYPOPITUITARISM

Failure of pituitary secretion may affect one or several hormones. Causes include:
(a) Pituitary tumour.
(b) Pituitary surgery/cranial irradiation.
(c) Head injury.
(d) Hypothalamic dysfunction, including craniopharyngioma.
(e) Inflammatory disorders/infections, e.g. sarcoid, tuberculosis, syphilis.
(f) Sheehan syndrome (post-partum hypopituitarism) is used as an example.

This syndrome is due to ischaemic necrosis of the pituitary following post-partum haemorrhage. The normally low pressure in the pituitary portal vascular supply increases the susceptibility of the gland. The results vary with the extent of necrosis and may include the following:

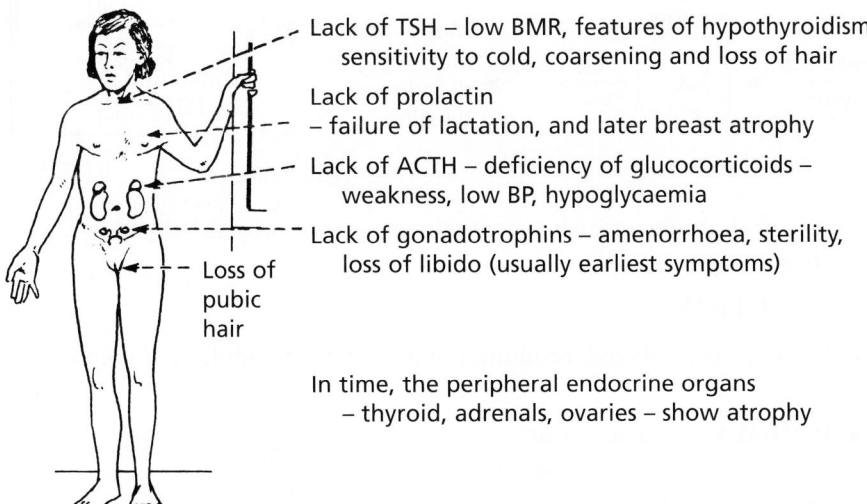

Lack of TSH – low BMR, features of hypothyroidism, sensitivity to cold, coarsening and loss of hair

Lack of prolactin – failure of lactation, and later breast atrophy

Lack of ACTH – deficiency of glucocorticoids – weakness, low BP, hypoglycaemia

Lack of gonadotrophins – amenorrhoea, sterility, loss of libido (usually earliest symptoms)

Loss of pubic hair

In time, the peripheral endocrine organs – thyroid, adrenals, ovaries – show atrophy

**In childhood,** growth hormone deficiency is a cause of dwarfism (pituitary dwarfism). Skeletal growth is diminished with retarded sexual development but normal intelligence. Hypothalamic GHRH deficiency may be responsible.

*Note*: Some individuals treated with human growth hormone have developed Creutzfeld–Jacob disease (p. 599).

**In adults,** growth hormone deficiency leads to lethargy, diminished muscle mass, obesity and premature atheroma.

# THYROID GLAND – UNDERACTIVITY

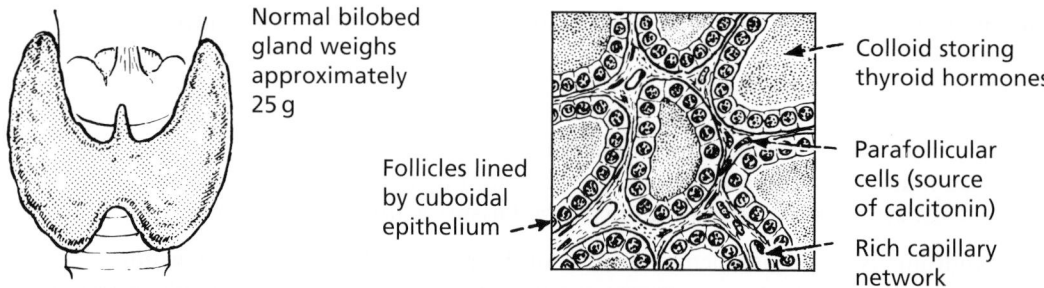

Normal bilobed gland weighs approximately 25 g

Follicles lined by cuboidal epithelium

Colloid storing thyroid hormones

Parafollicular cells (source of calcitonin)

Rich capillary network

The thyroid gland is under the control of the pituitary TSH (p. 623).

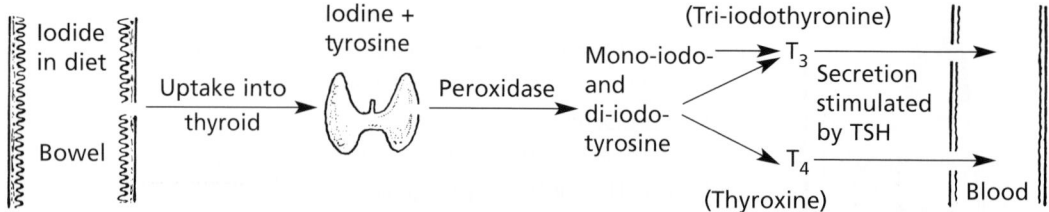

Iodide in diet

Bowel

Uptake into thyroid

Iodine + tyrosine

Peroxidase

Mono-iodo- and di-iodo-tyrosine

(Tri-iodothyronine)

$T_3$

Secretion stimulated by TSH

$T_4$

(Thyroxine)

Blood

$T_4$ can be regarded as a prohormone, which is converted to active $T_3$ by deiodination in liver, muscle and kidney.

## THYROID HYPOFUNCTION

Insufficient thyroid hormone is produced, resulting in myxoedema in adults and cretinism in children.

### ADULTS – MYXOEDEMA

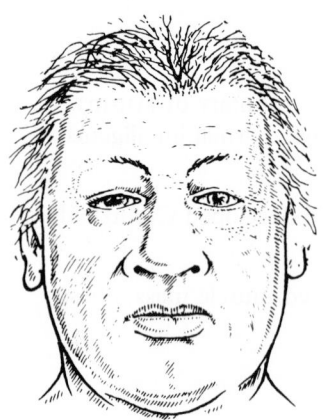

*Clinical signs*
Basal metabolic rate reduced, weight gain.
Body temperature falls, cold intolerance.
Lethargy and apathy.
Appetite reduced.
Constipation.
Respiratory and heart rates reduced.
Diminished libido.
Lack of ovulation.
Skin thickened, non-pitting oedema due to increase in mucopolysaccharide ground substance.
Hair brittle, dry and falls out.
Blood cholesterol is raised.
TSH secretion is increased.
$T_3$ and $T_4$ blood levels low.

# THYROID GLAND – UNDERACTIVITY

*Causes*

Hypothyroidism can be caused by any disorder which interferes with production of thyroid hormone. This includes:

1. Auto-immune thyroiditis.
    (a) Atrophic form – so-called **'primary myxoedema'** – the commonest cause of hypothyroidism.
    (b) **Hashimoto disease**.

2. Severe iodine deficiency.
3. Dyshormonogenesis – inborn errors in the formation of thyroid hormones.
4. Anti-thyroid drugs, e.g. lithium.
5. Excessive surgical resection of thyroid gland.
6. Treatment with radioiodine.
7. Hypopituitarism → reduced TSH.

*Pathological changes in primary myxoedema*

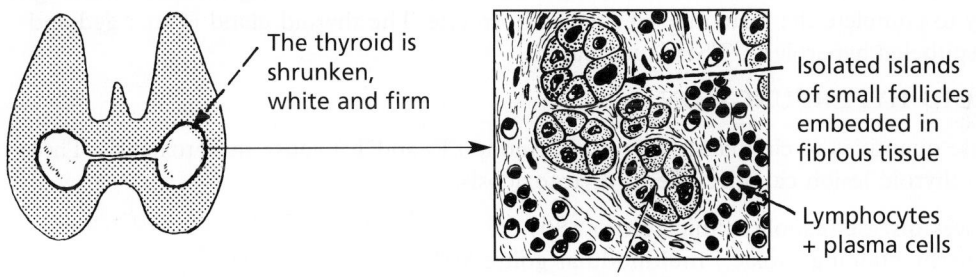

The thyroid is shrunken, white and firm

Isolated islands of small follicles embedded in fibrous tissue

Lymphocytes + plasma cells

Lack of colloid

## CHILDREN – CRETINISM

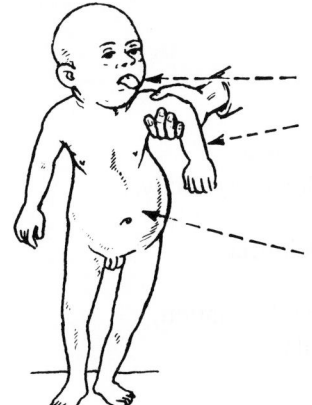

Infants are normal at birth, but abnormality appears within weeks.
*Clinical signs*
Protruding tongue

Growth retardation with short limbs
Coarse dry skin
Lack of hair and teeth
Mental deficiency

Pot belly – often umbilical hernia

Changes are irreversible unless treatment is given early. Two forms are recognised:

(1) Endemic and (2) sporadic cretinism.

# THYROID GLAND – OVERACTIVITY

### *Endemic cretinism*

This occurs in areas of the world where goitre is common due to iodine deficiency. The infantile thyroid is usually enlarged and nodular. Histologically, there are hyperplastic foci containing colloid which compress the intervening tissue. The incidence of this disorder has reduced following addition of iodine to salt.

### *Sporadic cretinism*

This is usually due to congenital hypoplasia or absence of the thyroid. Deaf mutism is often present.

### *Dyshormonogenesis*

In this condition, cretinism is due to a congenital familial recessive enzyme defect leading to inability to complete the formation of thyroid hormone. The thyroid gland is enlarged and shows epithelial hyperplasia. TSH is increased.

## THYROID HYPERFUNCTION

Excessive quantities of circulating thyroid hormone ($T_3$ and $T_4$) cause thyrotoxicosis. Three types of thyroid lesion can give rise to thyrotoxicosis.

1. Graves disease (exophthalmic goitre) >80%.
2. Hyperfunctioning ('toxic') multinodular goitre 10%.
3. Hyperfunctioning ('toxic') adenoma <5%.

### Graves disease (exophthalmic goitre)

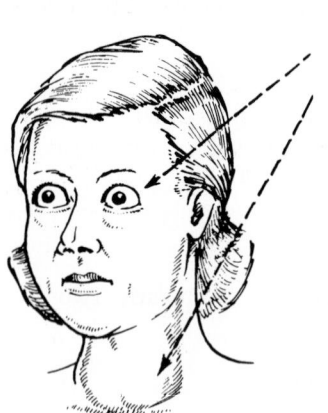

*Clinical signs:*
Exophthalmos.
Prominent thyroid.
*BMR increased.*
Skin warm and sweaty: heat intolerance.
Weakness, hyperkinesia and emotional instability.
Loss of weight.
Glucose tolerance diminished, glycosuria.
Rapid pulse.
Cardiac arrhythmia, especially atrial fibrillation, and heart failure in older patients.
TSH low.

# THYROID GLAND – OVERACTIVITY

**Graves disease**

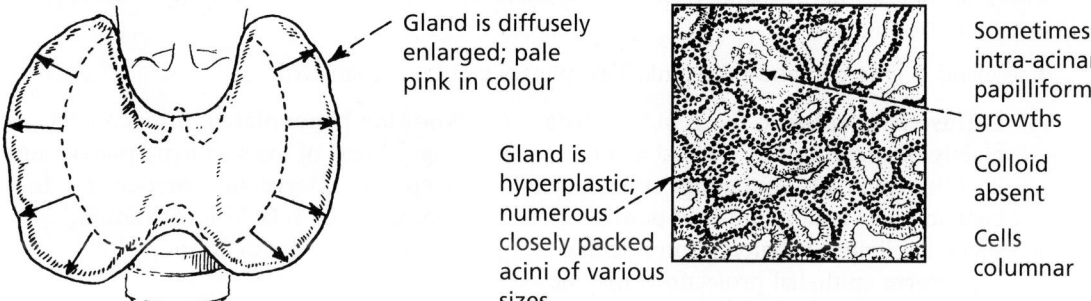

Gland is diffusely enlarged; pale pink in colour

Gland is hyperplastic; numerous closely packed acini of various sizes

Sometimes intra-acinar papilliform growths

Colloid absent

Cells columnar

In some cases there are foci of thyroiditis with lymphocytes and plasma cells.

*Other changes:*
1. Patches of myxoedema – usually on pre-tibial aspect of legs.
2. Exophthalmos, due to T cell mediated auto-immune damage to the eye muscles.

*Aetiology:*
1. Usually in females, peak 20–40 years.
2. Associated with HLA DR3.
3. More common in families showing high incidence of auto-immune disease, e.g. thyroiditis, pernicious anaemia.
4. The stimulation of the thyroid is due to an auto-antibody (thyroid stimulating immunoglobulin/TSH antibody also known as TRAb) which reacts with and activates the surface receptor for TSH on thyroid epithelium. Cyclic AMP is formed and this stimulates hyperplasia of the epithelium and increased formation of thyroid hormone. With the increase in hormone, the blood TSH falls.

**Hyperfunctioning ('toxic') adenoma**

Most adenomas are non-active; only a small proportion (1%) give rise to toxic symptoms. Most patients are women over 40 years.

There is usually only one large adenoma present. The histological features are follicles, which may be small or of normal size. Increased production of thyroid hormone by the adenoma, which is autonomous, causes a fall in TSH, and the remainder of the thyroid is inactive.

**Hyperfunctioning ('toxic') multinodular goitre**

This develops in some cases of non-toxic nodular goitre. Nodules of hyperplasia are interspersed with inactive tissue. The condition is more common over the age of 50, especially in women. Exophthalmos is absent. Cardiac arrhythmias and heart failure is common.

*Note:* The measurement of serum TSH is the most useful single screening test for hyperthyroidism, as TSH levels are decreased even at the earliest stages of the disease.

# THYROID GLAND

### Non-toxic goitre

This is a simple enlargement of the thyroid gland, not associated with increased secretion of thyroid hormone.

The gland is enlarged and pale pink. Two phases can be recognised:

(a) **Diffuse hyperplasia**: the gland consists mainly of small, closely packed acini lined by columnar epithelium and containing a small amount of poorly stained colloid. Occasional intra-acinar papilliform epithelial projections may be seen.

(b) **Nodular hyperplasia**: this is a later stage. Areas of marked hyperplasia cause atrophy of intervening parenchyma. It appears to be related to continuing severity of iodine deficiency.

Sometimes the enlarged gland is translucent and brown due to the large amount of stored colloid (colloid goitre).

This is common in women and appears at puberty or during pregnancy. There are usually no symptoms, but pressure symptoms develop if the thyroid is retrosternal, e.g. pressure on trachea causing stridor, pressure on recurrent laryngeal nerve → hoarseness.

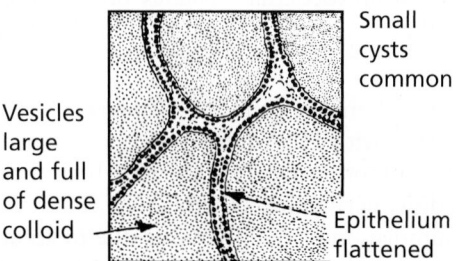

Vesicles large and full of dense colloid — Small cysts common — Epithelium flattened

*Aetiology*. In most regions the aetiology is unknown. Goitre is endemic in central areas of the world, mountainous regions remote from the sea – Switzerland, Himalayas, Andes, etc. There is a lack of iodine in the soil, hence in the food. Addition of iodine to salt has lowered the prevalence of goitre.

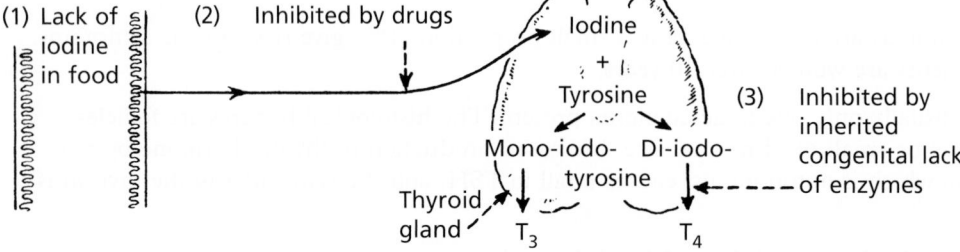

(1) Lack of iodine in food
(2) Inhibited by drugs
Iodine + Tyrosine
Mono-iodo- / Di-iodo-tyrosine
Thyroid gland $T_3$ $T_4$
(3) Inhibited by inherited congenital lack of enzymes

# THYROID GLAND

*Mechanism of goitre production*

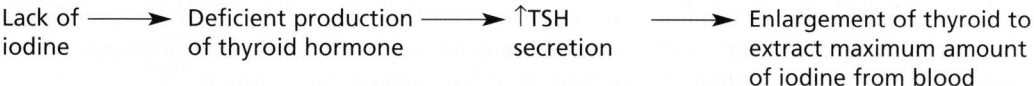

Lack of iodine ⟶ Deficient production of thyroid hormone ⟶ ↑TSH secretion ⟶ Enlargement of thyroid to extract maximum amount of iodine from blood

## THYROIDITIS

Inflammation of the thyroid gland can be caused by a variety of conditions.

1. **Chronic lymphocytic (Hashimoto) thyroiditis**

   This auto-immune thyroid disease is the commonest cause of hypothyroidism in parts of the world where there is sufficient iodine. It is commoner in women and in middle age.
   *Pathogenesis*: there is a breakdown in self-tolerance. There is CD8 T cell-mediated damage to thyroid epithelium. Anti-thyroid antibodies are also produced.
   There is an increased risk of developing non-Hodgkin lymphoma.

2. **Subacute granulomatous (de Quervain) thyroiditis**

   Occurs between 30 and 50 years and is more common in women. It is thought to be precipitated by a viral infection. It is characterised by neck pain. The gland shows inflammation with the formation of granulomas.

3. **Riedel thyroiditis**

   In this rare disorder there is extensive fibrosis of the thyroid gland and adjacent neck structures. This may mimic a thyroid tumour.

4. **Subacute lymphocytic thyroiditis**

   This presents as a painless neck mass in middle-aged women, sometimes following pregnancy (post-partum thyroiditis). It is thought to have an auto-immune basis.

# TUMOURS OF THYROID

### Follicular adenoma

This fairly common benign tumour is usually single and is encapsulated with compression of the surrounding gland. Very occasionally there is hypersecretion with thyrotoxicosis. Degenerative changes including haemorrhage into the tumour are common.

**MALIGNANT TUMOURS** are uncommon. Five forms are recognised:

1. *Papillary carcinoma*, 60–70%. This affects particularly young women; the tumours are usually small and may be multiple within the thyroid. They metastasise readily to local lymph nodes and the first clinical sign may be an enlarged cervical lymph node containing metastatic papillary tumour. Remote spread is unusual. Associated with chromosomal rearrangement of RET oncogene.

   The histological appearances are typical:

   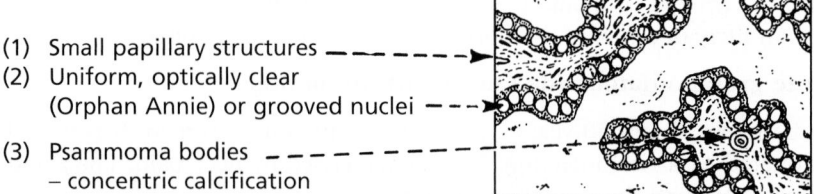

   (1) Small papillary structures
   (2) Uniform, optically clear (Orphan Annie) or grooved nuclei
   (3) Psammoma bodies – concentric calcification

2. *Follicular carcinoma*, 15–20%. These tumours have their highest incidence in women over middle age. They present in two forms:

   (a) Minimally invasive, well encapsulated and can only be differentiated from adenoma by invasion of the capsule and/or veins.

   (b) As a tumour of varying degrees of follicular differentiation, which spreads widely in the thyroid and invades venules.

   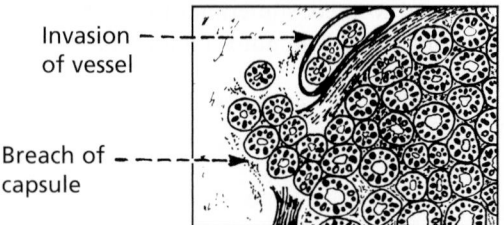

   Invasion of vessel

   Breach of capsule

   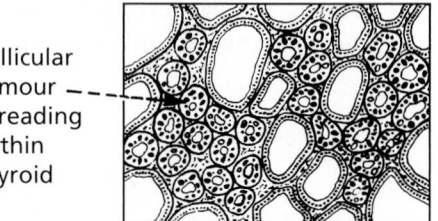

   Follicular tumour spreading within thyroid

   Blood spread, particularly to BONES and LUNGS, is usual in follicular carcinoma. Associated with PAX8/PPARG fusion genes.

3. *Medullary carcinoma*, 5–10%. This is a rare neuroendocrine tumour arising from the calcitonin-producing cells of the thyroid. Blood calcitonin is high. Amyloid deposits may be seen. In addition, there may be production of other hormones resulting in a carcinoid or Cushing syndrome. There is a familial form in which there are multiple tumours of a number of endocrine organs (MEN 2, p. 691).

4. *Anaplastic carcinoma.* This occurs in the elderly and may cause stridor. Distant metastases are common. The prognosis is very poor.

5. *Lymphoma.* B cell lymphoma occasionally arises in long-standing auto-immune thyroiditis (particularly Hashimoto disease).

# ADRENAL GLAND

The adrenal gland has two parts and several functions.

These are:

1. Cortex, secreting
   - glucocorticoids
   - mineralocorticoids
   - androgens

2. Medulla, secreting
   - catecholamines

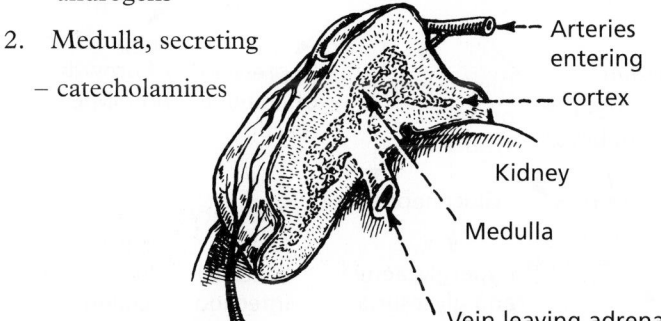

Arteries entering

cortex

Kidney

Medulla

Vein leaving adrenal

**Mineralocorticoids**

The main one is aldosterone. It is involved with the renin–angiotensin system and ADH in the maintenance of blood volume. The mechanism is as follows:

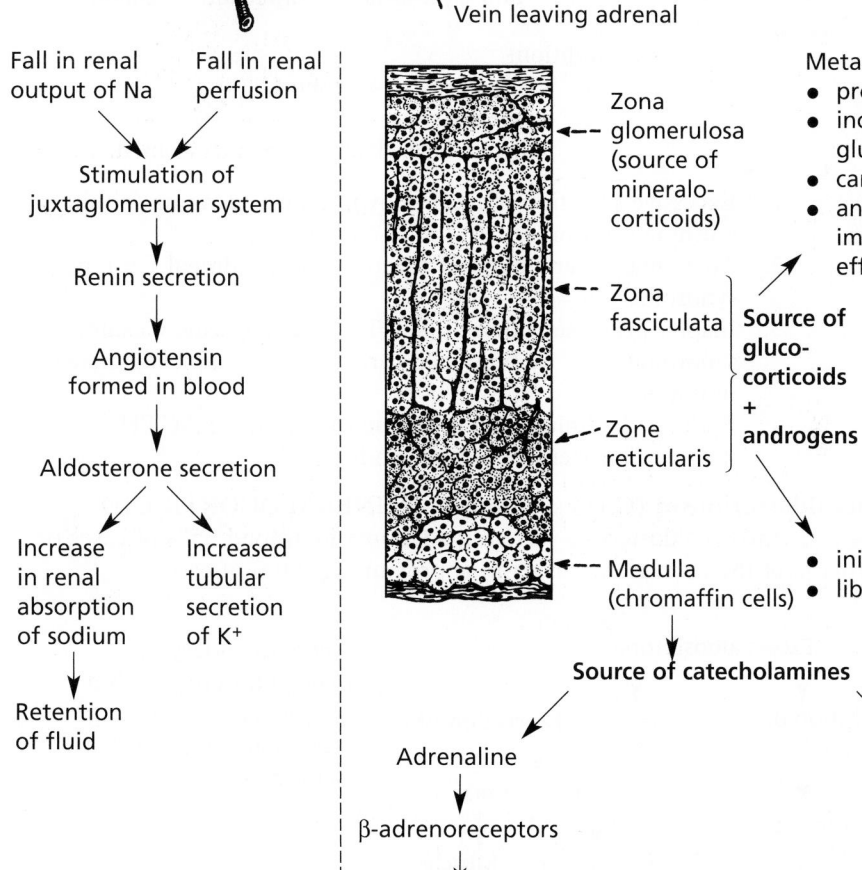

Fall in renal output of Na

Fall in renal perfusion

Stimulation of juxtaglomerular system

Renin secretion

Angiotensin formed in blood

Aldosterone secretion

Increase in renal absorption of sodium

Increased tubular secretion of $K^+$

Retention of fluid

Zona glomerulosa (source of mineralo-corticoids)

Zona fasciculata

Zone reticularis

**Source of gluco-corticoids + androgens**

Medulla (chromaffin cells)

Metabolic effects, e.g.:
- protein catabolism
- increased gluconeogenesis
- cardiovascular effects
- anti-inflammatory plus immunosuppresive effects

- initiation of puberty
- libido (in females)

**Source of catecholamines**

Adrenaline

β-adrenoreceptors

↑ Heart rate
Vasodilatation
Insulin resistance

Noradrenaline

α-adrenoreceptors

Vasoconstriction

↑ Blood pressure

681

# ADRENAL CORTEX – OVERACTIVITY

Overactivity manifests itself in three ways:

1. **Cushing syndrome** (hypersecretion of cortisol) – CORTICOSTEROID EXCESS. This condition is commonest in women, but occurs also in men and rarely in children.

**Clinical effects**

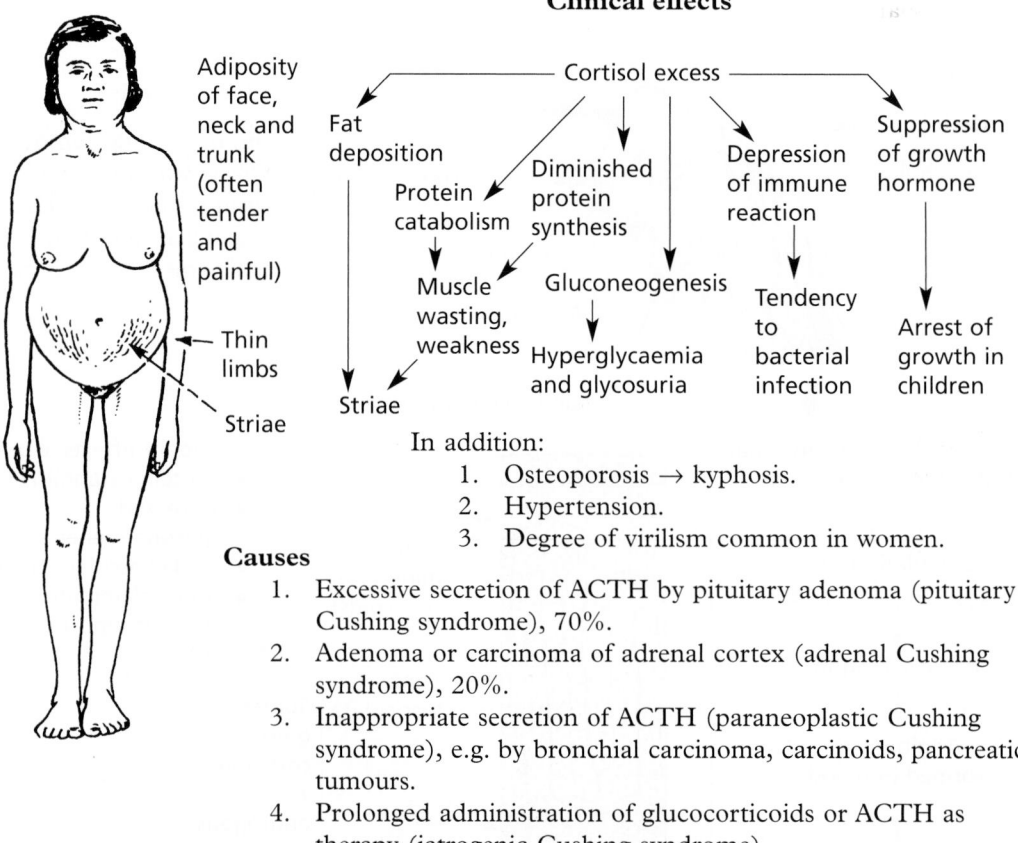

In addition:
1. Osteoporosis → kyphosis.
2. Hypertension.
3. Degree of virilism common in women.

**Causes**
1. Excessive secretion of ACTH by pituitary adenoma (pituitary Cushing syndrome), 70%.
2. Adenoma or carcinoma of adrenal cortex (adrenal Cushing syndrome), 20%.
3. Inappropriate secretion of ACTH (paraneoplastic Cushing syndrome), e.g. by bronchial carcinoma, carcinoids, pancreatic tumours.
4. Prolonged administration of glucocorticoids or ACTH as therapy (iatrogenic Cushing syndrome).

2. **Primary hyperaldosteronism** (Conn syndrome) – MINERALOCORTICOID EXCESS. This is due to an aldosterone-secreting adenoma in around 35% of cases or bilateral hyperplasia of the zona glomerulosa in approximately 60% of cases.

**Effects**

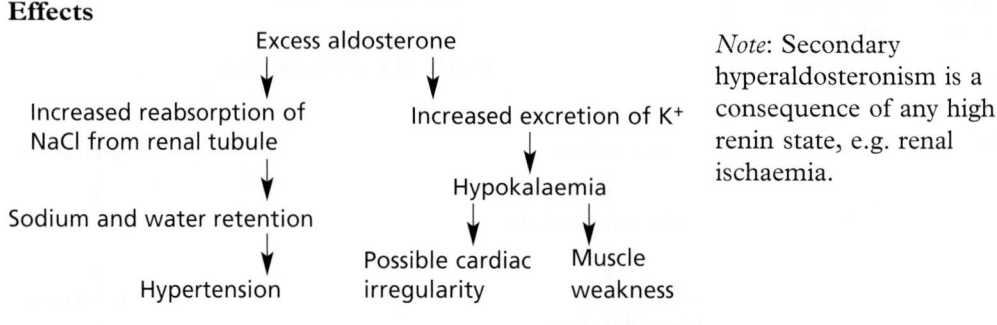

*Note*: Secondary hyperaldosteronism is a consequence of any high renin state, e.g. renal ischaemia.

# ADRENAL CORTEX – OVERACTIVITY

3. **Excessive sex hormone secretion (adrenogenital syndromes)** – ANDROGEN EXCESS. This can occur occasionally with adrenal cortical neoplasms (carcinomas more commonly than adenomas) whereby excessive androgens are secreted. It can also occur in the setting of congenital adrenal hyperplasia – an uncommon group of autosomal recessive disorders with defects in steroid synthesis (see p. 684). (a) In children it causes precocious puberty; (b) in adult females – virilism, oligomenorrhoea.

# ADRENAL CORTEX – HYPOFUNCTION

Adrenal cortical insufficiency may be primary or secondary to pituitary failure. Primary causes can be subdivided into acute causes and chronic ones as listed below.

**Acute adrenal failure**

**Causes**

1. Waterhouse–Friderichsen syndrome. This is usually due to *Neisseria meningitidis* septicaemia.
2. Sudden withdrawal of long-term corticosteroid medication.

**Chronic adrenal insufficiency (Addison's disease)**

**Causes**

1. Auto-immune adrenalitis. There is auto-immune damage to the adrenal gland. It is responsible for at least 75% of cases. Other auto-immune diseases affecting other endocrine glands may occur, e.g. thyroid, parathyroid, pancreas.
2. Tuberculous destruction of adrenals – remains an important cause, especially in developing countries. Other infections can also be involved such as *Histoplasma capsulatum*.
3. Metastatic neoplasms.

**Other features**

Muscular weakness and wasting.
Loss of weight.
Gastrointestinal upsets (vomiting, diarrhoea).
Anaemia.
Pigmentation of exposed and pressure areas of skin ($\uparrow$ MSH).
Dehydration.
Crises occur, especially if acute infection complicates the condition.
Administration of adrenal hormones restores individual to normal.

*Note*: In adrenal gland failure, a high level of ACTH results. Melanocyte stimulating hormone is derived from the same precursor POMC.

# ADRENAL CORTEX AND MEDULLA

**Congenital adrenocortical enzyme defects**
These are rare autosomal recessive disorders.
Each transformation step in the pathways of steroid formation in the adrenal cortex requires the activity of one or more enzymes. Deficiency of any enzyme will interfere with production of the end product.

**21 hydroxylase deficiency**
This is the commonest type, and the lack of this enzyme prevents the production of cortisol and aldosterone. The low blood cortisol activates ACTH secretion. Adrenal hyperplasia follows and, although cortisol is not formed, other steroids are produced in excess. The resulting clinical syndrome varies with the severity of the defect.

1. Symptoms of Addison's disease.
2. Lesser degrees of adrenal failure plus symptoms due to excess of sex steroids.
   (a) Pseudohermaphroditism in females; precocious puberty in males.
   (b) Virilism in female.
3. No signs of adrenal failure but sex disturbance, e.g. amenorrhoea, hirsutism.

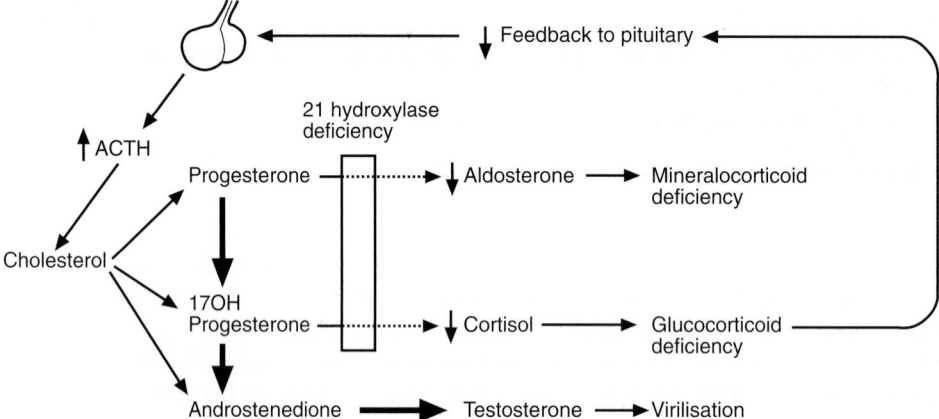

**ADRENAL MEDULLA**
Excess production of catecholamines may occur with some tumours of the medulla. Three are described:

1. **Phaeochromocytoma**. This tumour is composed of chromaffin cells. Symptoms are due to paroxysmal overproduction of the amines with hypertension, raised metabolic rate and blood sugar. Cerebral haemorrhage may occur. There is an increased risk of myocardial ischaemia and heart failure. About 25% of phaeochromocytomas are familial, 10% are bilateral and 10% are malignant. It is very difficult to predict behaviour on histological grounds.

   Familial cases may be associated with:   (a) MENS.
         (b) Neurofibromatosis.
         (c) Von Hippel–Lindau syndrome.
         (d) Germ line mutations of succinate dehydrogenase genes.

2. **Ganglioneuroma**: a benign tumour, composed of well-differentiated ganglion cells (p. 622).

3. **Neuroblastoma**: a very malignant tumour of primitive nerve cells, occurring in children.

# ENDOCRINE PANCREAS

The islets of Langerhans form 1–2% of the pancreatic tissue. Four types of cell make up the islets. The majority are β cells.

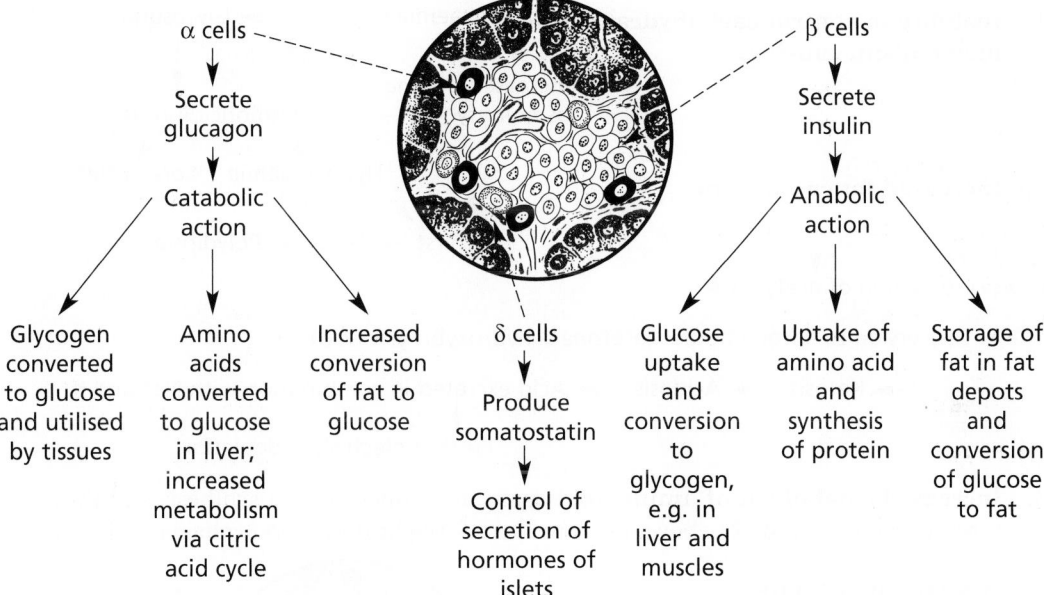

α cells
↓
Secrete glucagon
↓
Catabolic action

- Glycogen converted to glucose and utilised by tissues
- Amino acids converted to glucose in liver; increased metabolism via citric acid cycle
- Increased conversion of fat to glucose

δ cells
↓
Produce somatostatin
↓
Control of secretion of hormones of islets

β cells
↓
Secrete insulin
↓
Anabolic action

- Glucose uptake and conversion to glycogen, e.g. in liver and muscles
- Uptake of amino acid and synthesis of protein
- Storage of fat in fat depots and conversion of glucose to fat

Insulin also stimulates reabsorption of glucose from the renal glomerular filtrate.

Insulin and glucagon have virtually opposite actions. The action of insulin is also opposed by growth hormone and glucocorticoids.

The fourth type of cell is the pancreatic polypeptide (PP) cell, found in highest concentration in the head of the pancreas.

## DIABETES MELLITUS

This condition is due to an absolute or relative lack of insulin activity.

There are two main types:

Type 1 – immune mediated β cell destruction ⟶ absolute insulin deficiency.

Type 2 – adult onset due to insulin resistance, and β cell dysfunction and a range of rarer causes including genetic defects of β cell function and insulin receptors, diseases of the exocrine pancreas and gestational diabetes.

# ENDOCRINE PANCREAS

## BIOCHEMICAL CHANGES AND CLINICAL EFFECTS

The main results of lack of insulin are:

1. **Inability to control carbohydrate metabolism, causing:**

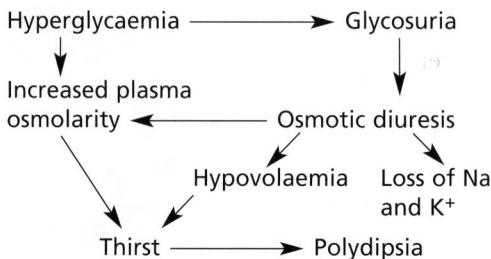

2. **Increased fat catabolism.**

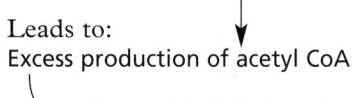

Leads to:
Excess production of acetyl CoA

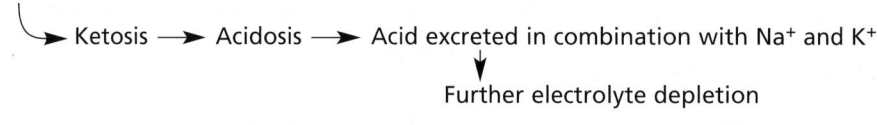

3. **Increased catabolism of amino acids** prevents proper protein synthesis and this, together with (1) and (2) above, leads to loss of weight despite polyphagia.

## TYPES OF DIABETES

### *Primary forms*
### TYPE 1 diabetes

This form is due to destruction of β cells in the islets of Langerhans.

The onset is acute and the peak of incidence is around 13 years. Factors of importance in the aetiology:

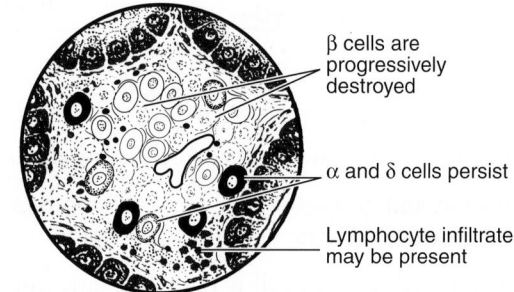

β cells are progressively destroyed

α and δ cells persist

Lymphocyte infiltrate may be present

1. There is a familial incidence and in 80% of cases there is an association with Class II HLA antigens (particularly HLA DR3, DR4).
2. Environmental factors, e.g. Coxsackie B virus may trigger islet cell destruction.
3. Cell-mediated immunity against islet antigens and humoral antibodies are present in most cases.

This has given rise to a theory of pathogenesis:

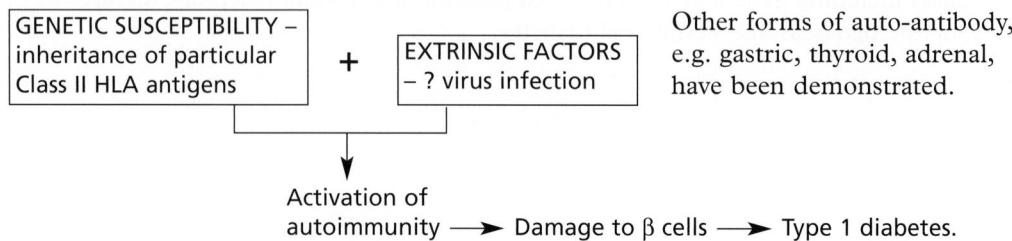

Other forms of auto-antibody, e.g. gastric, thyroid, adrenal, have been demonstrated.

# ENDOCRINE PANCREAS

## *Primary forms*
## TYPE 2 diabetes mellitus

This is the commonest form of diabetes, affecting 10% of adults over 65 years in Western society. It is commoner in Asians and Afro-Caribbeans within Western societies. It is more frequent in females and the incidence increases with age. In contrast to Type 1, the onset is slow and the changes in glucose metabolism mild. (Diet restriction to reduce OBESITY and oral hypoglycaemic drugs usually control the blood sugar.) Clinical presentation is often due to complications, particularly vascular. Often the disorder is detected by biochemical screening.

## Aetiology

This is a multifactorial disorder involving environmental and strong genetic factors. The basic mechanism is prolonged INSULIN RESISTANCE in the tissues leading eventually to inadequate secretion of insulin by β cells. The combination of obesity, Type 2 diabetes and hyperlipidaemia leads to an increased risk of cardiovascular disease.

The following theory accommodates the known facts:

| OBESITY | | | |
|---|---|---|---|
| **Adipocytes** | Free fatty acids | Cytoxins | Adipokines |
| **Islets** | | Compensation | Failure |
| **Insulin secretion** | Normal | Raised | Decreased |
| **Blood sugar** | Normal | Impaired glucose tolerance | Diabetes |

*Note 1*: The concordance rate for identical twins is up to 60% in some studies.
*Note 2*: β cells secrete islet amyloid protein along with insulin. **Amyloid** is deposited in islets in Type 2 diabetes, probably reflecting the prolonged β cell activity.

# ENDOCRINE PANCREAS

### *Secondary forms (Type 3)*

Diabetes may complicate:

1. A number of endocrine diseases (acromegaly, Cushing syndrome, phaeochromocytoma).
2. Metabolic diseases (haemochromatosis).
3. Drug therapy (steroids, thiazide diuretics).
4. Pancreatic inflammation, etc. (chronic pancreatitis, mumps, cystic fibrosis).

### Gestational diabetes (Type 4)

This is associated with glycosuria during pregnancy and the birth of overweight babies. Control of the maternal blood sugar reduces birth weight to normal. Permanent diabetes is apt to develop at a later date.

## COMPLICATIONS OF DIABETES

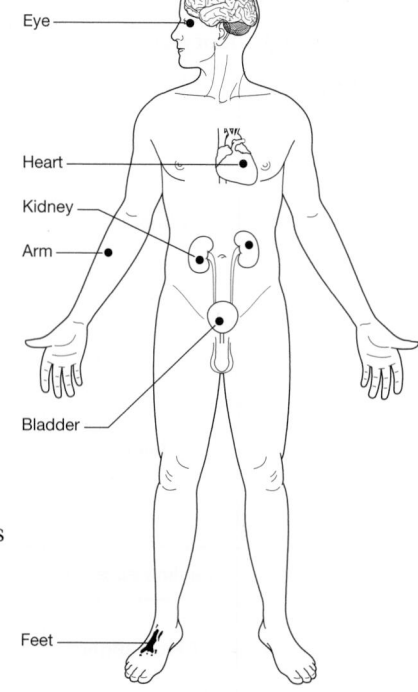

1. **Diabetic coma**. Two forms occur:
   (a) **Keto-acidotic coma**. This is common in Type 1 diabetes. Hyperosmolarity, hypovolaemia, acidosis and loss of electrolytes, if unchecked, lead to coma.
   (b) **Hyperosmolar non-ketotic coma**. This develops slowly in Type 2 diabetes. Hyperglycaemia builds up and produces profound dehydration.
2. **Hypoglycaemic coma**. This complication of treatment occurs when insulin intake is excessive for the amount of food consumed.
3. **Cardiovascular lesions**.
   (a) Atheroma develops at an earlier age and with increased severity. Coronary thrombosis is common.
   (b) Microangiopathy, causing occlusion of arterioles and capillaries. These vascular lesions are responsible for many of the clinical lesions, e.g. cardiac failure, retinopathy, neuropathy, gangrene of limbs, Kimmelstiel–Wilson lesions in the kidney.

The frequency of cardiovascular lesions can be minimised by tight control of blood glucose levels (usually by monitoring glycated haemoglobin) and blood pressure.

4. **Renal failure** is common. It may be due to glomerulosclerosis, but pyelonephritis and renal papillary necrosis are other causes.
5. **Infections**. There is an increased susceptibility to sepsis, fungal infections and tuberculosis.
6. **Neuropathy**. (a) Peripheral ⎤ Possibly due to direct metabolic damage
                 (b) Autonomic ⎦ ± microvascular occlusion

## PANCREATIC ENDOCRINE TUMOURS (ISLET CELL TUMOURS)

These are uncommon. Most are benign and are asymptomatic unless they secrete excess hormones. Ten percent are malignant. The clinical effects vary with the hormone produced.

1. INSULINOMAS arise from β cells and produce attacks of hypoglycaemia.
2. GASTRINOMAS cause multiple peptic ulcers (Zollinger–Ellison syndrome).
3. Glucagonomas and somatostatinomas induce diabetes.
4. Other hormones secreted, e.g. serotin and ACTH, leading to carcinoid syndrome, Cushing syndrome, etc.

These tumours may form part of MENS (p. 692).

# PARATHYROID GLANDS

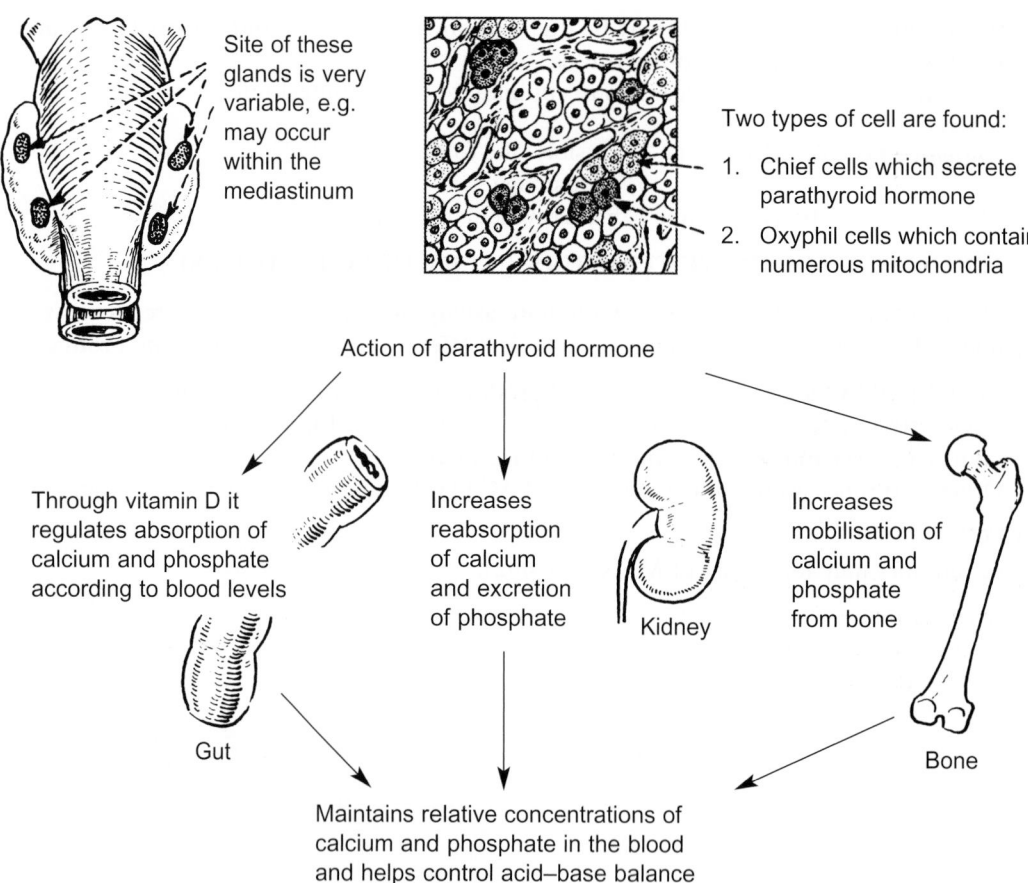

Site of these glands is very variable, e.g. may occur within the mediastinum

Two types of cell are found:

1. Chief cells which secrete parathyroid hormone

2. Oxyphil cells which contain numerous mitochondria

Action of parathyroid hormone

Through vitamin D it regulates absorption of calcium and phosphate according to blood levels

Gut

Increases reabsorption of calcium and excretion of phosphate

Kidney

Increases mobilisation of calcium and phosphate from bone

Bone

Maintains relative concentrations of calcium and phosphate in the blood and helps control acid–base balance

The parathyroids are four small glands lying posterior to the thyroid gland.

## HYPERPARATHYROIDISM (see p. 638)

There are three forms:

1. **Primary**

   This is due to **adenoma** (>80%), **hyperplasia** (approx. 15%) and **carcinoma** (approx. 2%).

   The **blood calcium** is **raised**.

   The effects are:

   (a) Formation of renal calculi sometimes leading to renal failure.
   (b) Parathyroid bone disease, now uncommon.
   (c) General muscle weakness.
   (d) Metastatic calcification.

# PARATHYROID GLANDS

2. **Secondary**

Parathyroid hyperplasia is a response to the low blood calcium from various causes as follows:

CHRONIC RENAL FAILURE ⎫
Malabsorption syndromes ⎬ HYPOCALCAEMIA ⟶ PARATHYROID
Vitamin D deficiency ⎭ HYPERPLASIA

3. **Tertiary**

In a few cases of secondary hyperparathyroidism an autonomous nodule develops in the hyperplastic gland and HYPERCALCAEMIA results.

*Note*: **Humoral hypercalcaemia of malignancy.**
Carcinomas, particularly of the lung and kidney may produce
**Parathyroid hormone-related peptide** (PTHrP) which causes **hypercalcaemia**.
This is not related to parathyroid disease.

## HYPOPARATHYROIDISM

This occurs in three circumstances:
1. Surgical removal, sometimes accidentally during thyroidectomy.
2. Auto-immune disease (very rare).
3. Congenital deficiency (e.g. DiGeorge syndrome).

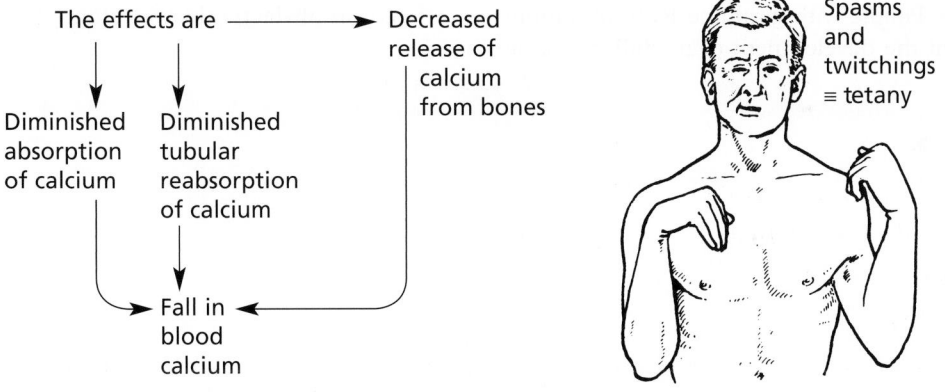

The effects are ⟶ Decreased release of calcium from bones

Diminished absorption of calcium

Diminished tubular reabsorption of calcium

Fall in blood calcium

Spasms and twitchings ≡ tetany

# MULTIPLE ENDOCRINE NEOPLASIA SYNDROMES (MENS)

This is a group of familial conditions (autosomal dominant inheritance) characterised by multiple endocrine tumours.

The main syndromes are:

**MEN 1** – Parathyroid adenoma, hyperplasia,
Pancreatic endocrine neoplasms,
Pituitary adenomas, especially prolactinomas.

This is due to mutation of the MEN 1 gene on chromosome 11, which encodes menin, a nuclear protein.

**MEN 2A** – Medullary carcinoma of thyroid,
Phaeochromocytoma,
Parathyroid adenoma or hyperplasia.

**MEN 2B** – Medullary carcinoma of thyroid (poor prognosis),
Phaeochromocytoma,
Mucosal 'neuromas',
Ganglioneuromas of gut and skin,
Marfanoid habitus.

These are due to mutations activating the RET oncogene on chromosome 10, which encodes a cell surface receptor with tyrosine kinase activity.

Genetic testing can now identify RET mutation carriers earlier and more reliably than before. People with germline RET mutations are offered prophylactic thyroidectomy to prevent the development of medullary carcinoma.